HANDBOOK OF
TEACHING
and LEARNING
for PHYSICAL
THERAPISTS

HANDBOOK OF
TEACHING
and LEARNING
for PHYSICAL
THERAPISTS

Gail M. Jensen, PT, PhD, FAPTA
Dean
Graduate School and University College
Associate Vice President
Academic Affairs
Professor of Physical Therapy
School of Pharmacy and Health Professions
Creighton University
Omaha, Nebraska

Elizabeth Mostrom, PT, PhD
Professor
Director of Clinical Education
Doctoral Program in Physical Therapy
School of Rehabilitation and Medical Sciences
Central Michigan University
Mount Pleasant, Michigan

ELSEVIER
BUTTERWORTH
HEINEMANN

THIRD EDITION

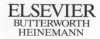

3251 Riverport Lane
St. Louis, Missouri 63043

Handbook of Teaching and Learning for Physical Therapists   ISBN: 978-1-4557-0616-7

Notices

Knowledge and best practice in this field are constantly changing. As new research and experience broaden our understanding, changes in research methods, professional practices, or medical treatment may become necessary.

Practitioners and researchers must always rely on their own experience and knowledge in evaluating and using any information, methods, compounds, or experiments described herein. In using such information or methods they should be mindful of their own safety and the safety of others, including parties for whom they have a professional responsibility.

With respect to any drug or pharmaceutical products identified, readers are advised to check the most current information provided (i) on procedures featured or (ii) by the manufacturer of each product to be administered, to verify the recommended dose or formula, the method and duration of administration, and contraindications. It is the responsibility of practitioners, relying on their own experience and knowledge of their patients, to make diagnoses, to determine dosages and the best treatment for each individual patient, and to take all appropriate safety precautions.

To the fullest extent of the law, neither the Publisher nor the authors, contributors, or editors, assume any liability for any injury and/or damage to persons or property as a matter of products liability, negligence or otherwise, or from any use or operation of any methods, products, instructions, or ideas contained in the material herein.

Library of Congress Cataloging-in-Publication Data

Handbook of teaching and learning for physical therapists / [edited by] Gail M. Jensen, Elizabeth Mostrom.
    p. ; cm.
    Rev. ed. of: Handbook of teaching for physical therapists / edited by Katherine F. Shepard, Gail M. Jensen. 2nd ed. c2002.
    Includes bibliographical references and index.
    ISBN 978-1-4557-0616-7 (pbk.)
    I. Jensen, Gail M. II. Mostrom, Elizabeth. III. Handbook of teaching for physical therapists.
    [DNLM: 1. Physical Therapy Specialty–education. 2. Curriculum. 3. Learning. 4. Physical Therapists–education. 5. Teaching–methods. WB 18]
    615.8′2071–dc23

2012016475

Content Strategist: Kathy H Falk
Content Development Specialist: Megan Fennell
Publishing Services Manager: Gayle May
Project Manager: Divya Krish
Designer: Margaret Reid

Printed in the United States

Last digit is the print number: 9 8 7 6 5 4 3 2 1

CONTRIBUTORS

J.B. Barr, PT, DPT, OCS
Associate Professor
Department of Physical Therapy
Creighton University
Omaha, Nebraska

Debra Brady, DNP, RN, CNS
Associate Professor of Nursing
School of Nursing
California State University Sacramento
Sacramento, California

Tracy Chapman, MEd
Executive Director, eLearning and Academic
 Technology
Creighton University
Omaha, Nebraska

Nicole Christensen, PT, PhD, MAppSc
Associate Professor
Physical Therapy Department
Samuel Merritt University
Oakland, California
Adjunct Instructor
Kaiser Permanente Orthopaedic Physical
 Therapy Residency and Fellowship
 Programs
Los Angeles, California

Teresa Cochran, PT, DPT, GCS, MA
Associate Professor
Department of Physical Therapy
Vice Chair, Director
Office of Interprofessional Scholarship,
 Service and Education
Creighton University
Omaha, Nebraska

Brenda Coppard, PhD, OTR/L, FAOTA
Associate Dean for Faculty Development
 and Assessment
Department of Occupational Therapy
Creighton University
Omaha, Nebraska

Jody Shapiro Frost, PT, DPT, PhD
Director
Department of Academic/Clinical Education
 Affairs
American Physical Therapy Association
Alexandria, Virginia

Julie Eshsner Gahimer, PT, HSD
Professor
Krannert School of Physical Therapy
University of Indianapolis
Indianapolis, Indiana

Judith R. Gale, PT, DPT, MPH, OCS
Associate Professor
Department of Physical Therapy
Creighton University
Omaha, Nebraska

Lisa K. Kenyon, PT, PhD, PCS
Assistant Professor
Department of Physical Therapy
Grand Valley State University
Grand Rapids, Michigan

David M. Morris, PT, PhD
Vice Chair and Associate Professor
Department of Physical Therapy
University of Alabama at Birmingham
Birmingham, Alabama

Diane E. Nicholson, PhD, PT, NCS
Associate Professor
Department of Physical Therapy
University of Utah
Salt Lake City, Utah

Terrence M. Nordstrom, EdD, PT
Chair, Associate Professor
Department of Physical Therapy
Samuel Merritt University
Oakland, California

Karen A. Paschal, PT, DPT, MS
Associate Professor
Department of Physical Therapy
Creighton University
Omaha, Nebraska

Brad Stockert, PT, PhD
Professor
Department of Physical Therapy
California State University
Sacramento
Sacramento, California

Carol Jo Tichenor, PT, MA, FAAOMPT
Director
Physical Therapy Fellowship in Advanced
 Orthopedic Manual Therapy
Kaiser Permanente
Hayward, California

EDITORS

Gail M. Jensen, PT, PhD, FAPTA, is Dean, Graduate School and University College, Associate Vice President in Academic Affairs, Professor of Physical Therapy, School of Pharmacy and Health Professions and Faculty Associate, Center for Health Policy and Ethics at Creighton University, Omaha, Nebraska. She holds a B.S. in education from the University of Minnesota, an M.A. in physical therapy and a Ph.D. in educational evaluation both from Stanford University. Dr. Jensen is a leader known nationally and internationally for scholarly contributions related to expert practice, clinical reasoning, professional ethics and educational theory and application. Dr. Jensen has served on several editorial boards including Physical Therapy and the Journal of Physical Therapy Education and is currently deputy editor for *Physiotherapy Research International* and Associate Editor for Physiotherapy Theory and Practice and on the Editorial Board of Qualitative Health Research. She has co-authored nine books, most recently, *Leadership in Interprofessional Health Education and Practice* (2009), *Expertise in Physical Therapy Practice* (2nd edition, 2007), *Educating for Moral Action: A Sourcebook in Health and Rehabilitation Ethics* (2005) and now the third edition of the *Handbook on Teaching for Physical Therapists* (3rd ed). During her career, she has held faculty appointments at Stanford University, Temple University, the University of Alabama at Birmingham, Samuel Merritt University, and Creighton University. She has served on multiple APTA consensus conferences, task forces and consultant groups, and is an accreditation reviewer for the Commission on Accreditation in Physical Therapy Education as well as the Higher Learning Commission of the North Central Association. She is a recipient of the American Physical Therapy Association's Jules M. Rothstein Golden Pen Award for Scientific Writing, the APTA's Lucy Blair Service Award, and was elected a Catherine Worthingham Fellow of APTA in 2002 and was the 2011 Mary McMillan Lecturer.

Elizabeth Mostrom, PT, PhD, is Professor and Director of Clinical Education, Doctoral Program in Physical Therapy, School of Rehabilitation and Medical Sciences at Central Michigan University in Mount Pleasant, Michigan. She received a B.S. in health education from West Chester State College, an M.S. in physical therapy from Duke University, and a PhD in educational psychology from Michigan State University. She has served on the editorial advisory boards of several professional journals and is past editor of the Journal of Physical Therapy Education. She is a past recipient of the APTA's Mary MacMillan Scholarship for doctoral students, a Foundation for Physical Therapy doctoral research grant, the Central Michigan University Excellence in Teaching Award, the APTA's 2007 Lucy Blair Service Award, and is the APTA Education Section's 2013 Polly Cerasoli Lecturer. Her research interests, publications, and professional presentations span the areas of student and professional learning and development, clinical education, and qualitative research. She has been a contributing author to several books including *Expertise in Physical Therapy Practice (1st and 2nd editions)*, *The Handbook of Teaching for Physical Therapists (2nd edition)* and *Educating for Moral Action: A Sourcebook in Health and Rehabilitation Ethics (2005)*.

Editor Emeritus

Katherine F. Shepard, PhD, PT, FAPTA, is Professor Emeritus and past Director of the PhD Program in Physical Therapy, Department of Physical Therapy, College of Health Professions at Temple University in Philadelphia. She received a Bachelor of Arts degree in psychology from Hood College, a Bachelor of Science degree in physical therapy from Ithaca College, and Masters degrees in physical therapy and sociology, as well as a Doctor of Philosophy degree in sociology of education from Stanford University. She is the recipient of the Temple University Lindback Award for Distinguished Teaching, the American Physical Therapy Association (APTA) Section for Education Award for Leadership in Education, the APTA Baethke-Carlin Award for Teaching Excellence, and the APTA Golden Pen Award for outstanding contributions to the journal Physical Therapy. She is a Catherine Worthingham Fellow of the APTA and the 38th Mary McMillan Lecturer. She has written and lectured extensively on academic and clinical education, the behavioral sciences, and qualitative research design.

FOREWORD

Understanding the essential concepts behind the acts of teaching and learning is critical for all physical therapists. There are any number of factors which can impact learning needs and preferences; generational and cultural differences are two examples. To be an effective instructor and achieve optimal outcomes, physical therapists in both the academic and clinical settings need be able to teach considering the learning needs and preferences of their students/patients and know how to modify their teaching to facilitate learning.

Part of facilitation is a learning process on the part of the clinician; a process of learning how health care professionals can work together in today's complex and dynamic health care environment to build a safer, patient-centered, community-oriented health care system. For optimal health outcomes, physical therapists' focus has to expand from individual patient care to encompass a wide range of interprofessional interactions and include an understanding of community and population health needs that might affect their patients health related quality of life.

The use of technology in health care is now mainstream, with electronic medical records, patient simulations, the advances of telemedicine, and the use of robotics in patient care. Whether digital natives (Generation X) or immigrants (Boomers), physical therapists need to understand how to effectively use technology to promote learning.

The third edition of *Handbook of Teaching and Learning for Physical Therapists* continues to address the foundational concepts of teaching related to contemporary physical therapy practice across the professional continuum—from student to novice practitioner to clinical or academic educator to advanced clinical practice—but it has also expanded the scope of inquiry from the first two editions to include the technological and interprofessional facets of modern clinical care mentioned above. With this text, leaders in physical therapy education become the readers' mentors by sharing their experience and expertise and promoting excellence in educating patients and the next generation of physical therapists.

PREFACE

The preface of a book is very important as it provides the reader with the authors' personal insights about what this book means. For us, we believe that there is nothing more important and central to the work of physical therapists (PTs) and physical therapist assistants (PTAs) than teaching and learning. We also subscribe to the notion that if there is no evidence of learning from patient, student, caregiver, or colleague then there is no evidence of teaching. In practice, we cannot succeed without the patient working with us as much of our practice relies on human performance as the ultimate outcome. As educators, the outcomes for our students lies in their learning and who they become and what they do.*

Every day PTs and PTAs are engaged in teaching and learning. They design and implement strategies to facilitate change in patients' health behaviors, demonstrate lifting techniques to family members, guide students through clinical internships or clinical residencies, present in-service programs or grand rounds to their health care colleagues, deliver professional presentations at local and national meetings, serve on curricular committees or program advisory boards, plan and implement health promotion programs for members of the community, and consult with teachers in the local school system. Perhaps no process other than teaching and learning so permeates the professional contributions made by members of the physical therapy profession.

Teaching is a skill that PTs often take for granted. We have all experienced many years of being taught; that is, we have been apprentices of teaching and teachers through our life experiences as learners. During these years, we have observed both effective and ineffective teaching. Ineffective teaching can leave teachers and students frustrated and alienated from learning more about teaching—or, at worst, learning more about anything at all. Few PTs and even fewer PTAs have been exposed to the substantial and informative body of knowledge, research and theory that exists in education. From observing expert teachers at work, we know that skill in teaching requires much more than knowing the material, illustrating lectures with PowerPoint, or learning how to construct a valid examination. Effective learning experiences are crafted by expert teachers, suffused with practical and theoretical knowledge, compellingly delivered with accurate insight into the needs of the learner, and constantly assessed and improved.

This handbook has emerged from an ongoing dialogue and reflection on our own experiences as PTs, educators, and educational researchers. Our interest and background in educational theory is tied to a specific belief and value about the central importance of teaching and learning to those practicing physical therapy. We believe deeply that evidence of *learning* is what matters most. We embrace learning as a threshold concept for the profession. By that we mean it is a portal or window that provides us with a new way of thinking about something and that new way of thinking results in a transformative experience. Our hope is that this third edition of the handbook will provide you with new insights and renewed perspectives on the critical importance of teaching and learning in physical therapy. (Jensen ref)

Consistent with lifelong learning, we ourselves are committed to providing the reader with a text that is driven by inquiry and reflection. We believe that one is always a teacher *and* learner in physical therapy practice. These roles are constantly interchanging. The PT and PTA must initiate and engage in both roles to do either one well. We also believe that teaching and learning within the clinic or classroom is always more chaotic and complicated than what theory may account for, and constant inquiry and adaptation are essential skills for understanding and improving teaching and learning. Theory does provide a framework for understanding practice, and practice yields ever more useful theory. Thus, a dedicated commitment to ongoing inquiry and deliberative reflection—that is, becoming a reflective practitioner *and* educator—is needed to teach and learn in chaotic settings and maintain an essential and iterative dialogue between theory and practice.

In an effort to link theory and practice in this text, we have invited expert contributors known for their practical experience in "the real world" as well as their theoretical understanding and expertise. By including these expert contributors, we are celebrating the learning community of scholars in physical therapy education who are reflective and responsible stewards of their work.

As qualitative researchers, we are committed to understanding teaching from the inside—that is, from the individual and collective experiences of learners and teachers. You will read stories from the "trenches" of practice in each chapter. We hope these examples of your colleagues at work as teachers will facilitate your intuitive understanding of some of the broader conceptual issues proposed.

Teaching and learning are perhaps the most important skills a PT and a PTA can acquire. Development of sound, practically relevant, theoretically based educational strategies can result in significant reform in our ability to perceive, understand, and foster expansion of knowledge, insight, and skills for students, patients, colleagues, and the public.

---

* Jensen GM. Learning:What Matters Most, 42nd Mary McMillan Lecture. Phys Ther. 2011;91: 1674–1689.

ACKNOWLEDGEMENTS

We have many people to thank for this book. First, thanks to our mentors at Stanford University in the Department of Physical Therapy (Helen Blood, Barbara Kent, Katherine Shepard) and School of Education (Lee Shulman, Elliot Eisner, Joan Talbert) and at Michigan State University in the Department of Counseling, Educational Psychology and Special Education and the College of Education (Christopher Clark, Susan Florio-Ruane, Penelope Peterson). Our doctoral experiences in education continue to have a profound effect on how we think, what we value, what we do, and who we are. We were urged to question, grapple with new ideas, and be intrigued with failures. These experiences set our course as teachers, learners and scholars. Thanks to our loved ones, colleagues, and friends (human and animal), who unconditionally accept us and our life journeys. You each know who you are. Thanks to Kathy Falk who steadfastly supported the third edition of the handbook and to Megan Fennell who was there for every step of the way in the editorial process and who with Divya Krish persistently and skillfully put this book together. Our grateful thanks to Dr. Katherine Shepard who is mentor to both of us in shaping our ideas. Kay is enjoying retirement but we insisted that we carry her name forward in key chapters and you will clearly hear her voice and influence.

Finally, thanks to all those to whom this book is dedicated—the many students and patients who have taught us so profoundly for so many years.

GMJ, EM and KFS

INTRODUCTION

Gail M. Jensen, Elizabeth Mostrom, and Katherine F. Shepard

"Good teaching comes in many flavors and colors. It occurs when a teacher leads you to a vista that changes forever the way you see. It happens when someone introduces you to a delicious idea that you can chew on for the rest of your life. It occurs when somebody helps you discover possibilities in yourself you didn't know were there. Good teaching is many things. It has no essential quality. It takes place through books, it occurs in classrooms, [in health care clinics and communities], it emerges in conversations and in the presence of those who give us a vision of how life in its large and small moments might be lived."*

"Try the experiment of communicating, with fullness and accuracy, some experience to another, especially if it be somewhat complicated, and you will find your own attitude toward your experience changing... The experience has to be formulated in order to be communicated. To formulate requires getting outside of it, seeing it as another would see it, considering what points of contact it has with the life of another so that it may be got into such a form that he [or she] can appreciate its meaning. ... One has to assimilate, imaginatively, something of another's experience in order to tell him [or her] intelligently of one's own experience. All communication is like art. It may fairly be said, therefore, that any social arrangement that remains vitally social, or vitally shared, is educative to those that participate in it. ... In the final account, then, not only does social life demand teaching and learning for its own permanence, but the very process of living together educates. It enlarges and enlightens experience; it stimulates and enriches imagination; it creates responsibility for accuracy and vividness of statement and thought."**

Purpose of the Handbook

For many students who learn in physical therapy academic settings, the experience is one of struggling to understand and remember an endless array of ill-connected, seemingly inert, knowledge bits. Many of these knowledge bits have a half-life of 3–5 years, and others already are outdated for physical therapy practice in today's constantly evolving health care system. Certainly, the strain of teaching and learning in academic settings is due in part to the knowledge explosion in the sciences as well as in the guiding principles and techniques of physical therapy practice, especially in the many and expanding clinical specialty

areas. Often arguments for "more content" lead to a call for more critical processes. Is there a point at which "less is more"? If so, how much less? What type of "less"? Shulman argues that what is held to be true by any individual or group is intrinsically incomplete and that knowledge is a process of continuous debate, dialogue, deliberation and reasoning.*

For many patients who learn in clinical settings, the experience is one of attempting to focus attention and grasp information under the most difficult of circumstances (i.e., while ill or in pain or experiencing devastating loss). Typically, patients are exposed to rapidly delivered sound bites of important, perhaps even lifesaving, information delivered by a multitude of fleeting health care professionals who are strangers (and who may not even understand or speak the patient's native language). Certainly, some of this strain of teaching and learning in health care settings is owing to the realities of health care delivery systems in which everyone labors under time restrictions that limit access to clinicians and shorten contact with patients and families.

The fragmented learning and embarrassingly limited outcomes that often occur with such experiences in academic and clinical settings are perplexing and sad. However, failures and crises also present us with opportunities to use our ingenuity and strengths as health care providers and teachers. When we find ourselves competing with time and costs to deliver the most effective health care possible, do we find ourselves teaching more? Are we involving the patient as well as family and caretakers much earlier in learning to assume health care tasks? Are we thinking about what we as physical therapists (PTs) and physical therapist assistants (PTAs) can do to facilitate and promote healthy practices in the community? And have we figured out what is essential for novice practitioners to know and how we can prepare them to acquire knowledge and new skills throughout their professional lives? With the continuing growth of clinical residencies and fellowship programs, what are the best ways to mentor therapists in advanced practice settings?

The primary purpose of this book is to stimulate the growth of the reader in teaching and learning by presenting theoretical concepts, current evidence grounded in sound educational research, and related practical applications that will improve skills in the educational processes used in academic, clinical and community settings. Again, we believe that learning is a threshold concept that is foundational in the practice of physical therapy and that learning is a life long process, central to professional development.

---

* Eliot Eisner, Professor of Education and Art, Stanford University. (Stanford *Educator*, Spring 1995;3)

** John Dewey (1916) *Democracy and Education*. New York, NY: The Free Press, pages 6–7.

---

* Shulman, pg 321;2004; Shulman L. The Wisdom of Practice: Essays on Teaching, Learning and Learning to Teach. San Francisco, CA: Jossey Bass Pub. 2004.

What is Teaching? What is Learning?

From the perspective of many experienced educators, effective teaching involves the following: (1) deeply *comprehending* the information to be taught, (2) being able to *transform* and present that information in such a way that students "get it," (3) engaging the student in *active collaborative* learning experiences, and (4) teaching the student how to learn by constant *inquiry and reflection,* which lead the student to acquire her or his own new knowledge and comprehensions. (This teaching process is discussed more thoroughly in Chapter 3.) Similarly, for students to learn, they must comprehend and transform ideas, information, and beliefs through inquiry and reflection during learning experiences in which they, the students, are active participants and collaborators. Such learning results in a change in students' store of information to hopefully become a framework of knowledge along with changes in behaviors, perceptions, feelings, and interactions.

Because teaching and learning are two inseparable sides of the same coin, designating one person as the teacher and another person as the learner is an artificial distinction, much like saying kinesthetic perceptions and functional movement should be considered as two separate and distinct entities. Just as teachers can shape learners and learning, learners can shape teachers and teaching. For either process to work well, both processes must work in concert. At any given moment, anyone can be the learner or the teacher—patients and families, students participating in formal academic programs or clinical education experiences, health care colleagues, community neighbors, and one's self.

Characteristics of Good Teachers and Learners

As Eliot Eisner stated, good teaching is many things and comes in many colors and flavors. We think, however, that there are three major components that must be present for good teaching and learning to occur:

1. **Teachers must understand deeply the topics that they are teaching and ceaselessly engage in adding to their knowledge stores.** Teaching is, indeed, an intellectual enterprise. To be continually learning requires curiosity, initiative and intellectual excitement about uncovering more and more about a specific topic or field. Learning means seeking out and engaging in experiences that foster learning—reading, clinical practice, conferences, research, talking with colleagues over coffee and, of course, being stimulated and challenged to learn even more by one's students. Reflecting on these experiences results in transformation of the knowledge so that it becomes an integral part of what and how one teaches and who one is as a teacher. Where there is no passion for the topic or for teaching, there is no thinking about what and how one is doing and how it might be done better; there is only the repetitive transmission of dusty, uninspired information from yellowed notes. As educational philosopher John Dewey cautioned, ". . .Only when it [communication] becomes cast in a mold and runs in a routine way does it lose its educative power."*

---

* Dewey J. Democracy and education. NY, NY:The Free Press. 1916. (page 6)

2. **Teachers must know about the students whom they are teaching.** This awareness and knowledge comes from listening to students speak—learning what they understand and feel as well as how they think and reason, through watching students' faces, postures, and gestures; observing students perform manual skills; reading student papers; and noting how students interact with people around them. The ability to effectively transform and transmit knowledge rests on understanding students. This understanding undergirds the teacher's ability to figure out ways to capture the students' curiosity and interest, to create experiences that challenge students to think and risk, and to persistently support students for the discipline, patience, and sometimes tedium it takes for learning to occur. In this way, teaching is also an emotional and relational enterprise.

The effective teacher remembers well what it is like to be a student. From this memory comes empathy for students in academic settings who must sit through hours of writing down new and often perplexing information, sitting in uncomfortable chairs, and not feeling allowed to move or to speak without permission. From this memory also comes sensitivity to a student's anxiety about undersupervision and frustration with oversupervision by the clinical instructor. Similarly, practitioners in clinical settings who have encountered illness or physical impairments or disabilities of their own have a greater tacit understanding of how to teach patients to achieve maximum recovery.

Knowing the student is not only easier but a highly pleasurable activity if the student is the only individual being taught, is open and verbal about his or her educational needs, is motivated by the desire and need to know, and is graciously responsive to the PT or teacher's interest and assistance. However, this situation is rare. The task of knowing a student is clearly daunting when faced with a classroom of 50 or 60 students or a minimally verbal patient who has no family advocate and is scheduled for discharge tomorrow. However daunting, without knowing something about one's students and how they think, what their values and goals are, and what anxieties or concerns they have about the information or skill to be learned, one cannot teach well. Simply put, if the information being delivered is insensitive or inflexible to the proclivities of the learner, little or no learning occurs.

3. **Teachers must be acquainted with a number of different theoretical approaches and techniques (pedagogy) that can facilitate learning for richly diverse groups of students.** The more one knows about these approaches and techniques, the more innovative, improvisational and flexible one can be in providing learning experiences that match the student's quest. The military model of teaching often prevails in academic and clinical settings. The military model involves the rigid, repetitive sequence of demonstrating a task to be accomplished, breaking the task into component parts, teaching the component parts, having the student master the component parts, and then putting the components together. This method is certainly effective in teaching a well-known task for which a right and wrong way is clearly demarcated—for example, learning how

to assemble and disassemble a rifle. However, it is highly questionable whether this method is responsive to most individual learning in academic or clinical settings, which inherently involves perceptions, attitudes, beliefs, prior learned behaviors, and building-block information that the learner may or may not hold.

There are many intriguing methods that one can use to teach and to assess teaching and learning—problem-solving cases, journals, peer teaching, virtual classrooms and discussions, portfolios, interactive laboratories with experts, stories, community activities, simulations and so forth. By presenting a wide variety of teaching-learning techniques, we hope to engage readers in learning more about them and expanding their teaching, learning, and assessment repertoires.

Overview of the Handbook

This edition of the handbook is generally divided into two main sections. In the first section of the book (Chapters 1 to 7), the focus is on education in the academic environment. All chapters have undergone major revision and updating. This section includes two new chapters, Chapter 6 on Authentic Assessment: Simulation-Based Education and Chapter 7: Strategies for Planning and Implementing Interprofessional Education. The second half of the book, (Chapters 8 to 16), the focus is on education in practice environments. In addition to substantial updates and major revisions to chapters included in the second edition, in this section we have three new chapters: Chapter 10 on What Makes a Good Clinical Teacher, Chapter 11 on Facilitating the Teaching and Learning of Clinical Reasoning, and Chapter 12 on Patient Education and Health Literacy. Although each chapter is designed to be read independently of all other chapters, in some cases understanding will be greatly enhanced if several chapters are read together. For example, the reader would benefit from reading the chapter on preparing to teach (Chapter 2) before reading about teaching and learning in academic settings (Chapter 3). Likewise, preparation for teaching in clinical settings (Chapter 8) will greatly add to one's understanding of teaching techniques used in the clinical setting (Chapter 9) and the discussion of what makes a good clinical teacher in chapter 10.

One final addition is that each chapter has two threshold concepts listed at the conclusion of the chapter.

A threshold concept is one that leads to a transformative change in the way the learner understands an area.* Threshold concepts are essential for learners moving on; that is, to cross a threshold at the doorway to deeper understanding. For our purposes we have asked chapter authors to identify two of these concepts for their chapters as a way to signal the MOST important areas of learning in the chapter.*

The Scholarship of Teaching and Learning

Teachers need to find ways to bring teaching and learning, which are primarily private and hidden activities, into the arena of public and community property. The visible scholarship of teaching and learning needs to continue to grow and flourish in physical therapy. Shulman argues that this scholarship of teaching and learning should be motivated by a spirit of faithfulness or fidelity. This fidelity should include integrity of the discipline; the learning of students; the society, community, and institution where one works; and the teacher's sense of self as scholar, teacher, and valued colleague.**

Our hope is that this *Handbook of Teaching and Learning for Physical Therapists* will continue to evolve over time with the sharing of educational research, intuitive ideas, and practical experiences that are part of the community property of physical therapy education in all of its dimensions. The work of the educational community in physical therapy transcends the ability of any one person and rests with all the members of the community as their work and ideas are critically examined and shared. If the readers of this book grapple with, enjoy, debate, and muse over the concepts presented in this handbook and then share the ongoing development and assessment of their own educational endeavors, we will have come a long way toward creating a true community of educational scholars that will contribute to the learning and development of future physical therapists and the positive growth of the profession of physical therapy itself.

---

*Meyer JF, Land R. Threshold concepts and troublesome knowledge: Epistemological consideration and a conceptual framework for teaching and learning. Higher Education. 2005; 49: 373–388.
**Shulman, 2004. Teaching as Community Property: Essays On Higher Education., San Francisco,CA; Jossey-Bass, 2004.

CONTENTS

PART I

EDUCATION IN THE ACADEMIC ENVIRONMENT

CHAPTER 1

CURRICULUM DESIGN FOR PHYSICAL THERAPY EDUCATIONAL PROGRAMS

Gail M. Jensen ☼ Karen A. Paschal ☼ Katherine F. Shepard

CHAPTER OUTLINE

Dr. Katherine Shepard shared this story, which has a powerful moral for all educational programs, in previous editions of this text and revisited the story in her McMillan lecture.[1] "In 1983, the physical therapy program at Stanford University was suddenly and without warning told by the Stanford Medical School that we were to terminate the program." The physical therapy program at Stanford University had been associated with the University since the 1920s and had advanced degree programs since 1940. As a young faculty member in the early 1970s, I assumed we belonged at Stanford just as much as any other department in the university. I never realized how changing the philosophy, mission, and expectations in other parts of the university could affect the very existence of our program. In 1982, the School of Medicine changed its mission from developing physicians to developing physician-researchers (MD-PhDs) and covertly designated the land on which the physical therapy building was located as the new center of Molecular Genetic Engineering. Subsequently, an all-physician review committee informed us that we didn't belong in the School of Medicine because we didn't have a PhD program and weren't producing "scholars." While meeting with the university president on an early spring evening to plead our case, he informed us that if we were to be considered scholars we should be publishing in the Journal of Physiology (his field was physiology) and not Physical Therapy (a technical journal by his standards). It was devastating to belatedly realize how the pieces were being put in place to discontinue our program. Our own mission statement, philosophy, and program goals were essentially ignored because they were now incongruent with the new university-sanctioned "direction" of the medical school. The Stanford University Board of Trustees acted to close the program with the graduating class of 1985.[1] The moral of this story is that the philosophy and goals of any physical therapist or physical therapist assistant program must be in concert with the philosophy and goals of the program's institution or the program will not survive.

LEARNING GOALS

After completing this chapter, the reader will be able to:

1. State the core questions that guide curriculum design[2] and describe the three-phase process of how faculty engage in curriculum development.[3]

2. Defend the need for a clearly stated program philosophy and goals to guide curriculum planning. Demonstrate how program philosophy and goals can be articulated and integrated with institutional mission, societal needs, and professional expectations and functions.

3. Distinguish the formal from the informal curriculum, applying the concepts of implicit, explicit, null, and hidden curricula to the specific educational setting.

4. Describe the role of curriculum alignment as an organizing strategy for program development.

5. Discuss main trends in health professions education that affect curriculum development and dynamic reform, including perennial challenges (and opportunities) between the curricular needs of health care professional programs and liberal arts education, growing demands for teamwork and interprofessional collaboration, and health professions' role in meeting societal needs.

6. State the purpose of professional accreditation and outline the process of accreditation used by the Commission on Accreditation in Physical Therapy Education (CAPTE).

CURRICULUM DESIGN

Everything depends on the quality of the experience that is had. The quality of any experience has two aspects. There is an immediate aspect of agreeableness or disagreeableness, and there is its influence on later experiences. The first is obvious and easy to judge. The effect of an experience is not borne on its face. It sets a problem to the educator. It is the educator's business to arrange for the kind of experiences that, although they do not repel the student, but rather engage the student's activities are, nevertheless, more than immediately enjoyable because they promote having desirable future experiences. Hence, the central problem of an education based on experience is to select the kind of present experiences that live fruitfully and creatively in subsequent experiences.[4]

For educational experiences to be coherent and enjoyable to the individual student, as well as relevant to the desired performance of the program graduate, an all-embracing framework for educational experiences—a curriculum design—must be in place. *Curriculum design* refers to the content and organization of the curricular elements of philosophy, goals, coursework, clinical experiences, and evaluation processes. There is a rational assumption that what drives the curriculum designed for the education of physical therapists and physical therapist assistants is preparation for practice in the health care arena, which involves the development of knowledge, skills, attitudes, and values that undergird competent physical therapy practice that can meet societal needs.

A curriculum design reflects input, directly or indirectly, from literally thousands of people. People with health care needs, regulatory bodies, such as regional and professional accreditation groups and state board licensing agencies, members of the American Physical Therapy Association (APTA) who establish and act on professional standards,[5] physical therapy clinicians, faculty and administrators in the college or university in which the program is located, and each generation of students have an impact on curriculum design. A curriculum design must be steadfastly relevant to the current tasks and standards of physical therapy practice and dynamically responsive to rapidly changing practice environments and human health care needs.

DEVELOPING A CURRICULUM

Eliot Eisner noted that the word *curriculum* originally came from the Latin word *currere*, which means "the course to be run." He states, "This notion implies a track, a set of obstacles or tasks that an individual is to overcome, something that has a beginning and an end, something that one aims at completing."[6]

TYLER'S FOUR FUNDAMENTAL QUESTIONS

Four fundamental questions identified by Ralph Tyler in 1949 are useful in deciding how to develop a "racecourse."[2] These four questions are rediscovered by each generation of faculty seeking to develop a physical therapy curriculum.

1. What educational purposes or goals should the school seek to attain?
2. What educational experiences can be provided that are likely to attain these purposes?
3. How can these educational experiences be effectively organized?
4. How can it be determined whether these purposes or goals are being attained?

These questions and their answers should be interrelated, with each question and answer building on the preceding questions and answers. The easiest, and often first place, for a group of novice faculty to begin, however, is with the second and third questions. Faculty can confidently produce and organize educational experiences based on

their own personal experiences in physical therapy education and practice. However, if curricula are designed in such a way that the answers to questions 2 and 3 are not directly related to question 1, it is like setting sail without plotting a course. That is, despite knowing everything about sailing a ship, sailing with no clear destination may be disastrous. The result of an analogous educational program is haphazard curricular growth, which, at the least, is perplexing to faculty, students, and clinical educators and, at most, can produce graduates who are ill-focused and perplexed about their role in the health care system.

In designing a curriculum, the elements must be logically ordered. This logic can be obtained by thinking about how each level is directly responsive to the levels above and below. As illustrated in the curricular design column in Figure 1–1, the content of a physical therapy educational program (i.e., coursework, learning experiences, and evaluation and assessment processes) is based on meeting program objectives designed to fulfill the program's goals. The program goals reflect the philosophy of the program and the mission of the institution. Evaluation of the program and assessment of student learning and graduate performance therefore demonstrate the success or lack of success of the program's ability to build a curriculum that meets its stated goals.

Tyler's Question 1: Program Philosophy and Goals

Macro Environment

A good strategy for looking at the macro environment is to engage in an environmental scan. This includes a look at trends and issues outside of the discipline of physical therapy as well as other external influences that need to be considered in being responsive and dynamic. Figure 1–2 demonstrates how the philosophy and goals of any physical therapy curriculum are imbedded in a global (macro) environment that includes society, the health care environment, regulatory agencies, the higher education system, the institution in which the program resides, and the knowledge supporting the discipline of physical therapy.

When any component of this macro environment changes, it is necessary to engage in reflective, deliberative discussion and consider potential changes in the physical therapy curriculum. Looking both inside and outside the profession is part of an environmental scan that is important in designing a socially responsive curriculum. Here are some examples to consider. Historical changes outside the profession (e.g., medical discoveries such as the Sabin polio vaccine or the role of the genome) and inside the profession (e.g., the creation of the physical therapist assistant and the continued growth of clinical specialization) and national initiatives (e.g., patient safety or increasing importance of public health) have led to curricular changes.[7–9] More than 20% of the U.S. population will be older than 65 years in 2030.[10] Advances in technology and care along with pressures for reduced costs have resulted in decreased patient care stays in acute care and rehabilitation hospital settings. Physical therapy direct-access state laws have spawned curricular changes in entry-level and advanced coursework for physical therapists and physical therapist assistants. Other changes

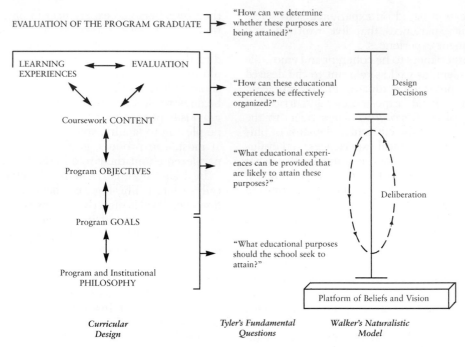

FIGURE 1–1 Relationship between curriculum design, Tyler's fundamental questions, and Walker's naturalistic model.

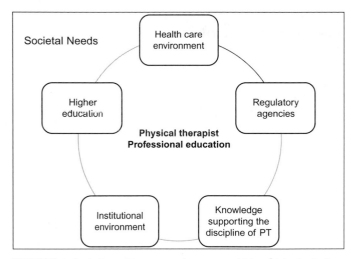

FIGURE 1–2 A view of systems environment within which physical therapy education exists.

include the federal government support of health and health promotion and prevention activities seen in *Healthy People 2020*, which outlines a 10-year agenda for improving the health of the nation.[7] Social determinants, such as employment, level of education, and living environment, all contribute to health outcomes. There is increased emphasis on preparation of health professionals who are collaboration ready, can work on teams, and understand the need for promoting health in communities as well as with individuals.[11,12] The focus on health and wellness rather than disease, interprofessional team competencies, and community health are captured in Chapters 7, 12, and 15. There are many sources for performing environmental scans that range from looking at trends in higher education through the media and other literature to a regular look at health policy changes and new initiatives. The Institute of Medicine issues position papers[13] and panel documents on critical health issues, which are excellent sources of information.

An example of important work in professional education is the Carnegie Foundation for the Advancement of Teaching's comparative study of five professional fields (law, engineering, the clergy, nursing, and medicine).[14–18] This research was grounded in a shared conceptual framework applicable to all professions that focused on the three major dimensions of professional education: knowledge (habit of mind), both theoretical and practical; practical skills (habit of hand), and professional identity (habit of heart). One of the most critical findings was that, given the lack of public trust in some professions, professional education must be clear about its social contract and engaged in cultivating the life of the mind for the public good (Figure 1–3). What the student is to know (i.e., the language of the discipline and the ways of science) is only part of what people who engage in curriculum design must include. Students must also be prepared to reason, to become sensitive and responsive to cultural diversity and society's needs, to undergird decisions and actions with empathy, and to begin a quest for knowledge that will last throughout their professional lives.[19] Professional education is the portal to professional life and an essential component of laying the groundwork for professional formation.

Health professionals must better organize professional education around what actually happens, as well as what *should* happen, in clinical practice. For example, students must be taught thinking and insight skills, such as reflection-in-action and reflection-on-action, and intellectual humility as well as social responsibility to prepare them for the complex, unique, uncertain, and challenging

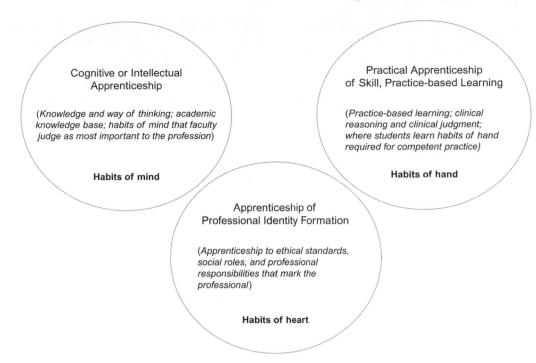

FIGURE 1–3 The conceptual framework used in the Carnegie comparative study of the professions.

health care situations they will face.[19,20] Students need to be "collaboration ready" to work on interprofessional teams. Clearly, the knowledge, critical thinking and practical reasoning skills, humanistic skills, and professional responsibility and obligations and the ability to take moral action could be incorporated into the goals of any physical therapist or physical therapist assistant program.

Macro Environment: Body of Knowledge Related to Physical Therapy

The APTA monographs, *A Normative Model of Physical Therapist Professional Education: Version 2004*,[5] which incorporates the document "Professionalism in Physical Therapy; Core Values," and *A Guide to Physical Therapy Practice*,[21] continue to provide a grounding structure for physical therapy educators. These monographs help educators define the body of knowledge related to physical therapy. In addition, the APTA vision statement for the profession is another foundational element for curriculum consideration.[22]

One of the main functions of the *Normative Model* is to "provide a mechanism for existing, developing, and future professional education programs to evaluate and refine curricula and integrate aspects of the profession's vision for professional education into their vision."[5]

The *Normative Model* is based on 23 practice expectations that define the expected entry level performance of a physical therapist. Educators can use this monograph to review how their coursework in Foundational and Clinical Sciences relates to examples of content, terminal behavioral objectives, and related instructional objectives in academic and clinical settings suggested by content experts. Although certainly not exhaustive, the suggestions can be extremely helpful, especially in guiding novice physical therapy instructors as well as those program faculty who are not physical therapists (Box 1–1).

BOX 1–1   Example of Information in the Normative Model of Physical Therapist Professional Education

Primary Content	Examples of Terminal Behavioral Objectives *(After the completion of the content, the student will be able to...)*	Examples of Instructional Objectives
Adaptations to regular exercise of various types (aerobic or endurance training, interval or anaerobic training, muscle strengthening programs) Exercise specificity Effects on cardiovascular and pulmonary systems, metabolism, blood lipid levels, and skeletal, connective tissue, hormonal systems Hormonal changes with exercise and aging	Describe neural and muscular adaptations that occur as a result of resistance exercise training based on age, gender, and culture.	Describe changes in maximal oxygen consumption, submaximal heart rate and blood pressure, and maximal and submaximal ventilation that occur as a result of endurance exercise training. Describe changes in capillary density, oxidative enzymes, and mitochondria that occur as a result of endurance exercise training. Discuss the effects and side effects of the use of hormones and steroids for improving muscle strength. Differentiate the effects of aging and gender and exercise on hormones, including cortisol, estrogen, testosterone, and insulin.

Data from American Physical Therapy Association Education Division. A Normative Model of Physical Therapist Professional Education: Version 2004. Alexandria, VA: American Physical Therapy Association; 2004.

A Guide to Physical Therapy Practice presents the current practice of physical therapy by outlining common practice roles and defining the types of tests, measures, and treatment interventions commonly used by physical therapists.[21] In addition, preferred practice patterns are offered for four body systems: musculoskeletal, neuromuscular, cardiopulmonary, and integumentary. Each of the sections on preferred practice patterns contains the patient/client diagnostic group being considered; *International Classification of Diseases, Tenth Revision, Clinical Modification* (ICD-10-CM) codes[23]; types of examinations, tests, and measures; anticipated prognosis; expected number of visits per episode of care; patient care goals and related physical therapy interventions and anticipated outcomes; and prevention and risk factor reduction strategies. Thus, the guide is rich with information that can be used by educators teaching and students learning clinical course content. In addition, *Vision 2020*, the APTA's official vision statement for the future of physical therapy, provides several key strategic elements for the profession (e.g., educational preparation, direct access, professionalism).[22]

Another important document is the *International Classification of Functioning, Disability and Health* (ICF).[23] The domains in this model are classified from body, individual, and societal perspectives and provide a means to look at an individual's functioning and disability in a context that includes environmental factors such as social support. The ICF model is the World Health Organization's framework for measuring health and disability and an important concept for physical therapy.

Together, the *Normative Model, Guide to Physical Therapy Practice*, and ICF model are extremely useful resources for any physical therapist, clinical, or academic educator who carries the responsibility of transmitting the core knowledge of physical therapy to the next generation. In addition to these APTA-conceived documents, the *Journal of Physical Therapy Education* presents a steady stream of ideas and special issues directed toward physical therapist and physical therapist assistant educators as well as a growing number of education-specific journals across the health professions (e.g., *Academic Medicine, Teaching and Learning in Medical Education, Medical Teacher, American Journal of Pharmacy Education, Journal of Nursing Education, Journal of Dental Education*).

Micro Environment

Although there are shared expectations and standards for physical therapist and physical therapist assistant education, there is also the unique imprint of the institution and the program faculty that distinguish graduates across programs. Table 1–1 demonstrates two examples of how the mission and values of the institution are seen aligned across all levels (institution, school, and department). In the private institution example, the philosophy of the physical therapy curriculum at Creighton University reflects the "inalienable worth of each individual." It also shows the emphasis on moral values in mission statements of the university and the school in which the physical therapy program is located. The public institution example reveals the connection that the School of Physical Therapy and Rehabilitation Sciences has as part of the College of Medicine.

The philosophy, mission, vision, and core values provide a foundation for the explication of educational outcomes for students. Box 1–2 lists the educational outcomes for a Doctor of Physical Therapy (DPT) program that are divided into Professional Core Abilities and Physical Therapy Care Abilities. The Professional Core Abilities

TABLE 1–1 Two Examples Demonstrating Alignment of Missions across Institution, School, and Department

Private, Faith-based Institution	Public, Research Institution
From mission statement: Creighton University Creighton exists for students and learning. Members of the Creighton community are challenged to reflect on transcendent values, including their relationship with God, in an atmosphere of freedom of inquiry, belief, and religious worship. Service to others, the importance of family life, the inalienable worth of each individual and appreciation of ethnic and cultural diversity are core values of Creighton.	**From mission statement: University of South Florida** USF is committed to promoting globally competitive undergraduate, graduate and professional programs that support interdisciplinary inquiry, intellectual development, knowledge and skill acquisition, and student success through a diverse, fully-engaged, learner-centered campus environment.
From mission statement: School of Pharmacy and Health Professions at Creighton University The Creighton University School of Pharmacy and Health professions prepares men and women in their professional disciplines with an emphasis on moral values and service to develop competent graduates who demonstrate concern for human health. This mission is fulfilled by providing comprehensive professional instruction, engaging in basic science and clinical research, participating in community and professional service, and fostering a learning environment enhanced by faculty who encourage self-determination, self-respect, and compassion in students.	**From mission statement: School of Physical Therapy and Rehabilitation Sciences** The mission of the University of South Florida, School of Physical Therapy and Rehabilitation Sciences, is to prepare doctors of physical therapy who have a strong foundation in the basic and clinical sciences, and who demonstrate excellence in patient/client management, critical thinking and professionalism.
From Creighton's departmental program philosophy The faculty of the Department of Physical Therapy affirm the mission and values of Creighton University and the School of Pharmacy and Health with the recognition that each individual has the responsibility for maintaining the quality and dignity of his/her own life and for participating in and enriching the human community.	**From statements of educational philosophy of the School** We believe interprofessional experiences enhance the future collegiality of healthcare professionals. Respect for individual and cultural differences is necessary for professional effectiveness in a global society.

From Department of Physical Therapy, School of Pharmacy and Health, Creighton University, Omaha, NE; University of South Florida, School of Physical Therapy and Rehabilitation Sciences, Tampa, FL.

BOX 1-2   Example of Educational Outcomes for a Doctor of Physical Therapy Program

Professional Core Abilities

1. *Professional Formation and Critical Self-Reflection.* The student shall utilize a process of deliberative self-reflection to enhance understanding of self and engage in continued professional formation. Formation of professional identity is based on the following core values: accountability, altruism, compassion, excellence, integrity, professional duty and social responsibility.
2. *Communication Skills.* The student shall read, write, speak, listen, and use media and technology to communicate effectively. The student shall demonstrate respectful, positive and culturally appropriate interpersonal behaviors in the counsel and education of patients and families, and in communication with other health care professionals.
3. *Critical Thinking and Clinical Judgment.* The student shall acquire, comprehend, apply, synthesize, and evaluate information. The student shall integrate these abilities to identify, resolve, and prevent problems and make appropriate decisions. The student shall demonstrate the behaviors of the scholarly clinician by developing and utilizing the process of critical thinking and systematic inquiry for the purpose of clinical reasoning, decision making, and exercising sound critical judgment.
4. *Learning and Professional Development.* The student shall consistently strive to expand his/her knowledge and skills to maintain professional competence and contribute to the body of professional knowledge. The student shall demonstrate the ability to gather, interpret, and evaluate data for the purpose of assessing the suitability, accuracy, and reliability of information from reference sources.
5. *Ethical Foundation and Moral Agency.* The student shall practice in an ethical manner, fulfilling an obligation for moral responsibility and social justice. The student shall identify, analyze, and resolve ethical problems.
6. *Social Awareness, Leadership, and Advocacy.* The student shall provide service to the community and to the profession. The student will assume responsibility for proactive collaboration with other health care professionals in addressing patient needs. The student will be prepared to influence the development of ethical and humane health care regulations and policies that are consistent with the needs of the patient and society.

Physical Therapy Care Abilities

1. *Patient Examination.* The student shall perform: (a) thorough patient interview with appropriate medical history and review of systems; (b) physical examination utilizing appropriate tests and measures.
2. *Patient Evaluation and Physical Therapy Diagnosis.* The student shall: (a) interpret results of the physical therapy examination and other diagnostic procedures; (b) synthesize pertinent data; (c) formulate an accurate physical therapy diagnosis. The process of evaluation also may identify the need for consultation with or referral to other health care providers.
3. *Patient Prognosis.* The student shall predict the patient's level of optimal improvement that may be attained through intervention within a given period of time.
4. *Patient Intervention.* The student shall design an appropriate plan of care to produce changes consistent with the physical therapy diagnosis and prognosis. The student shall develop a customized plan of care in collaboration with the patient's/family's expectations and goals. The student shall also assume responsibility for delegation and supervision of appropriate human resources engaged in patient care activities.
5. *Patient Re-examination/Re-evaluation.* The student shall perform an accurate re-examination and re-evaluation to determine changes in patient status and to modify or redirect physical therapy intervention. The process of re-examination and re-evaluation also may identify the need for consultation with or referral to other health care providers. Patient re-examination and re-evaluation may also necessitate modification of delegation and supervision of appropriate human resources engaged in patient care activities.
6. *Patient Outcomes.* The student shall track the results of physical therapy management, which may include the following domains: pathology; impairments; functional limitations; participation; risk reduction/prevention; wellness; community and societal resources; and patient satisfaction.
7. *Systems Management.* The student shall identify the specific contribution of physical therapy management within the health care system and the influence of health care policy on that system. In addition, the student shall demonstrate knowledge and be able to effectively interact within the independent framework of the health care team in a complex society. The student shall extend his/her responsibility for physical therapy care beyond individual patients to include care of communities and populations.

From Creighton University, Doctor of Physical Therapy Program, Omaha, NE.

---

are shared across three health professions in the School (physical therapy, occupational therapy, and pharmacy) and reflect many of the core values of a Jesuit institution.

Faculty time spent considering macro-level and micro-level philosophy and goals is time well spent. Developing program goals and outcomes and related curricular themes together encourages academic and clinical faculty members to reflect on and explicate their own philosophy and goals and come to a common shared understanding of their profession's and college's or university's philosophy and goals. Such an activity unifies and grounds academic and clinical faculty as a community in their work as educators.

Tyler's Question 2: Educational Experiences

Once goals and philosophy are understood, the next question to be answered is what educational experiences (classroom, laboratory, and clinical) are needed to achieve these purposes. Coursework in physical therapist and physical therapist assistant programs consists of foundation sciences, including both basic and applied across biological, physical, and behavioral sciences; and clinical sciences, including knowledge, skills, and abilities across body systems to understand diseases that require the direct intervention of physical therapists for management as well diseases that affect conditions managed by physical therapists and clinical education. The actual coursework designed and offered depends on the program's practice expectations and the type and depth of prerequisite coursework. Matrices or tables can be very effective tools for mapping out the integration and implementation of courses and course sequences linked to the curriculum model.[24] Box 1–3 provides an example of an integrative curriculum model designed to address future practice that matches curricular threads with specific content.[25]

Within each course, written objectives identify specific attitudes, behaviors, and skills that the instructor expects each student to develop. The APTA *Normative Model* maps out the following sequence: content, terminal behavioral objective (TBOs) (behaviors expected at the conclusion of the educational unit), and instructional objectives (IOs), which are specific objectives for the classroom or clinically based activities. Included in these objectives are expectations that directly relate to the program's philosophy and goals. For example, if one of the program's goals is to develop critical thinking skills, each instructor should present objectives and related learning experiences to

---

BOX 1–3   Example of Curricular Threads and Links to Content Areas

Medical and Behavioral Sciences	Practice Environment	Examination, Evaluation, Diagnosis	Plan of Care, Intervention, Outcome
Anatomy	Ethics	Musculoskeletal	Musculoskeletal
Physiology	Communication	Neuromuscular	Neuromuscular
Kinesiology	Psychosocial	Cardiopulmonary	Cardiopulmonary
Biomechanics	Cultural	Integumentary	Integumentary
Pharmacology	competence	Medical	Medical
Neuroscience	Leadership	screening	screening
Pathology	Professional	Gait	Gait
Nutrition	practice		Therapeutic
Diagnostic	Business		exercise
imaging	practice		Physical agents
Psychology	Health care		
Research/	administration		
evidence-based			
practice			
Teaching/learning			
Motor learning			

From Weddle M, Sellheim D. An integrative curriculum model preparing physical therapists for Vision 2020 practice. J Phys Ther Educ 2009;23:12-21.

---

stimulate development of students' abilities to reflect, critically analyze, and make rational decisions. Figure 1–4 shows a logical connection between an element of a program's philosophy or mission and how a course in pediatrics presents this element in course objectives, required

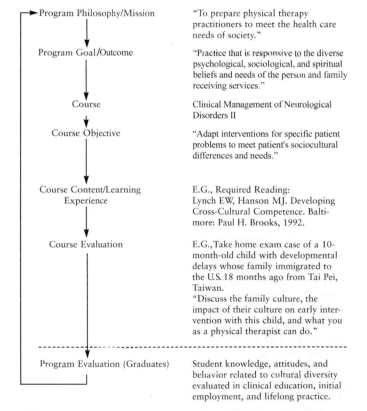

Program Philosophy/Mission	"To prepare physical therapy practitioners to meet the health care needs of society."
Program Goal/Outcome	"Practice that is responsive to the diverse psychological, sociological, and spiritual beliefs and needs of the person and family receiving services."
Course	Clinical Management of Neurological Disorders II
Course Objective	"Adapt interventions for specific patient problems to meet patient's sociocultural differences and needs."
Course Content/Learning Experience	E.G., Required Reading: Lynch EW, Hanson MJ. Developing Cross-Cultural Competence. Baltimore: Paul H. Brooks, 1992.
Course Evaluation	E.G., Take home exam case of a 10-month-old child with developmental delays whose family immigrated to the U.S. 18 months ago from Tai Pei, Taiwan. "Discuss the family culture, the impact of their culture on early intervention with this child, and what you as a physical therapist can do."
Program Evaluation (Graduates)	Student knowledge, attitudes, and behavior related to cultural diversity evaluated in clinical education, initial employment, and lifelong practice.

FIGURE 1–4 Example of the logical connection between program philosophy, program goal/outcome, course objective, course content and learning experience, and program evaluation.

readings, and stimulation of student thought during an examination.[26] Further information on designing coursework is provided in Chapters 2 and 3.

Tyler's Question 3: Organization

Tyler suggests three factors to consider in organizing educational experiences: continuity, sequence, and integration.[2] *Continuity* refers to the vertical reiteration of curricular elements, that is, providing continuing opportunities for students to practice and develop the cognitive, affective, or psychomotor skills they have learned. For example, teaching students good body mechanics in an early basic skills laboratory is followed by attention to, and reinforcement of, these same skills throughout clinical laboratory courses.

Sequence is related to continuity but moves beyond the reiteration and development of a single skill. Thus, sequence is the process of having each experience build on prior experience while moving increasingly broader and deeper into the material. For example, students assume greater and greater responsibility for patient care through each successive clinical internship. It would be considered poor sequencing to have a student spend the same amount of time observing the instructor during the last clinical internship as during the first internship.

Integration refers to the horizontal relationship of learning experiences. For example, a kinesiology course and an anatomy course might be placed together so that the same body segments are covered within similar time periods, and knowledge gained in one course could overlap and clarify knowledge gained in the other course.

Obviously, proper continuity, sequence, and integration can be extraordinarily helpful in assisting the student to master curricular content. However, there are many structural constraints to organizing a curriculum. The primary consideration is the academic calendar of the college or university in which the program is located (i.e., the length of each semester or quarter and how many units of work are normally expected of students within that institution within the given time frame). Consideration must also be given to availability of clinical sites—it would be impossible to expect clinical internships to occur only in the summer when the usual academic year is not in session (and clinics may have the greatest number of staff on vacation). In addition, faculty and clinical expertise must be juggled across classes in different years of the program, with available laboratory space factored in as a major structural constraint. One can see how easy it would be to organize a curriculum based on structural constraints alone!

In addition to these resource and structural constraints, the faculty who design physical therapy curricula are concerned about what students *must* know before their first clinical experience. Faculty often desire that students know at least a little about nearly everything before entering their clinical internships. This is strongly reinforced by clinical instructors who, faced with examining and treating patients within dwindling time periods, want students to know at least something about typical clinical problems they will be treating and common evaluation and treatment strategies that will enable them to be immediately useful. Because of the pressures of the clinical environment, most clinical administrators are understandably more receptive to accommodating students during their last clinical internship compared with the students' first internship. This desire to have immediately useful patient care skills even during an initial clinical assignment may result in a curricular organization that is antagonistic to the program's overall philosophy and goals. For example, a common strategy to "get it all in" is the presentation of foundation science courses (i.e., biological and physical science courses) and clinical skill courses as early as possible in the curriculum. Courses deemed less relevant to hands-on patient care (e.g., the behavioral sciences, clinical management, and research courses) are taught late or last in the curriculum. In sacrificing long-term goals for short-term goals, faculty must realize they are also giving students a strong implicit message about what they consider most important in physical therapy practice.

Figure 1–5 illustrates how one physical therapy program that is using a problem-based learning approach (PBL) explicates its view of the relatively balanced approach across the foundation sciences (Biological/Physical/Clinical Sciences; Behavioral Sciences), clinical management, research, clinical reasoning, and clinical practice by presenting all these educational components in almost every semester of a 3-year physical therapy program with strong links to the five main curricular threads—professional reflection, physical therapy reasoning, foundational sciences, patient/client management, and professional topics/formation. The reader should be able to identify elements of continuity, sequence, and integration in this curricular organization.

In summary, the organization of educational experiences should relate directly to fulfilling the program's philosophy and expected outcomes for its graduates. Thus, it is more important for the faculty member to concentrate on how each student will perform after graduation than to concentrate on how many technical skills the student has before the first clinical internship.

Tyler's Question 4: Evaluation

If the objectives, content, and learning experiences of each course or clinical experience relate to the program's philosophy and goals, then student and instructor evaluation of each course and clinical component will give the faculty a good sense of whether the program's goals are being attained. Of course, the ultimate measure is how the graduates perform in clinical practice.

Program evaluation should cover all general and specific curricular goals. See Figure 1–4 for a specific example of how program evaluation provides a feedback loop so that faculty can determine how successfully the student has been taught to achieve a program goal. Regular and systematic

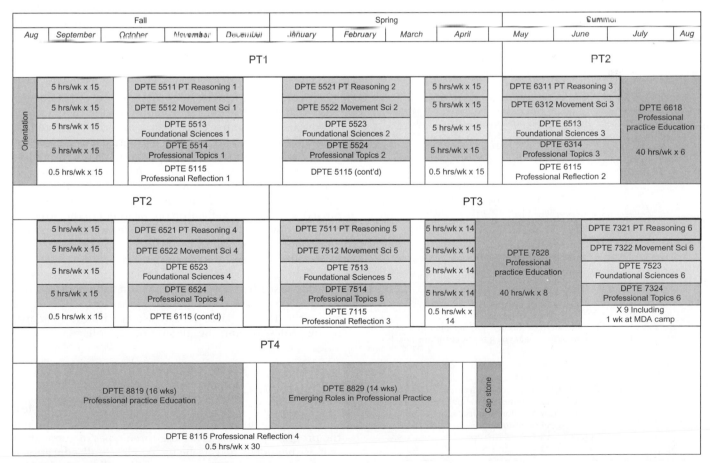

FIGURE 1–5 Example of a balanced approach to courses and curricular threads in a problem-based curriculum in a developing program. (From the University of Incarnate Word, San Antonio, TX.)

assessment of student performance at the end of every semester is an excellent strategy for integrating performance assessment of critical learning outcomes across all courses. Ask: What can the student do at the end of a designated semester or year? How can the student's ability to integrate knowledge and skills across courses be evaluated? These integrated assessments can include written components that help students develop test-taking skills as well as practical, laboratory performance and self-assessment and reflective skill development. Faculty collaborations in these kinds of accountability activities are rich resources for scholarly work. Chapter 5 on assessment provides much more detail in this area. Regular systematic evaluation of recent graduates by indirect assessment measures, such as surveys, interviews, or focus groups, will assist the program faculty in completing the curriculum design connections and answering the most important curricular question: Did the educational program achieve what it stated it would achieve in the program's philosophy and goals (outcomes)?

See Table 1–2 for examples of a variety of sources that might be tapped for meaningful program evaluative information. The data retrieved can be aligned with the

TABLE 1–2　Examples of Program Evaluation Data

Sources	Examples of Types of Data
Students	Recruitment activities Admissions (prerequisite course work required, grade point averages, cultural diversity profile; personal statements) Academic performance (timely feedback to students, remediation activities; tracking of performance across program) Student retention issues
Faculty	Resumes (preparation for teaching; scholarship [publication and grants]; service to department, university, and profession; practice and consultation activities; honors and awards) Faculty development plans
Academic curriculum	Course syllabi (content, types of learning experiences, level of evaluation) Minutes of faculty retreats and planning sessions Assessment accountability reports/forms Student ratings of course instruction (course evaluations) Faculty and peer evaluations
Clinical curriculum	Development of clinical sites Types and length of clinical rotations Student evaluation of clinical instructors and learning opportunities Clinical instructor evaluation of student clinical performance
Environment	Support services (library holdings, computer laboratories, financial aid opportunities, health care services provided)
Graduates	Alumni surveys (clinical positions held; continuing education courses taken; specialist certifications awarded; participation in local, state, and national professional activities; participation in research and publications; community volunteer activities) Licensure examination scores Employer satisfaction surveys Patient satisfaction surveys

Adapted from Diamond R. Designing and Assessing Courses and Curricula, ed 3. San Francisco: Jossey-Bass, 2009.

philosophy and goals of any particular physical therapist or physical therapist assistant program.

THE DYNAMIC CURRICULAR PLATFORM

Decker Walker[3] proposed a naturalistic model of how faculty *really* go about developing a curriculum. He suggests that faculty discussions that culminate in a shared vision for a program form the platform on which all deliberations and eventual decisions about the program rest (see Figure 1–1). Walker[3] states, "the word *platform* is meant to suggest both a political platform and something to stand on. The platform includes an idea of what is and a vision of what ought to be, and these guide the curriculum developer in determining what he should do to realize his vision."

This process of deliberation in curriculum development is well documented. It is not an orderly progression from goals to objectives to content and then to evaluation, as was suggested by Tyler, but instead is a process of deliberation whereby faculty move back and forth between all these elements.[27] This deliberation informs the design decisions. We believe the Tyler and Walker models are useful in helping faculty understand the process of curriculum development. Tyler delineated the component parts of the process, and Walker described how faculty actually discuss, debate, and negotiate to arrive at a curriculum.

It is useful for all academic and clinical faculty members to have the agreed-on program philosophy and goals (a synthesis of the platform) in front of them when preparing their academic or clinical course objectives and related learning experiences. During this preparation time, faculty can use the philosophy and goals as a guide in their planning. The program philosophy and goals/outcomes that provide the platform on which the physical therapy program rests should be discussed and revised, if necessary, every year before curriculum planning for the following year (that is, before Tyler's second and third questions are discussed and answered). Furthermore, every student in the physical therapy or physical therapist assistant program could benefit from having a copy of the program's philosophy and goals/outcomes, and an opportunity to discuss these philosophy and goals/outcomes with the faculty early on as well as during her or his academic program. Such discussion and reflection on the intent of the program can be a powerful tool in helping students understand the coursework and required educational experiences, as well as socializing them into the profession.

For an example related to physical therapist assistant education, see Box 1–4. In this mission statement, a physical therapist assistant program has clearly stated what the student will be prepared for consistent with the standards of the profession and the mission of the college.

IMPLICIT, EXPLICIT, AND NULL CURRICULUM

Throughout the design and implementation of a physical therapy curriculum, the faculty can gain insight about the program by considering the three types of curriculum that Eisner identified as being taught in all educational programs: the *implicit*, *explicit*, and *null* curriculum.[6,28] The explicit curriculum is publicly stated and is available

BOX 1–4 Physical Therapist Assistant Program Mission: Clarkson College

Mission: Preparing students to professionally provide high-quality, ethical, and compassionate health care services

- Values
  - **Learning:** The lifelong process of education through both structured and unstructured experiences
  - **Caring:** An empowering relationship through an attitude of empathy, compassion, and respect for those with whom we interact and serve
  - **Commitment:** Dedication to the shared mission of Clarkson College
  - **Integrity:** Adherence to moral and ethical standards in personal, professional, and organizational actions
  - **Excellence:** A level of performance in which all individuals strive for extraordinary quality

Physical Therapy Assistant (PTA) Program mission and philosophy: The PTA program at Clarkson College utilizes high-quality, well-integrated, contemporary curricula to prepare students to deliver professional, ethical, competent, and compassionate health care. Physical Therapy (PT) is a healing profession. It focuses on the restoration of musculoskeletal and neuromuscular function, the promotion of physical wellness, and a commitment to service to others. PTAs are individuals who play an integral role as part of the patient care team by assisting the physical therapist in patient care. Involvement with patient care in PT requires an educated individual who possesses a basic insight into human nature and who places a strong moral value on human life. PTAs are influential professionals who advance the field of PT as clinic administrators, faculty members, clinical instructors, and clinicians—and by participating in professional organizations at the state and national levels. They are educationally and technically trained health care professionals concerned with improving the well-being of all humankind and empowered to make a positive difference.

From Clarkson College, Physical Therapist Assistant Program, Omaha, NE

to everyone. The implicit curriculum, which is more subtle and potentially more powerful, is known especially by students and graduates of the program. The term *hidden curriculum* is also used in referring to this informal learning that is such an important but often unrecognized aspect of the learning environment.[29] The null curriculum may be known to only a few or to no one because it includes the elements that are left out of the explicit curriculum, and it is a potential blind spot in planning.

EXPLICIT CURRICULUM

The explicit curriculum includes those explicitly defined and publicly shared aspects of the curriculum that are found in university catalogues, program brochures, and course syllabi. Explicit curricular elements include, for example, the prerequisite courses, the program's stated philosophy and goals/outcomes, course objectives and required readings, the sequence and type of clinical affiliations, and the faculty's credentials.

Physical therapy students often identify the type of program they want to enter based on this explicit curriculum. Explicit elements, such as the location, length, and cost of the program, as well as the type of degree awarded, guide the applicant's choice of programs. Faculty are acutely attuned to the explicit curriculum as they discuss and alter various aspects in yearly or biyearly curriculum planning sessions. Clinical instructors receive explicit curricular information on student preparedness for their clinical affiliations (e.g., description of coursework completed by the affiliating students). When program outcomes are assessed, alumni are often asked to state their level of satisfaction with specific courses they completed. One easily might consider the explicit curriculum to be the only curriculum. However, students, alumni, clinicians, and new faculty can often distinguish and discuss the presence and power of a second type of curriculum, the implicit curriculum.

IMPLICIT CURRICULUM

The implicit curriculum includes the values, beliefs, and expectations that are transmitted to students by the knowledge, language, and everyday actions of the academic and clinical faculty. The faculty themselves may be less aware of these values, beliefs, and expectations than students and alumni of the program. As we wrote in our 1990 article, "...students regularly receive from faculty members implicit messages about the relative importance of certain types of knowledge, what types of patients are most interesting and challenging, and what personal and professional behaviors are acceptable and unacceptable"[28] (Table 1–3).

Clinical and academic faculty are often unaware that every time they appear before students they are demonstrating behaviors they consider appropriate and professional. These often unconscious behaviors, for better or for worse, are powerful socializing elements that mold the future professional behaviors of students. For example, how faculty members engage in their own lifelong learning, make off-hand comments about patients and families or other faculty or students, participate in the concerns of professional organizations, and demonstrate caring are all absorbed by students as templates on which to model their own professional values, attitudes, and behaviors.

The implicit curriculum is also the basis for many decisions made about the explicit curriculum. For example, as discussed earlier, the sequence of coursework in a program (e.g., biological sciences first and social sciences last) and the length of time devoted to certain topics (e.g., prevention and wellness versus acute and chronic pathologic conditions) can give students a strong implicit message about what information is considered more or most important to the practice of physical therapy and what is considered less or least important. In fact, every aspect of explicit coursework contains an implicit message. For example, do the objectives of a course in clinical procedures include an emphasis on professional behaviors or dispositions (routine or habitual behaviors) as well as on specific manual techniques? Do instructors expect the same careful draping techniques when students are working with each other in laboratories as when they are working with patients? Do examinations include clinical problems that challenge the student to think about the individual person who is receiving treatment as well as about the specific impairment problems they are treating? The most critical point about the implicit or hidden curriculum is that the less distance and greater congruence between the explicit curriculum (formal) and the informal curriculum, the greater is the chance of facilitating a consistent professional identity.[28] Engaging your faculty in this kind of critical reflective conversation that uncovers strong messages in the informal curriculum is an important aspect of a dynamic curriculum process.

TABLE 1-3 Examples of Implicit Curriculum in Physical Therapist and Physical Therapist Assistant Programs

Curriculum Component	Example
Courses considered most important versus those considered least important	Courses that receive scheduling priorities for class time, location, and optimal examination times
Modeling of effective stress management	Faculty members* demonstrate calm and resiliency in response to no-show patients or guest lecturers, broken audiovisual equipment, sudden scheduling changes
Critical thinking considered inherent in professional behavior	Faculty members critically analyze information, brainstorm ideas, and demonstrate tolerance for ambiguity
Modeling of effective, professional behaviors	Faculty members demonstrate and expect of students courtesy, initiative, respect for other viewpoints, and willingness to act as moral agents
Expectations for lifelong learning	Faculty members display a continual quest for the latest evidence and knowledge, integrate references into their teaching, share ideas from their research, attend and make presentations in health care settings and at clinical conferences
Respect for and trust in one's colleagues	Faculty members demonstrate enthusiasm for team teaching and treating and express fascination with alternative viewpoints. Faculty members demonstrate respect for other health care professionals and are engaged in interprofessional teaching and practice activities on campus or in the community.
Openness to innovation	Faculty members encourage students to explore alternative health care philosophies and models of practice (e.g., acupuncture, Feldenkrais method, Alexander technique)
Respect for and sensitivity to patients	Faculty members refer to patients as individuals characterized by complex and unique physical, social, and behavioral characteristics rather than by diagnosis or body parts
Expectations for lifelong service to the profession	Faculty members participate in committees and task forces and on boards at district, state, and national level of the American Physical Therapy Association and other organizations
Professional commitment to our social contract with society	Program has a dynamic curriculum that is responsive to societal needs; the program and faculty are connected in meaningful ways to the communities (institutional, local and regional).

The term faculty members implies academic and clinical faculty members.
Adapted and revised from KF Shepard, GM Jensen. Physical therapist curricula for the 1990s: Educating the reflective practitioner. Phys Ther 1990;70:566.

NULL CURRICULUM

The null curriculum includes those elements of physical therapy practice that are missing from the curriculum. Some elements are missing because there is no voice to champion their inclusion. This becomes a blind spot and

is especially true about areas of physical therapy practice in which fewer physical therapists are currently engaged. For example, how much information do students receive about the role of physical therapists in obstetrics-gynecology care, hospice care, pro bono work with the homeless, or contributions that could be made in hospital emergency rooms and during times of disaster?

The null curriculum has the same impact on the professional attitudes and behaviors of students as the explicit curriculum and implicit curriculum. If, for example, students are never exposed to centers for adults who are developmentally delayed or well-elderly centers during their clinical internships, who will elect to seek a position in such a setting as a first choice after graduation?

Some curricular elements are missing because there simply is no time to teach any more information. Every academic and clinical faculty member grapples with how best to spend the limited time available for teaching. "More is better" is not the answer. Cramming more and more material into an unexpandable time sequence encourages rote memorization and repetition of tasks, drives out analytical and creative thinking, and, worst of all, snuffs out a desire to learn by setting unattainable goals that leave the students awash in fatigue and frustration.

Faculty must carefully consider and consciously weigh what to include and what to exclude from each course. Faculty need to remember that they are helping students develop their knowledge structure or scaffold, a central point in facilitating student learning. This building of the knowledge structure is not downloading information but rather is the careful selection of critical components of knowledge that are part of the need to know. Time for reflective thought and integration of concepts and ideas, as well as time for being presented with new information, must be consciously and deliberately built into the curricula structure from the beginning. In the same manner, clinical instructors must weigh whether to expose the student to an extensive potpourri of diagnoses and potential physical therapy treatment techniques or to teach students in-depth assessment and treatment skills for the most common clinical problems the student will encounter in practice. Trying to do both in depth will only promote anxiety and end in frustration for the clinical instructor and the student.

Decisions concerning the null curriculum are not easy to make. Two guideposts faculty might use in deciding what not to include are the current skills demanded in clinical practice and what skills students can attain after they are practicing in the field. To use the first guidepost, academic faculty benefit enormously from visiting students at clinical sites and having clinicians from different settings participate in curriculum planning sessions. For example, how much time are physical therapists and physical therapist assistants spending on hands-on care in comparison with teaching the patient and family to manage their own health care needs? The related curriculum issues are how much curricular emphasis is placed on teaching students to teach patients and families compared with how much time is devoted to presenting students with an ever-increasing array of manual skills. What skills are physical therapists and physical therapist assistants currently performing? Are they working as teams? The related curriculum questions are: (1) Does the physical therapy curricula contain information on physical therapists' and physical therapist assistants' roles, supervision, and the basic elements of effective teamwork? and (2) Do clinical education experiences allow guided experiences in physical therapist–physical therapist assistant teamwork?

The second guidepost, an emphasis on lifelong learning, can relieve the time constraint frustrations experienced by academic and clinical faculty and students. If faculty believe that the degree-granting educational program is only the start of the student's career and that the program provides only the most basic building blocks of that career, then attention can be turned from *what* to learn to *how* to learn. Thus, if students are taught how to gather and analyze information, to incubate ideas, to constantly reflect on their decisions and clinical performance, and to identify their learning needs (and observe academic and clinical faculty doing this), then they will become lifelong learners, learning as much each year in practice as they did during their matriculation in an academic program. The development of students' meta-cognitive skills, that is, their ability to think about their thinking, is perhaps the most important component of professional education. A program cannot teach everything, but it can teach to the needs of the current clinical climate and prepare students to learn for all the years of their lives.

An effective educational program for physical therapists and physical therapist assistants is one in which the explicit, implicit, and null curricula are known to the faculty and are complementary. Faculty can identify strategies that will allow them to garner periodic input about their implicit, as well as explicit and null, curricula from students, alumni, clinicians, and on-site accreditation teams. Being able to assess and understand the power, influence, and outcome of one's curricular efforts through input from multiple parties is an intellectually challenging, rewarding, and joyful endeavor.

BRIDGING THE LIBERAL ARTS AND PROFESSIONAL EDUCATION

In 1974, Lewis Mayhew and Patrick Ford first described the inevitable conflicts that arise between educational programs for professionals (e.g., medicine, education, engineering, and law) and the traditional long-standing liberal arts educational programs (e.g., biology, English, philosophy, and physics).[30]

Many of these issues are still unresolved, which is a testament to the long-standing conservatism and resistance to change that characterizes American higher education. Elizabeth Domholdt included many of these issues, which she calls "sins of professional programs," in her 2007 Cerasoli Lecture.[31]

The conflicts stem from the different educational outcomes that liberal arts programs and professional programs seek to attain. The goal of traditional liberal arts colleges is to create a learned person who has a grasp of many aspects of the world through development of both the analytical mode of thinking and the more contextual or narrative mode of thinking through the humanities, whereby one learns about making sense of situations, understanding diversity of meaning and views, and prepares to go out into the world to continue to learn. The focus is on discourse,

theory, and the need to reason, argue, create, and, as graduation speakers exhort, "to make a difference in the world." The goal of professional programs, in general, and physical therapy programs, in particular, is to graduate students who will be prepared to function as professionals in a specifically defined field of endeavor. The focus is on attainment of practical skills, behaviors, and attitudes that reflect the ethos and functions, as bestowed by society, of that profession.

Here are some of the continued areas of tension between liberal arts programs and physical therapy programs located within the same institution:

Perceptions of curriculum content. The curricular content of most physical therapy education programs is contested by college and university academicians and physical therapy practitioners. Academic faculty from liberal arts departments who have a strong voice on college and university curriculum committees often argue that physical therapy curricula focus too much on practical application and not enough on the theoretical underpinnings of knowledge. Conversely, clinicians chide physical therapy faculty for spending too much time on theory and not being responsive to the "real world" of clinical practice. (An unfortunate refrain often echoed by students returning from clinical internships.) If the physical therapy faculty member has recently come from the clinical setting, she or he is more likely to teach clinical knowledge, knowledge that has been transformed by experience. Thus, these novice educators present students with a rich potpourri of clinically relevant information, only some of which can be found in textbooks. In contrast, the longer faculty members have been in the academic setting, the more socialized they are to the traditions of academia, and the more theory and critical analysis will play a prominent role in their courses. Of course, both perspectives are important and relevant to physical therapy curricula. However, conflict arises because there simply is not time to teach both perspectives in depth. Thus, the collective faculty continually struggle with (and faculty meetings are often permeated with) arguments about these somewhat antagonistic perspectives.

Graduates as agents of change. The university has traditionally been perceived as an agent of change in society. It is a place in which new ideas, skills, materials, and methods are created and shared with the world. However, to produce practitioners who must work in today's demanding health care environments, faculty must first ensure that their graduates are ready to practice. That is, they must focus their attention on codifying and transmitting the conventional lore that is accepted by the profession and will be tested by national licensing examinations. Creating new knowledge clearly has a secondary place in professional programs. This fact has placed many professional graduate physical therapy programs at odds with graduate curricular and promotion and tenure committees.

Role of prerequisite courses. All physical therapy programs rely on the liberal arts programs of colleges and universities to supply prerequisite coursework for their entering students. The breadth and level of many of these prerequisite courses in the biological, physical, and social sciences are an anathema to physical therapy educators. Professional programs, of course, have little say in the content of these prerequisite courses, and similarly titled courses at community colleges, small private colleges, and large public universities yield strikingly dissimilar educational backgrounds among students in an entering physical therapy class. Teaching students who enter with different levels of prerequisite coursework is frustrating to faculty (and the students themselves), who must continually readjust the foundation science, clinical science, and transcurricular content of their coursework to meet a low to middle level of student knowledge.

Role of clinical education. The clinical education portion of the curriculum that takes place outside the walls of the university is not well understood nor particularly well supported by most institutions of higher education. Although students do pay a fee for clinical education coursework to the college or university to cover costs (e.g., salary for the academic coordinator of clinical education, travel to site visits, legal fees for preparation of clinical contracts, and administrative costs for maintaining student records), the clinical education site receives little or no compensation for its participation in physical therapy student education. The cries of clinical educators and administrators within health care environments who must figure out how to absorb the cost of clinical education programs long have fallen on the deaf ears of university administrators. As a result of current health care economics, many health care facilities have downsized or eliminated their student education programs. In response to the loss of clinical sites, different models of clinical education are being created that are more cost-effective to health care organizations than the time-honored, effective but expensive model of one instructor to one student teaching. See Chapter 8 for further discussion of this issue.

Faculty integration into the academy. Tenure and stability for any faculty member (and the program in which the faculty member teaches) come as a result of proven performance in three traditional areas of academic engagement: scholarship, teaching, and service. Of these three, scholarship, or success in developing a research program that garners external grants and provides the grist for research papers (creation of knowledge) acceptable for publication in peer-reviewed professional journals, is the area that has traditionally counted most toward tenure in universities. Most university arts and sciences faculty begin their academic careers with a doctorate degree in hand and their own well-defined and productive area of research. For these faculty, it is difficult, but not impossible, to juggle these three areas of endeavor with a high level of competence.

As Patrick Ford states, "Because physical therapy educators have, by and large, been socialized and mentored into a profession different from the profession of college and university teaching, they bring to the academy an ethos and a set of values and expectations that are frequently quite at odds with the prevailing value structure within higher education."[32] That is, physical therapy faculty are generally more than ready to teach students about clinical practice and to maintain their own clinical competence. However, many are exceedingly ill prepared to embrace the traditions

of scholarship that are expected and needed for full acceptance in the academic world. Physical therapy faculty who teach in the clinical sciences must, of course, keep their clinical skills and knowledge updated. Many faculty work at least part-time in clinical settings, thus squeezing a fourth area of engagement into their busy academic schedules. It is difficult enough to do three things well (teaching, research, and service), but it is nearly impossible to do four things well (teaching, research, service, and clinical practice). Many excellent clinician-educators have found themselves outside the university walls after 6 years because they were unable to fulfill the three classic tenure requirements.

Of course, knowing that these inevitable conflicts exist in the university is the starting place for resolution. At the heart of this resolution is the development of physical therapy educational programs that attract scholars who fit the traditional liberal arts model of excellence in teaching and research, as well as experienced clinicians who provide students with excellence in teaching and exposure to excellence in clinical practice. Creative thinking about ways to keep these clinical educators within the university has prompted such solutions as the development of faculty-run clinical practices and consultation and service contracts with nearby health care agencies and creation of clinical faculty appointment lines in schools of health professions.

Finally, a powerful argument is made for bridging our worlds of liberal arts and professional education by William Sullivan.[33] He argues that the practical, field experiences that are central in most of professional education are a missing dimension in liberal arts education. In turn, he argues that the professions are at risk with their dominant emphasis on analytical thinking when there is a need for deeper training in understanding the context, values, and meanings that are part of the fabric of human interaction that comes with a sound liberal arts background. He believes that health care professionals need to further develop their practical reasoning ability, which includes bringing the analytical skills together with the concern and understanding of human well-being so that they can make judgments in uncertain conditions that are part of everyday practice. This situation is ideal for more intentional faculty development and discussion across a campus, and the bridge between the liberal arts and the professional schools can be helpful in enhancing both areas. He argues the need for educators to explore, "How to educate for integrity as well as competence, how to impart the fundamentals of good professional judgment, and how to teach complex skill so that students not only master the technical craft of the profession but also develop analytical skills and learn generalizable principles that make possible creative solutions to new situations." (p 84)

PROFESSIONAL ACCREDITATION FOR PHYSICAL THERAPIST AND PHYSICAL THERAPIST ASSISTANT PROGRAMS

Accreditation is an American invention—in fact, it is uniquely American. Because it is a peer-review process carried out by volunteers and, at least as originally conceived, voluntary and nongovernmental, it is not only American by invention but also in principle. Like American democracy, it is not a perfect system, but also like American democracy, no one has found a better way to do what it does. To our knowledge, every other nation in the world has a federal ministry of education that governs who shall teach what, and often who shall study what and at what level. That we in the United States rely on a nongovernmental, voluntary system of quality assurance is partly because our founding fathers rejected the notion of a federal education system. They respected choice and recognized the importance in an ideal democratic society that the intelligentsia not be controlled by the government.[34]

The primary function of accreditation is to set and ensure performance standards within disciplines across colleges and universities. Review Box 1–5 to gain an understanding of the breadth of purposes that support this quality assurance function.

Academic programs are judged by performance standards that include quantitative criteria and qualitative analysis. Quantitative criteria might include, for example, national licensure examination scores of program graduates and professional qualifications of the faculty. Qualitative analysis might include the type of learning experiences students are engaged in and how these experiences affect the performance of the program graduates. These qualitative judgments can only be made by other people, and thus an on-site peer review visit is common practice. In this way, the public is assured that the institution meets or exceeds the general standards set for similar programs and institutions.

Judging quality is not easy. It cannot be reduced to quantitative indices or formulas. Such judgments are made by gathering appropriate information about an institution or program and by having knowledgeable people appraise it. This is the essence of accreditation.[35] The Council for Higher Education Accreditation lists these core steps in the U.S. accreditation process[35]:

- Accrediting organizations develop standards that must be met to be accredited.
- Institutions or programs undertake self-studies based on these accreditation standards.
- Institutions and programs are then subject to peer review that include site visits and team reports.

- Accrediting organizations make a judgment based on standards through their decision-making commissions or board and grant (or do not grant) accredited status.
- Institutions and programs undergo periodic review by accrediting organizations to maintain accredited status.
- Accreditation is a standards-based, evidence-based, judgment-based, peer-review process.

Physical therapy educational programs can achieve accreditation through a process established by CAPTE.[36] The mission of CAPTE is to serve the public by establishing and applying standards that assure quality and continuous improvement in the entry-level preparation of physical therapists and physical therapist assistants and that reflect the evolving nature of education, research, and practice. The mission is carried out by a 29-member commission composed of physical therapy educators who are basic scientists, curriculum specialists, and academic administrators; physical therapy clinicians and clinical educators; administrators from institutions of higher education; and public representatives assisted by a cadre of more than 250 trained on-site reviewers and a seven-member staff in the APTA Department of Accreditation.

Since 1983, CAPTE has been the sole accrediting agency recognized by the U.S. Department of Education and the Council on Higher Education Accreditation to accredit entry-level physical therapist and physical therapist assistant education programs. As the sole accrediting agency, CAPTE makes autonomous decisions regarding the accreditation status of physical therapist and physical therapist assistant programs.

Although accreditation of physical therapy education programs is considered a voluntary process because there are no federal laws requiring a program to be accredited, all viable physical therapy education programs in the United States are accredited or in the process of becoming accredited. The reason, beyond assuring students and the public that the program conforms to general standards for the education of competent practitioners, is that all 50 states, the District of Columbia, and Puerto Rico require graduation from an accredited program as a prerequisite for acquiring a practice license.

The development of a new program does not occur overnight. APTA Accreditation Department staff and physical therapy educational consultants are available to work with an institution from the time it first inquires about developing a program. The preaccreditation, or candidacy, phase begins when an institution has employed a qualified, full-time program director. During this phase, the program submits substantive documentation 6 months before enrolling students. This documentation contains a comprehensive prospectus that includes an overview of the entire curriculum plan and identification of faculty, clinical sites, college or university resources (e.g., budget, space, and libraries) in place or needed to support the program, and a plan for evaluating performance of the graduates. This documentation is thoroughly reviewed and evaluated by a Candidacy Reviewer, who then makes a visit to the institution to further review the program's progress in development. The Candidacy Reviewer prepares a report that is discussed with the program director, faculty, and

---

BOX 1–5   General Purposes of Accreditation

1. To foster excellence in postsecondary education through the development of criteria and guidelines for assessing educational effectiveness.
2. To encourage improvement of institutions and programs through continuous self-study and planning.
3. To assure other organizations and agencies, the educational community, and the general public that an institution or a particular program (a) has clearly defined and appropriate objectives, (b) maintains conditions under which its achievement can reasonably be expected, and (c) accomplishes its goals and continues to do so.
4. To provide counsel and assistance to established and developing programs and institutions.
5. To encourage the diversity of American postsecondary education and allow institutions to achieve their particular objectives and goals.
6. To endeavor to protect institutions against encroachments that might jeopardize their educational effectiveness or academic freedom.

From Young KE, Chambers CM, Kells HR, et al. Understanding Accreditation. San Francisco: Jossey-Bass, 1983, p 23.

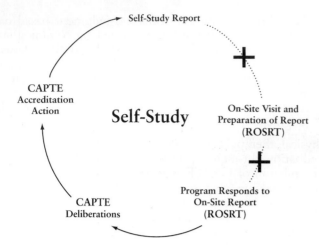

FIGURE 1–6 Ongoing self-study by the educational program is central to the accreditation process. (*CAPTE*, Commission on Accreditation in Physical Therapy Education; *ROSRT*, report of the on-site review team.)

college administrators and, along with updated materials, is forwarded to the commission for its decision regarding candidacy status. Candidacy status is required for a program to move forward in seeking accreditation status.

SELF-STUDY REPORT

The accreditation process is somewhat parallel to the pre-accreditation process in that a program prepares and submits a detailed self-study report. The self-study process is a continual cycle fundamental to accreditation (Figure 1–6). During a self-study, the program's faculty is encouraged to use a system of ongoing review and evaluation for all program aspects.

With respect to the previous Council on Postsecondary Accreditation quotation, in physical therapy accreditation, "gathering appropriate information" would refer to the self-study report, and the "knowledgeable people" would be the members of the on-site review team as well as members of CAPTE.

The program is guided in its ongoing program review and development of the self-study report by the Evaluative Criteria for Accreditation of Educational Programs for the Preparation of Physical Therapists or a comparable set of evaluative criteria for the physical therapist assistant program.[36] The evaluative criteria are periodically revised by CAPTE with input and feedback from many sources to reflect current standards of professional practice.

Reviewing these criteria will provide the reader with an excellent overview of the standards against which comparable physical therapy educational programs are assessed.[34,35] These criteria can be used on an ongoing basis by faculty for program evaluation. Reading these criteria also gives one an appreciation for the amount of extensive documentation regarding all phases of the program that is contained in a self-study report and reviewed and evaluated by the faculty as well as CAPTE.

The process of preparing a self-study report allows academic and clinical educators to review in depth all components of the curriculum to determine what is done and done well, what is done to an adequate or less than adequate degree, what is missing that should be included, and what can be omitted to update and strengthen the

program. Thus, the process of developing a self-study report is the first and most important aspect of ensuring and enhancing the quality of a physical therapy or physical therapist assistant educational program.

The self-study report contains extensive information in two major areas: (1) institution and program integrity and capacity (including program mission, goals, and expected outcomes; program faculty; and program resources), and (2) curriculum plan, evaluation, content, and outcomes. The most important of these areas are the data that substantiate the outcome performance of the program graduates. All physical therapist and physical therapist assistant programs are urged to collect, compile, and review performance outcome data at frequent intervals. These data may include national physical therapy and physical therapist assistant licensing examination scores, surveys of graduates regarding their opinions about the strengths and weaknesses of the educational program, information that reflects the ongoing professional growth of graduates, input obtained from employers, and patient satisfaction surveys. Review Table 1–2 for a more complete list of examples of potential program evaluation data.

The self-study report is reviewed by a three-member on-site review team. The team consists of at least one physical therapist (or physical therapist assistant) educator and one physical therapist (or physical therapist assistant) clinician. The third team member may be a higher education administrator or basic scientist or educator from another health discipline. The purpose of the on-site visit is to confirm the information presented in the self-study report, to describe the qualitative aspects of the program that cannot be determined by simply reading a paper document, and to provide summary information and consultation to the program.[34] The on-site review team's knowledge of the program by the conclusion of the visit enables team members to provide expert consultation in areas where the program may wish to enhance quality and is not included in the team's written report to the commission. The report of the on-site review team functions as a powerful "snapshot" of the program at the time of the site visit. The program's self-study report, along with the report of the on-site review team and any updated information the program wishes to present as a result of the report, is reviewed by members of CAPTE. Based on this review, the program is granted one of three general types of accreditation status: accreditation, probationary accreditation, or withdrawal of accreditation. This intensive process is currently scheduled to occur 5 years after initial accreditation and then every 10 years, with smaller annual accreditation reports containing updated program information due to CAPTE each year.

Mary Jane Harris, MS, PT, Director of the APTA Department of Accreditation, states, "CAPTE accreditation is all about fostering quality physical therapy education by encouraging program enhancement. In that way, CAPTE helps to assure that graduate physical therapists and physical therapist assistants are competent to enter the profession."

Faculty, clinicians, students, graduates, and administrators who have the opportunity to become involved with any aspect of the accreditation process are encouraged to do so with enthusiasm. In doing so, one witnesses an amazing process in which a community of professional peers works with unusual dedication to constantly strengthen and improve the educational foundations of physical therapy practice.

SUMMARY

This chapter has given the reader an overview of the rational yet dynamic process of curricular design and has identified macro- and micro-level factors that influence curricular content. The three components of all curricula—implicit, explicit, and null—have been identified, as well as factors that have the potential to support or hinder implementation of a coherent, meaningful curriculum. Historical and pervasive conflicts between liberal arts and professional programs have been outlined and several strategies for resolution and opportunity identified. Finally, this chapter has presented a synthesized overview of accreditation, which is an engaging process that provides a stimulus and benchmark for quality physical therapy and physical therapist assistant education. The focus of all these efforts is to ensure excellence in clinical practice and provide learning experiences that will, as John Dewey states, "live fruitfully and creatively in subsequent experiences."[4]

THRESHOLD CONCEPTS

Threshold Concept #1. The power of the implicit or hidden curriculum is well known across educational programs. We know that 5 years from graduation our graduates are much more likely to remember elements of the implicit curriculum than the explicit or formal curriculum. Much of the formation of professional identity or professional formation stems from this informal or implicit curriculum.

Think about strategies you can use to identify and expose elements in the core curriculum. Can you integrate more reflective questions into your evaluation or assessment processes? Perhaps you can look at focus group data from your graduates. What about the platform of beliefs and values of your core faculty? What are they, not on paper, but in action?

Threshold Concept #2. Accreditation is an important multidimensional tool for not only accountability but also quality enhancement. Educational leadership is critical to the success of this process centered on self-evaluation.

If you were entering into the self-evaluation process to prepare a self-study report for accreditation by CAPTE, how might you conceptualize and carry out a process to accurately assess your program? How would you involve multiple stakeholders? How could the process be designed and implemented to enhance outcomes?

ANNOTATED BIBLIOGRAPHY

American Physical Therapy Association Education Division. *A Normative Model of Physical Therapist Professional Education: Version 2004.* Alexandria, VA: American Physical Therapy Association; 2004.

This normative model originally was developed as a result of a series of national curricular conferences sponsored by the APTA Education Division. Using a framework of 23 practice expectations for entry into the field of physical therapy, this monograph contains examples of suggested curricular content in foundation and clinical sciences along with examples of terminal instructional objectives for classroom and clinical settings. Planned ongoing revisions of this model ensure responsiveness to changing practice, education, and health care environments. Physical therapy educators can glean many useful ideas for providing relevant classroom and clinical learning experiences from this monograph.

Commission on Accreditation in Physical Therapy Education. *Accreditation Handbook.* Alexandria, VA: American Physical Therapy Association; 2010.

A "must" online document or book for all physical therapy faculty. This handbook contains the evaluative criteria for all physical therapy and physical therapist assistant programs. Interpretive comments and guidelines provided under the criteria are very useful in helping faculty to understand all relevant components of a physical therapy educational program and what is important to focus on to meet national standards. Several position papers are included on areas such as faculty scholarship, faculty credentials, and distance education.

Diamond RM. *Designing and Assessing Courses and Curricula: A Practical Guide,* revised ed. San Francisco: Jossey-Bass; 1998.

This classic text provides several detailed examples of how to map out content and design of curricula. The book is written to be a helpful tool for faculty. It covers everything from aligning or linking program goals and courses to designing learning experiences.

Kern DE, Thomas PA, Howard DM, eds. *Curriculum Development for Medical Education: A Six-Step Approach.* 2nd ed. Baltimore: Johns Hopkins University Press; 2009.

This second edition continues to do an excellent job of explaining a simple six-step approach to curriculum development that includes problem identification, needs assessment, goals and objectives, educational strategies, implementation and evaluation, and feedback. The authors provide several helpful tables and charts for mapping the relationship between goals and objectives, objectives and educational methods, and strengths and weaknesses of evaluation tools. This is an excellent resource for anyone who is involved in curriculum work with health professions faculty.

Tyler R. *Basic Principles of Curriculum and Instruction.* Chicago: University of Chicago Press; 1949.

This small (124 pages), classic book suggests ways to go about finding answers to the four questions Tyler posed as fundamental to curriculum development. The methods proposed to seek these answers have stood the test of time. The author provides an easy-to-read, enlightening, commonsense approach to curriculum design.

REFERENCES

1. Shepard K. 38th Mary McMillan Lecture. Are you waving or drowning? *Phys Ther.* 2007;87:1543–1554.
2. Tyler RW. *Basic Principles of Curriculum and Instruction.* Chicago: University of Chicago Press; 1949.
3. Walker D. The process of curriculum development: a naturalistic model for curriculum development. *School Rev.* 1971;80:51
4. Dewey J. *Experience and Education.* New York: Collier Books; 1938.
5. American Physical Therapy Association Education Division. *A Normative Model of Physical Therapist Professional Education: Version 2004.* Alexandria, VA: American Physical Therapy Association; 2004.
6. Eisner EW. *The Educational Imagination: On the Design and Evaluation of School Programs.* 3rd ed. New York: Macmillan; 1994.
7. U.S. Department of Health and Human Services. Healthy People 2020. Available at: http://www.healthypeople.gov/2020/about/default.aspx. Accessed 5.08.2011.
8. Siller C. Exploring the ethos of the physical therapy profession in the United States: social, cultural and historical influences and their relationship to education. *J Phys Ther Educ.* 2000;14:7–15
9. Institute of Medicine. Quality and Patient Safety Report. Available at: http://www.iom.edu/Global/Topics/Quality-Patient-Safety.aspx. Accessed 5.08.2011.
10. Centers for Disease Control and Prevention. State of Aging and Health in America Report. Available at: http://apps.nccd.cdc.gov/SAHA/Default/Default.aspx. Accessed 5.08.2011.
11. Core Competencies for Interprofessional Collaborative Practice. Report of an Expert Panel. Interprofessional Education Collaborative. Available at: http://nnlm.gov/bhic/2011/05/26/core-competencies-interprofessional. Accessed 3.08.2011.

12. Sullivan K, Wallace J, O'Neill M, et al. A vision for society: physical therapy as partners in the National Health Agenda. *Phys Ther.* 2011;91:1664–1672.

13. Institute of Medicine Reports of the National Academies. Available at: http://www.iom.edu/About-IOM.aspx. Accessed 5.08.2011.

14. Foster C, Dahill L, Golemon L, Tolentino BW. *Educating Clergy: Teaching Practices and Pastoral Imagination.* San Francisco: Jossey-Bass; 2006.

15. Sullivan WS, Colby A, Wegner JW, et al. *Educating Lawyers: Preparation for the Profession of Law.* San Francisco: Jossey-Bass; 2007.

16. Sheppard S, Macatangay K, Colby A, Sullivan W. *Educating Engineers: Designing for the Future of the Field.* San Francisco: Jossey-Bass; 2009.

17. Benner P, Sutphen M, Leonard C, Day L. *Educating Nurses: A Call for Radical Transformation.* San Francisco: Jossey-Bass; 2010.

18. Cooke M, Irby D, O'Brien B. *Educating Physicians: A Call for Reform of Medical School and Residency.* San Francisco: Jossey-Bass; 2010.

19. Schön DA. *Educating the Reflective Practitioner: Toward a New Design for Teaching and Learning in the Professions.* San Francisco: Jossey-Bass; 1987.

20. Sullivan W. *Work and Integrity: The Crisis and Promise of Professionalism in America.* 2nd ed. San Francisco: Jossey-Bass; 2005.

21. American Physical Therapy Association. Guide to Physical Therapist Practice. Available at: http://guidetoptpractice.apta.org. Accessed 5.08.2011.

22. APTA Vision Sentence and Vision Statement for Physical Therapy 2020. Available at: http://www.apta.org/Vision2020; Accessed 5.08.2011.

23. World Health Organization. International Classification of Functioning, Disability and Health (ICF). Available at: http://www.who.int/classifications/icf/en/. Accessed August 5, 2011.

24. Prideaux D. Curriculum design: ABC of learning and teaching in medicine. *BMJ.* 2003;326:268–270.

25. Weddle M, Sellheim D. An integrative curriculum model preparing physical therapists for Vision 2020 practice. *J Phys Ther Educ.* 2009;23:12–21.

26. Kern DE, Thomas PA, Howard DM, Bass EB. *Curriculum Development for Medical Education: A Six-Step Approach.* Baltimore: Johns Hopkins University Press; 2009.

27. Harris I. Conceptual perspective and the formal curriculum. In: Hafler JP, ed. *Extraordinary Learning in the Workplace: Innovation and Change in Professional Education.* NY: Springer Science and Business Media; 2011:3–16.

28. Shepard KF, Jensen GM. Physical therapist curricula for the 1990s: educating the reflective practitioner. *Phys Ther.* 1990;70:566.

29. Hafler JP, ed. *Extraordinary Learning in the Workplace: Innovation and Change in Professional Education.* NY: Springer Science and Business Media; 2011.

30. Mayhew LB, Ford PJ. *Reform in Graduate and Professional Education.* San Francisco: Jossey-Bass; 1974.

31. Domholdt E. 2007 Pauline Cerasoli lecture: sins of the professional programs. *J Phys Ther Educ.* 2007;21:4–9.

32. Ford PJ. The nature of graduate professional education: some implications for raising the entry level. *J Phys Ther Educ.* 1990;4:3.

33. Sullivan WM, Rosin MS. *A New Agenda for Higher Education: Shaping the Life of the Mind for Practice.* San Francisco: Jossey-Bass; 2008.

34. Glidden R. The Contemporary Context of Accreditation: Challenges in a Changing Environment. Council for Higher Education Accreditation. In: *Keynote address for 2nd CHEA "Usefulness" Conference*; 1998:35 Washington, DC; June 25.

35. Council on Postsecondary Accreditation. Available at:http://www.chea.org/ Accessed August 6, 2011.

36. Commission on Accreditation in Physical Therapy Education. *Accreditation Handbook.* Available at:Alexandria, VA: American Physical Therapy Association; 2011. *http://www.capteonline.org/AccreditationHandbook/* Accessed 6.08.2011.

FROM CURRICULAR GOALS TO INSTRUCTION:
PREPARING TO TEACH

Gail M. Jensen ☼ Elizabeth Mostrom ☼ Katherine F. Shepard

CHAPTER OUTLINE

I remember well my first teaching experience in physical therapy education. I was assigned a "student teaching experience" to do a lecture and laboratory on the kinesiology and functional anatomy of the foot and ankle. I spent an entire holiday break preparing for my two hour lecture and one hour laboratory session. I read volumes of materials—articles, books and reviewed previous teaching materials. When I finally got to the point of preparing the objectives and teaching materials I struggled with decisions on how much, what depth, what applications, do I need to cover all of these conditions? By the end of the holiday break, I had proudly finished my lecture outline, handout materials, and accompanying visuals (in this case, about 50 slides). The next phase was a meeting with the faculty member who was supervising my teaching. Her first question was—just how much time did I think I had to teach this material? She reminded me that this was ONE lecture and laboratory session not an entire course on the foot and ankle. Patiently, she helped me downsize and focus on the key learning objectives and accompanying materials for a lecture and laboratory session. Even with that expert guidance and advice, I still found myself with TOO much material and too many expectations when I actually taught the class. This is a typical novice experience. You have to prepare with such breadth and depth and then want to put all of what you have learned into your teaching experience. It does not fit. Experienced teachers are able to make decisions about enduring knowledge—what students absolutely need to know.

LEARNING GOALS

After completing this chapter the reader will be able to:

1. Identify and discuss the characteristics of five different philosophical orientations to curriculum design and give specific examples of how each applies to physical therapy or physical therapist assistant curricula.

2. Describe four broad categories of learning theories that are based on different views of how students can learn: (1) behaviorism, (2) cognitive learning theory, (3) experiential/problem solving, and (4) social-cultural learning theory. Give specific examples of course materials that could best be taught by using each learning theory.

3. Discriminate among three major learning domains (i.e., cognitive, affective, and psychomotor) by citing elementary to complex levels within each that can be used to guide design of course content and assessment of student learning.

4. Identify the four learning styles described by Kolb[5] and give examples of student behavior that may be manifested by a high and low interest in each learning style.

5. Discuss construction of and specify the use of three different types of objectives that can be used to guide student learning: (1) behavioral, (2) problem solving, and (3) outcome.

6. Demonstrate how the delivery of course material, design of significant learning experiences, and evaluation of students is linked to the larger concepts of teaching and learning for enduring understanding through the processes of philosophical orientations, learning theories, learning domains, student learning styles, and course objectives.

7. List the items that could be included in a course syllabus.

8. Prepare a syllabus concept map that demonstrates the linkages across course key concepts.

Getting ready to teach a class or a course for the first time is almost always a perplexing situation. Where to start? Educators have suggested there are at least three kinds of knowledge essential to teaching effectively: (1) knowledge of the subject matter, (2) knowledge of the learners, and (3) knowledge of the general principles of teaching (i.e., knowledge of pedagogy).[1-4] This chapter presents an overview of the type of knowledge that physical therapy and physical therapist assistant educators are most often missing—knowledge of pedagogy.

PREACTIVE AND INTERACTIVE TEACHING

In 1967, a yellow paperback book titled, *Handbook for Physical Therapy Teachers*, was printed and distributed by the American Physical Therapy Association (APTA).[6] This small book was developed by a publication committee composed of Ruth Dickinson at Columbia University, Hyman L. Dervitz at Temple University, and Helen Meida at Western Reserve University. This book was the only source of information regarding physical therapy education at the time and included information on how to develop, organize, and teach a physical therapy curriculum across academic and clinical settings. The teaching focus of that pioneering book and this chapter is preactive teaching.

The terms *preactive* and *interactive* teaching were coined by psychologist Phillip Jackson.[7] *Preactive teaching* refers to those elements one considers when preparing to teach a course. Such activities include reading background information, preparing course syllabi, developing media, and even arranging the furniture in the classroom. These activities are highly rational—that is, the teacher reads, weighs evidence, reflects, organizes, relates the current class content to past and future classes the students are involved in, and creates an optimal environment for learning. Like the first-year teacher who was grappling with how to organize a 2-hour lecture, most of these activities occur when the teacher is alone and in an environment that allows for quiet, deliberative thought. Preactive preparation allows the teacher time to think through the breadth and depth of information that is to be presented (subject matter knowledge) to a particular group of students (knowledge of learners) as well as the most coherent and understandable way to present the information (pedagogical knowledge).[1,2]

By contrast, *interactive teaching* refers to what happens when the teacher is face to face with students. Interactive teaching activities are more or less spontaneous—that is, when working with large groups of students, the teacher tends to do what he or she feels or knows is right. In the chaotic milieu of a classroom, laboratory, or clinic, little time is available to reflect on what are appropriate and useful teaching strategies. Obviously, experienced teachers are considerably more skilled in interactive teaching and reflection-in-action than novice teachers.[8] This is similar to experienced clinicians who seem to know the right thing to do with patients with an ease and confidence that amazes novice clinicians. However, thoughtful preactive teaching preparation can allow even the novice teacher the freedom to focus on student understanding and learning rather than remain tightly tied to one's lecture notes. Preactive teaching elements are covered in this chapter. Chapter 3 focuses on interactive teaching elements.

PREACTIVE TEACHING GRID

This handbook assumes that the teacher is extraordinarily competent regarding the subject matter to be taught (subject matter knowledge) and is a physical therapist or physical therapist assistant who has a good knowledge of the students to be taught and what information they need for competent clinical practice. However, to organize and present material in a manner that is responsive to the program mission and desired student outcomes, the teacher is urged to think through the components identified in the preactive teaching grid (Figure 2–1). This grid is useful whether designing a whole course or a single class. When all components of the grid have been identified and are related to each other in a coherent fashion, the delivery of the course content also tends to be coherent to student and teacher. Note that the grid encourages the teacher to think through how much percentage in time and effort each of the elements contributes to the presentation of a particular content area.

PHILOSOPHICAL ORIENTATION

Eliot Eisner conceived of five philosophical orientations that can be used to guide curriculum design: development of cognitive processes, academic rationalism, technology, societal interests (social adaptation and social reconstruction), and personal relevance.[9,10] These orientations are based on what teachers think the aims of a curriculum, course, or class should be—that is, why they are teaching what they are teaching.

Cognitive Processing-Reasoning

The philosophical orientation of cognitive processing-reasoning focuses on teaching students to develop and refine their intellectual processes (e.g., how to gather and analyze data, how to pose and solve problems, how to infer, how to hypothesize, and how to make judgments based on limited information). The concern of the educator is on the *how* rather than the *what*. Little emphasis is placed on acquiring facts because the development of cognitive processing-reasoning orientation proposes that by teaching students how to think, reason, and use resources, they will be able to identify, locate, evaluate, and apply whatever information they might need.

Problem-based learning (PBL) is the centerpiece of problem-based curricula. PBL scenarios that are based on key cognitive processes needed by physical therapists are developed by faculty and form the basis of the core curriculum. Students then use "triggers" from the problem case scenario to define their own learning processes and then engage in independent, self-directed study before returning to the group to discuss and build their knowledge base. The building of a knowledge structure or scaffold is an essential component of all learning. Students must build that structure for themselves, and the PBL approach is

Teacher_____   Institution_____   Audience_____   Class Size_____   Date/Time_____

Philosophical Orientation +	Learning Theory +	Domain of Learning +	Student Learning Style +	Objectives
(%)	(%)	(%)	(%)	Behavioral
__Cognitive Processing-Reasoning	__Behaviorism	__Cognitive	__Concrete Experience	1._____
__Academic Rationalism	__Cognitive Structure	__Affective	__Reflective Observation	2._____
__Technology	__Experiential-Problem Solving	__Psychomotor	__Abstract-Conceptualization	
__Social Adaptation	__Social-Cultural	__Perceptual	__Active Experimentation	Problem Solving
__Social Reconstruction		__Spiritual		1._____
__Personal Relevance				2._____
				Outcome
				1._____
				2._____

Format of Delivery +	Teaching Aids +	Student Evaluation +	Teaching Environment +	SUBJECT BACKGROUND PREPARATION
(%)	A. Audiovisual	(%)	__Room Arrangement	(secure reference sources, evaluate and synthesize content, order the sequence, prepare questions for class, set time allotted for each section, identify skills to be demonstrated, etc.)
__Lecture	__Computer generated	__Practical exam	__Room Environment: temperature, light, acoustics, cleanliness	
__Laboratory	__Chalk or pen board	__Written short answers		
__Seminar-Discussion	__Overhead projector	__Written essay	__Teacher Materials: podium, chalk/pens, media setup, computer setup	
__Independent study	__Slides	__Report or project		
__Web based	__Digital Media	__Journal		
		__Portfolio		
	B. Handouts			
	__Lecture outline			
	__Laboratory exercises			
	__Small group tasks			
	__Take home assignments or pre-class work			
	C. Online Interactions			
	__Listserve or chat rooms			
	__Blogs, wikis			

THE LEARNING EXPERIENCE

FIGURE 2–1 The preactive teaching grid.

one that emphasizes a knowledge-building process that is centered on clinical reality. See Table 2–1 for an overview of the steps in a PBL tutorial process.[11,12]

In a problem-based curriculum, the entire curriculum is composed of clinical problems. For example, rather than a class of students sitting in traditional physical therapy courses, such as anatomy, pathology, therapeutic exercise, and health care policy, students in small groups guided by a mentor discuss patient problems. With any given patient problem, students learn to seek out, analyze, and act on the information they need. That is, students gather information from a variety of sources, including anatomy, pathology, therapeutic exercise, and health care economics because these sources relate to the patient problem under consideration. For an excellent overview of the advantages and disadvantages of problem-based learning, read *The Challenge of Problem-Based Learning* by Boud and Feletti.[11]

Of course, in any class or any course in any curriculum one could be working toward the development of cognitive processes and reasoning. For example, you might ask students to use their "hunch" regarding the outcome of a patient care problem. Students could then identify and analyze what data their hunch was based on and what additional data they would need to confirm their hunch. By this process, the student is introduced to the cognitive processes of inductive and deductive thinking and how both processes are used in health care decision making. As another example, students could be presented with a clinical problem that represents a moral dilemma. Analyzing such a problem involves the cognitive processes of identifying the student's own values, comparing and contrasting these values with the principles contained in a professional code of ethics, and working out a rational, empathetic decision. Because time to evaluate and treat patients has declined in all health care settings, teaching students to think rationally, humanely, creatively, and quickly is time well spent in every course.

Academic Rationalism

The philosophical orientation of academic rationalism focuses on traditional areas of study that faculty think represent the most intellectually and artistically significant

---

TABLE 2–1 Steps in the Problem-based Learning Tutorial Process

Step	Process
Step 1	Identify and clarify terms in the case scenario that are unfamiliar
Step 2	Define the problem or problems to be discussed (all views should be considered)
Step 3	Discuss the problem(s) at brainstorming sessions. Suggest possible explanations based on prior knowledge. Students draw on each other's knowledge; identify areas of incomplete knowledge
Step 4	Review steps 2 and 3; move explanations to tentative solutions; record explanations and restructure if needed
Step 5	Formulate learning objectives; group works toward consensus of learning objectives; tutor makes sure learning objectives are focused, achievable, comprehensive, and appropriate
Step 6	Private study (all students gather information related to each learning objective)
Step 7	Group shares results of private study (students identify their learning resources and share their results); tutor checks learning and assesses group (scribe records key findings during each step of the process)

Adapted from Cantillon P, Wood D. ABC of Learning and Teaching in Medicine, 2nd ed. West Sussex, UK: Wiley-Blackwell, 2010.

ideas within the field they are teaching. This approach relishes the history and the careful inquiry that have led to formulation of universal principles and philosophical, scientific, and artistic concepts useful in today's world. In this type of orientation, more time is spent on theory and less on practical application. The belief is that once students learn of the great ideas created by the most visionary people in their field (and related fields), they are able to perform as educated men and women. As Eisner states, "The central aim is to develop man's rational abilities by introducing his rationality to ideas and objects that represent reason's highest achievement."[9] Thus, college classes based on the works of great thinkers, such as Darwin, Emily Dickinson, Einstein, Ghandi, Picasso, and Martin Luther King, would have as their focus academic rationalism.

Obviously, no health care curriculum could be based solely on academic rationalism because too much health care information and related patient care intervention strategies are outdated within a decade or less. However, physical therapy and physical therapist assistant educators struggle with how much academic rationalism to put into curriculum. For example, in the neurological rehabilitation area educators may grapple with how many students should be exposed to historical perspectives such as Margaret Rood, Maggie Knott, Berta and Karl Bobath, and Signe Brunnstrom, when compared with the time devoted to the current theories of motor control and motor behavior. In research on stroke rehabilitation, Jette found that therapists now are using more eclectic intervention techniques to address impairments and compensate for functional limitations. Therapists report that their interventions are grounded in motor control and motor learning theories.[13]

All disciplines need linkages to what has come before them. The historical roots and context of the discipline is an important dimension of the profession necessary for fully understanding and addressing answers to questions the profession continues to face.

Technology

The philosophical orientation of technology focuses on practical or technical behaviors that the student should attain to become proficient in her or his field. Using this orientation, a curriculum or a course would consist of a series of clearly delineated behavioral objectives the student is to master. The underlying approach is essentially a stimulus-response-reinforcement model. Computer-assisted instruction is an example of this orientation. The answers are predetermined to be clearly right or wrong, and students receive immediate corrective feedback. Using computer-assisted instruction, the student can repeat material until a certain proficiency level is attained.

In physical therapy and physical therapist assistant programs, there are many areas of content and skill knowledge that lend themselves to the technology orientation. For example, in anatomy there are clearly right and wrong answers, and the teacher's task is to determine how much anatomy, at what level, and what approach can be used that will help students memorize and apply the material accurately. Practical skills knowledge, such as the biomechanics of lifting or the steps involved in a wheelchair transfer, are often taught using this philosophical orientation.

Social Adaptation and Social Reconstruction

The philosophical orientation of social adaptation and social reconstruction focuses on societal interests. This is a two-pronged orientation, with one prong being social adaptation and the opposite prong being social reconstruction. Social adaptation curriculum orientation focuses on knowledge and skills students need to function in today's world—that is, on what society needs to maintain the status quo. Under this orientation, for example, physical therapy and physical therapist assistant students would be taught the information and technical skills that are needed to immediately fill those areas of practice with the greatest number of job vacancies.

In contrast, the philosophical orientation of social reconstruction focuses the curriculum on identifying the changing composition and projected needs of society and the skills that will be needed in the future to be responsive to these changes. Such skills might include working to change certain aspects of society, such as intolerance to ethnic and cultural differences, environmental pollution, or the rise of homelessness. For example, in a physical therapy or physical therapist assistant curriculum, students would be engaged in experiences designed to develop their tolerance for working with patients whose heritage and lifestyles differ considerably from their own, become involved in environmental health groups, embrace participation in pro bono services for the homeless, or engage in community health initiatives and needed health policy changes. Thus, although social adaptation and social reconstruction have different aims, they are tied by the common philosophical belief that societal needs should guide curriculum. The social reconstruction approach is one that would underlie a curriculum philosophy of change agents. Although many programs espouse such an outcome, one needs to ask: Do the courses have learning outcomes that challenge students in this direction?

Personal Relevance

The philosophical orientation of personal relevance focuses on what is personally relevant to the student. In this orientation, the teacher and the student jointly plan educational experiences that are meaningful to the student. Probably the archetype of this orientation is portrayed is A. S. Neil's famous boarding school, Summerhill, founded in England in 1921 and designed to "make the school fit the child instead of making the child fit the school."[14]

This orientation is challenging to entry-level physical therapist and physical therapist assistant educators who have little enough time to teach groups of students the basic tenets and tasks of their profession without responding to the individual personal relevance requirements of each student. Although one sees a version of this approach in discussions about addressing generational differences. How are generation X or millennial students different from faculty who are mostly baby boomers, and does this matter in how faculty teach?[15] The personal relevance orientation is very much in evidence in continuing education programs as well as post-professional graduate degree programs that must consider adult learners. The most successful continuing education programs appear to be those that offer clinicians knowledge and advanced skills (e.g., in manual therapy), which can be immediately applied in an individual clinician's health care setting. The most successful post-professional graduate programs appear to be those that offer the student a great deal of latitude in what she or he chooses to pursue and where the faculty is dedicated to encouraging and supporting students in their individual pursuits.

Using the Five Curriculum Orientations to Guide Curriculum Design and Course Development

There are two useful ways to use these five curriculum orientations in developing a whole curriculum or a single course. In working with an entire curriculum design, the five philosophical orientations can be used to review the multiple courses that make up the curriculum and to identify what philosophical orientation the curriculum emphasis is built on. Faculty might realize that they are spending too much time on technology or academic rationalism and not enough time on developing cognitive processes and reasoning. You might find that the social reconstruction orientation is a nice thread throughout the curriculum, or it may be left out altogether. This is an enjoyable and often revealing activity for individual faculty as well as the collective faculty. It will clarify the faculty's own values and beliefs about the mission, structure, and outcomes of physical therapist or physical therapist assistant education as well as how any group of faculty envisions the present and future practice of physical therapy.

In using the five philosophical orientations to develop a course, the teacher would first specify the goals of the course and then identify how much of each philosophical orientation will be used to help student reach those goals. For example, for a course in basic skills, the teacher probably wants a high percentage of class time devoted to technology (e.g., 60%). He or she might also want to teach students how to think about applying basic skills in a wide variety of clinical situations, so the teacher may plan to devote 20% of class time to stimulating cognitive processing-reasoning. Finally, the teacher might focus on some skills students will need to use immediately in clinical practice, such as taking blood pressure or performing bed-to-wheelchair transfers. Thus, the remaining 20% of the time might be used for laboratory sessions organized around common clinical problems in which students can learn basic skills that are immediately applicable in their next internship. Going through the process of thinking about philosophical orientations related to the goals for each class can be an eye-opening experience, which can guide teachers in reapportioning classroom and laboratory time appropriately. Such a process can also ensure that all class time is not devoted inadvertently to a single philosophical orientation or an orientation that does not have a coherent fit with the overall curriculum design.

In Chapter 5, the Teaching Goals Inventory is presented and discussed. At that point, you will be able to see how the curriculum philosophy you are using is tied directly to your specific teaching goals.

LEARNING THEORIES

The next column in the upper part of the preactive teaching grid contains learning theories (see Figure 2–1). Theories about how people learn have been discussed at least since the time of the Greek philosopher Plato (428-347 BC). Plato postulated that knowledge was innate—that is, in place at the time of birth. The function of a teacher was to help the learner "recall" what one's soul had already experienced and learned. Nearly 2000 years after Plato, the British philosopher John Locke (1632-1704) proposed an opposite view of the learner. Locke postulated that infants were born with the mind a blank slate, a *tabula rasa*. The teacher's role was to provide experiences that would fill this blank slate with knowledge.[16]

There are many ways to classify learning theories. We use four broad categories (Table 2–2)[16–19]:

- Behavioral learning theories
- Cognitive learning theories
- Experiential/problem-solving learning theories
- Social-cultural learning theories

Learning theories provide the teacher with ideas about how to present students with different types of knowledge and skill in a way that reinforces the underlying philosophical orientations the teacher is focusing on.

Behavioral Learning Theories

The behaviorism theory was developed in the first half of the 20th century as a result of numerous experiments, primarily on animals and birds, by the experimental psychologists E. L. Thorndike[20] and B. F. Skinner.[21] The basic theory of behaviorism rests on their observations that behaviors that were rewarded (positively reinforced) would reoccur. For behaviorists, the process of learning involves rewarding correct behavior until the behavioral change is consistently demonstrated.[16,17]

Physical therapists and physical therapist assistants use behavioristic principles continually in patient care to teach psychomotor skills. For example, patients are reinforced with enthusiastic praise for attempting and subsequently achieving self-care activities or gait training. In classrooms, acquiring accurate knowledge (i.e., knowing the right answer) is rewarded by receiving high grades and praise from faculty. Lack of responsiveness to acquiring the knowledge presented is quelled by poor grades and perhaps even failure to proceed in the program. Computer-assisted instruction is based almost exclusively on this learning theory. Students receive immediate feedback contingent on the accuracy of their responses. Clearly, many psychomotor skills and specific facts that need to be memorized are successfully taught using behavioristic principles. For a teacher whose main philosophical orientation to a course is technology, the predominant learning theory of choice would be behaviorism. The behavioral approach works well when teaching a skill with a measurable action.[17,18]

Cognitive Learning Theories

Cognitive learning theory focuses on the development of knowledge structures, abstract problem presentation, and problem solving that are critical elements of clinical

TABLE 2-2   Common Categories of Learning Theories

Learning Theory	Key Concepts	Examples of Application
Behavioral learning theory	Based on the concept that behavior could be influenced by the consequences (that reinforcement could help shape the desired behavior) Useful for teaching skills with measurable actions Foundation for performance-based education Some behavioral checklists may be inadequate for some professional competencies	Mastery learning, where you have the opportunity to practice the behavior and receive feedback on performance until mastery is achieved Often used for teaching technical patient care skills Can be used for assessing clinical competencies (particularly skills)
Cognitive learning theory	Emerged when limitations of behavioral theory were discovered Learning is an active process of meaning making whereby the organization or structure of knowledge is a critical element Addresses the use, such as information processing and retrieval and transfer of knowledge into practice settings	Foundation for building knowledge in the learner's memory Knowledge that is connected to a clinical context bolsters retention Building a strong knowledge structure is necessary for developing reasoning and clinical judgment skills
Experiential/ problem-solving learning theory	Experience and reflection on that experience are central to learning Students must learn not only *what* but also *how* to apply what they know Reflection-in-action is necessary for building practice-based knowledge	Designing learning opportunities whereby learners are engaged in active learning Creating learning experiences in which there is a structure that facilitates learner reflection on the learning Experiential learning is well suited to clinical or community settings
Social-cultural learning theory	Learning occurs in the social or practice setting The learning is situated in the community of practice as the learner engages in participation with others Meanings are socially constructed in these communities of practice	Clinical practice settings are powerful examples of social-cultural learning The social learning community needs to build self-efficacy in learners to allow them to have incremental success and enhanced participation Role models and mentors can have a powerful effect on the learners

reasoning. Cognitive learning theory development stemmed from the perceived inadequacy of stimulus-response behavioral theories of learning that did not account for advanced knowledge and skill development that is so critical in professional education.[17,18] Jean Piaget's well-known research demonstrating the influence of the environment on the cognitive development of children and the stages of the learner as he or she is developing cognitive schema.[22,23] Building on the work of early theorists, Ausubel[24] asserted that learners construct meaningful knowledge by being able to connect new concepts or knowledge to what they already know.[24] Learners need to build that structure, not just have information poured in.

Cognitive learning theories also address the most important aspect in learning, that of transfer of knowledge to actual practice settings that require problem solving and decision making. Experience with clinical cases is a very important element in building a knowledge structure (cognitive schema) that students will remember and be able to apply. Teachers need to remember to build from typical cases to more complex cases in building this structure.

Robert Gagne proposes a hierarchy of learning that begins with the simple and concrete and moves to the complex and abstract.[25] The ideas contained within stages of a hierarchy suggest that higher-order cognitive abilities build on lower-order cognitive abilities. That is, students must master lower-order abilities before they can master higher-level ones. Gagne suggests the following hierarchy: (1) facts, (2) concepts, (3) principles, and (4) problem solving. Thus, for example, students should be able to identify the muscles, nerves, and connective tissues involved in the shoulder rotator cuff (facts) before they can understand conceptually how these structures fit together. After they understand how the structures are related, they can understand the biomechanical principles involved in the rotator cuff mechanism. After understanding these principles, they can solve problems related to rotator cuff injuries. If a student missed any one of these steps, it would be difficult to proceed to the next step. For example, if the student did not understand conceptually how the various tissue structures are related, then it would be difficult to understand the biomechanics of movement. Thus, cognitive structure learning theories are very useful in thinking about ways to organize and present information. For a teacher whose main philosophical orientation to a course is academic rationalism, the predominant learning theory of choice would be cognitive learning theories.

Albert Bandura's work in social learning theory and more recently social-cognitive learning theory has led to the development of several models and frameworks for understanding the underlying values and beliefs that are part of health behaviors and facilitating behavior change.[26] Much of this work is focused on applied behavioral theory and adherence (see Chapter 13).

Experiential/Problem-Solving Learning Theories

John Dewey (1859-1952), who has been called America's greatest educational philosopher, expanded on the experiential learning theory or learning through context and experience.[17] For Dewey, the issue of activity (i.e., students being actively involved in an authentic experience from which they could learn) was essential.[27]

This principle of learning through experience clearly operates in clinical practice and academic settings. Physical therapists, who in the past prepared patients for functional activities by working on strength and endurance of specific muscle groups, now ascribe to modern motor learning theories in which teaching movement within meaningful functional patterns hastens the acquisition of motor skills (see Chapter 14). In academic settings, it is known that students need a framework for information so that the knowledge "makes sense." For example, the tedious process of memorizing anatomic origins and insertions of muscle groups in an anatomy class has long been seen as an absolute necessity to the practice of physical therapy. However, students are quick to point out that learning this anatomic information is greatly enhanced by acquiring corresponding knowledge of the function of muscle groups in a kinesiology class and learning how to assist patients to improve the function of muscle groups in a therapeutic exercise class. In this manner, students learn and understand the origin and insertion of muscle groups in the context of muscle function and in the context of the use of this information in patient care. Thus, memorization of anatomic structures is easier because it has a useful experiential context and therefore "makes sense."

Dewey described the process of human problem solving, reflective thinking, and learning in many slightly different ways because he knew that intelligent thinking and learning is not just following some standard recipe. He believed that intelligence is creative and flexible—we learn from engaging ourselves in a variety of experiences in the world. However, in all of his descriptions, the following elements always appeared in some form: Thinking always gets started when a person genuinely feels a problem arise. Then the mind actively jumps back and forth—struggling to find a clearer formulation of the problem, looking for suggestions for possible solutions, surveying elements in the problematic situation that might be relevant, drawing on prior knowledge in an attempt to better understand the situation. Then the mind begins forming a plan of action, a hypothesis about how best the problem might be solved. The hypothesis is then tested; if the problem is solved, then according to Dewey something has been learned.[17-19]

Both in the classroom and in the clinic, when teachers present students with clinical problems to solve, they are following the traditions of John Dewey. Perhaps even more important, Dewey illuminates how we learn from our experience in clinical practice. His postulation that learning occurs from actively solving meaningful problems explains the accumulated wisdom of experienced practitioners that is far beyond the knowledge contained in current textbooks. The concepts of *reflection-in-action* and *reflection-on-action* described by Donald Schön and elaborated on in Chapter 3 of this book are the present-day versions of this experiential learning theory that was first articulated by Dewey.[8] For a teacher whose main philosophical orientation to a course is development of cognitive processing-reasoning, the predominant learning theory of choice would be the experiential.

Social-Cultural Learning Theories

Social-cultural learning theories are robust examples of what is called constructivist learning theories. These are theories that focus on learning that occurs in social or practice settings. These theories are central to what occurs in clinical education and practice settings. Social-cultural learning theories have emerged because both the behavioral and cognitive learning theories have not explained the learning that occurs in the community of practice. Social-cultural learning theories focus on the importance of situated learning in which learners construct meaning in the community of practice. For example, when students return from their clinical experiences and are full of excitement as they relate much they have learned about the actual performance of physical therapy, this is situated learning. Suddenly, the knowledge from the classroom or laboratory seems to pale in comparison to what they have just experienced in a clinical practice setting. From the academic perspective, if this new situated learning is based on evidence and good practice, we are happy, but if the situated learning is based on tradition or philosophical beliefs about what works, then we are distressed.

The learning that occurs in the community of practice is powerful, enduring, and critical for all health professions education. Although we may see some evidence of social-cultural learning theory in the classroom or laboratory, it is much more visible in actual practice settings. We are constantly working to build a better bridge between our learning communities. Teaching and learning in the clinical environment is the focus of Chapters 8 to 11.

Thinking through the Relationship between Philosophical Orientations and Learning Theories

When the learning theory used is not compatible with the underlying philosophical orientation, course materials tend to be jumbled, leaving students and teachers frustrated with the teaching-learning process. For example, suppose a teacher believes strongly in the development of cognitive processing-reasoning (philosophical orientation) and regards that as the aim of teaching. In fact, the teacher sets up examinations in the format of patient cases about which he or she asks a series of open-ended questions. The questions are designed to require students to use cognitive reasoning skills. However, suppose the material was actually taught using the behaviorism learning theory. Behaviorism is the learning theory that has predominated classroom life for most students since first grade, and they are well prepared for memorizing and parroting information. Does it seem that these students would be ready and able to take specific facts for which they know correct and incorrect responses and apply these facts without having had some learning that involved the patient care context—that is, experiential problem-solving experiences? This "miss" between how the material has been taught and how the students are asked to apply it on a test is often apparent. The miss represents a discrepancy between the teacher's philosophical aim of the course and the learning theory that guides instruction.

Looking at the preactive teaching grid (see Figure 2–1), one can see that if a large percentage of the philosophical orientation to the material is technology (wanting students to learn specific facts and skills within a hierarchy of facts-to-principles involved), then the learning theories of behaviorism and cognitive structure could logically guide the presentation of the material. Likewise, if a teacher is interested in the social reconstruction philosophical orientation, then the experiential problem-solving learning theory approach could be a useful way to present course materials. Remember that seldom is only one philosophical orientation and learning theory used in a class. However, just thinking through the emphasis to be placed on each orientation and learning theory and their resultant compatibility will help guide teaching and evaluation efforts in a way that will help students learn rather than be frustrated.

DOMAINS OF LEARNING

The third column in the upper part of the preactive teaching grid identifies the domains of learning (see Figure 2–1). In considering aspects of being human that are subject to growth and development and, thus, have implications for teaching and learning, at least five domains of learning can be identified:

- Cognitive (thinking)
- Affective (feeling, willing)
- Psychomotor (purposeful movement, doing)
- Perceptual (involving all the senses, including vision, olfactory, auditory, taste, and kinesthetic)
- Spiritual (faith)

The first three domains, the cognitive, affective, and psychomotor, are well known to physical therapy educators because clinical practice obviously involves knowledge and skill in all three areas. These are the domains that have been most well defined and developed for educators.

In 1956, Benjamin Bloom and associates wrote the first book in this area entitled, *Taxonomy of Educational Objectives, Handbook I: The Cognitive Domain.*[78] A companion book (*Handbook II: Affective Domain*) was produced by Krathwohl, Bloom, and Masia in 1964 and was revised in 2002 by Krathwohl.[29,30] In the 1970s, several books appeared on the psychomotor domain, one of the most useful being that by Simpson.[31] The primary reason these books have been so useful to teachers is that they clearly define lower-order and higher-order thinking, psychomotor, and affective abilities. Thus, the domains of learning provide a guide for student development when acquiring knowledge and developing psychomotor skills and values.

Cognitive Domain

The six levels of the cognitive domain are depicted in Figure 2–2.[28,30] The upward progression of steps illustrates that students must acquire some basic knowledge of the material before they can comprehend it, and they must comprehend the material before they can apply it. The three higher levels illustrate that it is easier for students to analyze information than to synthesize it, and only after achieving a sufficient understanding of analysis and synthesis can one learn to evaluate the material. The list of verbs under each level identifies the kind of behaviors students might exhibit when learning in that domain. For example, in learning how the center of mass is a key to moving one's body through space, the student might learn logically through the following steps in the cognitive domain:

1. *Knowledge:* Define the center of mass.
2. *Comprehension:* Describe principles of the center of mass involved in body movement.
3. *Application:* Demonstrate how center of mass relates to balance.
4. *Analysis:* Compare how center of mass differs in maintaining sitting, stooped, and standing postures.
5. *Synthesis:* Design a wheelchair-to-car transfer that uses the principles involved in the body's center of mass.
6. *Evaluation:* Compare several different wheelchair-to-car transfers and determine which is the safest using the principles of the center of mass.

Thus, knowing the various levels of the cognitive domain and deciding at which level the student is ready to learn will help the teacher ensure that students have not missed any level of a knowledge component that would lead to full understanding. Similarly, the teacher can review examinations to determine whether students are being asked to respond at the same domain levels that have been taught. This is similar to the need for coherency between philosophical orientation and learning theories in teaching and evaluation.

In 2002, Krathwohl revised Bloom's taxonomy table by beginning the taxonomy with remembering versus knowledge, replacing comprehension with understanding, and then keeping application, analysis, and evaluation and removing synthesis and making the highest dimension creating (Table 2–3). He also articulated more clearly the categories of knowledge formation and added another category, metacognitive knowledge. This revised taxonomy has

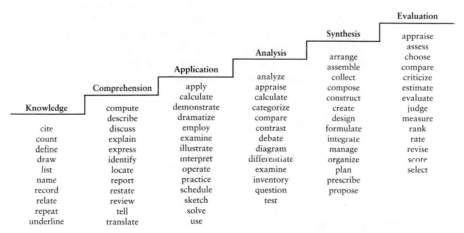

FIGURE 2–2 The six levels of the cognitive domain. (From Ford CW [ed]. Clinical Education for the Allied Health Professions. St. Louis: Mosby, 1978.)

TABLE 2–3 Revision of the Cognitive Domain of Bloom's Taxonomy

Cognitive Process	Learner Action
Remembering: retrieving facts, information, relevant knowledge from long-term memory; done mostly with recall	Recognizing Recall
Understanding: determining the meaning of instructional messages (oral, written, and graphic communication); translating material to a new form, often done with explanation	Interpreting Exemplifying Classifying Summarizing Inferring Comparing Explaining
Applying: Using a procedure in a given situation; starting to transfer the knowledge	Executing Implementing
Analyzing: Breaking the material down into parts; detecting how the parts relate to each other or to the overall purpose or structure	Differentiating Organizing Attributing
Evaluating: Making judgments based on criteria and standards; assessing or providing a critique	Checking Critiquing
Creating: Putting elements together to form an innovative whole or to make an original product	Generating Planning Producing

From Krathwohl D. A revision of Bloom's taxonomy: an overview. Theory Prac. 2002; 41: 212-217.

TABLE 2–4 Structure of Knowledge in a Revision of Bloom's Cognitive Domain

Knowledge Dimension	Examples
Factual knowledge: basic elements that students must know in a discipline, required to solve problems	Knowledge of terminology Knowledge of specific details and elements
Conceptual knowledge: interrelationships among the basic elements within a larger structure that ensures they function together	Knowledge of classifications and categories Knowledge of principles and generalizations Knowledge of theories, models, and structures
Procedural knowledge: how to do something; methods of inquiry, criteria for using skills, algorithms, techniques, and methods	Knowledge of subject-specific skills and algorithms Knowledge of subject-specific techniques and methods Knowledge of criteria for determining when to use appropriate procedures
Metacognitive knowledge: knowledge of cognition; awareness and knowledge of one's own cognition	Strategic knowledge Knowledge about cognitive tasks that includes contextual and conditional knowledge Self-knowledge

From Krathwohl D. A revision of Bloom's taxonomy: an overview. Theory Prac. 2002; 41: 212-217.

much to offer health professions education in which the focus is on the development of reasoning, meta-cognitive skill development, and decision making (Table 2–4).[29]

Affective Domain

The affective domain, which includes student interests, attitudes, appreciation, and values, is obviously more difficult to teach and evaluate.[26,29] Basically, behaviors in this domain are taught and measured by approach-avoidance tendencies, meaning positive attitudes are believed to exist if a student approaches and grapples with an issue rather than avoids it.

The levels of the affective domain are depicted in Figure 2–3. In this domain, the first step is to attend to an issue or "receive" it. After receiving an issue, one responds to that issue and subsequently may demonstrate that the issue is of value to her or him. The highest levels of organization and characterization include deciding the importance of that issue given other competing issues and acting consistently according to the value one places on the issue. The following is an example of how the affective domain could be used in physical therapy education regarding the issue of valuing diversity and embracing nondiscrimination:

1. *Receiving:* Realize that health care professionals may treat patients and families differently because of race, gender, or lifestyle.
2. *Responding:* Discuss how responding differently to patients because of race, gender, or lifestyle might affect treatment outcomes.
3. *Valuing:* Defend the right of each patient and family to receive the best health care possible regardless of race, gender, or lifestyle.
4. *Organization:* Judge, or decide, when patients and families are being treated differently by health care professionals because of their race, gender, or lifestyle.
5. *Characterization:* Internalize the belief in individual patient and family rights regardless of race, gender, or lifestyle, and act consistently with those beliefs.

Krathwohl and associates[29,30] note that there is a good deal of hesitancy by teachers to evaluate students in the affective domain. Teachers, as well as students, often see it as inappropriate to grade on interest, attitudes, or character development, all of which are regarded as personal or private matters. Furthermore, education in the affective domain may be seen as indoctrination—that is, persuading or coercing students to adopt a particular viewpoint, act in a certain manner, or profess to a particular value or way of life.[29] Certainly, the issue of professional socialization, now more commonly referred to as *professional formation*, is who students become as professionals and the expectations that exist for professional behavior. These behaviors are part of the affective domain. In physical therapy and physical therapist assistant curricula, clinical educators are regularly called on to evaluate students in affective areas, such as enthusiasm, dependability, judgment, and sensitivity in patient-family care. Clinical educators also evaluate how well students adjust to a department, how well they work with colleagues, how receptive they are to new ideas, and how they react to constructive criticism. Now all educators are responsible for assessing students' professional behaviors.

Assessment of the generic abilities (critical thinking, problem solving, interpersonal communication, communication skills, professionalism, responsibility, commitment to learning, effective use of time and resources, use of constructive feedback, and stress management) involves a common set of expectations that many physical therapist education programs use to monitor students' professional behavior.[15,32] Table 2–5 provides an example of how one health professions school has a consensus-based

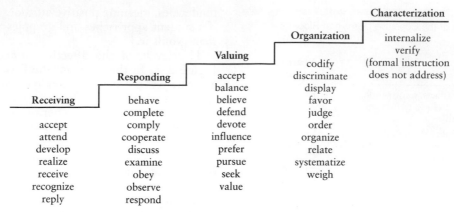

FIGURE 2–3 Five levels of the affective domain. (From Ford CW [ed]. Clinical Education for the Allied Health Professions. St. Louis: Mosby, 1978.)

TABLE 2–5   An Example of Tracking Professional Behaviors

Core Professional Ability: Critical Thinking and Clinical Judgment (Physical and Occupational Therapy)

- The student shall acquire, comprehend, apply, synthesize, and evaluate information.
- The student shall integrate these abilities to identify, resolve, and prevent problems and make appropriate decisions.
- The student shall demonstrate the behaviors of the scholarly clinician by developing and utilizing the process of critical thinking and systematic inquiry for the purpose of clinical reasoning, decision, making, and exercising sound clinical judgment.

Core Professional Ability: Critical Thinking (Pharmacy)

- The student shall acquire, comprehend, apply, analyze, synthesize, and evaluate information.
- The student shall integrate these abilities to identify, resolve, and prevent problems and make appropriate decisions.
- The student shall understand the research process.

Critical Thinking and Clinical Judgment Reflect the Core Value of Excellence

Entering Student	Developing Student	Senior Student

1. Demonstrates initial stages of clinical reasoning and problem solving
  a. Begins to recognize and prioritize problems
  b. Generates potential solutions to problem
  c. Identifies resources needed to develop solutions
  d. Begins to examine multiple solutions to problems
  e. Raises relevant questions
  f. Considers all available information
  g. Demonstrates an understanding that knowledge is always evolving
	1. Applies clinical reasoning and problem-solving processes to patient care decisions
	  a. Clarifies problems using a broad source of information
	  b. Identifies contributors to the problem
	  c. Identifies areas of uncertainty in problem solving. Articulates risks and benefits of possible solutions given uncertainties in current knowledge
	  d. Considers consequences of possible solutions
	  e. Constructively critiques hypotheses and ideas
	  f. Formulates new ideas and alternative hypotheses
	2. Prioritizes responsibilities
	3. Uses time effectively
		1. Determines deliberate actions to be taken
		2. Evaluates the effects of his/her actions using measures known to be reliable and valid
		  a. Accepts responsibility for implementation of solutions
		  b. Assesses issues raised by contradictory ideas
		  c. Demonstrates proactivity in seeking current scientific and clinical information to support clinical decisions
		  d. Recognizes appropriate solutions in presence of cognitive dissonance
		  e. Justifies solutions selected
		  f. Adapts plan of care to manage dissonant situations (to capture the key elements of handling uncertainty and adapting the plan of care)

From School of Pharmacy and Health Professions, Creighton University, Omaha, NE. Available at: http://spahp2.creighton.edu/oasa/Polices,Procedures%20.aspx.

document for ongoing assessment of professional behaviors. Students can be cited for both negative and positive behaviors.

For affective behaviors to be seen as legitimate in the academic setting, teachers must determine before the class begins what clinically related behaviors are acceptable or unacceptable and explicitly notify students that such behaviors will or will not be supported and will be evaluated.

Psychomotor Domain

The stages of the psychomotor domain are noted in Figure 2–4. The steps of these stages are self-evident, especially to the many physical therapy educators and students who have participated in sports. In fact, remembering how skill in a specific sport was acquired may be an excellent guide to teaching patients motor skills. (For more on the specific topic of learning motor skills, see Chapter 14.)

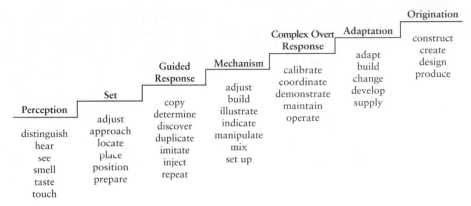

FIGURE 2–4 Seven levels of the psychomotor domain. (From Ford CW [ed]. Clinical Education for the Allied Health Professions. St. Louis: Mosby, 1978.)

The following examples of psychomotor domain stages could be applied to most sports as well as to patient tasks, such as gait training:

1. *Perception:* Distinguish among various maneuvers.
2. *Set:* Position oneself to engage in each maneuver.
3. *Guided response:* Duplicate the maneuver a skilled performer presents.
4. *Mechanism:* Adjust the maneuver to the needed response.
5. *Complex overt response:* Coordinate various maneuvers to accomplish successful play or task.
6. *Adaptation:* Adapt maneuvers to obtain the most successful response.
7. *Origination:* Create new maneuvers.

As with the other domains, thinking through the steps in the psychomotor domain before teaching, as well as before an evaluation such as a practical examination, helps the teacher determine at what levels he or she is presenting and requiring students to demonstrate motor skills.

Another useful visual tool in thinking about the performance of skills is Miller's triangle. Here you see a progression of skill development from knowing what to knowing how (usually classroom or didactic teaching) to showing how (laboratory demonstration) to doing, or the actual performance (Figure 2–5).[33,34]

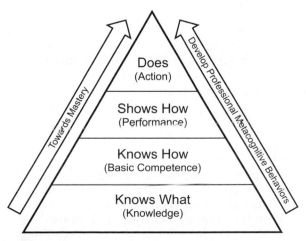

FIGURE 2–5 Progression of performance skills.

Perceptual and Spiritual Domains

Neither the perceptual nor the spiritual domain has yet been fully described or classified in a series of learning steps, as has been done with the cognitive, affective, and psychomotor domains. However, neither of these domains should be neglected in physical therapy education. Clearly, the perceptual domain involving use of the senses plays a dominant role in how patients receive and use information regarding components of movement. For example, the psychomotor skill of balance is clearly enhanced with the use of kinesthetic proprioception and vision. Think about how the perceptual domain can be incorporated into classes with content in motor learning and motor control.

The spiritual domain appears to be very comfortable or very uncomfortable for health care professionals in their work with patients and families. The same is true of academic and clinical faculty in their work with students. The degree of comfort in presenting and discussing various beliefs related to spirituality with students appears to be directly related to one's own exploration and understanding of spirituality, as well as to how colleagues support or dismiss attention to this domain. Certainly, this domain of learning plays a significant role in how patients and families perceive disease and manage illness within their lives and across their lifespan. Perhaps as we become more open to and comfortable with, and begin to introduce students to, complementary and alternative health care practices, spirituality issues will enter the physical therapy curriculum naturally.[35,36]

Thinking through the Relationships among Philosophical Orientations, Learning Theories, and Domains of Knowledge

Think about teaching a class in physiology of exercise. It is likely you will use some mix of philosophical orientations (e.g., technology [60%], cognitive processing-reasoning [30%], and academic rationalism [10%]). The predominant learning theories might be behaviorism (75%) and cognitive structure (25%). The learning domain might be the cognitive domain (100%). Contrast these choices with an approach to a class about sexuality of persons with spinal cord injury. For this class, you might choose to teach predominantly from a social adaptation philosophy using the experiential/problem-solving learning theory and attending to the affective and psychomotor domains as well as the cognitive domain. Is it clear how thinking through the preactive grid (knowledge of pedagogy) can lead to a course or class design that is as remarkably different as it is remarkably coherent.

STUDENT LEARNING STYLES

The fourth column in the upper part of the preactive teaching grid (see Figure 2–1) displays one example of how to think about student learning styles. Identifying your own learning style brings an understanding of how you prefer to learn. It is important for teachers to be aware that they are likely to teach using the learning style they are most comfortable with. For example, if the teacher likes to learn by reading, an extensive assigned reading list will probably be in the course syllabi. Conversely, if the teacher likes to learn by doing, the course syllabi will be peppered with practical learning experiences for students. Thus, it is important for the teacher to be aware of her or his predominant learning styles as well as the learning styles that she or he favors less. The less-favored learning styles may be ones that some students are most comfortable with and can learn the most from. Thus, one can become a more effective and appreciated teacher through devising activities that are responsive to a wide range of student learning styles.

Presented below is an example of one learning style inventory and how it can be used in academic and clinical teaching. (There are other inventories, such as the Myers-Briggs Type Indicator[37,38] and the Canfield Learning Styles Inventory,[39,40] both of which are used by health professionals.)

Kolb postulated a model of normal learning processes that was eventually developed into the Learning Styles Inventory.[5,41] As seen in Figure 2–6, learning is depicted as a recurring cycle consisting of four stages, beginning with a concrete experience. Most concrete learning experiences involve other people in everyday situations. This type of learning relies on feeling and intuition rather than logic and reasoning. The second stage, reflective observation, involves learning by observing what happens to oneself as

well as what happens to others during a concrete experience through observation and reflection. In this stage, no action is taken, but through observation one learns to understand situations from different points of view. The third stage, abstract conceptualization, involves logic and reasoning. In this stage, there is formation of abstract concepts, and generalizations are developed about what has been done and observed. Then actions may be taken and problems solved based on these theories. In the fourth and final stage, active experimentation, learning is through testing different approaches in new situations based on the concepts generated. In this stage, the practical use of ideas and concepts is evident.[38]

Physical therapists and physical therapist assistants use this cycle constantly in clinical practice when treating a patient (concrete experience), observing and reflecting on what happened to the patient as a result of that treatment (reflective observation), thinking about how a successful intervention with one patient may work on similar patients and theorizing why (abstract conceptualization), and then trying the intervention on other patients (active experimentation). By this learning process, clinicians create the ever-expanding knowledge base (tacit knowledge) they use in practice.

Kolb's Learning Styles Inventory[5] consists of a series of choices the respondent ranks according to his or her learning preference. For example:

"When I learn,
___I like to deal with my feelings." (Concrete experience)
___I like to watch and listen." (Reflective observation)
___I like to think about ideas." (Abstract conceptualization)
___I like to be doing things." (Active experimentation)

Completing this inventory takes 5 to 10 minutes, and it is available online.[42] You can then compute the scores and plot them on a grid comparing your individual scores with normative data using the self-scoring key. By looking at the grid, you can quickly see your most and least preferred learning styles.

In preparing for each class, think through the student learning styles that the presentation of material will most emphasize. That is, are students asked to observe, theorize, or engage in a practical activity? Whether one uses Kolb's Learning Styles Inventory or another learning inventory, the intent is to become aware of individual learning style preferences and how they influence teaching and student learning. The goal for academic and clinical educators is to expand their understanding and use of all possible learning styles or preferences so that individual students, as well as collective groups of students, can get the most out of each learning opportunity.

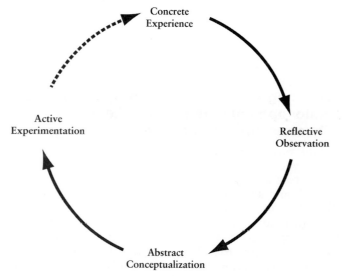

FIGURE 2–6 Kolb's learning styles. (From Kolb DA. Learning Styles Inventory. Boston: McBer, 1985.)

OBJECTIVES

The last column in the top of the preactive teaching grid contains objectives (see Figure 2–1). Objectives identify for student and teacher specifically what the student is to learn as a result of the class or course. There are three types of objectives: (1) behavioral, (2) problem-solving, and (3) outcome.[9,10]

Behavioral Objective

The most popular and most extensively used type of objective is the behavioral objective.[42] Traditionally the behavioral objective has been made up of four parts[43]:

1. *Audience:* In what situation is the student to perform?
2. *Behavior:* In what action is the student to engage?
3. *Criterion:* What is considered acceptable and unacceptable performance?
4. *Degree:* Degree of criterion for acceptable performance.

Another easy way to remember the component parts is the A, B, C, D approach. Here we have four parts: A, audience; B, behavior; C, condition; and D, degree of criterion for acceptable performance.[42]

An example of a behavioral objective is, "Given a patient immediate postop hip surgery (condition), the student will be able to identify and state the rationale (behavior) for three primary contraindications at a level of 90% accuracy or above (criterion)." The key to writing a behavioral objective is to specify an observable behavior, such as the behaviors identified under the cognitive, affective, and psychomotor domains in Figures 2–2, 2–3, and 2–4. Thus, the student is asked to engage in a behavior that can be seen and evaluated, such as describe (cognitive), demonstrate (psychomotor), or defend (affective). As more complex learning behaviors are required of students, action verbs in the higher levels of the three domains can be used to guide the teaching/learning content. By identifying specific behaviors rather than expecting students to "know" or "understand" material, the expected level of performance is much clearer to students and the teacher.

More recently the Gronlund and Brookhart's[33] approach to instructional objectives has focused on stating instructional objectives as learning outcomes, making certain that there is a performance or demonstration of the outcome of instruction. Can the student demonstrate what was learned?[33]

Even partial behavioral objectives, which identify at least the content area of knowledge to be acquired and the level of mastery (behavior) but not the grading criterion, are useful in identifying for the student what is to be achieved by her or his efforts. At the beginning of each chapter in this book, partial behavioral objectives are stated to identify for the reader what is to be gained from reading the chapter. Obviously, if the reader is able to perform the stated objectives, there is no need to read the chapter!

The problem with focusing teaching only on a list of behavioral objectives is that education is and should be more than the sum of a list of behavioral objectives. Along with behaviors that can be seen and measured, teachers also hope to stimulate and accentuate in students such behaviors as insight, curiosity, creativity, and tolerance. Additionally, students will encounter an endless number of situations in the chaotic world of clinical practice for which they would be ill prepared if the curriculum focused solely on the competencies stated in behavioral objectives. Teaching students to learn constantly from the clinical practice environment (lifelong learning) requires setting up the type of objectives that alert students to the complex skills required of them in clinical practice.

Problem-Solving Objective

The problem-solving learning objective poses a "problem" for the student to solve. In solving a problem, the student will be asked to move beyond specific predictable behaviors, demonstrate analysis of a situation, and provide a reasonable solution. Often, many different solutions or behaviors will solve a single problem. For example, students might be given a series of short clinical cases. For each case, students individually or in small groups might be asked to determine additional evaluative information they will need to treat this patient and give a rationale for why they need that information. Each student or group of students might identify somewhat different evaluative information—and all may be "right."

The following is an example of a problem-solving objective and a brief clinical case.

Problem-solving objective: Determine the additional evaluative information you need to provide treatment for the following clinical case and provide a rationale for your evaluation choices.

Mrs. Gonzales is a 76-year-old Hispanic female with a history of left hemiplegia of approximately 1 year. She fell 8 weeks ago and sustained a Colles' fracture of the right wrist. She was seen late last week by her orthopedist, Dr. Barbara Feigenbaum, who removed the cast and referred Mrs. Gonzales to physical therapy for evaluation and treatment.

Students at different levels of academic and clinical education will give different answers regarding evaluative information needed based on classroom materials and prior clinical encounters. Note that in stating a problem-solving objective, only general rather than specific student behaviors are identified. Thus, rather than focusing on a predetermined behavioral outcome, what is stressed is thinking through the materials or situations presented and "solving" the related problems.

Outcome Objective

Outcome objectives are comprehensive, broad-based objectives that specify practice expectations for students and teachers. The APTA's *Normative Model of Physical Therapist Professional Education* identifies 23 of these practice expectations, which can be used to guide course content and learning experiences for physical therapy students.[43] For example:

1. Demonstrate integrity in all interactions with patients/clients, family members, caregivers, other health care providers, students, other consumers and payers. (Practice expectation 4.1)
2. Use clinical judgment and reflection to identify, monitor, and enhance clinical reasoning in order to minimize errors and enhance patient/client outcomes. (Practice expectation 8.1)
3. Effectively educate others using culturally appropriate teaching methods that are commensurate with the needs of the learner. (Practice expectation 10.1)
4. Promote health and quality of life by providing information on health promotion, fitness, wellness, disease, impairment, functional limitation, disability,

and health risks related to age, gender, culture, and lifestyle within the scope of physical therapy practice. (Practice expectation 19.2)

Under each of these outcome objectives (called Terminal Behavioral Objectives in the APTA document), specific behavioral objectives (called Instructional Objectives in the APTA document) are used to identify the knowledge and skills needed by the student to achieve the outcome objective. See the example in Chapter 1, Box 1–1.

For any class, course, or curriculum, any number of behavioral objectives and problem-solving objectives could be created to guide the coursework and student learning to prepare students for practice expectations (outcome objectives). Academic and clinical educators can use objectives to clarify and order learning experiences for different levels of physical therapy and physical therapist assistant students. In addition, writing objectives is the final step in stimulating student learning behaviors that are congruent with how the teacher has conceived the philosophical orientations, learning theories, domains of learning, and student learning styles that will receive focus for any class, course, or clinical experience.

LOWER HALF OF THE PREACTIVE TEACHING GRID

As can be seen in the lower half of the preactive teaching grid (see Figure 2–1), the next steps are to consider the types of delivery format and prepare relevant computer based or audiovisual materials and handouts. The delivery formats selected should logically be related to the elements in the top half of the preactive teaching grid. Thus, for example, if the teacher was primarily interested in philosophical orientation of cognitive processing-reasoning, using the experiential/problem-solving learning theory, with a focus on the cognitive and affective domains of learning and emphasizing the abstract conceptualization student learning style, the format of delivery likely would be a seminar discussion focused on case materials rather than a lecture. A thorough discussion of classroom delivery formats is presented in Chapters 3 and 4.

The teacher also must start thinking about how to evaluate students' knowledge well before the first day of class. Evaluations of students are events when students and faculty see how well they have engaged the teaching-learning process. Evaluations should be consistently related to the elements in the preactive teaching grid and specifically guided by the course objectives that have focused the course content and student learning. A basic educational truth is that the better students perform on all types of evaluations, the better the teacher has thoughtfully employed the pedagogical aspects of teaching to best engage students in their own learning. Thus, student evaluations demonstrate the level of success of teachers as well as students. Suggestions for different types of student evaluation are presented in Chapter 3.

TEACHING ENVIRONMENT

Note that the last element in the preactive teaching grid before actually preparing the learning experience is attention given to the physical teaching environment. Preactive teaching includes content and format preparation well in advance as well as arriving at the classroom early to attend to the room arrangement and the room environment (including cleanliness and temperature) and being sure that all media and materials needed for teaching are available and working. Make sure you know how to work any form of media presentation, and you may even want a back up plan (see Chapter 4). Stand quietly in any empty classroom. Think of the impact on student learning when there are half-empty coffee cups and food wrappers from prior classes, dirty media equipment that is a rat's nest of electrical cords, bulletin boards that are empty or contain woefully outdated information, ceiling lights that have expired, and seating arrangements that make you invisible to students (and vice versa).

Make friends with the people from the housekeeping department, the media department, and administrative assistants in the dean's office. Work with them to create clean and inviting learning environments. Even if the classroom is used by many different faculty and student groups, assess and set up an effective learning climate for your students in your class. Your efforts, part of the implicit curriculum, will not go unnoticed or unappreciated by students or colleagues.

PREPARING A COURSE SYLLABUS

Preparing a course syllabus is an excellent way of dealing with the often paralyzing gap between what one would like to teach and the reality of the time available for teaching. From the students' perspective, a course syllabus provides a complete overview of the course content, course requirements, and timeline on the first day of class.[43] This overview allows students to organize their semester in a way that best promotes their learning and achievement. Box 2–1 contains a list of items that are often included in a course syllabus.

Remember that course requirements are the first thing students will want to see. You will want to make sure that you provide a clear discussion of these requirements in that first visit with your class. An important element in course syllabi is the linking and alignment of the course learning

---

BOX 2–1 **Contents of a Course Syllabus**

Commission on Accreditation in Physical Therapy Education (CAPTE) requires the following in course syllabi in this order:
- Course title and number
- Course description
- Instructor
- Credit hours
- Clock hours (lecture and laboratory)
- Course prerequisites
- Course objectives
- Outline of content
- Schedule of when content is taught in course
- Description of teaching methods and learning experiences
- Methods of student evaluation/grading
- Required and recommended readings
- Additional elements that are useful in a course syllabus:
- Teaching philosophy
- Attendance policy/expectations for professional behavior
- How much each assignment counts toward final grade
- Detailed information on the course assignments, including grading rubrics (content, length, due dates)
- Office hours/office location/access information

outcomes (objectives) with the program outcomes. A good technique for this alignment is having faculty identify the linkage between their course outcomes and the appropriate program outcomes. This kind of tracking is an important element in assessment and program evaluation (see Chapter 5).

Draw the student's attention to important items in your syllabus by bolding, bulleting, using graphics, color, and so forth. Early in the syllabus is also a good place to briefly share your classroom teaching philosophy and expectations for student presence and involvement in your class. The following example is from a course on the Psychology of Illness and Wellness Behaviors:

> **Philosophy and focus of this course related to your presence:** This class is about human beings—you and the people you interact with personally and professionally. The information presented and ideas exchanged during lectures or seminars and highlighted from required readings will be essential to the well-being of the patients and families you will treat and to your own health and effectiveness as a health care professional. As much active learning takes place during class time as during outside reflection and reading. A missed class means you miss stimulation for awareness of your personal attitudes, beliefs, and value judgments. You are urged to attend all lectures and seminar. You may miss one class during the semester for your personal "low-ebb day," which may be taken for any reason.
>
> **Class participation:** Each student is urged to participate freely and honestly in sharing the facts, impressions, and perceptions that constitute her or his reality. I believe that although students may hold some misinformation regarding their own and others' behaviors, there is very little right or wrong—only less effective and more effective ways to work with others. You will discover your own unique mode of effectiveness through active participation in class-related activities both in and out of the classroom setting.
>
> Many programs have adopted standard language for class attendance and professional behaviors and clearly the expectations that stem from school and the profession's standards. *Participatory attendance is an important aspect of your professional education and this course. An excused absence must be requested before the beginning of the class and must be validated by the course instructor. One unexcused absence will result in a reduction of your overall course grade. Other professional behavior expectations include coming to class prepared and on time, having done the assigned readings/ exercises; meeting assignment deadlines; actively participating in class and small group activities; and adhering to university/school honor code and the APTA Code of Ethics and School's Professional Behavior Policies.*

Model good intellectual behaviors in your syllabus. Remember the implicit curriculum. What are you telling students by presenting incomplete information for reference sources, including last year's dates and misspelled words? Thus, give *complete* and *consistent citations* for required and recommended readings (e.g., author, title, journal [or publisher], year of publication, volume number, page numbers). Carefully review your syllabus for accuracy—dates, spelling, sentence structure, and so forth. Remember that preparing a good course syllabus takes time and that being only "one step ahead of the students" is reserved for first-year novice teachers.

Finally, give students a sense of fun and adventure about the learning they are to engage in. For example, ending your syllabus with a statement such as, "I am delighted to be your guide on this journey we are about to embark on together!" rather than a "law enforcement" message regarding poor performance sets the stage for a respectful and enjoyable mutual teaching-learning adventure.

GRAPHIC SYLLABUS

A creative strategy used by many faculty developers is having faculty make a visual or graphic syllabus that shows the courses topics or units, how they are connected, and the overall flow of the course (Figure 2–7).[44] This is particularly helpful for new faculty because they may find it difficult to see the flow in their course. If it is difficult for faculty, imagine what the experience of the student may be.

SUMMARY

This chapter has provided a broad overview of the elements a physical therapist or physical therapy assistant educator should consider before, and in concert with, preparing the course content and conducting the academic teaching-learning experience. That is, it covers the preactive teaching elements or pedagogical principles, including philosophical orientations, learning theories, domains of learning, learning styles, and objectives that form the teaching-learning framework of a course. This chapter, along with Chapters 3, 4, and 5, suggests a number of ways (pedagogical knowledge) to think about organizing, conducting, and evaluating classes and courses in a manner that supports learning and learning to love learning.

THRESHOLD CONCEPTS

Threshold Concept #1: Student learning is central to the design and implementation of all teaching and learning experiences.

Without evidence of student learning, there is no evidence of successful teaching. This chapter provides an important foundation in seeing how understanding more about theories of learning is essential in the active of "preactive teaching." Planning for teaching and learning is not just about the "download" of what you know in the classroom or laboratory. The preactive planning process helps a teacher think more intentionally about aligning what they want to do with how they will go about designing that teaching experience.

Threshold Concept #2: Learning is an active process by which learners are constructing meaning all of the time both inside and outside of the classroom and laboratory.

We know that humans learn all of the time. As discussed in this chapter, the situated learning that occurs during the interactions in the community of practice, whether that be the academic setting or clinical setting, is an important aspect of student learning. Teachers need to be aware of helping students develop their knowledge structure, both inside and outside the classroom. Strategies that can be useful may include a graphic syllabus that shows the links across concepts or being aware that you need to move students from factual knowledge to more procedural knowledge to meta-cognitive knowledge.

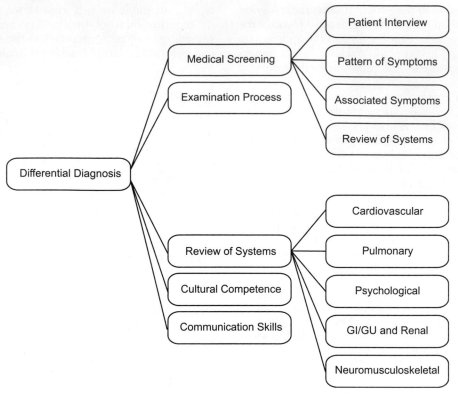

FIGURE 2–7 Graphic approach to connecting key concepts in a course syllabus.

ANNOTATED BIBLIOGRAPHY

Cantillon P, Wood D. *ABC of Learning and Teaching in Medicine.* 2nd ed. West Sussex, UK: Wiley-Blackwell; 2010.

    The ABC book is a succinct resource for beginning and experienced teachers. It is a compendium of short chapters on core concepts in health professions education. This book covers everything from course design, to teaching methods, to assessment.

Dent J, Harden R, eds. *A Practical Guide for Medical Teachers.* 3rd ed. New York: Churchill Livingstone/Elsevier; 2009.

    This text addresses all of the core components in teaching, including curriculum development, learning situations, educational strategies, teaching tools, and assessment. The chapters are easy to understand, and the important take-away points are highlighted.

Ende J, ed. *Theory and Practice of Teaching Medicine.* Philadelphia: American College of Physicians and Surgeons; 2010.

    This is one in a series of books from the American College of Physicians on teaching medicine. All the books in the series are written in a style that is reader friendly. This book addresses key theories of learning, applying the concepts to teaching novices in the classroom and clinic. Two chapters are devoted to providing tips for enhancing teaching.

Gronlund NE. *Writing Instructional Objectives for Teaching and Assessment.* 8th ed. Upper Saddle River, NJ: Merrill Education/Prentice-Hall; 2008.

    This is a classic paperback text for assisting teachers in writing instructional objectives. The book includes three major sections: (1) how to write instructional objectives, (2) writing objectives for various outcomes (across the cognitive, affective, and psychomotor domains), and (3) how to use objectives for teaching and assessment. The author provides extensive examples throughout the book, including a set of well-known appendices that give specific examples of objectives and "illustrative verbs" that can be used to identify student learning behaviors.

Phillips DC, Soltis JF. *Perspectives on Learning.* 5th ed. New York: Teachers College Press; 2009.

    This book, now in its fifth edition, remains one of the most interesting, readable, and concise overviews of learning theories.

Svinicki M, McKeachie W. *McKeachie's Teaching Tips.* 13th ed. Belmont, CA: Wadsworth; 2011.

No text on teaching would be complete without a reference to McKeachie's classic text for college and university teachers. This 13th edition covers the bases from essential information on getting ready to teach your first class to strategies for dealing with challenging students and sticky testing and grading issues. Consistent with the other 12 editions, the book provides an excellent reference list for each of the chapters.

REFERENCES

1. Shulman L. *Teaching as Community Property: Essays on Higher Education.* San Francisco: Jossey-Bass; 2004.
2. Grossman PL. *The Making of a Teacher: Teacher Knowledge and Teacher Education.* New York: Teachers College Press; 1990.
3. Skeff K, Stratos G, eds. *Methods for Teaching Medicine.* Philadelphia: American College of Physicians; 2010.
4. Irby D. What clinical teachers in medicine need to know. *Acad Med.* 1994;69:333–342.
5. Kolb DA. *Learning Styles Inventory.* Boston: McBer; 1985.
6. Dickinson R, Dervitz H, Meida H. *Handbook for Physical Therapy Teachers.* New York: American Physical Therapy Association; 1967.
7. Jackson P. *The Practice of Teaching.* New York: Teachers College Press; 1986.
8. Schön D. *Educating the Reflective Practitioner.* San Francisco: Jossey-Bass; 1987.
9. Eisner EW. *The Educational Imagination: On the Design and Evaluation of School Programs.* 3rd ed. New York: Macmillan; 1985.
10. Shepard K. Alternatives for curriculum design in physical therapy. *Phys Ther.* 1977;57:1389–1393.
11. Boud D, Feletti GE. *The Challenge of Problem-Based Learning.* 2nd ed. London: Kogan Page; 2003.
12. Schwartz P, Mennin S, Webb G, eds. *Problem-based Learning: Case Studies, Experience and Practice.* New York: Routledge; 2001.
13. Jette D, Latham NK, Smout RJ, et al. Physical therapy interventions for patients with stroke in inpatient rehabilitation facilities. *Phys Ther.* 2005;85:238–248.
14. Neil AS. *Summerhill: A Radical Approach to Child Rearing.* New York: Hart; 1960.

15. Stumbo T, Thiele A, York A. Generic abilities as rank ordered by baby boomer and generation X physical therapists. *J Phys Ther Educ.* 2007;21:48–52.

16. Phillips DC, Soltis JF. *Perspectives on Learning.* 5th ed. New York: Teachers College Press; 2009.

17. Ende J, ed. *Theory and Practice in Teaching Medicine.* Philadelphia: American College of Physicians; 2010.

18. Harris I. Conceptions and theories of learning for workplace education. In: Hafler JP, ed. *Extraordinary Learning in the Workplace.* New York: Springer; 2011.

19. Redman B. *The Practice of Patient Education: A Case Study Approach.* 10th ed. St. Louis: Mosby/Elsevier; 2007.

20. Thorndike FL. *Educational Psychology: The Psychology of Learning.* New York: Teachers College Press; 1913.

21. Skinner BF. *Science and Human Behavior.* New York: Macmillan; 1966.

22. Piaget J. *The Construction of Reality in the Child.* New York: Basic Books; 1954.

23. Ausubel DP. The use of advance organizers in the learning and retention of meaningful material. *J Educ Psychol.* 1960;51:267–272.

24. Bransford J, Brown A, Cocking R, eds. *How People Learn: Brain, Mind, Experiences and School.* Washington, DC: National Academy Press; 2000.

25. Gagne RM. *The Conditions of Learning.* New York: Holt, Rinehart & Winston; 1970.

26. Bandura A. *Social Foundations of Thought and Action: A Social Cognitive Approach.* Englewood Cliffs, NJ: Prentice Hall; 1986.

27. Dewey J. *Experience and Education.* New York: McMillan; 1938.

28. Bloom B, ed. *Taxonomy of Educational Objectives, Handbook I: The Cognitive Domain.* New York: David McKay; 1956.

29. Krathwohl DR, Bloom BS, Masia BB. *Taxonomy of Educational Objectives, Handbook II: Affective Domain.* New York: David McKay; 1964.

30. Krathwohl D. A revision of Bloom's taxonomy: an overview. *Theory Pract.* 2002;41:212–217.

31. Simpson EJ. *The Classification of Educational Objectives in the Psychomotor Domain.* Washington, DC: Gryphon House; 1972.

32. May W, Kontney, Iglarsh AZ. *Professional Behaviors for the 21st Century.* Available at: http://www.marquette.edu/physical-therapy/documents/ProfessionalBehaviors.pdf; Accessed 23.09.2011.

33. Miller GE. The assessment of clinical skills, competence and performance. *Acad Med.* 1990;65:S63–S67.

34. Dent J, Harden R, eds. *A Practical Guide for Medical Teachers.* Philadelphia: Churchill Livingstone; 2009.

35. Sargeant D. Teaching spirituality in the physical therapy classroom and clinic. *J Phys Ther Educ.* 2009;23:29–35.

36. Gillen M, English L. *Addressing Spiritual Dimensions of Adult Learning: What Educators Can Do.* San Francisco: Jossey-Bass; 2000.

37. Bezner J, Boucher BK. The influence of personality type on decision making in the physical therapy admission process. *J Allied Health.* 2001;30:83–91.

38. Harasym PH, Leong EJ, Juschka BB, et al. Myers-Briggs psychological type and achievement in anatomy and physiology. *Am J Physiol.* 1995;268:S61–S65.

39. Theis SL, Merritt SL. Learning style preferences of elderly coronary artery disease patients. *Educ Gerontol.* 1992;18:677–689.

40. Merritt SL, Marshall JC. Reliability and construct validity of alternate forms of the Canfield Learning Styles Inventory. *Adv Nurs Sci.* 1984;7:78–85.

41. Kolb DA. *Learning Styles Inventory. Version 3.1.* Available at: http://www.haygroup.com/leadershipandtalentondemand/ourproducts/item_details.aspx?itemid=55&type=7; Accessed 21.08.2011.

42. Mager R. *Instructional Objectives: A Critical Tool in the Development of Effective Instruction.* 3 rd ed. Atlanta: Center for Effective Performance; 1997.

43. American Physical Therapy Association. *A Normative Model of Physical Therapist Professional Education: Version 2004.* Alexandria, VA: American Physical Therapy Association; 2004.

44. Nilson L. *The Graphic Syllabus and the Outcomes Map: Communicating Your Course.* San Francisco: Jossey-Bass; 2007.

TEACHING AND LEARNING IN ACADEMIC SETTINGS

Gail M. Jensen ✪ Elizabeth Mostrom ✪ Katherine F. Shepard

CHAPTER OUTLINE

As you walk into the physical therapy classroom—also used as the laboratory—you are hoping you will be able to cover all your material in the next 50 minutes. The students drag into the room, having just finished a 3-hour anatomy dissection laboratory. They disperse all over the classroom and look like they could hardly stay awake for the next hour. You think to yourself: Thank goodness, I don't want too many questions anyway and just need to get through this material so that we can get on with laboratory session tomorrow. In this coming hour, you are to give the overview lecture for the upcoming laboratory session on clinical measurement. You are very

comfortable teaching the clinical examination skills but a bit nervous about having to cover measurement concepts in this overview lecture; therefore, you have included several definitions of terms in your handout. You begin going through a quick PowerPoint slide presentation that complements the handout. You try to ask a few questions, but the students appear to be dutifully taking notes and not very interested in interacting. So, you think to yourself: Well that is all right, I will just get through the material, and then we can have more interaction in the lab tomorrow, where I am far more comfortable teaching the clinical skills.

If you were in the teaching situation described in the preceding anecdote, what could you do? How might you learn from this experience? What is going on? What are your options? Before focusing on specific techniques for teaching in academic settings, let's think about how teaching techniques or tools are part of a larger process of teaching and learning in academic settings. This chapter revisits the essential elements involved in any teaching situation:

1. Content and knowledge that a teacher holds and must share with students,
2. Transformation (transforming what is known into material that can be taught to others),
3. Instruction (teaching performance), and
4. Reflective evaluation (learning from one's teaching experience), which leads to
5. New comprehension or understanding as one learns from experience (Figure 3–1).[1] The chapter then

focuses on basic teaching and evaluation tools for large groups in the classroom, including lectures and strategies for facilitating collaborative learning, teaching and evaluation tools for clinical laboratory performance, strategies for facilitating reflection and problem analysis, and a brief overview of teaching technologies.

A PRACTICAL MODEL FOR TEACHING AND LEARNING
KNOWLEDGE OF THE SUBJECT MATTER

Good teachers have a thorough knowledge of the subject matter that allows them to display more self-confidence and creativity in teaching. Investigations of teachers also demonstrate that teachers not only have information in the area but also understand how the key concepts or ideas are connected, as well as the ways in which new knowledge is created and validated.[1,2] Using the previous anecdote, remember that the instructor was nervous about having to cover measurement concepts and was unable to engage the students in any interaction during a lecture. The teacher ended up covering the material on the handout with little student interaction. Why did this happen? Perhaps the instructor, although very comfortable with teaching the clinical skills of measurement (i.e., goniometry and manual muscle testing), was much less certain of her or his knowledge of clinical measurement concepts; therefore, the instructor covered the content with little discussion. For example, in discussing the measurement concept of validity and manual muscle testing, a teacher with thorough knowledge of clinical measurement would move beyond the definition of validity to a discussion of the use of manual muscle testing for the assessment of muscle weakness. Use of muscle testing for assessing muscle strength raises a validity question.[3] Research on teachers supports this example; when teachers do not know the subject matter well, they tend to focus more on content, whereas teachers who know their subject well teach not

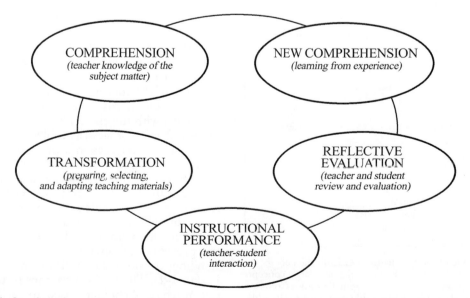

FIGURE 3–1 A model of teaching representing each of the key components in the teaching and learning process for teachers and students.

only the content but also the practical application of key concepts and the current controversies of what is known and not known about the subject.[1,2,4]

TRANSFORMATION

The transformation phase represents the teacher's ability to "transform" the material so that students can understand. As teachers, we need to get the "inside out"— that is, we need to know what is going on inside the heads of our learners.[5] There are teachers who are quite expert in certain subjects, yet they are dismal teachers. A second component of teaching is the teacher's ability to do good "preactive teaching." As detailed in Chapter 2, there is specific knowledge and skill involved in taking what is known and transforming it in preparation for teaching. First, one must review any instructional materials in light of what is known about the subject: Are there any errors? Have things changed? Has the thinking changed in this subject? A second step in transformation is thinking about how to go about presenting the content. What learning theories will you use and what type of objectives will you focus on? Will you use a clinical case, a focused small class activity, or visual aids? A final step is deciding how to tailor your understanding of the content to students' understanding. Students are not likely to have the breadth and depth of knowledge that the instructor has. The critical issue is for the instructor to adapt what he or she knows and come up with examples or representations that fit the students' present understandings of the content.[5] In the anecdote of teaching clinical measurement, one may be discussing range-of-motion measures as they apply to physical impairment measures and challenge students that they will ultimately need to address any functional limitations the patient may have. In doing so, the teacher also assumes that the students remember the International Classification of Functioning, Disability, and Health (ICF) model that had been presented and discussed the previous week (Figure 3–2).[6] The instructor quickly discovers that the students do not understand and therefore must backtrack, using the key model concepts and tying them in a simple and direct way to patient cases.

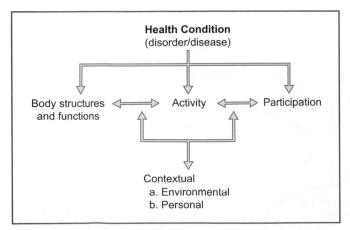

FIGURE 3–2 An example of the International Classification of Functioning, Disability and Health (ICF) model that uses larger concepts to represent specific data from a patient case. (From Towards a Common language for Functioning, Disability and Health: ICF. Geneva: World Health Organization, 2002, p 9.)

INSTRUCTION

Instruction is what is known as teaching, yet instruction is only the interactive phase or "performance" of teaching. It includes everything from pacing of the material, to classroom management, to asking and responding to questions. Many of the specific teaching tools discussed in this chapter are part of the instructional process. Active learning or learner engagement is frequently discussed as a key component of the instructional process.[5,7,8] Students must be engaged in their learning in order to learn. Some general characteristics of and strategies for active learning have been suggested by Barkley[7]:

- Be clear on your learning goals.
- Focus on the learning that results from the activity as opposed to the activity itself.
- Be clear on what your role is as teacher.
- Remember that teaching is not "telling."
- Help learners develop learning strategies such as linking concepts together, applying concepts to problems, or analyzing problems.
- Use strategies that will help learners transfer what they know to what they are learning.
- Teach for retention (here, an emotional connection is helpful, along with having the information make sense to the student and have meaning, such as a clinical case or context).
- Provide opportunities for guided practice and rehearsal.

REFLECTIVE EVALUATION AND NEW COMPREHENSION

This last component of the practical model for teaching is the ongoing process of learning from experience. This process of reviewing, reconstructing, and critically analyzing one's own performance and the class's performance is lifelong learning, a process that is central to teaching. For example, in the anecdote at the beginning of this chapter, the teacher found that after he or she presented the ICF model, followed by the patient clinical measurement data, the class looked perplexed and did not respond to questions. What could be done? The teacher could interrupt the class and admit that there appeared to be some confusion. The teacher might then begin to go through the model again by asking students to provide their understanding of the concepts and the clinical application. The teacher could clarify each concept while going through the model with the class. This is an example of reflection. In the reflection process, a problem arises with some uncertainty, so one engages in a process of thinking critically about what is going on and devising alternative solution strategies. The first step involves seeing the problem. In this case, the instructor stops the class because he or she recognizes that students are confused. Then the group reviews the ICF model, which can lead to a revised or new understanding with the instructor's guidance. The reflective process in this example is likely to lead to *new* understandings or comprehensions for students and teacher (see Figure 3–1). The last two sections of this chapter emphasize teaching techniques used to facilitate collaboration and reflection in the classroom.

CLASSROOM TEACHING WITH LARGE GROUPS

When thinking of a large class and limited time to cover a significant amount of material, the teaching tools that come to mind are lecture and discussion. If there is a great deal of content, there may be little discussion and a lot of lecture. This section addresses the formal, traditional lecture for large groups, including purposes, effective lecture design and delivery, and advantages and disadvantages of traditional lectures. This section is followed by active learning strategies for large groups, including discussion and questioning.

LECTURES

You need to remember that the lecture method is not just telling but involves carefully planning for organization and delivery. There is an old saying that lectures are a method of transferring the notes of the teacher to the notes of a student without passing through the heads of either.[9,10]

The lecture method of teaching was a prominent method for disseminating information before the invention of mass print in the 1600s. In these lectures, the instructor would talk, while the students wrote everything down—in effect, creating their own "texts." Why is it that the lecture remains such a significant part of our teaching repertoire in the midst of ready access to information through many sources?[9,11]

What Purposes Do Lectures Serve?

Lectures are often used to transmit a lot of information efficiently to large groups of students. McKeachie summarizes the skills of a good lecturer, saying "[e]ffective lecturers combine the talents of scholar, writer, producer, comedian, showman, and teacher in ways that contribute to student learning."[9] Research comparing the lecture to other forms of teaching demonstrates that the lecture is as effective as other methods for teaching knowledge. In addition to the cognitive component, lectures can also motivate. A skilled lecturer can stimulate interest, challenge students to seek more information, and communicate passion and enthusiasm for the subject matter. Lectures can also be used as an efficient method to consolidate and integrate information from a number of different printed sources. Lecture material can be specifically adapted or tailored to the class, and difficult concepts can be clarified in lecture. Finally, lectures can set the stage for discussion or other learning activities.[9]

Perhaps the most important use of lecture is that it is a powerful tool for building the bridge between student knowledge and the structures of the subject matter. For example, imagine that a teacher is lecturing about kinesiology of the shoulder complex. The students have a strong anatomic understanding of the subject matter and some understanding of the basic biomechanical principles and functional application. It is important in this case for the teacher to use the lecture as an opportunity to facilitate mutual levels of application and understanding when presenting how concepts from anatomy and kinesiology apply to a clinical problem. The lecture also can be used to explore and analyze specific concepts or ideas, and the teacher can demonstrate her or his problem-solving process. As most teachers find out, lecture preparation involves seeking a broad range of information and then analyzing, synthesizing, and integrating subject matter from various sources.

What Makes an Effective Lecture?

Planning

Teachers might plan a lecture as they approach writing a paper by thinking about the overall organization, the introduction, body, and conclusion. Good overall questions to start with when planning a lecture, in contrast to "covering the subject matter," are (1) What do you really want students to remember from this lecture over time? (2) How should students process the information? (3) Are you trying to be a conclusion-oriented lecturer, or is your aim to assist students to learn and think through a cognitive activity? (Review your preactive teaching grid [see Figure 2–1].)

One of the major concerns is keeping students' attention. One study reports that students recall 70% of the material covered in the first 10 minutes of class and only 20% of material covered in the last 10 minutes.[17] This finding about the serial placement of material remains constant. We remember best what comes first and second best what comes last and remember the least what comes in the middle.[7] How does the instructor capture the students' attention? One effective strategy is to announce that the information presented will be tested; however, there are also many other ways to stimulate students' thinking and actively involve them in learning.

Introduction

An effective introduction focuses and engages the students and outlines the specific topics that will be covered and the order in which the topics will be discussed. The introduction should also identify the gap between the students' existing cognitive knowledge and the topic, or it should raise questions. Pre-questions can be used to focus students toward the intent of the lecture. For example, imagine that the topic is an introduction to the role of culture in professional-patient interactions. One may begin the lecture by standing in the back of the room (not the front) to talk to the class. The teacher may ask the class to share observations about the traditional role of the teacher and then proceed to ask questions about students' meanings of classroom behavior—that is, the culture of the classroom. Another useful technique is to begin with a story or a case that highlights the relevance and importance of the lecture subject matter.[9]

Body

The body of the lecture should fit with the students' ability to process information. Perhaps the most common error of the novice teaching is to try to put too much information into the lecture. This occurs when the teacher overestimates the students' ability to grasp the information and see the relationship between concepts and applications. Russell et al.[12] demonstrated that increasing the density of a lecture reduces the students' retention of basic information. Often, trying to present too much information is the result of inadequate preparation in which the teacher has not clearly identified the key concepts.

The lecture should not be written out verbatim, but an outline can be very effective in guiding the body of the lecture. Color coding your notes can also be an effective procedural strategy. The use of graphic representations, computer flow charts, models or media clips can provide the class with a representation of the structure of the material presented. The instructor can also place cues in the lecture outline margins or notes that include learning strategies to be used along the way (e.g., the use of overheads, stimulating questions, different types of explanations, or brief dyad discussions among students).[9,11]

A single class usually represents a diverse group of learners. Some students may do better with a deductive process-that is, going from a sequence of generalizations to specific application—whereas other students may do better with a more inductive process—that is, moving from the specifics to the general concepts. The use of an outline and a visual structure provides cues for both groups.[13] An easy rule of thumb for a great lecture is a simple framework and lots of examples. Additional tips for facilitating student comprehension can be found in Box 3–1.[9]

Conclusion

The conclusion is a time to summarize the important points of the lecture by going back over the outline or key graphics. The teacher may also use this as an opportunity to have students summarize the material orally or in writing. Other strategies include having the students do a 3-minute writing exercise summarizing the major points of the lecture, or looking at student lecture notes to see what they are writing to determine whether they grasped key concepts. These methods provide additional information about the students' understandings of the lecture.[9,13]

Lecture Delivery: How Can You Maintain Attention?

Earlier in this chapter, we stated that instruction can be thought of as performance, and lecture delivery provides one of the most obvious chances to perform. Passion and enthusiasm for the subject matter are key aspects of any lecture. Although one of the most common strategies for getting students to pay attention is to say this will be on the test, there are also other strategies the teacher can use. The teacher is a powerful role model in front of the class and represents a thoughtful scholar to the students. Tips for improving lecture presentation can be found in Box 3–2.[9,10]

Perhaps the greatest advantage of the lecture is that it is economical, particularly when the teacher has lots of students and little time. The strongest disadvantages are the passive role of the students and the lack of student engagement in higher-order cognitive objectives (e.g., analysis, evaluation). One quick classroom assessment technique for determining whether students are attending to and grasping the lecture materials is called the *punctuated lecture*[14]:

- *Listen:* Students listen to the teacher's presentation.
- *Stop:* Teacher stops the presentation.
- *Reflect:* Students are asked to reflect on what they were doing while they were listening and how their behaviors enhanced or hindered their ability to listen and understand the material.
- *Write:* Students then write down their reflections (anonymously).
- *Feedback:* Students provide feedback to the teacher.

The use of personal response systems (computer-input devices) or clickers allows the teacher to interject questions or other activities and have students respond through the use of the handheld device. Refer to Chapter 4 for more on the role of technology.

BOX 3–2 Tips for Improving Lecture Presentation

- *Create movement.* Change your position in the room. Do not remain anchored at the podium.
- *Use visuals.* Use various visual teaching tools (e.g., overheads, the blackboard, charts, graphs). These visuals are particularly good for highlighting key points. Videotapes can be powerful tools for illustrating examples from the real world in the clinic or community.
- *Pay attention to the effect of the voice.* The voice can vary in terms of volume, rate, and tone. If your voice is not loud enough for the class to hear, a microphone may be necessary. Beware of avoiding a monotone delivery. Voice is one of the key ingredients for communicating enthusiasm to the students. The use of audiotape or videotape can be a helpful feedback mechanism for assessing how you use your voice.
- *Pay attention to body language.* In addition to the voice, teachers also communicate with students through nonverbal language. Be aware of nervous habits, such as playing with the pointer, jingling change, or any other persistent movement of the hands. Use body language to communicate points of emphasis and enthusiasm.
- *Pace the delivery and clarify the material.* As stated earlier, two common elements of excellent lectures are a simple plan with a structure and the use of numerous examples.[9] The structure of the lecture provides the foundation for pacing the delivery of the material. Observe the audience to see whether they are keeping up with note taking, are confused, or need more time for questions. Remember that attention in lectures declines after the first 20 minutes, so vary your activities. A second consideration is how to go about clarifying difficult concepts. In the previous section on transformation, we advocated that teachers are responsible for transforming ideas to assist learning. Ideas can be represented through analogies or metaphors. For example, performing a grade 1 mobilization movement can be described as having "a fly do deep knee bends" to overillustrate how small the movement it is. A metaphor can be useful for having students think expansively and creatively. For example, which metaphor best describes the work of a physical therapist or physical therapist assistant: teacher, gardener, business executive, or healer?

BOX 3–1 Tips for Facilitating Student Comprehension

- Use visual representations.
- Develop the idea or concept, then give examples. Reiterate your initial point.
- Pauses give students time to think—give periodic summaries in your lecture. You do not have to cover everything.
- Check for understanding. This is not just the standard, "Any questions?" If you want to check for understanding, give students a minute to write down a question. They can compare with their neighbor, and then you will get some questions from the class.

Another area for facilitating students' attention during the lecture is teaching students to be better listeners. This can be done by posing questions that can help them focus. What were the two most important points in this reading? You could have students listen to part of your lecture without taking notes and then write a brief summary or summarize the main points of the lecture.[9]

Should Students Take Notes during Your Lecture?

We know that note taking is an aid to your working or short-term memory. The critical component of note taking is that students need to be able to "chunk" or integrate the information. If they are madly taking notes trying to keep up, they run the risk of not integrating the information. Research demonstrates that for students with less background knowledge, note taking may limit their capacity for listening. Should a teacher distribute the lecture notes beforehand? In a recent study, students who received class notes before a lecture compared with after the lecture actually attended class more regularly and participated more in class. There is also research that supports giving students an outline that they must fill in.[15]

THE INTERACTIVE LECTURE: ROLE OF DISCUSSION AND QUESTIONING IN LARGE GROUP SETTINGS

Initiating the Class Discussion

Questioning and discussion are two tools for moving to a more interactive lecture within a large group. The teacher can move from lecture, to discussion, to questioning, and then back to lecture. Class discussion, however, is not something to do when the lecture material runs out or as a way to extend the lecture. A good discussion, just as the lecture, is done with planning and purpose.

- *Start with a question.* A discussion usually starts with a question. This question could be focused on a common experience (e.g., a reaction to a visual, a videotape, or a story).
- *Lead with controversy or a debate.* With this strategy, the class could be divided into two or more large groups and be given the task of developing a position.
- *Have students brainstorm.* When students brainstorm what they know about the topic, the teacher can use these ideas to build a framework consistent with the students' understandings and discuss with the group any misconceptions.[7,10]
- *Use the Socratic method of dialogue or discussion.* This approach has been used extensively in the education of lawyers. In this method, teachers focus on teaching from a known case to general principles, thus teaching students to think like a lawyer. The general questioning strategy is to use a known case to formulate general principles, and then to apply these principles to new cases; for example, you might begin by discussing the following with students[9]:

Imagine that your patient asks you to not document in the medical record that he has been playing softball, even though he is still unable to return to work with his low back pain. Ask students to identify all the factors that might lead a patient to ask a therapist to do that. Then ask the students what they would do if they were the therapist and why. Ask the students to talk about the importance of the medical record and the professional's responsibility to be honest. As you discuss this case, begin to introduce the general ethical principle of beneficence. Then you can move on and talk about deception and how the principle of beneficence would apply or not apply in this case. Then you might propose a second case wherein the therapist does not exactly record the "truth" in the medical record. Now the therapist is involved in deception because he or she wants to make sure the patient gets the additional rehabilitation that is necessary to get the patient back to work. These two cases are discussed, looking for the differences and then applying the ethical principle of beneficence.

Common Discussion Problems

The two most common discussion problems are students who talk too much or too little. There are a number of reasons why students may be silent in the classroom (e.g., fear of looking stupid, prior bad experiences such as being mocked or berated, or even shyness). What can be done about students who do not talk during discussion? A supportive classroom environment is a key element. It involves more than encourages students to participate. To have a supportive classroom environment, the teacher must create an emotional and intellectual climate supportive of risk taking. Suggestions for facilitating a supportive classroom environment can be found in Box 3–3.[7,9,13]

What about the student who talks too much and responds to every question? McKeachie[9] suggests the following options for large groups:

BOX 3–3 Tips for Facilitating a Supportive Classroom Environment

- Learn the students' names.
- Demonstrate a strong interest in students as individuals and be sensitive to subtle messages they give about the material or presentation.
- Respond to students' feelings about class assignments and be willing to listen.
- Encourage and invite students' questions and express interest in hearing their personal viewpoints. Consider having students write down their questions first, then ask them to share with the class.
- Demonstrate interest in the importance of students' understanding of the material.
- Encourage students to be creative and independent in reacting to the material. Begin by asking students to share their perceptions or ideas about general questions that do not have a right or wrong answer.
- If there is an argument or conflicting views in a discussion, turn this into an assignment for continued investigation with library work.
- If students are disputing what you know, give yourself time to think by listing the different perspectives on the board.
- Pay attention to the physical environment of the classroom. Even though you may be lecturing, you still want the physical environment to encourage active learning. For example, in traditional classrooms and auditorium-style classrooms where most lectures take place, think about having students sit so that they can easily participate in quick interactions in twos or threes as learning groups.[7]

- Ask the class if they would like the participation more evenly distributed.
- Audiotape a discussion and play it back for class analysis on how to improve the discussion.
- Assign class observers who observe participation and report to the class.
- Use a small group structure and assign roles for group members.
- Speak directly with the student outside of class.

What if students have not read the assignment? One strategy is to give students a set of questions they need to gather information on from the readings. You could use learning groups and assign different questions to different groups. Giving students a quiz at the beginning of class or before class through a web-based format is another strategy.

Finally, what kinds of actions have the potential to stifle discussion? Frequently, a teacher can slow a discussion by talking more than engaging in discussion with students. Here are a few tips to remember:

- Give students enough time to respond.
- Be careful not to phrase your questions as just requiring a "yes" or "no" response.
- Do not interrupt students.

Questioning

Questioning is an important teaching strategy that can facilitate the process of active learning. In questioning, students are asked to link concepts, evaluate ideas, or apply knowledge. Skilled teachers use questions to guide the student's thought process. To be able to ask effective questions, one needs to understand more about levels or types of questions and when to apply them.

One simple model classifies questions under three types: (1) concrete, (2) abstract, and (3) creative.[9] Concrete questions generally focus on a recall of facts, literal meaning, and simple ideas. These are the "who, what, where, and when" questions. Abstract questions have students generalize, classify, or reason to a conclusion about the facts presented. These are the "how" and "why" questions. Creative questions ask students to reorganize concepts into a new pattern that may require abstract and concrete thinking. The teacher may ask, "What would happen if?" or "How else could you go about?"

A helpful strategy is to think about the kinds of questions you would ask across the categories in the cognitive domain. In addition, you can include a column that identifies the knowledge dimension you are targeting (Table 3–1).[16,17]

Questioning Techniques

In addition to being aware of the type of question being asked, a teacher should attend to questioning technique or performance in the classroom (Box 3–4).[9,11]

STRATEGIES FOR FACILITATING COLLABORATIVE LEARNING

The best answer to the question, "What is the most effective method of teaching?" is that it depends on the goal, the student, the content, and the teacher. But the next best answer is, "Students teaching other students."[9] The retention rate for learning experiences and teaching methods that focus on learner engagement are impressive (Figure 3–3).

TABLE 3–1   Examples of Classifications of Questions in the Cognitive Domain

Category (Cognitive Domain)	Cognitive Requirement	Concept	Examples of Questions and Terms	Knowledge Dimension
Knowledge	Recall information	Memorization	What, when, who, which, list, name, describe	Factual knowledge
Comprehension	Understanding (questions can be answered by restating material in a literal manner)	Description Explanation Illustration	Compare, contrast, conclude, distinguish, explain, give an example of, illustrate	Conceptual knowledge
Application	Solving (questions involve problem solving in new situations)	Solution Application	Apply, build, consider, demonstrate (in a new situation), how, would	Procedural knowledge
Analysis	Exploration of reasoning (questions require the student to break the idea into its component parts)	Induction Deduction	Support your assumptions, what reasons, what evidence supports the conclusion, what behaviors	Conceptual knowledge Procedural knowledge
Evaluation	Judging (questions require students to make a judgment about something by using judgment principles)	Judgment Selection	Choose, evaluate in terms of, judge, select on the basis of, which would you consider, defend, which policy	Conceptual knowledge Procedural knowledge Meta-cognitive knowledge
Create	Creating (questions that get students to think about generating a novel solution or product)	Generating Producing	Think of a way, plan, create, propose, suggest	Conceptual knowledge Meta-cognitive knowledge

Adapted from Craig J, Page G. The questioning skills of nursing instructors. J Nurs Educ 1981;20:20; and Krathwohl D. A revision of Bloom's taxonomy: an overview. Theory Pract 2002;41:212-217.

BOX 3-4 Recommendations for Effective Questioning Techniques

- Use open-ended, not closed-ended (i.e., questions that can be answered with "yes" or "no"), questions.
- Plan ahead to have key questions that will provide structure.
- Avoid combining too many concepts or ideas and phrasing an ambiguous question.
- Ask your questions logically and sequentially.
- Use different levels of questions, going from simple to more complex, or higher-order, questions.
- Allow adequate thinking time for students—in other words, keep quiet. Research has shown that most teachers allow less than 1 second of silence before asking another question or reemphasizing, and that when teachers wait 3 to 5 seconds, the number and length of appropriate responses increases.[17]
- Follow-up with student responses by making a reflective statement or using deliberative silence.
- Try to ask and use types of questions that are aimed at broad student participation. For example, after a response, ask for additions to the response.

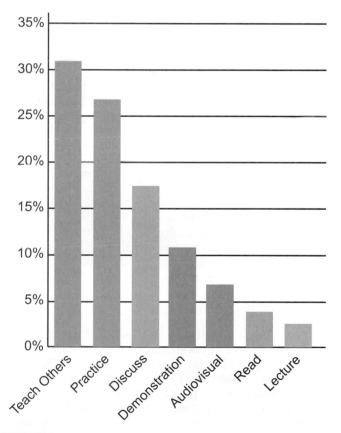

FIGURE 3-3 Average retention rate across difference teaching methods. (Adapted from Sousa D. How the Brain Learns. Thousand Oaks, CA: Corwin, 2006, p 95; and Barkley E. Student Engagement Techniques. San Francisco: Jossey-Bass, 2010.)

This section covers several teaching strategies that provide opportunities for collaborative learning. These collaborative strategies include small group work for learning tasks, discussions, seminars, tutorials, peer teaching, and other strategies.

SMALL GROUPS PROCESS: WHY GROUP WORK?

Group work is an effective teaching and learning strategy for achieving intellectual goals (e.g., conceptual learning, creative problem solving) and social goals (e.g., oral communication, decision making, conflict management). Working in groups is part of many professional workplace activities.[7,18] Two primary types of learning that lead to effective group work are collaboration and cooperative learning. Although not as much research on collaborative learning has been done in higher education, the findings from primary and secondary school research are relevant.[7,18] One of the most consistent findings is that students learn better through noncompetitive, collaborative group work than in classrooms that are highly individualized and competitive. A second element supporting group work is related to our understanding of knowledge. All knowledge, including scientific knowledge, has an element of "social construction" (i.e., knowledge includes the shared understandings within the group or discipline). Students need to experience that knowledge is not transferred from one person's head to another but rather is a consensus among members of a community of knowledgeable peers; it is dynamic understandings among people.

Learning in small groups provides the following[19]:

- A collective learning context
- Increased tolerance for complexity and uncertainty
- Opportunity to explore a diversity of views
- Development of learners' skills of giving and receiving feedback
- Opportunity for respectful listening for understanding

The role of the lecture and discussions in large class settings was discussed earlier. Small group work is another teaching strategy to engage students in large classes in active learning. In any small group process, there will always be issues of leadership, individual performance, and communication. Therefore, the use of small groups requires the same careful preparation and planning as a good lecture.

Preparation for Small Group Work

Students need to be prepared for successful group work. The following are two key concepts central to good small groupwork[18]:

1. *Learning to be responsive to the needs of the group.* Responsiveness to the needs of the group is a skill required for any cooperative task. Awareness of this skill can be facilitated through small group game activities, such as "broken circles," in which the group must cooperate to solve the group problem (see Appendix 3-A).[20]

2. *Developing a norm of cooperation and working toward equal participation.* Having students learn about working toward equal participation is another important norm for small groups, whether the group's task is discussion, decision making, or creative problem solving. Only when students believe that everyone in the group should have a say can any future problems of dominance be handled. Students need to appreciate that group leadership is a function

shared between group members.[7,18] A small group exercise called *Epstein's four-stage rocket*[21] is a good preparatory exercise for facilitating small group co-operative behaviors (see Appendix 3-B).

After students have gone through some initial group training, group work can be used as a teaching strategy. The following are basic ground rules for using small groups[18]:

- A group size of five to seven is optimal. Larger groups may be used when the task is so large that it needs to be subdivided.
- Groups should be diverse in terms of gender, academic achievement, and any other status characteristics that could influence group interaction. Allowing students to choose their own groups and work with their friends is usually not a good idea.
- The teacher must delegate authority and let go. The teacher is the direct supervisor who defines the task and suggests how the group might go about accomplishing the task, but the teacher is not in charge.
- If the overall goal is conceptual learning, then the learning task should require conceptual thinking rather than application of technique or information recall.
- The group must have the necessary resources to complete the tasks or assignments.

Group Expert Technique

The group expert technique is an extremely powerful tool that builds confidence and collegiality among group members and can cover several example cases. The technique involves two divisions of the class into small groups (Table 3-2). In the first division, each small group is given a different task (e.g., different patient cases to analyze). At this time, the teacher circulates around the class to make sure each group is on the right track. Each individual in the group must be an expert on solving the case because the class is then divided again, mixing representatives from each of the patient case groups. In this second division, each group member is an expert on a particular

TABLE 3-2 Steps Involved in Implementing the Small Group Expert Technique

Step	Process
Step 1: Initial Assignment	Each student is given a handout with a number and letter assignment (e.g., 1A, 1B, 1 C, 1D, 1E, 2A, 2B, 2 C, 2D, 2E).
Step 2: First Group Division	Class is divided according to numbers. Each group is given a patient case to analyze.
Step 3: Teacher Checks Out	Teacher circulates around to all groups to make sure each group has analyzed case correctly.
Step 4: Second Division of Groups	Class now divides a second time according to the letter assigned. This means each of the groups will have representation from each of the patient problems.
Step 5: Group Expert Discussion	All groups discuss each of the patient problems. Every group will have a resident expert (a member from the original group) who can facilitate the discussion.

Data from Cohen E. Designing Groupwork. New York: Teachers College Press, 1986.

patient case. The task for the second group division is to discuss each of the patient cases with the resident expert available to facilitate the discussion. This small group strategy provides the class with a variety of patient problems to discuss in a short amount of time and gives each student equal status as a group expert for one case.[22]

Seminars

The seminar is another small group teaching method usually associated with graduate study. The seminar also can be used in undergraduate and professional education after students master some content. The purpose of a seminar goes beyond discussion of an important topic and includes analysis, critique, and application of a topic. A seminar is not a class with small enrollment, nor is it an undirected or unfocused discussion of a topic. A seminar is a guided discussion in which students take the intellectual initiative.[9,13] Using seminars as a teaching method requires prior planning, explicit guidelines linked to objectives, and a clear structure for the students (Box 3-5).

Tutorials

A small group tutorial is a specific application of group work. In recent years, several of the health professions have begun advocating the central importance of problem-based learning, using a small-group tutorial as the teaching strategy aimed at solving patient cases. Essentially, each small group of generally no more than 10 students and one facilitator is a learning group. A faculty tutor assists students in moving from teacher-centered to student-centered learning.[10,19] The tutor is responsible for guiding the process of learning at the meta-cognitive level; that is, the tutor helps students in thinking about their thinking as they work through the learning process.[10,19,23] This type of learning group can be a very effective means for students to practice skills they will need as professionals. Using learning groups may require changes in faculty's teaching strategies as well as major or minor curriculum revisions. Tuckman's four stages of group development can be a helpful tool in working with small groups. (Table 3-3).

PEER TEACHING

Peer teaching is a critical tool for many of the collaborative learning experiences already discussed in this section. Peer teaching can be classified into five areas: (1) teaching or laboratory assistants, (2) peer tutors who work one on one with a student, (3) peer counseling involved in advising peers, (4) peer partnerships in which the partners alternate the roles of student and teacher, and (5) learning

BOX 3-5   Ideas for Structuring a Seminar

- Progress from teacher-led to student-led seminars.
- Assign topics or allow students to select from a list of suggested topics.
- Give responsibility for resources to students (e.g., a bibliography and readings).
- Use guidelines for presentation format (e.g., use of audiovisuals, responsibility for facilitating discussion with entire seminar group).
- Use peer evaluation.

TABLE 3–3   Tuckman's Four Stages of Group Development

Stage	Characteristics
Forming	Information is exchanged; group members' strengths and weaknesses are exchanged.
Storming	Conflict, dissatisfaction, and competition; can have interpersonal hostility; trust may be formed; group members may depart to another group.
Norming	Attempts are made to function by setting up rules and norms for behavior; clarity for roles and responsibilities; forming group identity.
Performing	Requires successful completion of the first three stages; perform at optimal level; focus on task as well as how everyone works; disagreements are accommodated within the group.

groups.[7] One particularly useful peer strategy is the "learning cell," a student dyad in which students alternate the role of teacher and student and ask one another questions. Use of learning cells in comparison to seminars, discussion, and independent study is a more effective teaching strategy regardless of class size, level, or the nature of the subject.[7,9]

Why does peer teaching and learning work? Remember that professionals read journals and attend conferences and seminars to stay up to date in their fields, yet most of the information is soon forgotten. If we run into a difficult case or problem, however, and have to read, consult colleagues or experts for advice, or research the literature for help, the information we gain is invariably far better retained.[7] Students are engaged in building a knowledge structure or scaffold for themselves as they find ways to organize what they know and how they can retrieve this knowledge.[1,5]

Peer teaching and learning provide the opportunity for elaboration of material so that students can put ideas in their own words. Successful peer interactions require that students question, explain, express opinions, admit when they are confused, listen, and correct misconceptions. Students are less threatened in peer settings, more likely to talk in small groups, and more likely to ask questions of their peers; thus, they are active participants in their learning process.[7,9]

OTHER USEFUL COLLABORATIVE STRATEGIES

Brainstorming

Brainstorming is a useful initial classroom strategy for quickly facilitating creative thinking and group participation. The following is an example of guidelines for a brainstorming process applied to a physical therapist assistant laboratory session on teaching gait training activities to patients whose first language is not English[7,9]:

1. *All ideas are fair game and should be recorded even if they seem off the mark.* The class generates a list of ideas, such as demonstrate the task, draw pictures, get a translator, just take the patient through the motions (don't talk), and demonstrate the task on another person first.
2. *There is no judgment rendered of the initial list of ideas until all the ideas have been generated.* That is, no one

in the class is allowed to judge any of the ideas until the class cannot come up with any more suggestions. This is the hardest part of brainstorming. Students have to be coached not to interrupt contributors with statements like "that won't work."

3. *The initial focus is on the quantity of ideas not the quality of ideas.* Again, keep the class focused on the number of ideas. Reward enthusiasm and creativity by cheering on the number of ideas that tumble forth.
4. *After the list is generated, combinations and transformation of ideas are encouraged.* After the list is complete, the class should discuss which of the ideas or combinations of ideas are the most practical and useful for the case. Then move the discussion to implementation.

Debate

Debate is a form of discussion that allows one to see the pros and cons of an issue. It can be helpful to encourage debate in the classroom by using specific examples, such as the issue of how to facilitate a supportive classroom environment or the issue of whether physical therapists or physical therapist assistants should support "cross-training" of health care workers—that is, individuals trained to perform skills for more than one discipline. Suggested steps for a debate framework can be found in Box 3–6.[24]

One criticism of debate is that it focuses on divergence and argument. Teachers may want students to assume positions that they are not committed to when making the initial group assignments. Remember that controversial issues work best for the debate format.

Examples of Other Student Engagement and Active Learning Experiences

Role-playing is a form of drama in which the students spontaneously act out roles without detailed scripts. Role-playing has been used in a variety of settings and most often deals with issues of human interaction and provides the opportunity for emotional engagement of the learner. Role-playing exercises should maintain student interest and provide students with experiences that they can use

---

BOX 3–6   Suggested Steps in a Debate

- *Step 1.* Divide the class into three groups—one group that supports cross-training, another group that does not support cross-training, and a third group that serves as a panel of debate judges.
- *Step 2.* The two debate groups meet to formulate a rationale in support of their position. Likewise, the panel of judges meets to discuss and formulate the criteria they will use to evaluate the debate. The criteria may include strength of the evidence, reasoning, rebuttal positions, flaws in the arguments, and so on.
- *Step 3.* The initial affirmative and rebuttal arguments are given, using time limits.
- *Step 4.* Debate teams meet briefly to formulate their strategy for the second round of the debate.
- *Step 5.* Teams present timed presentations.
- *Step 6.* Panel deliberates and presents findings.
- *Step 7.* Entire class discusses the process.

to analyze their own feelings. Role-playing can be used for the following purposes[9]:

1. *Illustrate principles from course content and provide students practice in the skills they have learned.* For example, in role-playing a therapist working with a difficult patient, the principles of active listening can be applied, and both students will be practicing nonverbal and verbal skills in their interactions.
2. *Develop insight into human relations problems that can be shared between students and can be used in class discussion.* After students perform a brief role-play, usually 3 to 5 minutes, they can each record their observations about the experience. These observations can be used for further analysis and discussion.
3. *Develop increased awareness of one's own and others' feelings that can initially be expressed under the guise of make-believe.* The role-playing exercise provides students with the opportunity to experience feelings in an engaging, yet controlled, setting.

Role-playing activities can be done with the entire class or with a few students as an example for the class. An essential aspect of role-playing is analysis and discussion in a small or large group setting.

Games and simulations are advantageous in that students are active participants rather than passive observers. They are usually engaging, stimulating learning activities. Educational games usually involve students in some form of competition in relationship to a goal similar to an old-fashioned spelling bee or television game such as *Jeopardy!* The use of games can be a refreshing change to traditional learning experiences, so long as the competition element does not facilitate negative behaviors among students. Whereas role-playing involves a form of drama in which the learners act out roles, simulation exercises involve a controlled representation of a part of a real situation. The learner can then manipulate key elements to better understand the real situation.[7] Simulations can be fun and interesting and usually require students to use creative and divergent thinking.[9] Perhaps the most frequently used simulation in physical therapy is a disability field exercise, in which students assume the role of having a physical disability in the community. Another well-known simulation is the aging game,[25] in which students experience the changes that occur with aging.

Expert panels are another teaching strategy in which students are able to hear first-hand from experts about their experiences. These expert panels can be used to represent a broad array of expertise (e.g., physical therapists and physical therapist assistants talking about working partnerships, patients living with physical challenges, or parents coping with a child with special needs). Barkley's book, *Student Engagement Techniques,* is an excellent resource for ideas on active learning strategies, many that engage students in collaborative learning.[7]

GRADING IN CLASSROOM TEACHING

For many teachers, making up tests, evaluating students, and assigning grades are difficult and, at times, unpleasant requirements of being an educator. Physical therapy teachers want students to be motivated to study and learn,

not because of grades, but in pursuit of the knowledge and skills that will make them sound physical therapy or physical therapist assistant practitioners. Teachers also want students to be lifelong learners who are motivated by their own thirst for knowledge and are able to evaluate their own learning.[9]

GRADING AS A TOOL FOR LEARNING

Appreciate the complexity of grading and use it as a tool for learning.[26]

No form of grading is absolutely objective, even multiple-choice tests are not, because the selection and design of questions are judgments made by the teacher. When people say that grading systems are socially constructed and context dependent, what they mean is that there is no absolutely right system by external standards. Grading is a form of communication. Teachers construct grading systems to meet the needs and constraints of the teaching environment and to communicate to several groups, including students, administrators, and employers. So what can you do to facilitate using grading as a tool for learning? Here are some relevant principles of grading to consider[26]:

- Consider substituting the term *judgment* for objectivity. Your role is to establish the most thoughtful criteria and standards you can.
- Distribute your time effectively; that is, do not spend all of your time trying to render perfectly objective grades. There are other aspects of student learning that need your time.
- Be open to change. The social meaning of grading is changing all of the time. In the mid-1900s, a C was the average grade, and today average is more typically a B.[9]
- Listen to and observe your students because grades have different meanings to various kinds of students. Remember it is the meaning that students attach to grades that most affects their learning.
- Communicate and collaborate with your students. Grading does not have to bring on antagonism. Aim to facilitate a spirit of collaboration with students toward common goals.
- Make grading an integral part of your classroom as much as planning and teaching.
- Seize teachable moments around grading issues. Grades are powerful because they shape the interrelationships among students and teachers and carry high stakes. Informal feedback and discussion about grades can affect student attitudes and learning.
- Student learning is the primary goal, and learning should be the most important goal of grading, not reports to outsiders. There are three conditions of excellence for student learning: (1) student involvement (the amount of time and energy invested in learning), (2) high expectations, and (3) assessment and feedback.[26]

Remember your role as a teacher or guide first and a gatekeeper last. Ask yourself, How do you allocate time? You would like your emphasis to be less on grading and more on guiding (Figure 3–4). A traditional function of public school education in the United States has been the gatekeeper role, in which grades are used to sort out those

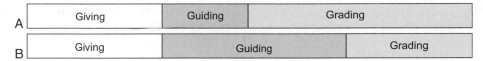

FIGURE 3–4 Distribution of teaching time. **A,** Distribution with an emphasis on grading. **B,** Distribution with an emphasis on guiding. (Adapted from Walvoord B, Anderson VJ. Effective Grading: A Tool for Learning and Assessment. San Francisco: Jossey-Bass, 1998.)

who are not "qualified" to advance. In professional education programs, teachers are gatekeepers at the end of the process, not the beginning. After we have demonstrated our belief in students, we figure out what they need and help them to learn, no matter what their backgrounds or academic history.

What do students, teachers, and employers want from grades? Students usually want to know how well they are doing and if they are succeeding in their pursuit of becoming a physical therapist or physical therapist assistant. For teachers, grading students is one of their required roles in academia. Grades provide information on how well the students are learning the material and provide a measure for assuring some minimal level of competence for preparing professionals. Employers may use grades as one factor in hiring decisions. How one feels about grades and grading is likely to depend on values and educational philosophy. Regardless of whether grades are seen as a motivator or a necessary evil, the following general guidelines should be considered[9]:

- Avoid grading systems that put students in competition with classmates by limiting the number of high grades. This is called *grading on the curve* or the *norm-referenced model.*
- Keep students apprised of their progress throughout the term.
- Emphasize learning, not grades.
- Consider allowing students some flexibility in selecting assignments for their grade (e.g., write a case report or create an educational module).
- Deal directly with students who are upset about their grades. Listen to their complaints, think about their request, and resist pressure to change a grade because of a student's personal needs.
- Keep accurate records of grades and use numerical grades for tests and assignments rather than letter grades whenever possible.

GRADING SYSTEMS
Criterion-Referenced Grading

Criterion-referenced grading is a common system based on the student's level of achievement compared with a fixed standard, which is set by the instructor. If all students obtained above 80 on the anatomy examination, they would all receive As or Bs. Institutions frequently set grading scales that schools and departments follow or have formulated their own numerical grading system.[9]

Norm-Referenced Grading

In norm-referenced grading, or grading on the curve, grades are assigned according to percentages of the class so that there is a normal distribution with few As, more

Bs, quite a few Cs, some Ds, and a few Fs. The strict application of this system has received a fair amount of criticism and is often labeled as educationally dysfunctional.[9]

The debate between grading on the curve (norm-referenced grading) versus criterion-referenced grading is centered on what the grade means. Do you want to identify the best students in the group, or do you want to indicate that students have achieved or met the certain standards?

Competency-Based Grading

Competency-based grading is used frequently in the professions in which educational programs are responsible for preparing students for safe practice of a profession. Students are held to a standard and must demonstrate competency in performing skills or demonstrate knowledge according to specified objectives. Students who do not achieve certain objectives continue to be assessed until they demonstrate "competence." Often, an 80% cutoff is established as a definition of minimal competence.[9]

Contract Grading

In the contract-grading approach, the student must fulfill the designated aspects of the contract to receive a designated grade. The requirements for the level of contract (e.g., A or B) differ. This grading system allows the student some flexibility and opportunity to participate in the grading process. However, it is difficult to design a system in which the grade is determined not only by the fulfillment of the assigned activities but also by the quality of the work completed.[9]

Self-Grading and Peer Grading

Providing students opportunities to engage in self-assessment and peer assessment should be an aspect of every professional educational program. Self-assessment and peer-assessment activities will certainly be part of the student's future as an employed therapist. Self-assessment can be included as a component of a course grade for any kind of course. Portfolio development, discussed later in this chapter, is a method for facilitating self-assessment throughout the educational program. Peer assessment is frequently used for group projects and presentations. Students will provide better assessments if given explicit criteria for evaluation and if each student evaluates each of the group members.[9,10]

TOOLS FOR STUDENT EVALUATION

How do you motivate students to aim for high learning expectations? You must tightly integrate grading with learning, engagement, and motivation. This takes us back to the central importance of carefully planned and delivered course goals. Evaluations of students are events when students and faculty see how well they have engaged the teaching-learning process. Evaluations should be consistently related to the elements in the preactive teaching grid discussed in Chapter 2. Remember the learning goals you have for your students are "operationalized" in your course objectives. These objectives focus on course content and student learning. Evaluations that closely follow the course objectives serve to reinforce this learning. A basic pedagogical truth is that the better students perform on tests, the better the teacher has organized the course materials and engaged students in their own learning. Thus, testing demonstrates the level of success of teachers as well as students.

As previously stated, the design and content of evaluation instruments should be thought through well before the first day of class. You might consider a number of different types of evaluation to give students a chance to shine in what they do best: short answer tests, essays, projects, individual and small group work, portfolios, and class participation can all be factored into a final grade. Approach evaluation as a chance for all students to be involved in one more learning activity rather than as an event in which a number of students could fail.

The next section presents some commonly used methods of written evaluation, such as short answer tests, essays, and quick checks. Later in this chapter, a section on facilitating reflection and problem solving covers newer and perhaps even more powerful methods of evaluation that can promote students' learning and growth (e.g., the use of journals and portfolios).

Think broadly about activities that can be evaluated that could facilitate professional growth and emphasize student learning. For example, you might have the students write a book review that could be sent to a professional journal or magazine for consideration of publication. You could have students attend a research symposium and write a critique of presentation styles, attend an American Physical Therapy Association district or chapter business meeting, or observe the work of a community support group for individuals with a chronic disease such as diabetes or arthritis and write a thought paper on one of the topics discussed. Evaluations should be filled with learning, fun, and professional growth whenever possible!

EXAMINATIONS ON COURSE CONTENT

One of the best ways to identify questions to be used in written evaluations is to make notes of possible questions in color in the margins of the lecture and laboratory materials. Cross-check these questions with your course objective to be sure they cover important concepts and are not shallow or nit-picking. Then, when it comes time to put together a test, you have already identified many good possible questions. Another strategy is to create a table of specifications. Here you cross-list the content areas with the instructional objectives and then construct test questions that are relevant to these objectives (Table 3–4).

A word of caution: Be sure that the questions posed in any evaluation are culturally sensitive and do not reinforce stereotypes. For example, avoid "cutesy" or derogatory patient names (e.g., Mrs. Badhip), occupational and gender stereotypes (e.g., women are always housewives, and men are always wage earners), and racial and socioeconomic biases (e.g., gunshot injuries are incurred only by Hispanic and African American males). Students read examination questions with great intensity and are vulnerable to absorbing, somewhat unconsciously, these destructive stereotypes.

Short Answer Questions

Short answer questions typically require a student to identify, distinguish, state, or name something. Answers can be free format, such as simple questions or fill-in-the-blank questions, or fixed format, such as true or false, multiple-choice, or matching questions (Table 3–5). Students can also be given a problem or case to read followed by a number of short answer questions.

Free Format Questions

The advantages of free format questions are that they minimize guessing, they give no clues as to correct response (testing recall not recognition), they are easy to write (alternative answers are not required as in multiple-choice questions), and they can accommodate a figure, graph, or map. The disadvantages are they can be difficult to score because many different types of wording, as well as content, can be arguably correct, and they work best for very specific subject matter, such as anatomy and biomechanics. Fill-in-the-blank questions are more difficult to

TABLE 3–4   Table of Specifications for Constructing a 40-Item Examination (Gronlund)

Content Area	1 Knowledge: Basic Terms	2 Comprehension: Concepts and Principles	3 Application of Concepts and Principles	4 Interpretation and Judgment
Code of ethics	3		2	
Ethical principles	4	2	4	
Ethical theories	4	2		
State practice acts	4	1		
Clinical cases			6	8
Total no. of test items	15	5	12	8

TABLE 3–5 Examples of Various Question Formats

Question Type	Example
Free-format questions	• Describe bucket-handle rib motion. • Label the parts of the thoracic vertebrae in the diagram below. • The type of justice concerned with every patient getting an appropriate share of the therapist's time is called _____ justice. • Diagram the components of a muscle spindle.
Fixed-format questions	
True or false	• T or F The extensor digitorum, extensor indices, and extensor digiti minimi are the main muscles responsible for extending the interphalangeal joints of the fingers. • T or F The legal concept in which offensive touching is done without the consent of the person being touched is called battery.
Multiple choice	1. Which assistive device requires the least amount of coordination? 　A. Tripod cane 　B. Walker 　C. Forearm crutches 　D. Axillary crutches 2. Patients with genu vara tend to develop degenerative changes at the: 　A. Medial facet of the patellofemoral joint. 　B. Medial aspect of the femorotibial joint. 　C. Lateral aspect of the femorotibial joint. 　D. Lateral facet of the femorotibial joint.
Essay test	• Read the research paper provided and give an assessment of the strengths and weaknesses of the method section. • Discuss at least four strategies that would be effective in modifying public attitudes toward persons who have physical disabilities. • Compare and contrast the major theories regarding therapeutic intervention in episodes of acute rheumatoid arthritis. • Read the following community hospital case. As a consultant, outline the recommendations you would make to the hospital administration.

write because there must be a sufficient, but not overabundant, amount of clues that direct the student to a one- or two-word response.

Fixed Format Questions

True or False Questions

The advantages of true or false questions are they are easy to write and can be answered quickly. There are two main disadvantages of true or false questions:

1. *When guessing, a student has a 50% chance of being right.* This can be remedied by asking the student to change a false item to read true, which decreases guessing.
2. *It is difficult to avoid ambiguity.* This can be remedied by thinking about the key point you want to make and focusing on the accuracy of key names, actions, or concepts rather than on obscure points, such as whether a fact should be singular or plural.

Multiple-Choice Questions

Advantages of multiple-choice questions are that well-constructed questions can measure knowledge and comprehension as well as application and analysis (i.e., higher levels of the cognitive domain), they are very easy to grade and can be scored by a computer, and a great deal of material can be covered quickly and in a single question.

The following are disadvantages of multiple-choice questions and possible solutions[2,9,13,15]:

- *It is difficult to write plausible distractors.* Try to think of at least three good distractors that are equal in length and parallel in structure to the correct answer. Do not overuse "all of the above" or "none of the above" for lack of inspiration in finding good distractors. Errors commonly made by students are a good source of distractors. Again, focus on major points related to your course objectives. Avoid triviality and irrelevance.
- *Refrain from using words such as "always," "never," "all," or "none."* Students know that few facts or concepts are always true.
- *A certain degree of success can be obtained through guessing or figuring out in what order the instructor is likely to put the correct answer.* Teachers are more systematic than they think. Given four choices in a multiple-choice question, the correct choice is most often in the middle (i.e., b or c). Use a table of random numbers to guide the placement of the correct response.
- *Avoid trick questions, such as those using negatively worded stems along with negatively worded choices that test semantics and logic rather than knowledge of the subject matter.*
- *The use of multiple, multiple-choice, also called type K questions, is strongly discouraged.* This is where you would have a list of possible answers, and then the multiple-choice distracters would focus on the combination of answers (e.g., "A, B, and C are correct"; "A and B are correct"; "Only A is correct"; and "A and C are correct"). These type of questions are made unnecessarily complicated in that the focus is not on evaluating knowledge but on sorting out the logic in the combination of answers.[9,10]

- *Key-feature approach questions is a format in which a clinical case or problem situation is followed by a number of questions that are focused on critical decisions.* Make sure that all of the important information is presented in the case, that the questions are directly linked to the case, and finally that the questions focus on essential decisions.

Essay Tests

Advantages of essay questions are that they are especially good for measuring the upper three levels of the cognitive domain (analysis, synthesis, and evaluation); the student is free to decide how to approach the problem, what information to use, what aspects to emphasize, and how to organize the response; it is the easiest type of question to write quickly; and the teacher can determine the student's depth of knowledge and the quality of the student's critical thinking abilities.

The following are disadvantages of essay tests and possible solutions:

- Scoring is difficult and time consuming, especially because writing comments on each paper regarding the strengths and weakness of the essay is imperative for student understanding and learning. Fatigue during grading can lead to grading inconsistencies. If you use a series of short essay questions, grade the same question on all the papers (without looking at the student's name) before going to the next question to increase the consistency of your response.
- Writing ability influences the grade received. Suggest to students that they read over their answers quietly to themselves looking for incomplete or run-on sentences and spelling and punctuation errors. Reviewing common errors with the class highlights the importance and necessity of good writing skills for health care professionals.

Good in-depth information on all types of written tests is given by Svinicki and McKeachie[9] (1993), Davis (2009),[13] and Gronlund (2008).[27] (See the Annotated Bibliography at the end of this chapter.)

Quick Checks

Quick checks are like pop quizzes with less anxiety and more learning imbedded in the process. Take the last few minutes of a class and ask students one short, focused question that will promote reflective thinking about the material that has just been presented, especially as it relates to the students' own thinking, feeling, or performing. The length of response should be no more than a few phrases or a couple of sentences. For example, you might ask students to give an example of one characteristic they exhibit that would promote effective physical therapist–physical therapist assistant interactions in the clinical setting and one characteristic they might consider working to change to avoid physical therapist–physical therapist assistant conflict. Quick checks also are one of many classroom assessment techniques that can be used for formative evaluation.[28]

Think about grading quick checks as "excellent," "good," or "try again." If the student receives a try again, he or she can do just that—hand in another response within the week. When the second response is reviewed, the student's grade may be moved up to a good. This method of grading avoids the stress of a one-shot pop quiz and puts the focus on students grappling with ideas and transforming knowledge. Quick checks are easy to grade quickly and give the instructor information about how individual students are absorbing the information presented. (See Chapter 5 for a broad range of assessment techniques that can be used to facilitate the teaching-learning process.)

CLINICAL LABORATORY TEACHING: DEVELOPMENT AND ASSESSMENT OF CLINICAL PRACTICE SKILLS

You remember well entering your first laboratory class session with 50 eager students just dying to learn the "real thing" from a real clinician. Of course, just a few months ago, you received a call from the director of the physical therapy program at your local university, and you were thrilled to be asked to coordinate this musculoskeletal assessment laboratory. After all, you have 15 years of clinical experience, have clinical specialty certification through the American Physical Therapy Association, and have served as a clinical instructor for several physical therapy students in the past. Now as you enter the laboratory for your first session, you realize this part-time teaching task may take much more of your time and energy than you imagined. You eagerly dive into the task, structuring your laboratory much like your own past experiences of learning clinical skills. You have picked up a few neat ideas along the way from your extensive continuing education background and wealth of clinical experience. Basically, you plan to demonstrate the skills to the class, have them perform the skills, and then circulate around the laboratory along with your other laboratory instructor, providing pairs of students with feedback on their skill performance. As you go around the laboratory, you notice that there appears to be some diversity of effort among the students—some are wonderfully task oriented, practicing diligently with their partners, whereas others do the activity once and are engaged in casual conversation. You also find students asking you to just tell them when to perform this or that technique. You think to yourself, How do I know what to do in my clinical practice? And then, How should I structure this laboratory so that I am not only teaching these extremely important clinical skills but also sharing my thinking and clinical knowledge with students as we go along? There must be a better way.

This anecdote describes the ultimate challenge of physical therapy faculty who teach in the clinical sciences. How do faculty in the professional education environment help students develop an effective system for learning that is responsive to practice needs and includes knowledge acquisition, problem solving, application of clinical judgment, and development of clinical skills? The profession of physical therapy is not alone here. The development of all aspects of professional competence, including clinical skills, knowledge, interpersonal attributes, problem-solving skills, clinical judgment, and technical and practice skills, is an ongoing challenge for faculty involved in all types of professional education.[29] It is certain that the field or clinical education portion of the programs is essential to the ultimate development of professional competence; however, teachers also have an obligation to begin developing all aspects of competence in the clinical laboratory. This section focuses on three critical concepts in laboratory teaching: (1) development of clinical practice skills, (2) development of clinical reasoning and judgment, and (3) performance of assessment strategies.

CLINICAL LABORATORY TEACHING: LEARNING PSYCHOMOTOR SKILLS

One of the major tasks in the clinical laboratory is to teach students new psychomotor skills, from the handling of their own bodies, to the handling of patients, to the sensing of changes of texture and mobility in soft tissue structures, to the ability to use touch as a way of communicating support and care. These tasks are an essential and fundamental aspect of professional competence. There is a growing body of literature in the area of motor learning that many therapists are applying to their work with patients.[30-32] Several of these concepts can also be applied to clinical laboratories. Chapter 14 covers the teaching of psychomotor skills in detail. This chapter highlights some key elements that can serve as a basic structure for planning the laboratory experience.

Phases of Skill Learning

Gentile[31] has a simple model for skill learning that includes two phases. The first phase is understanding the idea of the movement, which includes learning the skill that is specifically linked to the goal. After the skill is successfully performed, the learner can move to the second phase of refining the skill and committing the skill to memory. This phase is called the *stage of fixation and diversification*. In the learning process, the learner is exposed to many stimuli and needs to devote selective attention to the regulatory stimuli (i.e., those stimuli that affect accomplishment of the goal). These stimuli could be visual, verbal, written, tactile, auditory, and so on. Skills can also be categorized as closed or open. In a closed skill, environmental conditions and relevant stimuli remain stable throughout the performance. Consider the following example: You are teaching a lab in clinical measurement that starts with basic range-of-motion measurement with a goniometer. You would probably classify this skill as closed because the environment is the laboratory and the skill or measurement activity is being applied to a person with no limitation of movement. An open skill takes place in a changing environment, and the regulatory stimuli vary. Open skills are obviously more difficult for the learner because of the changing situation. After the learner can recognize and attend to the relevant stimuli, a plan for movement, or motor plan, that meets environmental demands can be formulated. When the skill or subset of skills is performed, the learner receives feedback on the skill execution. This feedback may be intrinsic (from the learner) or extrinsic (from the outside; a person or the environment).

Teaching a Skill

There are several strategies available to instructors when teaching students a new skill:

1. *Establish a problem that leads to a goal and ensures adequate learner motivation.* Students will know that they (most likely) do not know how to go about measuring the range of motion. In this way, the problem (i.e., they don't know) and the goal (i.e., they need to know) are presented.
2. *Attend to regulatory stimuli that will help the learner perform the skill.* In doing this, the teacher must decide how to help the learner recognize the stimuli. This could be done in any of the following ways:
   - Demonstrate the skill and give verbal instructions on the steps involved in performing the skill. (It is good to practice the skill ahead of time.)
   - Use a visual, media demonstration. This could be viewed before the laboratory session as well as used for continued review after the teaching session.
   - Use the guided-discovery approach, in which the students use a text or manual or other visual media to discover, through problem solving, the steps in the skill.
3. *Control the learning environment.* The teacher must decide how realistic the laboratory should be. There is some evidence that with nursing skills, when teaching open skills, the setting should be as realistic as possible. Teachers may provide students with different approaches they may try depending on a specific patient situation. Also, the laboratory can be structured to provide different stimuli (e.g., have students change partners, role-play).
4. *Provide feedback.* Each learner needs intrinsic and extrinsic feedback. Intrinsic feedback should be given before extrinsic feedback. Intrinsic, or internal, feedback allows the learner to learn how to learn from his or her own feedback to self. Extrinsic, or external, feedback is feedback from the teacher. This feedback is most effective when there is no interfering activity between the skill performance and the feedback. The more detail a learner can be given about an error, the more readily it can be corrected.[32] With large lab groups, the instructor may use periodic time-outs or teachable moments when common mistakes are discovered and address the common mistake to the entire group.
5. *Have the students practice.* The final stage for the teacher is to move students to the fixation and diversification stage in which the general motor pattern is practiced and refined. If one is teaching simple closed skills, students may move quickly to this stage and thus lose motivation to continue practice. To improve skills, continued practice also requires ongoing feedback. Repetition without feedback is not likely to lead to improvement. Feedback could come in ways other than the extrinsic expert form. Students could provide ongoing feedback for one another. They could also review media files of themselves or use other audiovisuals.

6. *Design effective timing and sequence of practice.* Is practice more effective if it is massed practice (no rest periods) or distributed practice (planned rest periods)? For motor skills, evidence supports that distributed practice is best. The rest periods must be short enough so that memory is not a problem, and reinforcement should follow after each practice session. After the learner reaches the fixation and diversification phase, then he or she is better able to attend to other stimuli in the environment.[31]

SUGGESTIONS FOR CLINICAL SKILLS DEMONSTRATIONS

In the clinical laboratory setting, instructors are frequently involved in demonstrating to students how to perform skills. The following are suggestions for clinical skills demonstrations:

- Plan and prepare ahead of time. Have the necessary equipment and practice the skill ahead of time. Determine how it will appear from the student's vantage point.
- Perform the procedure step by step and explain as you go along. The entire skill will be demonstrated more than once. If the skill is complex, you may wish to demonstrate the entire skill first and then break it down into the step-by-step procedures.
- It is best not to have students take notes so that they can concentrate on the demonstration. Have explanatory information in the text or a laboratory manual.
- You may wish to videotape your demonstration or have someone take slides or digital images of key teaching points. These materials could then be made available to students for independent study and practice.
- Ensure that the demonstration always adheres to fundamental principles of professional practice, such as proper body mechanics, patient positioning, and proper draping.
- Demonstrate the skill from different angles or sides so that students can see what the skill looks like from different perspectives. In many laboratories, there is access to a camera system that displays the instructor's demonstration.

SUGGESTIONS FOR TEACHING OPEN OR MORE COMPLEX PSYCHOMOTOR SKILLS

Graduated Practice

Psychomotor skills that are difficult may need to be broken into subcomponents; this process is known as *graduated practice.* This gives the student the opportunity to concentrate on the component steps. For example, in teaching students how to perform proprioceptive neuromuscular facilitation patterns, one might begin by having the students learn the movements on themselves. The students can then proceed to doing simple, straight-arm patterns on a fellow classmate. Finally, the students should be ready to apply a pattern to a specific patient condition. Each of these subtasks takes students through guided practice, that is, practice with each of the components.

Mental Practice

Mental practice, or imagery, is a technique that has been used by many athletes to help improve performance and reduce stress. For some clinical skills, students can learn by visualizing the sequence of steps involved in the mastery of the skill. The student would focus on mental rehearsal of a procedure (e.g., transferring a patient from a bed to a chair). With mental imagery, while students are waiting in the hallway for their practical examination, they can visualize themselves performing the steps and imagine the instructions they are giving the patient at each step.[31]

CLINICAL LABORATORY TEACHING: INTEGRATING DOING, THINKING, AND REASONING

When teaching in the clinical sciences, educators are interested not only in facilitating the development of students' psychomotor skills but also in developing the thinking skills (e.g., planning, analyzing, problem solving, evaluating, and decision making) that are essential to clinical reasoning and the decision-making process that are part of clinical practice.[32-34] They are "wise actions" that come from the professional's ongoing analysis, thinking, or reflection on practice. Such knowledge is frequently referred to as "knowing how," that is, knowing how to apply or do what you know. A second category of professional knowledge is "knowing that," that is, knowing about things. In professional education, students are exposed to increasing amounts of this kind of knowledge (knowing about things or facts), ranging from understanding how the body functions at cellular levels to understanding system functions and human actions. Educators are more likely to focus on "knowing that," with emphasis on students' cognitive abilities, than on "knowing how," which occurs when students analyze and give a rationale for their practical skills and actions.[33,34]

Shulman has created a taxonomy for learning, or what he calls the "table of learning" (Box 3–7).[2] This taxonomy demonstrates the complexity of learning as teachers move students from engagement to understanding, action, reflection, judgment, and commitment. He argues that learning is more about learner engagement than motivation; without engagement, there is no learning. The next element of understanding undergirds the element of knowledge: knowledge without understanding will not last. Although we tend to focus on performance, it is also the ultimate professional action that has meaning. We have long focused on critique and criticism when reflection is an essential

---

BOX 3–7   Shulman's Table of Learning

- Engagement and motivation
- Knowledge and understanding
- Performance and action
- Reflection and critique
- Judgment and design
- Commitment and identity

From Shulman LS. Making differences: a table of learning. Change 2002;34:36-44.

element for meaningful learning. Design provides us the opportunity to exercise understanding and apply skills, but it is judgment that is needed in considering multiple factors and values to make some evaluative judgment. Finally, we tend to emphasize identity as students embrace the concept of professional identity when it is much more about commitment that represents the inner values, character, and moral ways of being and must also be connected to outward action. The integration of these powerful elements of learning is central to teaching and learning in laboratory and clinical settings.

In the clinical laboratory, teachers need to find ways to teach students the performance of skills. However, teachers also need to develop the inquiry processes that allow students to continue to learn through experience. Physical therapists are not just technical problem solvers but must be able to respond to the complex, uncertain situations routinely found in clinical practice. Schön[33] argues that students can be taught to reflect on or inquire about situations that are uncertain and that professional educators should design laboratory experiences that are more representative of real-life, clinical settings. He draws the analogy that educators should move from the more traditional "follow-me" laboratory, in which technical skills are emphasized, to the "hall-of-mirrors" laboratory, in which students are challenged not only to perform the skill but also to discuss and critique the performance among peers.

Providing structure or a conceptual framework for analysis can be one way of facilitating a student's thinking or reasoning process in a hall-of-mirrors laboratory. For example, in the area of musculoskeletal dysfunction, application of concepts from a clinical reasoning model can be used to assist students to think about integrating evaluative skills with their interpretive, ongoing thoughts about the data. The teaching and learning involved in the development of clinical reasoning skills are the focus of Chapter 11.

CLINICAL LABORATORY TEACHING: ASSESSMENT OF CLINICAL SKILLS

It is your first experience with laboratory practical examinations. You remember how terrified you were as a student, but now you see the struggle from the other side, the tremendous number of hours that it may take to do a meaningful evaluation of students. How do you achieve consistency across evaluators? You remember again from your student days that sometimes these evaluation sessions can have a powerful effect on a student's self-confidence. How do you design an experience that provides the opportunity for a student's learning, demonstrates evidence of a student's competence and deficits, and can be done in less than 100 hours?

PRACTICAL EXAMINATIONS: DESIGN AND IMPLEMENTATION

The basic ingredients for designing and implementing practical examinations is a blueprint that includes a rationale (or aim of the evaluation), format, evaluation tools (including evaluators), and implementation.[10,19]

Rationale

What is the overall purpose of the examination? Are you just checking competence in select clinical skills? Are you interested in how students think on their feet, their decision-making skills, how they synthesize information? Are you using the examination process to look at information across courses? Should the examination include any elements of self-assessment or only evaluator assessment?

Format

The format of the practical examinations will follow from the overall purpose of the examination. If you use the practicals as a formative assessment strategy to check out the basic level of skill performance, you may want to use a simple check-out strategy. With this strategy, you should identify a list of psychomotor behaviors and develop a checklist of the skills involved. Students perform the tasks and are evaluated using the checklist. On the other hand, if the aim is to examine student performance of certain skills and the student's own analysis of the performance, you may choose to have the student create the "evaluation artifact" (e.g., videotape, audiotape, transcription, case description). For example, in looking at the patient interview process, you may want students to videotape their interview of another individual. They can do their own assessment of the tape, and, together, you and the students could do another assessment. Perhaps your faculty is interested in looking at student performance in a number of areas from the courses taught that semester. In this case, you may consider some form of examination stations in which each faculty member examines one area of performance, either by observing the student's performance or serving as the "standardized patient." If the faculty member serves as the patient, then she or he can experience the application of skills as well as assess the level of performance. This model is very similar to the objective structured clinical examination (OSCE) that has been used in medical education for assessing the clinical skills of medical students and residents.[10,19] Chapter 6 provides a comprehensive approach to using simulations for performance assessment.

Laboratory situations can also be used to stimulate students' thinking and assess their attitudes and ability to reason and make decisions in ambiguous situations. For example, one area of importance and recent investigation in professional education clinical assessment is assessing behavioral skills such as patient-centered interviewing and student awareness and sensitivity to diverse health beliefs. A study by Oh and colleagues[35] found that residents trained in patient-centered interviewing were more effective in handling patients' emotions and more skillful in gathering patient data. The assessment was done through video-recorded and scored interviews with standardized patients. The scoring tool, the Rhode Island Hospital Resident Interview Checklist, contained observable behaviors in core areas (opening of interview, exploration of problems, facilitation skills, and relationship skills).[36]

Another idea for working with students to assess their reasoning abilities and affective responses is use of a critical incident. See Table 3–6 for two examples of critical incidence techniques that can be used to look, not at what an individual can do, but at what an individual habitually does.[10]

TABLE 3-6 Examples of Critical Incidence Techniques

Technique	Example
Impossible dilemma: Provide the student with a realistic and relevant task that poses mutually exclusive alternatives that represent different value positions and that are more or less politically correct.	You are a member of the hospital's committee on health benefits. The committee must come up with recommendations for reducing the overall health plan by $3 million. Out of a list of provided services, you must now decide which of these services will no longer be part of the plan.
Role-play a situation in which a satisfactory resolution will be difficult to obtain.	You are a newly hired therapist in a large rehabilitation center. Steve, a patient well known to the department for his uncooperative behavior and substance abuse problems, is again being referred for physical therapy and is assigned to you. It is your task to establish a plan of care with Steve.

Evaluation Tools

Unlike a multiple-choice test that can be scored by machine, practical examinations require human beings as part of the evaluation process. The evaluator will have to render some judgment about student performance. Because the evaluation of clinical skills is more subjective than evaluating cognitive performance, one should be absolutely clear about specific expectations in the course syllabus. To assist with the evaluation process, you will need to create an evaluation form that identifies the behaviors (cognitive, psychomotor, and affective) that you wish to assess. This also would be the first step in demonstrating consistency across evaluators.[37] A drawback for the beginning teacher would be the lack of a data bank of experience regarding student performance. Even though your evaluation criteria are most likely criterion referenced on paper (i.e., identify the standardized expected behaviors of students to pass), there is likely to be an element of norm-referenced evaluation (i.e., student performance compared with other students who are taking the examination). When performing practical examinations, it is usually the case that you will judge not just the presence of a behavior but also the quality of the behavior. In such situations, it is important to have a more experienced teacher and mentor to consult to learn what is average or excellent student performance.

Implementation

A program strategy that facilitates curriculum integration as well as provides faculty with important information about how well students are integrating their knowledge and skill development is some form of comprehensive practical examination. This can be done in a station or OCSE format. Here the faculty must work together to design clinical cases and stations for the students. This kind of comprehensive examination can easily cross all coursework as computer stations with questions can also accompany the practical skill stations.

You may have wonderful ideas for your practical examinations, but are they realistic to implement? Time and personnel are perhaps the two biggest resources. Think creatively about how to stretch these resources. Perhaps there are clinical faculty who might love the idea of being involved in an assessment day or clinic. You may be able to recruit volunteers for patient role models (e.g., elders in the community, students from another year in the program, or students from other professions). If there are severe time constraints, you may want to provide students with the patient cases for the examination ahead of time. The students can then prepare and practice for all of the cases, even though they will only do selected elements in their examination time. However, because the students have prepared for all of the cases, your objective is accomplished. Also, think about ways to include peer assessment and self-assessment as part of the process.

STRATEGIES FOR FACILITATING REFLECTION AND PROBLEM ANALYSIS

None of us can ever teach students to think. We can, however, create experiences for students that will cause them to think and develop ideas. None of us can set thinking as our "terminal objective." Our obligation to the profession and to our students is to help them turn the wheel of their own minds with increasing power and ever clearer direction as they grow and learn.[5,9]

The greatest American philosopher of education, John Dewey, made many contributions to education. Perhaps one of his most important contributions was his writing about thinking—his "theory of inquiry."[8] Inquiry for Dewey was a combination of mental reasoning and action.[38] Schön[33] has furthered Dewey's theory in his writing on reflective practice. As discussed previously, reflection is the element that turns experience into learning. It is the process of purposeful thinking and inquiring about problems and how to solve them, that is, a process of deep and meaningful learning.[34] Physical therapist and physical therapist assistant students are faced with the challenge of many ill-structured problems in health care settings, for which the simple application of knowledge cannot produce a solution. How can teachers provide students with opportunities to "turn their own minds?"[39-43]

Recall that in Bloom's taxonomy, knowledge and comprehension are the beginning levels of cognitive ability, and synthesis and evaluation and creativity are the upper levels.[17] Language can be one way in which a teacher can structure the students' thinking and discussion. For example, terms like "argue," "explain," "hypothesize," "compare and contrast," and "provide evidence" all provide students with a more engaged and active image of how to think about their thinking. A key term used in the thinking and learning process is *meta-cognition*. Cognition is the construction of meaning, whereas meta-cognition is the awareness and monitoring of one's own thinking and learning process. The teacher's role is to facilitate this meta-cognition process through the instructional process.[39-43] This section discusses two strategies for facilitating this process: the use of case method and concept mapping.[44-47]

CASE METHODS

Educators have long been critical of academic programs dominated by the twin demons of lecture and textbook, each a method designed to predigest and deliver a body of key facts and principles through exposition to a rather passive audience of students.[44]

Case methods are widely used in business and law courses. The case method of teaching should be differentiated from a case report (usually a description of an intervention with a patient) or a case study (usually third-person accounts of detailed descriptions in which the focus varies from people to things). Cases are used in teaching to stimulate thought and discussion, often using Socratic questioning. In business, cases are used to train students to know and to act. Cases are used to help lawyers sharpen their analytical skills, and in case discussions, students are challenged to defend their argument. Cases are frequently developed from problems in the field and are often constructed to represent a particular principle or problem.[9,44,45]

As discussed earlier in this chapter, cases have been used in problem-based learning in which small group tutorials work on the patient case. This requires that the group identify and gather the information necessary to analyze the case. In other words, the group must use processes of problem identification, problem solving, and analysis. The facilitator does not lead the group but rather questions and probes for student reasoning and analysis. Case formats can vary from a written paper case, to a media file case, to a simulated or real patient.[9,44,45]

A critical dimension of case method is the formulation of the case as it relates to the broader issues of general principles and concepts. The case writer should ask, "What is this a case of?" Business education has perhaps the most detailed approach for assisting case writers. For the health professions, cases may go beyond the notion of the patient or client and include any number of real-world practice problems (e.g., management issues, staff problems, ethical dilemmas, reimbursement issues).

Writing cases that are grounded in real-life experience gives students and faculty the opportunity to address complexity of practice. Cases that are developed from practice or are adapted from situations in practice challenge faculty and students to move from a course orientation to integration and application of many courses (Box 3–8).

The case study in Box 3–8 presents a patient case developed so that students would synthesize information learned in biological, physical, clinical, and behavioral science courses during the semester and integrate this information with prior knowledge. Student groups were given specific questions for each area (i.e., clinical medicine, physical therapy procedures, and psychosocial and cultural factors) to guide their case analysis (Table 3–7).

In designing a challenging case, one may want to gather and present data beyond the usual written patient cases. This might include information gathered from interviewing, documents, or the media or artifacts provided as part of the case (e.g., documentation and videotape). A critical element in the formulation of the case is consideration of the thinking dimensions stimulated by the case (e.g., knowledge, analytical thinking, and conceptual thinking).[44] A physical therapy clinical management case is used as an example in Case 3-1 (Box 3–8).

BOX 3–8 Example of a Patient Case Used by Students to Integrate Information across Courses in the Curriculum

CASE STUDY 3-1

Betsy is a 27-year-old former fifth grade teacher referred to physical therapy for examination of bilateral lower extremity pain due to a peripheral neuropathy secondary to acquired immunodeficiency syndrome (AIDS).

Social and Medical History

No one is aware of her diagnosis except health care workers involved with her treatment and immediate family members. Her husband is also human immunodeficiency virus (HIV) positive, and his work associates are unaware of the patient's or the husband's diagnoses. The couple has a 2-year-old daughter who is HIV positive. They live in a one-story home with two bedrooms and a small bathroom. The patient has around-the-clock care and supervision when her husband is not home. Her husband and caregivers express concern over her declining function and their lack of knowledge of how to best help her. Previous medical history was negative before the diagnosis of HIV in 2001. Patient has had *Pneumocystis jiroveci (carinii)* pneumonia twice, mycobacterial tuberculosis, and candidiasis. She was recently hospitalized for a deep vein thrombosis in her lower left extremity.

Current Medical Status

The patient is in the advanced stage of AIDS and requires 24-hour supervision. She requires assistance to transfer and is able to ambulate for very short distances with a walker and frequent verbal cueing to keep her knees and hips extended. She has periods of lethargy and confusion.

Medications

The patient takes Bactrim (antibiotic used to prevent recurrence of *Pneumocystis jiroveci [carinii]* pneumonia), ciprofloxacin hydrochloride (Cipro; antibiotic), ethambutol hydrochloride (Myambutol, antitubercular agent), fluconazole (antifungal agent), sertraline (Zoloft, antidepressant), anticonvulsant, gabapentin (Neurontin, used for neuropathic pain), and a multiclass combination of antiretroviral drugs (Atripla—efavirenz, tenofovir, and emtricitabine).

Physical Therapy Examination Findings

Arrived in clinic in wheelchair assisted by her caregiver
Chief complaint: pain and weakness in legs
- Range of motion: grossly within functional limits
- Strength:
  - Shoulder elevation 4/5
  - Triceps 4/5
  - Biceps 4/5
  - Hands 5/5
  - Hip flexors 3/5
  - Hip extensors 2/5
  - Knee extensors 3/5
  - Ankle dorsiflexors 4/5
  - Ankle planter flexors 2/5
- Transfers: supine to sit with maximal assistance of 1; sit to stand with maximal assistance of 1.

From J Gale, K Paschal. Patient Case Materials. Omaha: Creighton University Department Physical Therapy, 2011.

TABLE 3–7 Example Questions Used in the Case Analysis for Case 3-1

Clinical Medicine (Cognitive Domain)	Physical Therapy Intervention	Psychosocial and Cultural Factors
How did the patient's medical diagnosis affect your evaluation and intervention?	What methods would your evaluation include? What is your justification for those methods?	What is your assessment of the patient's social support structure?
Could preventive measures, early intervention, or environmental adaptations minimize functional limitations?	Generate a problem list.	How would you go about establishing a therapeutic relationship with this patient?
What other health care professionals might this patient benefit from working with?	What is the working hypothesis?	Identify any cultural variations that may have an effect on your interaction with the patient and caregivers.
Strategies	List your short- and long-term functional goals and your plan of care.	What specific verbal and nonverbal strategies would be most effective with this case?

From Paschal K, Gale J. Patient Case Materials. Omaha: Creighton University Department of Physical Therapy, 2011.

As stated earlier in the section on tutorials, cases engage the way in which practitioners think and continue to learn. As an instructional strategy, cases allow students to be actively involved in the information gathering, problem solving, and decision making that are applied to real practice problems.[45]

A second case example is the use of a small group process that works with clinical case data and simulates an actual committee process. In this example it is the simulation of an ethics committee that uses a deconstructed case process for the teaching and learning. The basic components of the deconstructed case process are found in Table 3–8.[48]

CONCEPT MAPPING

Concept mapping is a multipurpose, fun graphic technique that can be used to see how students "build what they know" (i.e., how they structure their prior knowledge). A concept map is an illustration of relationships between concepts and facts developed by moving from a general idea to specific instances. The technique can be used by teachers and students to identify the structure of prior knowledge, to organize or present new information, or to assess progress and change.[46,47] Figure 3–5 compares a student's concept map of evaluation to a clinical instructor's concept map.

There are many creative uses for concept mapping, from thinking about course design to mapping out faculty rank and tenure progress. Refer to the Annotated Bibliography for more information on technology for creating concept maps.

NARRATIVE: A TEACHING TOOL FOR REFLECTION

The best physicians have always blended their understanding of psychology and culture with their biomedical knowledge as they diagnosed health problems and treated patients. And they have called on the resources of their faiths or philosophies, their senses of the meaning of the human experience, to give them the tensile strength to be healers and physicians rather than simply biomedical consultants.[49]

TABLE 3–8 Components in the Deconstructed Case Process

Component	Description
Component 1: Use of an authentic clinical case	Each case was an authentic clinical case encountered by members of the faculty. The data for each case were presented as they would be found in a patient's medical record with identifying information altered.
Component 2: Ethics advisory committee	Each of the six student groups acted as an ethics advisory committee, similar to a hospital ethics committee, by reviewing and analyzing the cases. This structure allowed the students to have exposure to the role of an ethics committee, focused on professional interactions, and fostered the resolution of issues.
Component 3: Student facilitators	The small groups were led by assigned student facilitators or student ethics committee co-chairs. Faculty moderators were present but served solely as background moderators; they answered questions as needed, redirected student discussion when necessary, and assisted students down a proper pathway.
Component 4: Stakeholder viewpoints	The fourth major component of the process was the inclusion of stakeholder viewpoints. Rather than focusing on an ethics case from a single reference point, this forced students to consider a case from various angles and increased awareness of a variety of ethical issues.

Hughes M, Laubscher K, Black L, Jensen GM. Use of Deconstructed Cases in Physical Therapist Ethics Education : An Assessment of Student Learning. Journal of Physical Therapy Education. 23 (1):22-28, 2009

One of the assumptions of this book is that clinical practice in physical therapy demands expertise in all domains of learning: cognitive, affective, psychomotor, perceptual, and spiritual. A student's identity as a physical therapist or physical therapist assistant depends not only on integrating the knowledge and skills of the discipline but also on developing self-knowledge through self-reflection. A very powerful teaching tool for facilitating this process of self-knowledge is the use of narrative, through one's own

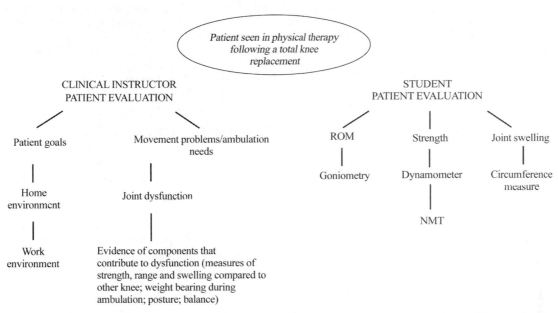

FIGURE 3–5 A comparison of clinical instructor and student concept maps for an evaluation of a patient with a total knee replacement. *NMT*, neuromuscular tension; *ROM*, range of motion.

writing or the stories of others.[50] Experiences of therapists and patients provide insight in understanding the meaning of experiences, decisions, or events. For example, a student may be asked to write an account of a time in the clinic when he or she was confused. In this account, the student addresses questions such as, What really happened here? Why did you do what you did? Would you do anything differently? What have you learned? Or, as other examples: You may have a patient with a terminal illness—how can you respond empathetically in the face of suffering and death? What inner resources can we develop to help us deal with our own limitations? The student may also want to listen carefully to the patient's story and write a similar account.

Stories are useful as a vehicle for expressing one's thoughts, but they can also be read aloud in class. The reading aloud of narrative (stories or poems) brings yet another opportunity for students to hear and think about the meanings embedded in the narrative. Jerome Bruner[51] describes two different patterns of thinking: analytical (the dominant pattern), in which thinking, things, and events are somewhat detached from everyday life as we look for general patterns of cause and effect; and narrative, in which significance is found in understanding the context of meaningful interaction. The analytical approach to thinking has strong ties to academic disciplines and is quite visible in physical therapy curricula.

An important tool for helping students develop their narrative thinking skills is phenomenology. By this we mean helping students formulate questions that are driven not only by filling in their evaluation structure but also by working to understand what patients experiencing and the meaning and perspectives they hold. This comes through designing learning experiences that engage students in "thick descriptions" of their experiences and those of their patients. Thick

descriptions are narratives that describe in rich detail the unfolding of events and human interactions.[52]

There are many learning exercises teachers can use to facilitate the role of narrative, such as journal writing, short free-writing or 5-minute writing exercises, reflection or reaction papers, and the sharing of short stories or poetry. All these tools provide students the opportunity to seek meaning in the experiences of themselves and patients.[22,50]

EVALUATION METHODS THAT PROMOTE REFLECTION

One of the central themes of this book is the role of educators in facilitating the development of "reflective practitioners." Dewey defined reflective thinking as a state of doubt or perplexity in which thinking originates and a process of inquiry begins that is aimed at finding ways to resolve the doubt or problem.[8] Schön, in studying several different professions, recognized reflection as an important vehicle for acquiring all types of professional knowledge.[33] More than a decade of research, dialogue, and writing has transpired since Schön's *Educating the Reflective Practitioner* struck the educational community. One recurring element is the use of structure to promote reflection, such as the use of portfolios and journals.[5,7,10]

Student Portfolios

Student portfolios can be useful tools as formative and summary evaluation measures to assist students to investigate their own learning experiences. It is important to provide some guidelines for students to follow in creating their portfolios. For example, you might ask students to include papers, reflective journal entries, and a self-assessment. The rule is variety; neither limit nor prescribe what the evidence must be in each of these categories.[53] Thus, the portfolio gives students permission to do creative self-assessment. One additional reflective strategy you might think about integrating into the portfolio process is Van Manen's levels of reflection.[53] He describes three levels of reflection:

1. *Technical*. "How to" questions—thinking about application of technical skills and knowledge
2. *Interpretive*. "What does this mean" questions—thinking about interpretation of words and actions
3. *Critical*. "What ought to be" questions—thinking about the worth and nature of social conditions

By encouraging students to question themselves and reflect on their classroom and clinic experiences at the three levels of reflection, the teacher can assist students to link their knowledge and skills with deliberate and moral actions.[54,55] Students can be given structured questions so that they can think more deeply (reflect) on their work.[56]

- Which item or element is your best work? Why?
- What is your most important work and why?
- What is your most satisfying work and why?
- What is your most unsatisfying work and why?
- Where did you take the greatest risk?
- What does this portfolio say about you as an emerging physical therapist?
- What are your professional development goals for the next 2 years?

Student Journals

Writing is an essential tool in the reflective process. Journal writing is a common learning activity used often in conjunction with clinical education experiences. Again, adding structure to the journal process is helpful in facilitating reflection.[57,58] For example, you may want to have students deliberately think about key aspects of a clinical environment—what they learn from patients, their views of the health care system, and how their clinical instructor teaches. The three levels of reflection (technical, interpretive, and critical) provide another structure students can use to facilitate reflective thinking and journal writing. Generally, students in the health professions write too infrequently given the requirements for a strong science background. Writing provides opportunity for achievement in that highest level in the revised cognitive domain—creativity.

TRADITIONAL INSTRUCTIONAL TECHNOLOGY

What about the use of traditional instructional technology? The most commonly used instructional media include handouts, chalkboards, overhead transparencies, web-based materials, media slides, and DVDs. The use of visual representation in the teaching and learning process remains an essential element in the act of teaching.

Chalkboards

Chalkboards (and white felt-tip pen boards or computer-supported smart boards) have been in the front of classrooms for many generations of students. A writing surface in front of a class allows spontaneity of visual representation of words, phrases, or concepts. Some tips for the use of chalkboards include the following: (1) write legibly and large enough for the class to see, (2) read aloud while writing on the board, (3) use the most visible parts of the board for critical points, (4) be selective in writing down only key principles, and (5) try to structure the board work with numbers or sections.[13]

Overhead Projection (Transparencies or LCDs)

Overhead transparencies and now liquid crystal displays (LCDs) can be used as a chalkboard for spontaneously writing down ideas or outlining content. Two positive features of using overhead projection are that (1) written materials can be made larger, and (2) the teacher can face the class while emphasizing key points. In addition, the classroom does not have to be dark as with slides, and the teacher can highlight words or phrases on the projection surface while he or she is talking. Overhead projection devices also are excellent tools for making copies of diagrams or drawings from texts. In general, use the same principles for writing on a chalkboard with overhead projection. A few additional tips for using overhead projections include the following: (1) prearrange the materials in the order in which they will be used; (2) when projecting a list, reveal only one item at a time; (3) after displaying an overhead, wait briefly before speaking; (4) make sure the material is not too busy and that the letters are legible; and (5) do not look at the screen—stand to the side of the projector.[13]

Digital Slides

Teaching with digital imagines through the use of PowerPoint or some other software has become part of most teaching environments. In teaching some topics, slides may be essential to helping students understand the necessary detail of the visual image. Digital slides are easy to create and store, and the teacher can easily talk while presenting the slides. The biggest disadvantage of slides is that the room must be dark, which makes class interaction difficult.[13] The same disadvantage (dark room and little chance to interact with students) is present when a teacher uses computer technology to generate and display visual material. Slides can be generated quickly and multiplied rapidly with the advent of various software programs and the ability to run visual displays from a "smart" classroom. One caution: more slides, fancier slides, and multimedia slides, in and of themselves, will not result in more engaged student learning and better outcomes. The role of the media display should be linked carefully and thoughtfully to your learning goals for students.

Digital Media

Digital media can be used to bring a sense of reality into the classroom. Again, as with slides, one large disadvantage is that students are passive viewers of the media unless they have been prepared to be active viewers. This means that students need to know what the expectations are for viewing the video or film. The teacher, of course, is responsible for setting the stage for follow-up activities and discussion.[13] Social video repositories such as YouTube can store a wide variety of short videos. The driving purpose must be connected to key learning goals in the classroom.

Finally, visual teaching tools, such as flip charts, chalkboards, overhead transparencies, and computers, can be useful instruments for sharing small group tasks or results. For example, small group assignments can be posted on a course platform or website. The use of computer laptops or other handheld devices provides many options for small group work in the classroom. Chapter 4 has more in depth coverage of the role of instructional technology.

SUMMARY

There are many educators who say that teaching methods have not changed much in the last 100 years—that is, the students sit, and the teacher stands in front and uses a blackboard or another visual to dictate information to students. Most faculty find the traditional methods of teaching more comfortable because they provide the greatest control, and that is the way that they themselves were taught. Common barriers that inhibit change in the classroom include the following: (1) the work setting is stable, (2) the teacher's definition of self resists change, (3) the feedback cycle is stable, (4) innovative ideas cause feelings of discomfort and anxiety, and (5) faculty like to think aloud and lecture. However, the biggest barrier of all is risk. Active learning for students and teachers requires learning new skills and taking risks.

In closing, Shulman[1] sums up the challenges in learning to teach well here:

> One of the reasons learning to teach is so difficult is because, unlike other professions where your discipline is the basis for your practice, in teaching the disciplines play a dual role. They are both the basis for practice and they are what you practice.... And all who teach are obligated to think about how they teach, as well as the content they teach. The stakes are too high for us to tolerate anything less. (p 125)

THRESHOLD CONCEPTS

Threshold Concept #1: Students' learning is along a continuum from knowing facts and information (declarative knowledge, or "knowing that"), to knowing how to apply information or knowledge (procedural knowledge, or "knowing how"), to applying what they know in clinical situations as they learn to make decisions and take actions.

Teachers are challenged in the classroom to find ways to engage student learners as they build a knowledge structure or schema that students can continue to develop and enhance along with their technical skills and their thinking and reasoning skills. There are many factors in education that keep us focused on the technical aspects, the linearity of linking goals and objectives, and the alignment of curricula and courses, yet we know that our students will practice in what Schön[33] calls the "swampy lowland of professional practice." How do we balance this need for alignment and

accountability with preparation for uncertainty? Here is where the powerful concept of reflection weighs in. We need to think explicitly about how we all (students and faculty) gain insight and further understanding of students' metacognitive skills. Students need to be able to "think about their thinking" and self-regulate so that they can change course when needed. Our educational systems tend to push up to certainty, but we also need to think about how we employ teaching methods that encourage the development of students' ability to handle uncertainty when there is no one right answer.

Threshold Concept #2: Grading is an important tool for learning, with an emphasis also on guiding, not just grading.

Grading is not just a process of grading the examination or giving the final grade but rather is a complex process that has a context in which good teachers assess and shape student learning over time. We all know that we do not want to teach directly to the test; however, if the test is properly designed, it should assess the central learning goals of the course. One could ask, Why would you not test and grade students on what we have taught them? Grading in a course needs to set high expectations, and the instructor needs to help students meet those expectations. The course syllabus is the road map that shows students just how the tests and other assignments meet those course learning goals. Remember that grading has four roles: evaluation, communication, motivation, and organization.[26]

ANNOTATED BIBLIOGRAPHY

Barkley E. *Student Engagement Techniques.* San Francisco: Jossey-Bass; 2010.
> The entire book is focused on techniques to keep students actively engaged in their learning. The book is written in a user-friendly style so that one can easily refer to various teaching methods for learner engagement. There is an excellent chapter on the conceptual background and framing for the text.

Bligh DE. *What's the Use of Lectures?* San Francisco: Jossey-Bass; 2000.
> This classic work addresses the strengths and limitation of lectures. It is well documented with clear explanations and examples.

Concept Mapping Resource. Available at: http://cmap.ihmc.us.
> The CmapTools is a tool that is being used in schools and universities around the world. The IHMC CmapTools client is free for use and available at: http://cmap.ihmc.us/

Davis BJ. *Tools for Teaching.* 2nd ed. San Francisco: Jossey-Bass; 2009.
> This book is a wonderful resource for quick reference on specific teaching tools. The book covers everything from traditional teaching tools to educational technology. There is an excellent chapter on the use of instructional media.

Shulman L. *Teaching as Community Property: Essays on Higher Education.* San Francisco: Jossey-Bass; 2004.
> This book of Shulman's essays focus on his research to improve teaching and learning in higher education. There are very practical chapters in the text that provide ideas for peer review of teaching and building models for the scholarship of teaching and learning.

Shulman L. *The Wisdom of Practice: Essays on Teaching, Learning and Learning to Teach.* San Francisco: Jossey-Bass; 2004.
> This book is a collection of Shulman's essays on teaching, learning, and learning to teach. The essays provide a rich conceptual background for any educator. There is no more thoughtful writer who brings to life the ideas of Dewey, Schwab, Schön, and others along with his own extensive research.

Svinicki M, McKeachie W. *McKeachie's Teaching Tips.* 13th ed. Belmont, CA: Wadsworth; 2011.
> This book was listed for Chapter 2 and now again in Chapter 3. There is no substitute for the classic McKeachie book. It provides quick, up-to-date information and supportive research for a number of teaching methods. This book is essential reading for any faculty member.

Walvoord B, Anderson VJ. *Effective Grading: A Tool for Learning and Assessment.* San Francisco: Jossey-Bass; 1998.

This book provides more essential reading for every physical therapy education department. Similar to the classroom assessment text, it includes multiple examples of strategies that teachers can design and implement to enhance student learning through their grading process.

REFERENCES

1. Shulman LS. Knowledge and teaching: foundations of the new reform. In: Shulman L, ed. *Teaching as Community Property: Essays on Higher Education.* San Francisco: Jossey-Bass; 2004:84–114.
2. Shulman L. Making differences: a table of learning. In: Shulman L, ed. *Teaching as Community Property: Essays on Higher Education.* San Francisco: Jossey-Bass; 2004:63–82.
3. Rothstein JR, Ecternach J. *Primer on Measurement: An Introductory Guide to Measurement Issues.* Alexandria, VA: American Physical Therapy Association; 1993.
4. Hafler J, ed. *Extraordinary Learning in the Workplace. Vol. 6: Innovation and Change in Professional Education.* New York: Springer; 2011.
5. Shulman L. *The Wisdom of Practice: Essays on Teaching, Learning and Learning to Teach.* San Francisco: Jossey-Bass; 2004.
6. World Health Organization. *International Classification of Functioning, Disability and Health.* Geneva: Author; 2001.
7. Barkley E. *Student Engagement Techniques.* San Francisco: Jossey-Bass; 2010.
8. Dewey J. *How We Think.* Buffalo, NY: Prometheus Books; 1991.
9. Svinicki M, McKeachie W. *McKeachie's Teaching Tips.* 13th ed. Belmont, CA: Wadsworth; 2011.
10. Dent J, Harden R. *A Practical Guide for Medical Teachers.* 3rd ed. New York: Churchill Livingstone; 2009.
11. Bligh DE. *What's the Use of Lectures?* San Francisco: Jossey-Bass; 2000.
12. Russell I, Hendrieson W, Herbert R. Effects of information density on medical school achievement. *J Med Educ.* 1984;59:881.
13. Davis BJ. *Tools for Teaching.* 2nd ed. San Francisco: Jossey-Bass; 2009.
14. Cross P, Steadman MH. *Classroom Research: Implementing the Scholarship of Teaching.* San Francisco: Jossey-Bass; 1998.
15. Babb K, Ross C. The timing of online lecture slide availability and its effect on attendance, participation, and exam performance. *Computers Educ.* 2009;52:868–881.
16. Craig J, Page G. The questioning skills of nursing instructors. *J Nurs Educ.* 1981;20:20.
17. Krathwohl D. A revision of Bloom's taxonomy: an overview. *Theory Pract.* 2002;41:212–217.
18. Cohen E. *Designing Groupwork: Strategies for the Heterogeneous Classroom.* 2nd ed. New York: Teachers College Press; 1994.
19. Cantillon P, Wood D. *ABC of Learning and Teaching in Medicine.* 2nd ed. Hoboken, NJ: Wiley-Blackwell; 2010.
20. Bavelas A. The five squares problem: an instructional aid in group co-operation. *Stud Personn Psychol.* 1973;5:29.
21. Epstein C. *Affective Subjects in the Classroom: Exploring Race, Sex and Drugs.* Scranton, PA: Intext Educational; 1972.
22. Gandy J, Jensen G. Group work and reflective practicums in physical therapy education: models for professional behavior development. *J Phys Ther Educ.* 1992;6:6.
23. Skeff K, Stratos G. *Methods for Teaching Medicine. American College of Physicians Teaching Medicine Series.* Philadelphia: ACP Press; 2010.
24. Fields E. Use of debate format to facilitate problem solving skills and critical thinking. *J Phys Ther Educ.* 1992;6:3.
25. Dempsey-Lyle S, Hoffman T. *Into Aging: Understanding Issues Affecting the Later Stage of Life (simulation game).* Thorofare, NJ: Slack; 1990.
26. Walvoord B, Anderson V. *Effective Grading: A Tool for Learning and Assessment.* San Francisco: Jossey-Bass; 1998.
27. Gronlund N. *Writing Instructional Objectives for Teaching and Assessment.* 8th ed. Upper Saddle Creek, NJ: Pearson-Prentice Hall; 2008.
28. Angelo TA, Cross KP. *Classroom Assessment Techniques: A Handbook for College Teachers.* 2nd ed. San Francisco: Jossey-Bass; 1993.
29. Epstein R, Hundert E. Defining and assessing professional competence. *JAMA.* 2002;287:226–235.
30. Winstein C, Knecht HG. Movement science and its relevance to physical therapy. *Phys Ther.* 1990;70:759.
31. Gentile A. A working model for skill acquisition with application to teaching. *Quest.* 1972;17:3.
32. Schmidt R, Wrisberg C. *Motor Learning and Performance: A Situation-Based Learning Approach.* 4th ed. Champaign, IL: Human Kinetics; 2008.
33. Schön D. *Educating the Reflective Practitioner.* San Francisco: Jossey-Bass; 1987.
34. Jensen GM, Gwyer J, Hack L, Shepard K. *Expertise in Physical Therapy Practice.* 2nd ed. St. Louis: Elsevier-Saunders; 2007.
35. Oh J, Segal R, Gordon J, et al. Retention and use of patient-centered interviewing skills after intensive training. *Acad Med.* 2001;76:647.
36. Novack DH, Dube C, Goldstein MG. Teaching medical interviewing: a basic course on interviewing and the physician-patient relationship. *Arch Intern Med.* 1992;152:1814.
37. Riolo L. Reliability of assessing psychomotor tasks in physical therapy curricula. *J Phys Ther Educ.* 1997;11:36.
38. Glassman M. Dewey and Vygotsky: society, experience and inquiry in educational practice. *Educ Res.* 2001;30:3.
39. Ende J. *Theory and Practice of Teaching Medicine.* American College of Physicians Teaching Medicine Series. Philadelphia: ACP Press; 2010.
40. Bereiter C, Scardamalia M. *Surpassing Ourselves: An Inquiry into the Nature and Implications of Expertise.* Chicago: Open Court; 1993.
41. Sullivan WM, Rosin MS. *A New Agenda for Higher Education: Shaping a Life of the Mind for Practice.* San Francisco: Jossey-Bass; 2008.
42. Cooke M, Irby D, O'Brien B. *Educating Physicians: A Call for Reform of Medical School and Residency.* San Francisco: Jossey-Bass; 2010.
43. Benner P, Sutphen M, Leonard V, Day L. *Educating Nurses: A Call for Radical Transformation.* San Francisco: Jossey-Bass; 2010.
44. Shulman J. *Case Methods in Teacher Education.* New York: Teachers College Press; 1992.
45. McGinty SM. Case-method teaching: an overview of the pedagogy and rationale for its use in physical therapy education. *J Phys Ther Educ.* 2000;14:48.
46. Beissner K. Use of concept mapping to improve problem solving. *J Phys Ther Educ.* 1992;6:22.
47. Vacek J. Using a conceptual approach to concept mapping to promote critical thinking. *J Nurs Educ.* 2009;48:45–48.
48. Hughes M, Laubscher K, Black L, Jensen GM. Use of deconstructed case in physical therapy education: an assessment of student learning. *J Phys Ther Educ.* 2009;23:22–35.
49. Caelleigh AS, Dittrich LR. Preface The humanities and medical education. *Acad Med.* 1995;70:758.
50. Engel J, Zarconi J, Pethtel L, Missimi S. *Narrative in Health Care.* New York: Radcliffe; 2008.
51. Bruner J. *Arts of Meaning.* Cambridge, MA: Harvard University Press; 1990.
52. Greenfield BH, Jensen GM. Understanding the lived experience of patients: application of a phenomenological approach to ethics. *Phys Ther.* 2010;90:1185–1197.
53. Van Manen M. Pedagogy, virtue, and narrative identity in teaching. *Curriculum Inquiry.* 1994;24:135.
54. Jensen GM, Paschal KA. Habits of mind: student transition toward virtuous practice. *J Phys Ther Educ.* 2000;14:42.
55. Jensen GM, Richert AR. Reflection on the teaching of ethics in physical therapy education: integrating cases, theory and learning. *J Phys Ther Educ.* 2005;19:78–85.
56. Suskie L. *Assessing Student Learning: A Common Sense Guide.* 2nd ed. San Francisco, CA: Jossey-Bass; 2009.
57. Jensen G, Denton B. Teaching physical therapy students to reflect: a suggestion for clinical education. *J Phys Ther Educ.* 1991;5:33.
58. Hayward L. Becoming a self-reflective teacher: a meaningful research process. *J Phys Ther Educ.* 2000;14:21.

Appendix 3-A Cooperative Group Training Exercise: Broken Circles*

Instructions

Step 1. Divide the class into small groups (three to six persons per group). Give each person an envelope with different pieces of a circle.

Step 2. The goal is for each student to put together a complete circle. To do this, students must exchange some of the pieces.

Step 3. Rules of the game include:

- No talking. The game is done in complete silence.
- A student may not point or signal any other player with his or her hands.
- The focus of the game is giving. Students may give pieces one at a time. They may not place a piece in another person's circle. Students can hand a piece to a player or place it beside the other pieces in front of him or her.
- Students must complete their own puzzle.

Step 4. This is a group task. Each group has 15 to 20 minutes.

- After the time is up, the class should discuss the game using the following questions:
  - What do you think the game was about?
  - How did you feel as a group member?
  - What helped your group be successful in solving the problem?
  - What made it harder?
  - What could the group do differently?

Directions for Making Materials for Playing Advanced Broken Circles

1. *Make a set from heavy cardboard.* Cut the circles approximately 20 cm in diameter. Each set of six circles should be a different color, with letters and numbers marked on the back of each piece. Numbers indicate the group size, and letters indicate the proper envelope. If a piece does not have a number on it, it remains in its lettered envelope regardless of group size.

2. *Angles used include: 60, 90, 120, 150, 180, 210, 240, and 270 degrees.* See the figure below.

3. *Placement of the other four pieces varies with the size of the group.* For example, if you have a six-person group, then 6-F (60-degree piece) goes into the F envelope, 6-E (150-degree piece) goes into the E envelope, 6-C (90-degree piece) goes into the C envelope, and 6-D (150-degree piece) goes into the D envelope. Repeat this pattern for each six-person group.

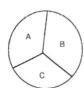

Angles (60,60,60)

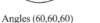
(240,120)

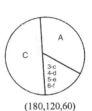
(180,120,60)

(270, 90)

(150, 150,60)

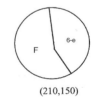
(210,150)

*Broken squares game developed by Bavelas A. The five squares problem—an instructional aid in group cooperation. Stud Personn Psychol 1973;5:29. Broken circles game developed by Graves T, Graves N. (Game) Santa Cruz, CA: 1985. May be purchased by writing from Graves, 136 Library St., Santa Cruz, CA 95060. Average class would need six to eight sets. Directions for preparation of game reprinted by permission of the publisher from Cohen EH. Designing Groupwork: Strategies for the Heterogeneous Classroom, 2nd ed. New York: Teachers College Press, 1994. ©1994 by Teachers College, Columbia University. All rights reserved.

APPENDIX 3-B COOPERATIVE GROUP TRAINING EXERCISE: EPSTEIN'S FOUR-STAGE ROCKET*

Group Activity

This training exercise involves having a small group discuss a topic that will generate interaction with different perspectives. The group is given a topic to discuss. As an example: For the next 20 minutes, you will discuss the role of research in physical therapy education. What should the role be? Consider you are a task force of students that is making recommendations to the faculty. Identify the driving and restraining forces and make a list of recommendations. Students can discuss what kind of research and scholarship they should do during their professional education (e.g., a literature review, a case report, a systematic literature review, a clinical research proposal, a full-blown research project), the amount of content and experience in the curriculum, and whether students should generate independent projects or group projects.

Ground Rules

There will be four stages and 4 minutes of group discussion to practice these skills at each stage.

1. *Conciseness.* Select a timekeeper who will watch the clock and keep time for the group. The timekeeper must make sure that each person talks for only 15 seconds. Do this for 4 minutes.
2. *Listening.* Select a new timekeeper. Now the timekeeper must make sure that each person waits 3 seconds after each person has spoken before he or she talks. Do this for 4 minutes.
3. *Reflecting.* Select a new timekeeper. Now the timekeeper must make sure each person talks for only 15 seconds, followed by 3 seconds of silence. The next person who speaks must begin by repeating to the group something that was said by the person who spoke before him or her. (The person who spoke before must nod his or her head to indicate if the repetition is correct.) Do this for 4 minutes.
4. *Everyone contributes.* Select a new timekeeper. All previous rules apply. In addition, no one may speak a second time until everyone in the group has spoken. Do this for 4 minutes.

Observers

The teacher can assign one or two observers to record examples of group members' skills for each of the four stages (conciseness, listening, reflecting, and contributions by all).

Debriefing Session

After the discussion, have the groups debrief using the following list of group behaviors as a structure for discussion.

Work Behaviors: Skillful Members

- Have new ideas for the group
- Ask for or give information
- Help explain better
- Pull ideas together
- Find out if the group is ready to decide what to do

Helping Behaviors: Helpful Members

- Get people together
- Bring in other people
- Show interest and kindness
- Be willing to change own ideas if someone makes a good argument
- Tell others in a good way how they are behaving

Troublesome Behaviors: Troublesome Group Members

- Attack other people
- Refuse to go along with suggestions
- Talk too much
- Keep people from discussing because they do not like the argument
- Show that they do not care about what is happening
- Let someone boss the group
- Do not talk and contribute to ideas
- Tell stories and keep the group from getting their work done

---

*Adapted from Epstein C: Affective Subjects in the Classroom: Exploring Race, Sex and Drugs. Scranton, PA: Intext Educational, 1972.

62

PHYSICAL THERAPY EDUCATION IN THE DIGITAL AGE
LEVERAGING TECHNOLOGIES TO PROMOTE LEARNING

Tracy Chapman ● Gail M. Jensen

CHAPTER OUTLINE

"If you are headed in the wrong direction, technology will not get you to the right place." Steven Ehrmann, 1995

Dr. Carter teaches two courses in the department of physical therapy. One of the courses, Research Methods for Health Care Providers, meets in the afternoon 3 days a week and includes didactic information delivered by lectures. Dr. Carter's course is one of the few required courses that students dread taking. End-of-course evaluations demonstrate students find the course boring and difficult, and do not see the applicability of the course information to physical therapy practice. Dr. Carter attributes the low student ratings of the research course to students' general dislike of research courses and therefore has not taken steps to make any changes to the course since he started teaching it 10 years ago. An observer standing at the back of the room during one of Dr. Carter's lectures will notice students using their laptops, iPads, iPods, and smart phones to take notes, post updates to FaceBook, send text messages, surf the Web, shop, and play games.

Dr. Carter recently received a major grant that will span 3 years, and therefore some of his teaching responsibilities will be assigned to a relatively new faculty member in the department, Dr. Martinez. The Chair of the Physical Therapy Department has told Dr. Martinez the research course must be restructured so that students are actively engaged and to help students understand the relevance of health sciences research to the practice of physical therapy.

Dr. Martinez will take over teaching the research course for Dr. Carter. Dr. Martinez has recently completed a postdoctorate program during which she had the opportunity to work with a faculty member fluent in the effective use of educational technology. Dr. Martinez is anxious to integrate technologies into Dr. Carter's course to create a blended course. Dr. Martinez envisions the possibilities of using technology to actively engage students during the course and to connect students with physical therapy practitioners and various practice environments.

LEARNING GOALS

After completing this chapter, the reader will be able to:
1. Describe a framework for selection of educational technology resources to facilitate and inspire student learning.
2. Describe processes for implementation of educational technologies in the face-to-face and virtual teaching environments.
3. Discuss the benefits and limitations of educational technologies in promoting student learning.
4. Discuss implications of cognitive load theory, situated learning, and learning engagement research for the use of educational technologies.
5. Describe the components of digital citizenship and the importance of including digital citizenship as part of health professions education.
6. Describe contemporary educational technologies and alignment with desired learning activities.
7. Describe opportunities for developing scholarship investigating student learning and the use of educational technologies.

Today's contemporary students depend on an assortment of technologies to stay connected with family and friends, to keep pace with current events, to navigate their physical environment, and to stay up to date with their education responsibilities. The ever-shifting technologic landscape,

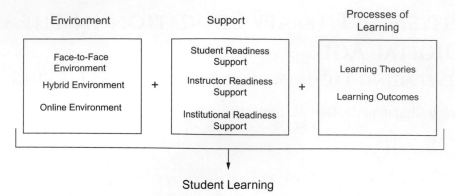

FIGURE 4–1 Diagram showing the interaction between the necessary factors for student learning.

including ubiquitous Internet access and mobile devices, is changing the way we access information, teach, learn, communicate, and socialize. These factors, combined with workforce globalization, highlight the importance of technology literacy—the ability to use technology fluently in our education, work, and daily lives. These circumstances present challenges and opportunities for instructors, students, and administrators.

The purpose of this chapter is to provide some theoretical foundation and practical advice for the selection, implementation, and evaluation of educational technologies within the context of traditional face-to-face, blended (combining face-to-face and online teaching), and online physical therapy education. Although the degree of technology integration varies across these learning environments, the core elements required to achieve student learning do not change. To engage the technology in a meaningful way, the use of technology must be shaped by learning theory and learning outcomes and supported by readiness on the part of the students, instructor, and institution (Figure 4–1). Implementing technology without these critical elements results in superficial use of technology, wasting the time, talent, and treasure of students, instructors, and the institution.

In the 10-plus years since the release of the second edition of *The Handbook of Teaching for Physical Therapists*, significant changes have occurred in the educational technology landscape. What was then new, innovative, and exciting is now part of the smorgasbord of learning resources expected by students. Digital presentation slides, posting of course materials online for 24 × 7 access, and the ability to use mobile devices inside and outside of class to access learning resources are part of the tapestry of teaching and learning tools students expect to be available.[1] Electronic books, new mobile devices, augmented reality, game-based learning, gesture-based computing, and learning analytics are some of the near-term and longer-term technologies expected to play a role in the educational setting.[2] To keep pace with these changes, the Association for Educational Communications and Technology (AECT) has rewritten its definition for educational technology. For the purposes of this chapter, AECT's updated definition will be used, "Educational technology is the study and ethical practice of facilitating learning and improving performance by creating, using, and managing appropriate technologic processes and resources."[3]

THE EDUCATIONAL ENVIRONMENT IN THE DIGITAL AGE: THE CONTEMPORARY STUDENT

A visit to any campus in the United States illustrates students' frequent use of technology. The omnipresence of cell phones, mobile computers, and iPod devices demonstrates the degree to which students have integrated technology into the routines of daily life. The most recent survey of student technology use conducted by the Educause Center for Applied Research (ECAR)[2] paints a profile of contemporary student use of technology for personal and educational purposes. Of the nearly 37,000 respondents, 89% indicated they own a laptop, nearly 63% have an Internet-capable handheld device, 94% use a library website regularly, and almost 80% use a learning management system at least weekly.

Regarding students' perceptions of educational technology, most students report using technology makes completion of course activities more convenient and positively impacts their learning; however, less than third believe the use of technology leads to more active engagement in courses.[2] Although students' use of technology in their personal lives seems to be ever present, they prefer a moderate amount of technology use in course activities. Perhaps this dichotomy is explained by students' perceptions of faculty's ability to use technology effectively. Forty-seven percent of students believe faculty use technology effectively, 49% think faculty have adequate preparation for using technology, and students report only 38% of faculty members provide adequate preparation for students to use course technology.[2,4]

Much has been written about factors that determine faculty adoption of educational technologies. Availability of support personnel, incentive structure, workload, technology and infrastructure reliability, training, and peer experiences are factors generally cited as determinates of adoption.[5,6] A key variable underpinning all these factors is the notion of digital natives and digital immigrants.[7] Students are generally digital natives, individuals who have grown up using technology; technology was present when they were born and they have used a variety of technology in many aspects of their lives. On the other hand, faculty tend to fall within the category of digital immigrants—those who were born in the predigital technology era and have assimilated into the digital teaching and learning landscape. Does this difference in digital status explain the variances in technology use rate between students and faculty? To what degree should use of technology be part of the physical therapy curricula? These questions are explored further in the following sections of this chapter.

NATIONAL EDUCATIONAL TECHNOLOGY STANDARDS FOR TEACHERS AND ADMINISTRATORS

The importance of technology fluency for faculty and students in the current educational environment is evident. To maximize the time, talent, and treasure invested in the use of technology, instructors and administrators must be prepared to make informed decisions in the selection and use of digital learning resources. Created by the International Society for Technology in Education (ISTE), the National Educational Technology Standards (NETS) are intended to serve as a guide for professional development of teachers and administrators in the use of educational technology.[8] NETS for teachers[a] are designed to provide a framework for the effective use of technology to advance student learning. NETS for administrators[b] are designed to define what administrators need to know and be able to do in order to fulfil their responsibility as leaders in the effective use of technology in educational settings. Faculty members and administrators are encouraged to incorporate the NETS into annual professional development plans as a means to keep student learning as the centerpiece of all instructional activities while adopting technology-rich educational environments. A listing of the NETS are found in Appendices 4-A (teachers) and 4-B (administrators).

LEARNING RESEARCH AND ITS IMPLICATIONS FOR EDUCATIONAL TECHNOLOGY

Grounding the selection and use of educational technology with learning theory will help ensure congruence between technology use and student learning outcomes. Particularly relevant to a discussion about educational technology and student learning is the ongoing debate about the degree to which the use of technology affects student learning as well as the concepts of student engagement and cognitive load theory.

TECHNOLOGY AND STUDENT LEARNING

The ability of technology use to directly impact student learning has been debated for decades. Some researchers argue that any change in student learning accompanying the introduction of technology can be attributed to the changes in instructional methods that occurred as a result of the introduction of technology, the novelty of the technology and therefore increased student interest, or more thoughtful design of the instruction.[9–11] Others suggest that, if the interactive nature of learning is taken into consideration, the use of technology can affect how something is learned. Therefore, the use of technology can, to some degree,

have a direct connection to student learning.[12–15] As the debate continues among educational researchers, most acknowledge that technology is a permanent and ever-changing fixture in the teaching and learning environment; therefore, employing instructional design principles to ensure the effective integration of technology-infused instructional methods is crucial. Revisiting Dr. Carter's and Dr. Martinez's course may serve as an example.

As previously noted, Dr. Carter employed a traditional, lecture-based teaching model. Students were expected to complete assigned readings before coming to class. Class time involved lecture peppered with questions to students about the reading assignment content. In realty, few students actually completed the preclass assigned readings. Dr. Martinez will be responsible for the same learning outcomes as she assumes responsibility for Dr. Carter's course. She is using the same textbook and other course readings; however, she will be using a combination of face-to-face and online learning activities. Using pre-recorded mini lectures, students will be expected to complete assigned readings, view mini lectures, and complete a quiz before coming to class. Class time will be used for discussion and application of the course concepts. If student grades are higher using this blended model, does that mean the introduction of technology in the course led to higher grades? Some educational researchers would argue that the change in instructional methods adopted as a result of the introduction of technology, not solely the introduction of the technology, resulted in the change in student grades. In other words, the addition of the technology made it possible to modify the instructional methods, but the technology itself did not directly affect student grades. Regardless of where researchers stand on the technology and student learning debate, general agreement exists on the importance of aligning course learning objectives, instructional design strategies, and technology selection.

COGNITIVE LOAD AND MULTIMEDIA LEARNING

Revisiting Dr. Martinez and her new teaching assignment, we see she is in the process of designing mini lectures for students to view outside of class. Each lecture is composed of audio and a PDF document containing the full text of the lecture audio as well as images to support the lecture information. Dr. Martinez has spent a significant amount of time creating the PDF documents. When a colleague asked why she was providing students both the audio and the text, Dr. Martinez replied that having both will help students learn by giving them the opportunity to hear and read the same information. This same colleague suggested using slides containing key points for the lectures in lieu of the PDF document. What do you think? Which strategy is better for student learning? The theory of multimedia learning addresses these questions.

Human working memory serves as a temporary storage and processing facility for new information. The capacity of working memory is limited to managing about seven elements of information at any given time. As information is processed and moved into long-term memory, it is filed away for permanent storage and on-demand retrieval. Learning complex information or tasks can be improved by employing instructional design strategies, which

---

[a] NETS for teachers: http://www.iste.org/standards/nets-for-teachers.aspx

[b] NETS for administrators: http://www.iste.org/standards/nets-for-administrators.aspx

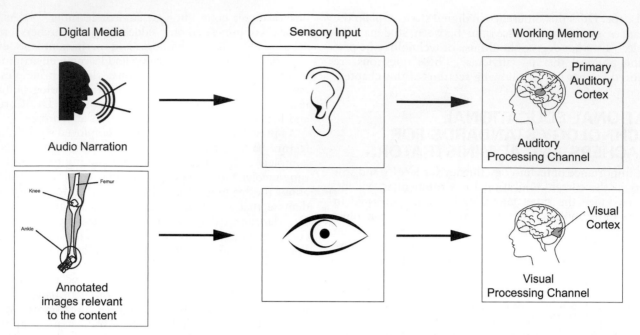

FIGURE 4–2 Effective use of auditory and visual channels of information processing.

effectively manage working memory and long-term memory capabilities.[16]

Cognitive load theory focuses on the capacity and role of working memory in processing information.[16] This theory suggests that cognitive load, or mental processing, is affected by intrinsic and extrinsic factors. Intrinsic cognitive load occurs as a result of the nature of the information being presented. For example, a problem requiring students to simultaneously process several elements would result in a high demand on working memory. Extrinsic cognitive load is determined by the way in which information is presented—the learning environment, instructional strategies, and design and quality of instructional materials. Using both text and images and placing them on separate pages requiring learners to constantly shift their focus between the text and images is an example of extrinsic cognitive load. Embedding the text directly in the image decreases extrinsic cognitive load and therefore expands working memory resources for other tasks.

The limited processing capacity of working memory is further explicated by the notion of separate channels for processing of auditory and visual information.[17] Each channel is limited in the amount of information that can be processed at any given moment (Figure 4–2); therefore, presenting the same information both visually and verbally does not make effective use of working memory—both channels are processing the same information. Learning can be increased by presenting complementary information visually and auditory.

The cognitive theory of multimedia learning was developed by applying cognitive load theory and the notion of dual channel processing to the use of digital media in educational environments.[18,19] This theory suggests instruction should be designed such that:

1. Only a single input of information per working memory channel (auditory or visual) is used,

2. Only relevant information is included, avoiding the use of decorative images and extraneous information, and

3. Words and graphics are included in the instructional materials.

Including unrelated information in one sensory channel is an inefficient manner of teaching; it can confuse the learner (Figure 4–3).

Providing both audio narration (words) and annotated images (graphics) ensures that both processing channels are used without overloading either channel. Embedding the text into the image allows students to easily make the connection between image and text, thus maximizing working memory devoted to processing the information presented.

Using both background music (regardless of how subtle) and audio narration overloads the auditory channel. Overload occurs as the student tries to discern the relevant information from that which is irrelevant, leaving less working memory available to process the relevant information. Including images not essential for teaching a concept adds unnecessary load to the visual processing channel of working memory as the student tries to relate the images to the audio narration. Multimedia theory suggests combining narration with relevant graphics or key words and phrases, thereby employing a single input into each working memory channel.

In summary, when designing digital media to support student learning:

- Use graphics and words to present information.
- Use only graphics and words essential for student learning.
- Place explanatory text directly next to or embedded in the graphic.
- Use audio to explain animations.

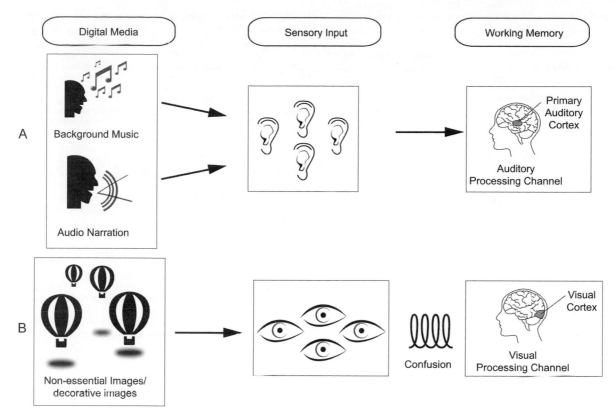

FIGURE 4–3 An inefficient teaching strategy. **A,** Two sets of data are being input through the auditory channel, meaning all information is being processed by the same cortex. **B,** Unrelated images are displayed as part of the lecture, causing confusion and distracting the student from the relevant information.

- Avoid extraneous sounds (e.g., background music).
- Avoid extraneous images (e.g., "fun" or decorative pictures not essential to understanding the content).

After reading about the use of digital media in education, Dr. Martinez decides to change her approach to the mini lectures. Instead of recording mini lectures by narrating the lecture notes handouts word for word, she decides to use a combination of audio and PowerPoint slides. The slides will contain bulleted text of key concepts and annotated images. She believes this design strategy will optimize students' use of their auditory and visual processing channels.

STUDENT ENGAGEMENT AND THE USE OF EDUCATIONAL TECHNOLOGIES

Chickering and Gamson's *Seven Principles for Good Undergraduate Education*,[20] first published in 1987 and based on decades of research about student learning, provides a basic set of guidelines for engaging students in the learning process. Although originally proposed for undergraduate education, the principles apply equally well to graduate and professional education. The availability of educational technologies provides opportunities to operationalize the seven principles in new and different ways.[21] Table 4–1 summarizes these principles and provides examples of ways in which technologies can be used to implement the principles.

Educational technologies afford instructors the opportunity to apply the seven principles as well as to reconsider the configuration of time and space for teaching and learning and increase student engagement.[22] Traditionally, students' first exposure to instructional content is in the classroom in the form of a lecture. Although students are often assigned readings to complete before class, the reality is that many (if not most) do not complete the readings, or do so at a very superficial level. Therefore, instructors find themselves spending class time lecturing, time they had planned to devote to learning activities. Technology allows us to shift the first exposure to content and concepts from inside to outside of the classroom, holding students accountable for completing the first exposure activities and thus allowing more in class time for applying the new information. Therefore, the application of new concepts occurs in the presence of the expert, the instructor, instead of outside of class, when students are separated by time and space from the content expert. Table 4–2 illustrates this notion of reconceptualizing the time and space for teaching and learning.

Revisiting Dr. Martinez's plans for Dr. Carter's course serves to illustrate this notion of shifting time and space. Her plans to combine prerecorded mini lectures and assigned readings for students to complete before class will prepare students for applying the information during in class discussions and learning activities. By adding a quiz or assigning a short summary of the key points to be completed before class, or at the beginning of class, Dr. Martinez's students are held accountable for completing the preclass

TABLE 4–1 Using Technology to Implement the Seven Principles

Principle: Summary	Potential Benefit of Using Technology	Examples of Activities and Technologies
1. *Encourage contact between students and faculty.* Frequent student-faculty contact in and out of classes is a critical factor in student motivation and involvement.	Engage students reluctant to speak during class. Increase access to faculty members. Ease communication for non-native English speakers.	Increase access to the instructor outside of class via the use of e-mail, text chat, or discussion boards. Use web conferencing to offer tutoring sessions during times convenient for students and instructors without requiring travel to campus.
2. *Develop reciprocity and cooperation among students.* Learning is enhanced when it is more like a team effort than a solo race. Good learning, like good work, is collaborative and social, not competitive and isolated.	Increase time available for collaboration. Ease communication for non-native English speakers.	Study groups and project collaboration can be accomplished by using electronic white boards contained in web-conferencing solutions or via virtual collaborative work spaces such as Google Docs. E-mail, discussion boards, text chat, and social networking tools can also provide avenues for collaboration.
3. *Encourage active learning.* Learning is not a spectator sport. Students must discuss what they are learning, write about it, relate it to past experiences, and apply it to their daily lives.	Increase opportunities for learning by doing and synchronous or asynchronous interactions.	Search for information using electronic databases available online via libraries or other resources. Increase access to experts in the profession through the use of web conferencing and discussion boards. Use virtual simulation environments to practice the application of new knowledge or skills. Provide opportunities for practice and formative feedback via self-grading electronic quizzes and practice examinations.
4. *Give prompt feedback.* Students need appropriate feedback on performance, opportunities to reflect on what they have learned and what they still need to know.	Increase timeliness and frequency of feedback opportunities. Increase ease of providing feedback.	Electronic submission of assignments and use of electronic portfolios increase the flexibility of time and space for practice (students) and feedback (instructor). Video captures of students' performance and use of video-commenting tools can provide opportunities for the student to review his/her own performance, for others to review and provide feedback, and for longitudinal review of performance. Screen-capture software provides the opportunity to quickly create mini tutorials and easily distribute them to multiple students.
5. *Emphasize time on task.* Learning to use one's time well is critical for students and professionals alike.	Increase efficiency of studying and ease of access to learning materials.	Recording lectures, tutorials, and instructional resources using lecture capture or podcasting and posting them online allows students to decrease the time spent commuting to campus, gives them the ability to review the materials when needed, and affords them the opportunity to shape their study time in a manner most beneficial to their learning needs. Shifting time and space for lectures and first exposure to information to outside of the classroom by recording lectures increases class time available for focused engagement in learning activities. Increase efficiency of study time by providing online access to study materials via the library or through the learning management system.
6. *Communicate high expectations.* Expecting students to perform well becomes a self-fulfilling prophecy; students will strive to achieve high expectations established by instructors and institutions.	Increases ease of providing formative feedback on drafts of assignment responses. Increases ability to provide multiple examples of high-quality work.	Collaborative work spaces such as Google Docs allow instructors or peers to provide feedback on draft of papers and presentations. Exemplars of completed assignments posted in the learning management system provide students examples of high-quality work.
7. *Respect diverse talents and ways of learning.* There are many roads to learning. Students need the opportunity to show their talents and learn in ways that work for them. Then they can be pushed to learn in new ways that do not come as easily.	Increases ability for students to represent their knowledge and skill in multiple formats. Provides multiple practice opportunities for students.	Multiple practice opportunities can be made available by posting lectures in the learning management system, creating practice quizzes and exams with automated feedback, using electronic flashcards. Using presentation software, inexpensive and easy-to-use video recorders, and freely available graphic creation and editing software presents the opportunity for students to demonstrate their knowledge and skills in a variety of ways.

Data from Allen IE, Seaman J. Class differences: online education in the United States 2010. Available at: http://sloanconsortium.org/sites/default/files/class_differences.pdf; Accessed 22.05.2011.

TABLE 4–2 Shifting Time and Space for Teaching and Learning

	Students with Teacher (In Class)	Student Study Time (Outside of Class)	Teacher (Outside of Class)
Traditional lecture method	First exposure to new content and concepts	Processing new information	Responding to students' application of new information
Reconsidering time and space	Processing new information. Responding to students' application of new information	First exposure to new content and concepts	Responding to students' application of new information

From Walvoord B, Laughner T. How to help faculty integrate technology and pedagogy. Workshop presentation. University of Notre Dame, June, 2002.

activities. These accountability activities will also highlight gaps in students' understanding of the content, which Dr. Carter can address with a mini lecture or short discussion during class. As a result most class time can be spent helping students apply the new concepts. Sometimes referred to as *just-in-time teaching*,[22] this model of leveraging technology increases the time students have with the content expert to process new information.

This discussion of cognitive load theory, multimedia learning, the seven principles, and reconsideration of time and space illustrates many opportunities available for leveraging a variety of educational technology to support student learning. Faculty members may choose from well-known and ubiquitous e-mail to leading-edge technology such as virtual simulations, and a host of options in between. The next section of this chapter provides suggestions and frameworks for selecting, implementing, and evaluating these educational technologies.

EDUCATIONAL TECHNOLOGY INTEGRATION: SELECTION, IMPLEMENTATION, AND EVALUATION

The ever-changing array of educational technologies available for use in the classroom or online provides a myriad of tools for instructors to create authentic, engaging, and meaningful learning experiences. Thus far in this chapter, we have examined some theoretical constructs to assist in designing technology-mediated instructional activities. Successful use of educational technologies to support instructional activities requires careful selection, planning and implementation, and evaluation.

SELECTION

Employing an intentional and outcomes-driven process to select technology can increase the chances of finding the right solution that is strategic and focused on supporting instructional methods to advance student learning. Resources for purchasing and supporting educational technologies should only be expended if they help to achieve the program's goals and objectives. Fragmented, inefficient, and ineffective efforts, wasting the time and energy of instructors and students, may result if factors other than learning outcomes drive technology selection. Figure 4–4 summarizes the key elements of educational technology selection.[23]

Six basic steps are employed to ensure that each technology selection element is considered (Table 4–3):

- Step 1: Identify instructional needs
- Step 2: Identify stakeholders
- Step 3: Develop selection criteria
- Step 4: Identify potential technologies
- Step 5: Determine the total cost of ownership (TCO)
- Step 6: Select the technology

Once the educational technology is selected, planning for implementation is the next step toward ensuring a successful integration with the teaching-learning environment and learning outcomes.

IMPLEMENTATION

As with most endeavors, planning leads to a greater chance for success. Using technology in the educational process is no different. Technology often exists on the periphery of an institution's instructional programming. Implementation conducted in a piecemeal fashion, perhaps when year-end "extra monies" are available, with little or no long-range plan, is a recipe for disaster. Following the four Cs of implementation maximizes the likelihood of successful technology integration.[24]

The Four C's of Implementation

Successful implementation of technology requires four Cs:

1. *Comprehensive* approach to planning
2. *Commitment* (of all stakeholders)
3. *Collaboration* (of all stakeholders)
4. *Continuity* (or "life cycle") planning

Comprehensive Approach to Planning

Introducing technology into the teaching and learning environment can be exciting and provide learning opportunities not previously available; however, success depends on planning for the obvious and the unexpected. A comprehensive approach to planning for implementation can increase your chances for success.

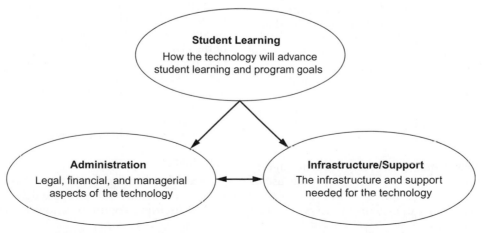

FIGURE 4–4 Key elements of educational technology selection.

TABLE 4–3   Basic Steps When Considering Technology Selection

Step	Process
Step 1: Identify instructional needs	Define the instructional activity or method and associated learning outcome or program goal the technology is expected to support. Describe what you as an instructor need to do that you cannot do without the technology or can do better with technology.
Step 2: Identify stakeholders	Include stakeholders to represent each of the three elements of educational technology selection: Student learning: Faculty colleagues, clinical preceptors, students, instructional support personnel Administration: Finance/budget personnel, representation from legal services Infrastructure/support: Help-desk, network, and infrastructure support representative
Step 3: Develop selection criteria	Selection criteria can be categorized as related to each of the three elements: Student learning: How well the technology appears to support the instructional activities, student learning outcomes, or program goals. How the technology affects cognitive load. How the technology helps facilitate good educational practices (see Table 4-1) Administration: Amount of training and support required for students, instructors, and support personnel; legal terms and conditions; alignment with the Family Education Rights and Privacy Act (FERPA) and other relevant regulations. Infrastructure/support: The technology's ability to run on multiple computing technology platforms (PC or Mac, different versions of operating systems, etc.) and on an average computer, network infrastructure requirements to use the technology, compatibility with existing technology used in the program or on campus, physical environment requirements (space, electrical power, etc.), reported reliability and maintenance time requirements
Step 4: Identify potential technologies	The instructor and stakeholders identify solutions to be evaluated using the criteria developed in step 3.
Step 5: Determine the total cost of ownership (TCO)	The TCO is calculated for each viable technology solution identified in step 4. TCO includes all costs associated with the implementation of a particular technology, including initial implementation costs and ongoing expenses. TCO calculations typically include: Licensing fees (initial fees and annual renewal if applicable) Maintenance and support fees Hardware and software required to host and run the technology Time spent to train faculty, students, and support personnel Time required to conduct the initial implementation Expected time required to maintain and support the technology
Step 6: Select the technology	Using the selection criteria and total cost of ownership information, stakeholders evaluate each of the technology solutions and select the technology that best fits the selection criteria.

Student Learning

Identification of instructional needs was addressed in the technology selection process. As you move into the implementation phase, detailed planning for incorporation of the technology into instructional methods will increase the chances for smooth implementation. Learning experiences should be shaped so that they take into account the tenets of cognitive load and multimedia theory. Students with disabilities may have difficulty interacting with the technology; therefore, proactive planning for accommodations is needed. Furthermore, the degree to which students have access to the technology tools necessary to carry out the technology-infused learning experience may vary. For example, some students may not own a computer or may not have an Internet connection at home. Therefore, steps must be taken to ensure these students are not placed at a disadvantage when completing course assignments. Establishing a plan for formative and summative evaluation of the technology used in your course will provide data that can be used to make adjustments, if necessary, before the end of the term as well as before the next time the course if offered. The Evaluation section of this chapter provides suggestions for data collection.

Administration

Terms and conditions contained in the contractual agreement with the technology provider may affect your use of the technology. As an example, some software providers allow a predetermined number of concurrent users, thus you may need to schedule times for students to use the software. It may be necessary to work with administrative personnel to understand potential Family Educational Rights and Privacy Act (FERPA) or other regulatory implications related to using the technology. Some applications store user-generated data on systems hosted and owned by the software provider. Such an arrangement may lead to privacy concerns. Google Documents is one example. Google Documents is a commonly used application for creating and sharing documents. Students can easily create drafts of papers to share with the instructor or group members. Instructors and peers can add comments to the draft documents. All Google Documents are housed on Google servers; therefore, instructors are cautioned to check with their institution's privacy administrators regarding the ability to include FERPA- or Health Insurance Portability and Accountability Act (HIPAA)-protected information as part of the project. Additionally, training for the instructor, support personnel, and students may be needed to ensure successful use of the technology. Furthermore, ensuring you are cognizant of the costs associated with the technology for the duration of its use will help optimize the financial investment. Data storage fees and number of software licenses used are areas in which cost overruns are easily overlooked.

Infrastructure

Proactively planning for the purchase of licenses, hardware, and software will mitigate delays in getting started. Use of multiple communication media (e.g., verbally in class, a document outlining the key points, posting information on the course website) to clearly inform students what is expected of them regarding the use of the technology is advised, including the type of computer, configuration, and network connection required to access and complete technology-enhanced course assignments. Making students a partner in the technology integration process by informing them about what the technology can and cannot do, acknowledging the introduction of technology may present some unexpected issues, ensuring students you will make allowances for unexpected technical problems so as to not affect their grades, and inviting their feedback and suggestions will increase student tolerance of unexpected technology glitches. Well before using the technology, practice, practice, practice with the same computer and in the same physical environment you will use for teaching with the technology. Anticipate what may go wrong and work with the technology support personnel to proactively mitigate these situations to the degree possible. Most important of all, have a backup plan for when the technology fails. It will fail at some point during your teaching, so it behooves you to have a fall-back plan ready.

Collaboration

Successful integration of technology into your teaching landscape requires a collaborative effort involving a variety of individuals from the across the institution. Faculty colleagues, students, instructional support professionals, and information technology support personnel all working together can create a rich, well functioning, and rewarding experience.

- You can leverage the lived experiences of faculty colleagues to learn from their success and mistakes.
- Students can provide you with insights into the use of technology not previously considered and with information about their computing capabilities and determine whether their computers have the ability to run the types of technology you plan to use and whether they have the bandwidth needed to use the technology.
- An instructional designer or instructional technologist can assist with (1) designing learning materials for delivery online, (2) designing online or blended courses, (3) helping faculty members identify technologies congruent with learning objectives and activities, (4) providing faculty and student training in the use of technologies, (5) assessing the impact of the technology on student learning, and (6) coordinating contact with other support personnel.
- Copyright librarians can assist with application of copyright laws to online and electronic learning materials and obtain copyright for materials to be provided to students electronically including online.
- Purchasing personnel may be able to leverage institution buying power; your institution may already own software licenses or have hardware available that you wish to use.
- The general counsel's office provides guidance on terms and conditions of contractual obligations, protection of data, and student information.

- The information technology (IT) help-desk personnel support faculty and students when they experience problems using the technology.
- Network technicians work to identify network infrastructure needs to support the technology and identify potential challenges due to infrastructure limitations and options to address limitations.
- Programmers and developers create applications to provide functionality needed to accomplish learning experience or add functionality to existing applications or electronic resources.
- Media production personnel generally encompass graphic design, photography, and video generation services.

Commitment

The commitment component of the four Cs of planning for implementation addresses the importance of ensuring those involved with your plan are committed to making it work. Success of technology integration requires commitment of those you are counting on for technical, administrative, and student learning support. Commitment stems from including stakeholders in all aspects of the planning and implementation process, formulating the overall goals and objectives as well as developing specific implementation plans.

Continuity

Technologies have a finite life cycle. What is new and innovative today is outdated and passé before we know it. Planning for implementation must take into account the technology's anticipated life cycle. Keeping current with updates and new versions maximize the life span of the technology you have worked so hard to integrate into your teaching activities. Continued collaboration with technology support personnel will provide an avenue to remain up to date and ensure your future students continue to benefit from the technology integration. However, at some point, the technology you are using will reach the end of its life span. Proactive planning for this eventuality will prepare you to re-engage in the selection process to identify more contemporary technologies to meet your needs.

Once implementation activities are complete, you are ready to put the technology to work in your teaching activities. Establishing a plan for assessing the impact of the technology will provide a means to collect data and make informed decisions regarding the need for modifications, either to the technology or how it is being used.

EVALUATION

Evaluation of the educational technology integration should take into account all aspects of the selection and implementation processes. Quantitative and qualitative data can be collected from stakeholders during and at the conclusion of the course to examine the degree of technology integration success. The matrix in Table 4–4 provides an example of evaluation items that can be used toward the end of the course. Formative data collection during the course can be as simple as asking students what is going

TABLE 4-4   Technology Integration Evaluation Matrix

	Stakeholders				
	Instructor	Students	Administrators	Instructional Support Personnel	Information Technology (IT) Support Personnel
The technology supported the instructional activity as expected.	X				
The right stakeholders were included in the technology selection process.	X	X	X	X	X
The calculation of the total cost of ownership was accurate.	X		X		
Effective instructional design of activities to optimize the technology features was achieved.	X	X		X	
Adequate preparation was in place to accommodate students with disabilities.	X	X			
Students had access to the necessary infrastructure and tools to effectively use the technology.	X	X			
Students were provided adequate training and preparation for using the technology.	X	X			
Legal terms and conditions for using the technology were acceptable (e.g., enough licenses were purchased)	X				
Instructor preparation and training resources for using the technology were adequate.	X				
The instructor engaged in sufficient practice before initial use of the technology.	X	X			
Adequate time was allocated for the process of purchasing the technology.	X		X		
Adequate time was allocated for obtaining copyright permissions.	X		X	X	
Adequate time was allocated for legal review of the technology.	X		X		
Adequate time was allocated for preparing to use the technology.	X				X
The network infrastructure was adequate to support the technology.	X				X
IT support personnel provided knowledgeable support.	X	X			
IT support personnel provided timely support.	X	X			

well, what is not going well, and what suggestions they have for change. As previously noted, technology is generally believed not to have a direct impact on student learning; rather, the changes in instructional methods that occur simultaneously with the addition of technology, novelty of the technology, and therefore increased student interest, or an increase in the efforts invested to design the instruction may affect learning outcomes. Therefore, evaluation of technologies must be careful not to suggest otherwise.

As Dr. Martinez prepares to reshape the research methods course she must identify the technologies to be used to create and deliver the mini lectures and accountability quizzes. She also wants to make sure she is accessible to students as this new course design model is implemented. To help with her planning, she uses tables to organize each of the components she must consider in selection (Table 4–5) and implementation (Table 4–6) of the technology.

PRIVACY AND DIGITAL CITIZENSHIP

Many technologies currently in use or on the verge of becoming a fixture in education can be categorized as either Web 1.0, Web 2.0, or Web 3.0 technologies. In contrast to Web 1.0, which only allows users to passively view content, Web 2.0 tools allow users to interact, collaborate, generate content, and engage in virtual community settings.[25] Web 2.0 tools are usually cloud based and available for free or at a low cost. Examples include wikis (Wikipedia), blogs (Twitter, Blogger), social networking sites (Facebook), and video-sharing sites (YouTube). Web 3.0, or the semantic web, is the next phase of the World Wide Web, which is predicted to be "smarter," capable of making connections between the user's online activities and automatically delivering relevant content to the user.[25] Web 3.0 is expected to help manage the deluge of information presented in results of online searches for information.

TABLE 4-5 Technology Selection for Research Methods for Health Care Providers

Step	Activity	Example
Stakeholders	Faculty members teaching other courses in the second year of the curriculum	Dr. Martinez wants to make sure her colleagues are aware of how she is reshaping the course and why she is doing so. She wants to learn from their experiences using technology. She will also be collecting data to gauge any changes in level of student preparation for spring semester courses in the PT2 year.
	Students: PT2 class officers will be part of Dr. Martinez planning and implementation team.	PT2 class officers will help Dr. Martinez understand students' readiness for using course technologies, help other students understand why the course is being redesigned, and help garner feedback from students.
	Instructional designer	Dr. Martinez has contacted the university's instructional designer team to seek advice and guidance in reshaping the courses. The designer assigned to work with Dr. Martinez will coordinate information flow and support services from the information technology personnel.
	Department chair	Dr. Martinez has informed the department chair about her course redesign plans and determined a small amount of funding is available to support her efforts.
Selection criteria	Compatibility with the university's learning management system	Students must be able to access the mini lectures and quizzes through the course's website in the university's learning management system.
	Alignment with cognitive theory of multimedia learning	Mini-lecture technologies must allow Dr. Martinez to provide an audio of the lecture that can be synchronized with visual aids, including PowerPoint slides containing key points and images. The technology must also allow Dr. Martinez to embed video clips and animations in her lecture.
	Self-grading quizzes using multiple-choice and short answer question types	For preclass quizzes
	Intuitive for students to use	Students should be able to access and use the technology with little or no training.
	Moderate amount of training for the instructor	Dr. Martinez is willing to devote a day or two to learning to use the technologies for creating the mini lectures and quizzes.
	Family Education Rights and Privacy Act (FERPA) compliant	Technology used to deliver and grade quizzes must be hosted in the university's data center to ensure compliance with FERPA regulations.
	Health Insurance Portability and Accountability Act (HIPAA) compliant	Mini lectures will contain references to actual clients and therefore contain information protected by HIPAA. As a result, the mini lectures must be housed in the university's data center to ensure compliance with HIPAA regulations.
	Mac and PC compatible	Students use both Mac and PC computers, so the technologies must run on both platforms.
	Compatible with computers in the student computer laboratory	The school has a student computer laboratory that is open 24 hours, 7 days per week during the semester. The mini lectures and quizzes must be able to run on the computers in the laboratory.
	Network support for high volume use of the mini lectures	Dr. Martinez expects that the mini lectures will be highly used in the days preceding an examination. Therefore, the university's network must be able to accommodate these spikes in use.
Identify potential technologies	Dr. Martinez contacts the stakeholders to invite them to be part of this project.	Contact each stakeholder and provide an outline of the project.
	Three meetings are planned with the stakeholders for this project.	*Meeting 1:* Overview of the project and selection criteria. Between meetings 1 and 2, stakeholders seek out potential technologies. *Meeting 2:* Overview of the potential technologies, including demonstrations from vendors or information technology (IT) personnel. Provide stakeholders access to technologies to allow them to explore the functionality offered by each. *Meeting 3:* Use selection criteria to rate potential technologies and identify the two or three that best fit the needs of the course.
Calculate total cost of ownership	IT personnel, instructional designers, student representative, and general counsel	Identify all aspects of costs associated with the technologies.
Select the technology	All stakeholders	Review ratings and total cost of ownership for each technology. Identify the technology that is the best value—the one that meets the needs of the course while aligning with the budget available to support the technology.

Although still in its infancy, Web 3.0 appears promising in its ability to help focus information presented on the Web to that which is most relevant.

With the introduction of technology into the educational environment, particularly social media and cloud computing tools, comes the responsibility on the part of faculty, administrators, support staff, and students to build awareness of legal implications and ethical practices in technology use. Cloud computing refers to the "practice of using a network of remote servers hosted on the Internet to store, manage, and process data, rather than a local server or personal computer."[26] Applications accessed through a Web browser are usually hosted in the cloud. Examples of cloud-based applications currently used in education include Google Docs for word processing, DimDim (Web meeting), Flickr for photo sharing, and

TABLE 4–6　Technology Implementation for Research Methods for Health Care Providers

Activity	Example
Securing licenses for the technology and ensuring compatibility	Dr. Martinez selected a lecture capture solution that records short lectures. The licensing allows her to run the software on one computer. She plans to download it onto her laptop provided by the university. Through the selection process, the information technology (IT) personnel determined the software was compatible with university's computing environment and Dr. Martinez's laptop.
Security of the lectures and data included in the lectures	The recorded lectures are saved to Dr. Martinez's laptop; she will then upload them to the server space she has obtained from campus IT. Dr. Martinez occasionally uses examples from actual patients (with their permission) during her lectures. By storing the recorded lectures on a server in the campus data center, Dr. Martinez is assured she is in compliance with Health Insurance Portability and Accountability Act (HIPAA) regulations for securing protected information.
Outline each module or lesson to identify how the technology will be used.	Dr. Martinez has the month of July to plan for the implementation of the technology. She is creating an outline of each course module, a PowerPoint for each lecture, and the quiz to accompany each lecture. Using the lecture capture technology, she will then record each lecture while sitting in her office. Each lecture will be no longer than 15 to 20 minutes. For training and guidance in creating the mini lectures, Dr. Martinez is working with a colleague at another institution that has experience with using recorded mini lectures as well as the instructional designer at her institution.
Contacting office of disabilities assistance	Before starting to record lectures, Dr. Martinez contacts the office of disabilities assistance to proactively plan for accommodations for students with disabilities.
Planning for student technology access	Dr. Martinez is working with campus IT to identify student computer laboratory resources for students who are not able to access the mini lectures and quizzes from home.
Coordinating with the IT help desk	The instructional designer working with Dr. Martinez has contacted the IT help desk to inform them about the technologies Dr. Martinez is using in her course and to ensure they understand the importance of students receiving timely assistance so they are able to prepare for class.
Editing course syllabus	Dr. Martinez is modifying her course syllabus to include explicit instructions for accessing the lectures and quizzes and a semester-long schedule for lecture availability dates and quiz completion deadlines. Also included will be information about HIPAA data security and the importance of limiting access to the lectures to only students enrolled in the course. The lectures cannot be downloaded, so storage will be limited to the campus data center.
Preparing students to use the technology	To ensure students are able to access the mini lectures and quizzes, Dr. Martinez will spend time during the first day of class demonstrating how to access the lectures and quizzes. She will also hand out instructions and place a copy of the instructions in the learning management system course website. The PT2 class officers have agreed to review and provide feedback on the first lecture and quiz as well as the instructions for accessing the lectures and quizzes Dr. Martinez is creating.
Backup plan for technology failure	If the lectures or quizzes are not available because of problems with the learning management system, the lecture capture technology, or other reasons, Dr. Martinez is prepared to provide the students copies of the lecture on DVD, and quizzes will be completed at the beginning of class on paper.
Grading for quizzes	The quizzes will account for a total of 20% of the students' overall course grade. Students are allowed to miss two quizzes during the semester without incurring a grade penalty.
Formative assessment of the technology and the teaching model	A formative assessment midway through the semester will be conducted. Dr. Martinez will be using a survey to gather feedback from students about their experience using the technology as well as their perceptions of the effectiveness of the teaching model being used for the course. The results of the formative assessment will be reported to the students along with plans to make any changes should the data indicate changes are needed.
Summative evaluation	A comparison of student grades for the course with those from previous semesters, and surveys to gather information from stakeholder groups will be conducted. The data will be reviewed before the next time the course is taught.

YouTube for video sharing. This type of technology provides faculty the autonomy to select and use technologies in their teaching without waiting for the myriad of "red tape" that can accompany institutionally purchased and hosted applications. Although cloud-based applications can help stretch the financial resources spent on technology as well as foster sharing and collaborative construction of knowledge, the types of information placed in cloud-based applications should be carefully considered. Because cloud-based applications are not housed in an institution's data center, the security of the data collected by these applications is not controlled by personnel responsible to the institution. Therefore, unintended and unrecognized violations of FERPA or of HIPAA can easily occur. Working with your institution's legal affairs or IT personnel to obtain guidance in the use of cloud-based applications is advised.

Social networking services are a specific type of cloud-based application designed to connect individuals who share common friendships, interests, and activities. Examples include Facebook, Twitter, and LinkedIn. Students' ubiquitous access to social networking services and the degree to which these have become assimilated into almost every aspect of students' daily life have created an environment ripe for misuse of technology. Students may have difficulty distinguishing between information that is appropriate and that which is inappropriate for sharing on social networks. As a result, *digital citizenship*, defined as "the norms of appropriate, responsible behavior with regard to technology use,"[27] has become a particularly important aspect of technology use in education. A concept that is of concern for educators around the world,[28] digital citizenship in the United States focuses on nine themes (Box 4–1).[27]

Students must be conversant with the ethics of technology use. Social networks such as Facebook have become the communication medium of choice for many students. Therefore, at times they post first and think later. For example, a student who had a particularly difficult day on a clinical rotation posts a "rant" to Facebook about an encounter with a patient using the patient's first name, referencing the patient's clinical diagnosis and the name of the clinical site. The student views this as venting to his friends, but the school or clinic sees it as a violation of HIPAA, which may lead to disciplinary action. Key considerations of digital citizenship within the context of physical therapy education include the following:

-   Ethical use of technology in the educational and clinical environments, including social networks, copyright infringement, plagiarism, and illegal downloading or sharing of music and other copyrighted materials
-   Ensuring students become fluent in the use of digital technologies to prepare them for the continued digitization of information and resources in health care environments, (e.g., electronic health records, professional journals, continuing education resources)
-   Ability to process information presented electronically and discern credible information from that which is not supported by trustworthy sources

Throughout the course of this chapter, we have examined many aspects of technology integration into the educational environment: a profile of the contemporary student; learning research as it applies to technology; student engagement; selection, implementation, and evaluation of technology; and privacy and digital citizenship. Next, application of these concepts is explored in the context of blended and online learning environments.

BLENDED LEARNING ENVIRONMENTS

The term *blended learning environment* refers to the integration of both face-to-face and online learning resources and activities within a course or program of study.[29] A commonly accepted definition of blended learning states that blended learning is a course in which 30% to 79% of the content or learning experiences are delivered online,

typically using online discussions, and having a decreased number of face-to-face meetings.[30] Dr. Martinez's reshaping of the research methods course is an example of a blended course.

Instructors choosing a blended approach to instruction typically do so for three reasons[29]:

1. Increased student learning potential
2. Increased convenience
3. Increased cost-effectiveness

Blended learning is often touted as the "best of both worlds." To fully realize the benefits of blended educational environments, however, instructors are encouraged to take a holistic approach, to reconsider the teaching and learning environment, and to examine how blending online and face to face can optimize the learning experience.[29] Convenience and cost-effectiveness should take a back seat to the transformational potential of blended learning. The description earlier in this chapter of reconsidering the time and space for teaching and learning is an example of a blended approach that has the potential of truly transforming the learning environment.

ONLINE LEARNING ENVIRONMENTS

In the Higher Education Opportunity Act,[31] the U.S. Department of Education defined online courses as those in which all or the vast majority (75% or more) of the instruction and interaction occurs through electronic communication or equivalent mechanisms, with the faculty and students physically separated from each other. Given the minimal level of face-to-face contact between instructors and students, designing and teaching online courses warrants some additional considerations beyond those previously discussed for technology integration into face-to-face and blended courses.

During the process of developing an online course, the instructor spends time reflecting on current pedagogical practices, reviewing materials used to teach the course, and discovering how these can be translated to the online classroom. Materials used in the face-to-face classroom cannot simply be copied into an online course. Instead, one must carefully architect student-student, student-content, and student-instructor interactions using tools and strategies designed for the online learner.

DEVELOPING COMMUNITY AMONG ONLINE LEARNERS

Community may be described as "a meaningful, association based on common interest and endeavor."[32] Effective learning in higher education requires the development of a community of learners that supports meaningful inquiry.[33] Furthermore, students who feel part of a community tend to have a higher persistence rate.[34] Development of community among online learners can be successfully facilitated using the Community of Inquiry model.[32] Comprising three interlocking elements (Figure 4-5)—social presence, teaching presence, and cognitive presence—the Community of Inquiry model presents a theoretical framework of online learning effectiveness.

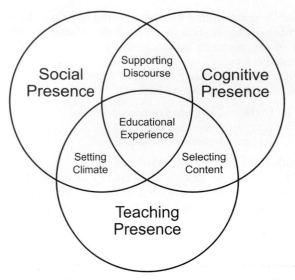

FIGURE 4–5   The Community of Inquiry model. (From McMillan DW, Chavis DM. Sense of community: a definition and theory. J Community Psychol 1986;14:6-23.)

Social Presence

Social presence is the degree to which students feel socially and emotionally connected.[35] Development of social presence requires a trusting environment in which students feel they are able to project their individual personalities and forge relationships with other students and the instructor. Online instructors can use a variety of strategies to foster the development of social presence, including establishing online etiquette (*netiquette*) standards for the class to create an environment in which students feel safe.[35]

To prevent or minimize misunderstandings among course participants and to promote respect of each other's work and contribution to the course, students should be aware of some basic, commonly accepted netiquette rules. Virginia Shea's book, *Netiquette*, and its related website, Netiquette Home Page,[36] are excellent sources of netiquette information. The core rules of netiquette as identified by Shea can be found in Box 4–2. Descriptions and examples of each rule, as well as a netiquette quiz, are available on the website.

Social presence is further developed by sharing feelings (e.g., inquire how others are doing), addressing students by name, using inclusive pronouns (we, us, our), and

---

BOX 4–2   Virginia Shea's Core Rules of Netiquette

- Rule 1: Remember the human being.
- Rule 2: Adhere to the same standard of behavior online that you follow in real life.
- Rule 3: Know where you are in cyberspace.
- Rule 4: Respect other people's time and bandwidth.
- Rule 5: Make yourself look good online.
- Rule 6: Share expert knowledge.
- Rule 7: Help keep flame wars under control.
- Rule 8: Respect other people's privacy.
- Rule 9: Don't abuse your power.
- Rule 10: Be forgiving of other people's mistakes.

BOX 4–3   Tips for Helping Students Learn to Work with Others Online

Educational experiences for most students have been predominantly lecture based in a face-to-face setting.[37] Instructors can help students acclimate to the online environment through a phased approach, gradually scaffolding students' level of engagement throughout the duration of the course.[36] Following is an example of such an approach.[36]

- During the first 1 to 2 weeks of the course, the instructor provides interactive activities that help learners get to know one another (e.g., students are requested to introduce themselves to each other, discussions are held to establish rules of engagement for the course).
- During the next 1 to 2 weeks, dyads of learners are created by the instructor, and activities requiring critical thinking, reflection, and sharing of ideas are assigned (e.g., discussion of assigned readings, peer review of assignments).
- Activities are assigned requiring small groups of students to collaborate, solve problems, and reflect on experiences during weeks 5 to 6 of a 15- to 16-week semester (e.g., discussion and debate of the course concepts, begin work on small group projects).
- During the later part of the course, students are ready for activities that are learner designed or learner led. Students take a more active role in setting the direction for discussions and interactions. The instructor participates as needed to correct misperceptions, refocus discussions that are veering off track, summarize discussions which are concluding, launch new conversations about course concepts, and provide feedback on projects (e.g., in-depth discussions, group project work advances, students bring forward their own ideas for projects).

---

employing an informal, conversational writing style.[35] Praising student work and their contributions to the course lets them know someone is paying attention; a human being is actually on the receiving end of their communication. Moreover, online instructors must be prepared to help students learn how to work with others online (Box 4–3).[38]

In addition to incorporating a stepwise approach to preparing students for working in the online environment, instructor immediacy has been shown to have a significant impact on developing a sense of community.[39-41] *Instructor immediacy* refers to the nonverbal behaviors that reduce physical or psychological distance between instructor and students.[41] Informal writing style and using students' first names and inclusive pronouns can promote immediacy. When immediacy of communication increases and formality decreases, social presence is amplified.[41,42]

Instructors must help students find the right mix of professionalism and informality to develop social presence. Students report that meeting face to face at the beginning of a class helps develop community among the student cohort.[39] However, if this is not possible, instructors are urged to consider using technologies that may provide a similar opportunity to jump-start development of community, such as Web conferencing.

Although a wide variety of communications tools are available for use in online courses, engagement of students in this environment has historically been accomplished through text-based discussion boards, e-mail, and text chat. These communication mechanisms take more time than face-to-face communication and pose a greater risk for misinterpretation. The limitations of text-based communications may be mitigated through the use multimedia and emerging technologies such as wikis, blogs, Web conferencing, and social networking tools.[43,44]

Teaching Presence

Teaching presence is defined as the "design, facilitation, and direction of cognitive and social processes for the purpose of realizing personally meaningful and educationally worthwhile learning outcomes."[33] Encompassing three components, teaching presence includes instructional design and organization, facilitating discourse, and direct instruction.

The instructional design and organization aspect of teaching presence includes "planning and design of the structure, processes, interaction, and evaluation aspects of the online course."[45] The design of an online course plays a critical role in its success and requires careful consideration of the activities and spaces to be used to develop community.[46] The following instructional design and organization considerations are presented as a means to help instructors plan for the design or their online course.

Instructional Design Teams

Historically, instructional design has been the component of teaching presence most likely to be performed exclusively by the instructor.[47] However, the growth of online education has been accompanied by an unbundling of faculty roles,[48] and instructional design is becoming a shared activity often performed by a team consisting of an instructional designer, faculty member as the content expert, and others as dictated by the needs of the course.[49] If instructional designers or other assistance is not available, faculty members are urged to seek out colleagues who are effective online instructors, faculty development seminars, and online instructional design literature. The culture shift required to form successful instructional design teams should not be overlooked.[50] The transition from putting a course together independently, in which the processes and time table are the purview of the instructor, to working within a team structure can result in feelings of tension and loss of locus of control.[51] Faculty may find the transition less troublesome if they approach it as an opportunity to become more aware their teaching and to try new approaches with a team supporting the effort.

Course Organization

A well-organized course structure employing a consistent layout is critical to the success of an online course.[52] Consistency in course layout allows students to maximize their focus on learning and minimize the time spent figuring out how to navigate the online course environment. Some pragmatic considerations of design consistence include the following:

1. Keeping due dates the same each week
2. Maintaining the same course layout among all course modules, including the location and structure of learning materials and location for student submission of assignments
3. Keeping consistent office hours during which distance students are able to reach you[53]

Explicitness

One of the most frustrating aspects of an online course for students, as well as instructors, is confusion about the course's administrative processes (e.g., due dates, turning

---

> **BOX 4–4   Basics of an Online Course Syllabus**
>
> 1. A policy on late assignments
> 2. Time-zone-based due dates and times for all assignments,
> 3. Virtual office hours
> 4. Instructor response time expectations
> 5. Writing style expectations (e.g., degree of formality for various writing activities)
> 6. Technologies to be used in the class, how to access them, and resources for training
> 7. E-mail format guidelines (e.g., subject line)
> 8. File types acceptable for assignment submission
> 9. Technical and administrative support contact information
> 10. A suggested sequence for each week's or each module's activity
> 11. Expectations for participation (frequency, netiquette)
> 12. Suggestions for effective participation
>
> Data from Paloff RM, Pratt K. Building Online Learning Communities: Effective Strategies for the Virtual Classroom. San Francisco: Jossey-Bass, 2007; Ko S, Rossen S. Teaching Online: A Practical Guide. New York: Routledge, 2010; Smith RM. Conquering the Content: A Step-by-Step Guide to Online Course Design. San Francisco: Jossey-Bass, 2008.

---

in assignments, contacting the instructor). Course management tasks that are easily accomplished in the face-to-face classroom during class must be clearly defined in writing for the online students. A well-designed syllabus for an online course will provide the structure and information needed to mitigate confusion.[50]

In addition to a course description, learning objectives, grading scale, and other syllabus components that may be required by a department or program, a syllabus for an online course should include all of the elements discussed in Box 4–4.

In addition to instructional design, development of a sense of teaching presence among online learners requires effective facilitation of discourse, with focused and sustained deliberation.[54] As with online course instructional design, promoting discourse in the online environment requires specialized knowledge and skills that may be new to many online instructors. The following guidelines are designed to help you master the art and science of facilitating discourse among online learners[37,38,49]:

- Don't drop out. Students notice when the instructor disappears. If you will be traveling or out of touch for more than a day or two, let students know.
- Keep an eye out for marginalization. Sometimes, group dynamics cause certain students to be marginalized. Their comments go disregarded; their posts are not responded to. Bring them into the fold, with a comment or question aimed to bring others to respond to them. On the same note, make sure the instructor does not fall into a trap, regularly engaging with the same students time and again and not relating to others.
- Don't be the first to respond. As a rule, try to avoid being the first to respond to a student's primary post. This can cut off or narrow the scope of the conversation that students might have developed. It is often better to rechannel, a little later on after discussion has developed, than to channel and limit ahead of time.
- Review discussions frequently to ensure the students are on track, and redirect the discussion if needed.

- Questions are better than comments. An instructor's comment can effectively end a discussion thread, no matter how lively. A comment with a question at the end can keep it going. Try to always include questions in your posts.
- Do not respond to each student's posting, the discussion will become a conversation between the instructor and each student.
- At the end of every week or every thread, summarize the discussion themes, adding an insight or two, connecting it to next week's material, and inviting students to add their own comments.
- Establish beginning and end dates for each discussion.
- Early in the course, praise and encourage postings; the need to do so decreases as students become comfortable with the discussion environment.
- Encourage concise, thoughtful responses.
- Establish a schedule for managing the discussion, then hang a sign on your office door that states you are "in class" during the time set aside for doing so.
- Establish a discussion board strictly for questions so that off-topic questions don't make their way into weekly discussion forums.

Direct Instruction

The direct instruction component of teaching presence encompasses many of the strategies addressed within the context of social presence and facilitating discourse. Direct instruction consists of the instructor serving as the subject matter expert through the presentation of content, summarizing discussions and injecting relevant information, assessing student work and providing feedback, identifying and correcting misperceptions, and using personal experiences to illustrate concepts and content.

Cognitive Presence

Cognitive presence has been defined as the "extent to which learners are able to construct and confirm meaning through sustained reflection and discourse in a critical community of inquiry."[33] Development of cognitive presence leverages many of the strategies employed within the contexts of social and teaching presences to guide students through the phases of practical inquiry: a triggering event, exploration, integration or meaning construction, and resolution.[40] Table 4–7 summarizes the phases of practical inquiry.

Using the Community of Inquiry model's three components as a framework for building an online course will provide a strong foundation on which to facilitate student learning as well as increase the likelihood of student persistence and success. Creation of a successful online learning community requires examination of traditional instructional practices and careful, thoughtful adoption of proven strategies to effectively engage and advance learning in this relatively new setting.

Regardless of the teaching environment (online, blended, or face to face), the infusion of technology allows for increased flexibility in structuring learning resources and activities, raising the level of student engagement, and extending student access to learning resources. This process of integrating technology into a course is rich with opportunities for scholarly examination of the processes and outcomes.

TABLE 4–7   Practical Inquiry Phases

Phase	Description
Triggering event	Piquing students' curiosity with a learning challenge, issue, problem, or dilemma arising during discourse or via an assignment. As a result, students are motivated to explore the content further.
Exploration	Students gain an understanding of the nature of the problem through critical reflection and discourse. Online discussions are frequently used as a means to help students appreciate different perspectives related to the problem.
Integration and meaning construction	Students construct meaning from ideas and information gained in the exploration phase. The instructor identifies misperceptions, asks probing questions, and provides additional information for the purpose of moving students from exploration to critically thinking about problem. Students combine pieces of new information to construct explanations and solutions.
Resolution	Students engage in authentic application of new knowledge and apply knowledge created during the course to the non-class-related activities, including the practice environment.

SCHOLARLY INVESTIGATION OF TECHNOLOGY INTEGRATION

Advancing teaching practices, including the use of educational technologies, by investigating student learning in a scholarly manner and making the results public is part of a rapidly growing movement, namely the scholarship of teaching and learning (SoTL).[55] The ubiquitous presence of technology in today's teaching and learning environments, coupled with the financial and human resources allocated to supporting these technologies, makes scholarly investigation of student learning outcomes in technology-infused learning experiences imperative. It is the responsibility of instructors and administrators to ensure the efforts devoted to educational technology are truly helping to advance student learning.

SoTL research typically includes qualitative data-collection methods such as case studies, interviews, focus groups, observations, and quasi-experiments.[56] Dissemination of findings may be accomplished in SoTL-focused journals such as the *Journal of the Scholarship of Teaching and Learning* (JoSOTL) or the *International Journal for the Scholarship of Teaching and Learning*. Additionally, findings may be promulgated through discipline-specific publications and scholarly presentations. Appendix 4-A contains several resources to support SoTL work.

SUMMARY

The ever-changing landscape of technology presents a myriad of opportunities for enhancing students' educational experiences. Face-to-face, blended, and online learning environments each offer unique opportunities for leveraging technology to increase student engagement and create meaningful learning experiences. Regardless of the educational setting or the type of technology used, learning outcomes and learning theory must underpin the selection and implementation of educational technologies. Cognitive load theory, the theory of multimedia learning, and the community of inquiry framework provide key factors critical for ensuring technology adoption is centered on student learning.

Given the rapid and ongoing changes in the educational technology landscape, any discussion of specific technology applications risks obsolesce by the time this book goes to press. However, instructors should not fall prey to paralysis by analysis, waiting to find out what will be released next month or next year before making the decision to integrate technology into the classroom. Using the selection and preparation processes described in this chapter will allow educators to employ educational technologies in a manner that is both effective and sustainable. Employing the four Cs of technology planning and the National Educational Technology Standards for instructors and administrators helps ensure successful technology integration. Accompanying the addition of technology to teaching and learning settings is the responsibility to ensure privacy of student and patient information and to prepare students to be good digital citizens. Web 2.0 and 3.0 technologies increase the availability of interactive, flexible technologies but also present significant risk for the unanticipated exposure of confidential information.

As instructors incorporate educational technologies into their toolbox of teaching strategies, they are encouraged to consider engaging in scholarly examination of the outcomes. The amount of resources expended to incorporate any educational technologies warrants investigation of the results to ensure effective and efficient allocation of time, talent, and treasure.

THRESHOLD CONCEPTS

Threshold Concept #1: Good teaching is good teaching. This chapter began with a quote from Steven Ehrmann, "If you are headed in the wrong direction, technology will not get you to the right place." In other words, the addition of technology will not 'fix' poor teaching. Effective teaching practices are applicable regardless of the venue or tools used in the teaching and learning process. One of the challenges faced by instructors seeking to either integrate technology into a classroom setting or to move their class online is the tendency to focus on the technology and abandon effective teaching strategies.

Successful instructors know they must encourage active learning, provide prompt and meaningful feedback, encourage frequent contact among students and instructors, help students work collaboratively, set high expectations for their students, provide student multiple means to learn and demonstrate their learning, and emphasize the important of staying on task and learning to use time wisely. When technology is introduced into the teaching and learning environment, or when a course is translated for the online classroom, instructors must carefully and intentionally identify the ways in which they will assure the principles for good teaching are driving the use of technology. This can be accomplished by:

A. Routinely conducting formative assessments throughout the semester, ask students to provide feedback regarding the use of principles for good teaching. This can be done through anonymous surveys of students or focus groups of students.
B. Compare the formative assessment results to feedback received from your students in courses taught without the technology or in courses taught in a face-to-face classroom.
C. Ask a colleague who is recognized as an effective teacher to conduct a peer observation of your course using Chickering and Gamson's 7 Principles for Good Education as a framework.
D. Periodic self-assessment. The instructor can periodically review the principles for good teaching and rate the degree to which she is adhering to the principles.

Threshold Concept #2: Successful integration of technology in teaching and learning requires the involvement of a wide variety of stakeholders. Instructors who have successfully incorporated a new technology into their teaching repertoire realize the involvement of stakeholders is crucial to this success. They cannot imagine planning for the addition of a technology without seeking the collaboration of everyone from the IT hardware/software support folks to the individuals who can assist with assessing the impact on student learning.

An instructor can certainly acquire and use a technology in her/his teaching without the involvement of the budget personnel, the purchasing department, the IT network team, the IT student support folks, and others. However, without the collaboration of these and several other stakeholders, the instructor risks unexpected interruption in the technology functionality. Including relevant stakeholders in the technology integration process helps assure the new technology will not exist just on the periphery of the teaching and learning environment; but will be recognized by the institution as a teaching tool and therefore supported as such. The four Cs of Implementation (starting on page 69 of this chapter) highlight the value of stakeholder planning.

ANNOTATED BIBLIOGRAPHY

Clark RC, Mayer RE. *E-Learning and the science of instruction: proven guidelines for consumers and designers of multimedia learning.* San Francisco: John Wiley; 2003.

Clark and Mayer team up to provide well-reasoned principles and concrete examples for designing multimedia learning experiences underpinned by sound research on student learning. The first two chapters summarize the science behind how people learn. Each subsequent chapter describes an instructional design principle in easy-to-understand language, includes illustrations of the principle in action, and concludes with a useful checklist of the principle's key design elements.

Ko S, Rossen S. *Teaching Online: A Practical Guide.* New York: Routledge; 2010.

This book is an essential read for faculty new, or relatively new, to teaching online. In its third edition, *Teaching Online* is full of advice and practical examples grounded by proven best practices for teaching online. Part 1 helps the reader take inventory of his/her readiness to teach online as well as institutional resources available to support the endeavor. Part 2 walks the reader through the process of putting together an online course. Part 3 provides no-nonsense suggestions for teaching in the online classroom. Preparing students to be online learners, facilitating student learning in the online environment, classroom management, and blended courses are addressed. This easy-to-read reference is a valuable addition to your personal library. Novak G, Gavrin A, Christian W, Patterson E. *Just-in-Time Teaching: Blending Active Learning with Web Technology.* Upper Saddle River, NJ: Prentice Hall; 1999.

This book is designed to serve as a getting-started guide as well as a resource book for instructors seeking to leverage a blended approach to their teaching. Preclass assessments of students' comprehension of web-based assignments are used to structure in-class time with students. Classroom time is spent on learning activities to help students master and apply course concepts. Sections One (Strategy) and Two (Implementation) provide the framework needed to implement the Just in Time Teaching strategy in almost any subject or discipline. Section Three includes resources that are specific to the study of physics; however. application to other disciplines is apparent.

Select journals are relevant to educational technology, blended learning, and online courses. Given the ever-changing nature of the educational technology landscape, providing a selection of journals in lieu of additional book annotations will provide readers with a set of resources to help them remain current in this area. The University of Wisconsin-Madison maintains a listing of distance education/education technology focused journals at www.wisc.edu/depd/html/mags3.htm.

Journals not requiring a fee-based subscription:

Educational Technology and Society is an online, peer-reviewed journal published by the International Forum of Educational Technology and Society. The journal's broad purpose is to help educators use technology to enhance individual learning as well as to increase access to education. Additionally, the journal seeks to help align developers and researchers in the area of educational technology with the needs and requirements of typical teachers. Available at: www.ifets.info/others/.

EDUCAUSE Quarterly (EQ) is an online, peer-reviewed journal from Educause focused on the use of technology in higher education environments. Articles are generally focused on practical issues and applications of technology. EQ's online format includes graphics, live links, audio, and video as well as tools to connect readers with each other and professionals in the field of educational technology. Available at: www.educause.edu/eq/about.

EDUCAUSE Review examines current developments and trends of technology in the higher education environment and implications of these trends at the institutional level as well as for higher education in general. Both *Educause Quarterly* and *Educause Review* are publications of the Educause organization, whose purpose is to advance higher education by promoting the intelligent use of information technology. In addition to the journals, the Educause website provides a wealth of information about technology and higher education. Available at: www.educause.edu/er/about.

International Review of Research in Open and Distance Learning (IRRODL) disseminates scholarly knowledge in open and distance learning theory, research, and best practice to distance education practitioners and scholars. The referred e-journal is published by Athabasca University. Available at: www.irrodl.org/index.php/irrodl.

Online Journal of Distance Learning Administration is a peer-reviewed electronic journal published by the State University of West Georgia. Authors are generally practitioners and researchers, and articles focus on implications for the management of distance education programs. Information provided in the journal is pragmatic and should be of interest to novice and experienced users of educational technology. Available at: www.westga.edu/~distance/jmain11.html.

Journals not requiring a fee-based subscription:.

American Journal of Distance Education (AJDE) is a peer-reviewed journal of research and scholarship in the field of American distance education. Currently, the journal's focus is on research related to the World Wide Web, on-line learning, e-learning, distributed learning, asynchronous learning, and blended learning. Specifically, articles report on findings in areas such as (1) building and sustaining effective delivery systems, (2) course design and application of instructional design theories, (3) facilitating interaction between students and with instructors, (4) factors influencing student achievement and satisfaction, (5) the changing roles of faculty and changes in institutional culture, and (6) administrative and policy issues including cost-effectiveness and copyright. Available at: www.ajde.com.

Educational Technology Research and Development is a bimonthly, peer-reviewed publication of the Association for Educational Communications and Technology. The journal includes rigorously documented articles of research studies and applied theory on the use of educational technology as well as the design and development of learning systems. Each issue also includes reviews of books relevant to the field. Available at: www.springer.com/education+%26+language/learning+%26+instruction/journal/11423.

The Internet and Higher Education is a peer-reviewed journal published quarterly that addressed contemporary issues and anticipated future developments related to online learning, teaching, and administration on the Internet in postsecondary settings. The journal's broad scope encompasses innovations or best practices in online teaching, learning, management, and administration. Available at: http://www.journals.elsevier.com/the-internet-and-higher-education/.

Journal of Asynchronous Learning Networks (JALN, a publication of the Sloan Consortium) publishes original work describing research-related to asynchronous learning networks (ALN), including online and blended learning environments. Articles provide practical information, backed by data, about best practices for teaching in the online environment. Submissions are double-blind peer-reviewed and articles containing quantitative data are encouraged. Available at: http://sloanconsortium.org/publications/jaln_main.

REFERENCES

1. Johnson L, Levine A, Smith R, Stone S. *The 2010 Horizon Report.* Austin, TX: The New Media Consortium; 2010.
2. Smith SD, Caruso JB. *The ECAR study of undergraduate students and information technology, 2010.* Educause Center for Applied Research; 2010. Available at: http://net.educause.edu/ir/library/pdf/EKF/EKF1006.pdf. Accessed 10.05.2011.
3. Januszewski A, Molenda M, eds. *Educational Technology: A Definition with Commentary.* Association for Educational Communications and Technology; 2004. Available at: *http://www.aect.org/publications/Educational Technology/* Accessed 2.05.2011.
4. *Professors' use of technology in teaching. Chronicle of Higher Education.* Available at: http://chronicle.com/article/Professors-Use-of/123682/; July 25, 2010 Accessed 15.05.2011.
5. Ensminger DC, Surry DW, Porter BE, Wright D. Factors contributing to the successful implementation of technology innovations. *Educ Technol Soc.* 2004;7:61–72.
6. Moser FZ. Faculty adoption of educational technology. *Educause Q.* 2007;1:66–69.
7. Prensky M. Digital natives, digital immigrants. *On the Horizon* 2001;9(5) Available at: http://www.marcprensky.com/writing/Prensky%20-%20Digital%20Natives,%20Digital%20Immigrants%20-%20Part1.pdf. Accessed 1.06.2011.
8. International Society for Technology in Education. National Educational Technology Standards Project. Available at: http://cnets.iste.org; 2001. Accessed 23.05.2011.
9. Clark RE. Confounding in educational computing research. *J Educ Comput Res.* 1985;1:137–148.
10. Clark RE. Media will never influence learning. *Educ Technol Res Dev.* 1994;42:21–29.
11. Clark RE, Salomon G. Media in teaching. In: Wittrock M, ed. *Third Handbook of Research on Teaching.* Chicago: Randy McNally; 1986:464–478.
12. Cobb T. Cognitive efficiency: toward a revised theory of media. *Educ Technol Res Dev.* 1997;45:21–35.
13. Kozrna RB. Learning with media. *Rev Educ Res.* 1991;6:179–211.
14. Kozma RB. Will media influence learning? Reframing the debate. *Educ Technol Res Dev.* 1994;42:7–19.
15. Ullmer EJ. Media and learning: are there two kinds of truth? *Educ Technol Res Dev.* 1994;42:21–32.
16. Sweller J. Cognitive load theory, learning difficulty, and instructional design. *Learn Instruct.* 1994;4:295–312.
17. Paivio A. Dual coding theory: retrospect and current status. *Can J Psychol Rev.* 1991;45:255–287.
18. Mayer RE, Moreno R. Nine ways to reduce cognitive load in multimedia learning. In: Bruning R, Horn C, PytlikZillig L, eds. *Web-based Learning: What Do We Know? Where Do We Go?.* Greenwich, CT: Information Age Publishing; 2003:23–44.

19. Clark RC, Mayer RE. *E-learning and the science of instruction: proven guidelines for consumers and designers of multimedia learning.* San Francisco: John Wiley; 2003.
20. Chickering AW, Gamson ZF. Seven Principles for Good Practice in Undergraduate Education. *AAHE Bulletin.* 1987;39(7):3–7.
21. Chickering A, Ehrmann S. Implementing the seven principles: technology as lever. *AAHE Bull.* 1996;49:3–6.
22. Novak G, Gavrin A, Christian W, Patterson E. *Just-in-Time Teaching: Blending Active Learning with Web Technology.* Upper Saddle River, NJ: Prentice Hall; 1999.
23. Lambert S, Williams R. *A model for selecting educational technologies to improve student learning.* Paper presented at HERDSA Annual International Conference, Melbourne, Australia; July 1999:3.
24. Steathelm HH. Common elements in the planning process. In: Carlson RV, Awkerman G, eds. *Education Planning: Concepts, Strategies and Practices.* New York: Longman; 1991:267–278.
25. Wahlster W, Dengel A. *Web 3.0: Convergence of Web 2.0 and the Semantic Web. Technology Radar, Volume: II.* Berlin, Germany: German Research Center for Artificial Intelligence (DFKI). Available at: http://www.mendeley.com/research/web-30-convergence-of-web-20-and-the-semantic-web/; Accessed on 22.05.2011.
26. *Cloud Computing* [Web page]. Wikipedia website. Available at: http://en.wikipedia.org/wiki/Cloud_computing; Accessed 24.05.2011.
27. Ribble M. *Digital Citizenship: Using Technology Appropriately* [homepage]. Available at: http://www.digitalcitizenship.net/Home_Page.html; Accessed 5.04.2011.
28. O'Brien T. Creating better digital citizens. *Aust Educ Leader* 2010;32(2).
29. Graham CR. Blended learning systems: definition, current trends, and future directions. In: Bonk CJ, Graham CR, eds. *Handbook of Blended Learning: Global Perspectives, Local Designs.* San Francisco: Pfeiffer; 2006:3–21.
30. Allen IE, Seaman J. *Class differences: online education in the United States 2010.* Available at: http://sloanconsortium.org/sites/default/files/class_differences.pdf; Accessed 22.05.2011.
31. U.S. Department of Education. *Higher Education Opportunity Act (Public Law 110-315).* Washington, DC: National Academy Press; 2008. Available at:http://www2.ed.gov/policy/highered/leg/hea08/index.html Accessed 8.04.2011.
32. McMillan DW, Chavis DM. Sense of community: a definition and theory. *J Community Psychol.* 1986;14:16–23.
33. Garrison DR, Arbaugh JB. Researching the community of inquiry framework: review, issues, and future directions. *Internet Higher Educ.* 2007;10:157–172.
34. Tinto V. Dropout from higher education: a theoretical synthesis of recent research. *Rev Educ Res.* 1975;45:89–125.
35. Lehman RM, Conceicao SCO. *Creating a Sense of Presence in Online Teaching: How to "Be There" for Distance Learners.* San Francisco: Jossey-Bass; 2010.
36. Shea V. *Netiquette.* San Francisco: Albion Books; 1994.
37. Conrad RM, Donaldson JA. *Engaging the Online Learner.* San Francisco: Jossey-Bass; 2004.
38. Paloff RM, Pratt K. *Building online learning communities: Effective strategies for the virtual classroom.* San Francisco: Jossey-Bass; 2007.
39. Conrad D. Building and maintaining community in cohort-based online learning. *J Distance Educ.* 2005;20:1–20.
40. Rovai AP. A preliminary look at the structural differences of higher education classroom communities in traditional and ALN courses. *J Asynchron Learn Netw.* 2002;6:41–56.
41. Arbaugh JB, Cleveland-Innes M, Diaz SR, et al. Developing a community of inquiry instrument: testing a measure of the Community of Inquiry framework using a multi-institutional sample. *Internet Higher Educ.* 2008;11:133–136.
42. Tu C, McIsaac M. The relationship of social presence and interaction in online classes. *Am J Distance Educ.* 2002;16:131–150.
43. Beldarrain Y. Trends: integrating new technologies to foster student interaction and collaboration. *Distance Educ.* 2006;27:139–153.
44. Nippard E, Murphy E. Social presence in the web-based synchronous secondary classroom. *Can J Learn Technol* 2007;33(1): Available at: http://www.cjlt.ca/index.php/cjlt/article/viewArticle/24/22 Accessed 10.11.2011.
45. Anderson T, Rourke L, Garrison DR, Archer W. Assessing teaching presence in a computer conferencing context. *J Asynchron Learn Netw.* 2001;5(2).
46. Stodel EJ, Thompson TL, MacDonald CJ. Learner's perspectives about what is missing from online courses. *Int Rev Open Distance Learn.* 2006;7(3).
47. Naidu S. Designing instruction for elearning environments. In: Moore MG, Anderson WG, eds. *Handbook of Distance Education.* Mahwah, NJ: Lawrence Erlbaum; 2003.
48. Neely PW, Tucker JP. Unbundling faculty roles in online distance education programs. *Int Rev Res Open Distance Learn.* 2010;11(2).
49. Shea PJ, Frederickson EE, Pickett AM, Pelz WE. A preliminary investigation of "teaching presence" in the SUNY learning network. In: Bourne J, Moore JC, eds. *Elements of Quality Online Education: Practice Direction.* Needham, MA: Sloan Center for Online Education; 2003:279–312. Sloan C Series 4.
50. Ko S, Rossen S. *Teaching Online: A Practical Guide.* New York: Routledge; 2010.
51. Boettchner JV, Conrad RM. *Faculty Guide for Moving Teaching and Learning to the Web.* Phoenix, AZ: League for Innovation in the Community College; 2004.
52. Swan K. Learning effectiveness: what the research tells us. In: Bourne J, Moore JC, eds. *Elements of Quality Online Education: Practice and Direction.* Needham, MA: Sloan Center for Online Education; 2004:13–45. Sloan C Series 4.
53. Smith RM. *Conquering the Content: A Step-by-Step Guide to Online Course Design.* San Francisco: Jossey-Bass; 2008.
54. Anderson T, Rourke L, Garrison DR, Archer W. Assessing teaching presence in a computer conferencing context. *J Asynchron Learn Netw* 2001;5(2).
55. Bass R. Scholarship of Teaching: What Is the Problem? *Creat Think Learn Teach* 1999;1(1) Available at: http://doit.gmu.edu//Archives/feb98/rbass.htm Accessed 10.11.2011.
56. International Society for the Scholarship of Teaching and Learning (ISSOTL). Available at: http://www.issotl.org/; Accessed 10.11.2011.

APPENDIX 4-A SCHOLARSHIP OF TEACHING AND LEARNING RESOURCES

- *Journal of the Scholarship of Teaching and Learning* (JoSOTL): https://www.iupui.edu/~josotl/
- The International Society for the Scholarship of Teaching & Learning (ISSOTL): http://www.issotl.org/
- *Transformative Dialogues: Teaching and Learning Journal:* http://kwantlen.ca/TD.html
- *International Journal for the Scholarship of Teaching and Learning:* http://academics.georgiasouthern.edu/ijsotl/index.htm
- Illinois State Univ SoTL website: http://sotl.illinoisstate.edu/
- Carnegie Foundation for the Advancement of Teaching: http://www.carnegiefoundation.org/scholarship-teaching-learning
- Carnegie Foundation's Knowledge Media Laboratory: http://www.carnegiefoundation.org/previous-work/knowledge-media-lab
- Indiana Univ SoTL website: http://citl.indiana.edu/programs/sotl/index.php
- Visible Knowledge Project and Index: https://commons.georgetown.edu/blogs/vkp/
- Univ of Wisconsin System SoTL website: http://www4.uwm.edu/sotl

ASSESSING AND IMPROVING THE TEACHING AND LEARNING PROCESSES IN ACADEMIC SETTINGS

Brenda M. Coppard ☉ Gail M. Jensen

CHAPTER OUTLINE

Did you ever express or hear comments like these?

Well, you have to be careful about putting too much time into your teaching. Good teaching takes time away from the things you need to do to get tenure and promotion at this institution. What really matters are research, grant writing, and publications.

Isn't program assessment the function of the curriculum committee? Besides, I was hired as a neuroscientist, not an educator. I know what the students need to know; that's why I need one more semester hour in my course to cover the material. Whatever you do, don't volunteer for the self-study task force; leave those accreditation activities to the educators. Sure, I evaluate my course. All students fill out an evaluation form the last day of class. I have good assessment data for my teaching, just look at my final student grades. They all achieved the learning outcomes as demonstrated by their grades.

Assessment techniques are used to assess one's teaching with the goal of improving student learning (curriculum) and the overall program. Essentially, there are two types of assessments: student learning outcomes and program effectiveness.[1] Assessment helps answer the question, How well do we do what we say we're going to do? Classroom educators purposefully focus on designing, evaluating, and revising the particular courses they teach. Intent on the subject matter they teach, educators often disconnect their teaching roles from the ongoing assessment and thoughtful scholarship of how their teaching actually influences student knowledge, understanding, attitudes, values, and behaviors. In this chapter, we explore practical mechanisms and tools that all educator-scholars can use for assessment and improvement of their teaching and resultant improvement in student learning.

LEARNING GOALS

After completing this chapter, the reader will be able to:

1. Define and give examples of the three main learning problems that students experience: amnesia, fantasia, and inertia.
2. Distinguish between assessment and evaluation.
3. Describe the relationships between assessment and student learning across educational settings, including classroom, program, and institution.
4. Identify the four pillars of transformative assessment and describe how and why they undergird program assessment activities.
5. Articulate principles of best practice for assessing student learning, including didactic and clinical student learning and performance, professional behaviors, and clinical reasoning.
6. Recognize the utility of the Teaching Goals Inventory and its relationship with the preactive teaching grid. (See Appendix 5-A.)
7. Describe processes that are intended to improve teaching: classroom assessment techniques (CATs), small group instructional diagnosis (SGID), quality circles, peer coaching, and end of course student ratings.
8. Describe how curriculum mapping can provide an alignment structure for the assessment process.
9. Distinguish between scholarly teaching and scholarship of teaching.

ASSESSMENT

What is assessment? Is it that periodic bother that comes once every so many years when a program goes through a self-study and accreditation process? Is it the course evaluations that students fill out at the end of the semester? Is it a formal program review that institutions and regional accreditors require of each department or program every few years or when a new president or provost is hired? Is it collecting data from graduates and alumni? Assessment pertains to all of these major activities. But notice that all these activities are summative—that is, they occur *after* a teaching-learning experience has been completed. However, formative assessment activities, which occur *during* a teaching-learning experience, have equal or more importance in improving one's teaching skills and resultant student learning. It is these formative assessment techniques that are the focus of this chapter.

The terms *evaluation* and *assessment* are often used interchangeably. However, for the purposes of this chapter, we make the following distinction: *Evaluation* refers to an end point, determining whether an action is right or wrong (e.g., answers to questions on a classroom examination). *Assessment* refers to looking closely at teaching events with a central emphasis on student learning and considerations of how to improve student outcomes.[2]

The assessment movement in education has been stimulated at the federal level by both institutional and specialized (professional) accreditation agencies. This movement is having a powerful influence on higher education. The central focus is on accountability of the educational program related to student learning outcomes.[2-4] The Association for the Assessment of Learning in Higher Education (AALHE; http://www.aalhe.org) is an organization that focuses on using effective assessment practice for purposes of improving student learning. AALHE offers members opportunities to join in discussions about assessment practices and hosts an annual assessment conference. Publications from the Council on Higher Education Accreditation (CHEA;http://www.chea.org) should be regular reading in physical therapy and physical therapist assistant programs for those interested in assessment. Why is ongoing educational assessment, which helps us determine ways to improve our teaching and resultant student outcomes, so important to physical therapy educators that we allocate an entire chapter to address it? The answer lies in the learning problems students bring with them when they enter physical therapy programs.

STUDENT LEARNING PROBLEMS

Students come to our physical therapy programs with well-ingrained learning problems that hinder both the acquisition and retention of information. Lee Shulman[5] identifies three of these common problems as amnesia, fantasia, and inertia. For those of us teaching the next generation of health care professionals, these problems with student learning are an anathema.

Amnesia refers to students' learning material for an examination but forgetting it immediately afterward. This happens when our physical therapy programs are packed with courses with little time built in for students to reflect, integrate, and apply the information they are receiving. Students learn to survive such programs by focusing on whatever examination is next. Thus, for instance, cramming for an anatomy examination is followed by "dumping" the information to cram for a pathology examination. This practice might not have severe consequences in an undergraduate liberal arts program in which a biology course is not connected to an English course. However, amnesia obviously has serious consequences for students in health professional programs, in which inter-relating and building on information is a well-imbedded assumption of the faculty.

Fantasia refers to illusions students have about how things in the world work and how people behave. Cognitive psychologists have long argued that new learning grows out of prior learning; that is, learning will occur only when new information is linked to existing knowledge. Thus, Shulman points out that the misconceptions students hold hinder the appropriate reception of new information. For example, if a student believes in "no pain, no gain" from her or his past athletic experiences, how will that belief influence her or his understanding of pain management and ability to work with patients who have painful, chronic, debilitating conditions?

Inertia is the student's inability to apply what is known. This occurs when students are taught piecemeal facts that they cannot organize or use in a problem-solving situation. For example, students who are asked to memorize origins and insertions of muscles without a functional movement context are very likely to forget this anatomic information by the time they are asked to assess gait deviations.

Seasoned faculty are familiar with these problems of learning. For physical therapy faculty, these problems must be dealt with in order for students to successfully attain the knowledge, skills, and values of a professional practitioner. Each new group of students enters our programs having done well in their prior academic endeavors despite exhibiting amnesia, fantasia, and inertia. Students may even believe they performed well because of amnesia, fantasia, and inertia! How do we deal with these three common learning problems, as well as the unique learning problems individual students bring with them (e.g., fear of asking questions in the classroom, competitiveness and the related unwillingness to share knowledge with peers, and the student-versus-teacher mentality)? A concerted, programmatic effort must be in place to diminish as much as possible these students' learning problems and give students the insights and skills they need to guide their own lifelong learning. In simple terms, we want to have further insight and understanding of how students are thinking and learning—we want to "get the inside out." Use of the assessment ideas and tools presented in this chapter is a powerful method to help teachers improve their teaching so that students learn and, equally important, find enjoyment in learning.

PILLARS FOR TRANSFORMATIVE LEARNING

Angelo states, "[D]o assessment as if learning matters most."[6] Assessment affects all levels of education, from individual classrooms and laboratories to programs and the institution in which the programs reside. Angelo argues that there are four essential components, or pillars, for transformative assessment (Figure 5–1). The term *transformative* is used with specific intent. It means that something actually will happen within an institution that leads to a change in the institutional culture. This change is facilitated through individuals who share common beliefs and values, work together to develop guidelines, and act on those guidelines. An example of transformative change in higher education is the current emphasis on student learning, which is visible in many venues (e.g., highlighted in conference topics, discussed and debated in the research literature, and emphasized in accreditation documents).

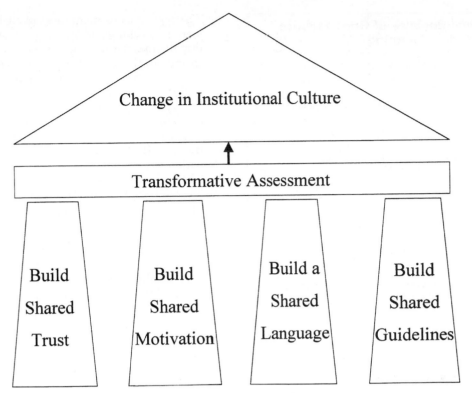

FIGURE 5–1 Angelo's four pillars of transformative assessment. (Adapted from Angelo T. Doing academic development as though we value learning most: transformative guidelines from research and practice. In James R, Milton J, Gabb R. Research and Development in Higher Education 22. Melbourne, Victoria: HERDSA, 2000.)

The four pillars for transformative assessment are as follows:

1. *Build shared trust.* This is done through the faculty's building a productive learning community in which the faculty involved in assessment trust one another. All persons must feel respected, valued, and safe to share their experiences.
2. *Build shared motivation.* There have to be collective goals worth working toward and problems worth solving. This means a shift for some faculty because faculty often focus on what they will teach rather than on what students will learn; students, in turn, often focus on getting through the program.
3. *Build a shared language.* Faculty need to develop a collective understanding of new concepts needed for transformative changes. Although assessment may mean only student course evaluations or standardized testing—and time wasted to some faculty members—a collaborative model would focus on assisting the entire faculty to see the broader conception of assessment that focuses on formative assessments and student learning and successful achievement of program outcomes.
4. *Build shared guidelines.* Faculty will benefit from a short list of research-based guidelines that can be used for assessment to promote student learning. An example of a research-based guideline in physical therapy or physical therapist assistant education might include gathering formative assessment data on the ability of students to demonstrate critical professional behaviors or ability-based outcomes. For example, do

students demonstrate empathy across the curriculum? What evidence do students provide in support of their clinical decision-making skills?

Angelo's assessment vision includes the formation of learning communities that include groups of faculty and students working toward shared, significant learning goals. He proposes that assessment should be seen as less of a technical data collection process and more of a monitoring and problem-solving process. Assessment is an ongoing process of quality improvement. Moving from a focus on summative evaluation to formative assessment requires the faculty to think about and distinguish between these two concepts. Think about the last time your department went through an accreditation process. What type of approach did your department use in providing information?

Nine principles of good practice for assessing student learning (Box 5–1) serve as a good starting point for thinking about your current assessment activities.[7(p 23)] You might want to examine these nine principles and see which of them are included in the assessment activities in your classroom, program, or institution. For example, do your assessment activities attend equally to the teaching-learning experience and the learning outcomes?

ASSESSMENT OF STUDENT LEARNING
Classroom Assessment

Learning can and often does take place without the benefit of teaching—and sometimes even despite it—but there is no such thing as effective teaching in the absence of learning. Teaching without learning is just talking.[8(p 3)]

(box source)

BOX 5–1   Nine Principles of Good Practice for Assessing Student Learning

1. Assessment of student learning begins with educational values.
2. Assessment is most effective when it reflects an understanding of learning as multidimensional, integrated, and revealed in performance over time.
3. Assessment works best when the program has clearly, explicitly stated purposes.
4. Assessment requires equal attention to outcomes and to the experiences that lead to those outcomes.
5. Assessment works best when it is ongoing and not episodic.
6. Assessment fosters wider improvement when representatives from across the educational community are involved.
7. Assessment makes a difference when it begins with issues of use and illuminates questions that people really care about.
8. Assessment is most likely to lead to improvement when it is part of a larger set of conditions that promote change.
9. Through assessment, educators meet responsibilities to students and to the public.

Adapted from AAHE Assessment Forum. Principles of Good Practice for Assessing Student Learning. In Maki PL. Assessing for Learning: Building a Sustainable Commitment Across the Institution. Sterling, VA: Stylus, 2004.

All of us in higher education, regardless of whether we are in a professional school or a graduate department, aim to produce graduates who achieve the highest possible quality of learning. As educators, our greatest reward is the success of our graduates. As we teach, we are constantly engaged in an "informal" process of classroom assessment—that is, determining what students know, do not know, need to learn, do, and become.[9] To do this, we ask students questions, observe and react to body language that depicts confusion or boredom, and listen carefully to students' comments. In response to this input, we may speed up, slow down, review material, or change in other ways to react to student learning needs.

We infrequently, however, undertake systematic and formal classroom assessment. As previously stated, classroom assessment techniques are well suited to formative assessment—that is, getting specific feedback from the entire class as we move through the course, thus gaining insight into student learning so that changes can be made to enhance the learning process *before* the end of the course.

Angelo and Cross's well-known classic book on classroom assessment techniques is an excellent resource for faculty.[8] This book is a practical guide for designing and implementing classroom assessment techniques for *any* faculty member, regardless of his or her background. Their model of classroom assessment is built on the following assumptions about teaching and learning: The quality of student learning is directly (not exclusively) related to the quality of the teaching. One of the most promising ways to improve learning is to improve teaching.[4,8,9] To improve effectiveness, teachers first must make their goals and objectives explicit and then obtain feedback to determine the extent to which students are achieving such goals. (See the preactive teaching grid in Chapter 2.)

- To improve learning, students need to receive appropriate and focused feedback early and often. They also need to learn how to assess their own learning.

- The type of assessment most likely to lead to improvement of teaching and learning is that conducted by faculty themselves, in which they formulate the questions specific to their own teaching concerns.
- The processes of systematic inquiry are an intellectual challenge and an important source of motivation for faculty. Classroom assessment provides this kind of challenge.
- Classroom assessment does not require specialized training. It can be carried out by any dedicated teacher within any discipline.
- Through collaborating with colleagues and actively involving students in classroom assessment efforts, faculty can enhance learning and personal satisfaction.

Teaching Goals Inventory

A useful way to initiate classroom assessment planning is for each faculty member to complete the Teaching Goals Inventory (TGI).[8] The TGI is a questionnaire designed to assist faculty in identifying and ranking the relative importance of their teaching goals for any class. With one particular class in mind, the faculty member rates the importance of 52 teaching goals across six clustered areas: higher-order thinking skills, basic academic success skills, discipline-specific knowledge and skills, liberal arts and academic values, work and career preparation, and personal development. The complete TGI is available in Appendix 5-A. You will see that there are many parallels between the TGI and the philosophical orientations to curriculum discussed in Chapter 2.

The primary role of the TGI for classroom assessment is for teachers to identify what goals they view as important so that they can target their assessment efforts toward those teaching goals. Secondarily, the collective faculty can share its teaching goals across classes within a semester or across the entire curriculum to assess where its collective teaching and learning focus lies. As with sharing one's philosophical orientation and learning theory emphasis, sharing teaching goals is often an eye-opening experience.

Classroom Assessment Techniques

CATs, as proposed by Angelo and Cross, have the following characteristics[8]:

- The focus is on observing and improving *learning* rather than on observing and improving *teaching*.
- The individual teacher decides what and how to assess and how to respond to the information. Autonomy and professional judgment are respected because the teacher is not obligated to share the results of her or his CATs with anyone else.
- Faculty improve their teaching by constantly asking themselves three questions: "What are the essential skills, knowledge and values I am trying to teach? How can I find out whether students are learning these skills? and How can I help students learn better?"[9(p 5)]
- Student learning is reinforced by doing CATs, as students are asked to reflect on what they are learning, give examples of how to use the information, and indicate points of confusion that can be clarified long before a midterm or final examination.

- As formative assessments with the purpose of improving the quality of student learning, CATs are usually anonymous as well as ungraded. Thus, students can focus on and provide honest feedback about what and how they are learning rather than searching for "the right answer." Students as well as teachers learn to enjoy CATs as both an intriguing and an intellectual process.
- Each class of students presents with a unique and diverse mix of student backgrounds, learning attitudes and skills, and learning problems, and as such, each class develops a unique microculture. Thus, CATs need to be used sensitively and specifically with each different class being taught. A CAT that is successful for one teacher in one class with one group of students at one time of the year will not necessarily be similarly successful if any one of these variables changes.
- Use of classroom assessments is an ongoing process throughout the semester.

What does a CAT look like? Here is a simple example of an introductory assessment technique for looking at student learning. Let's say you are teaching a unit in a neuromuscular course on motor learning. You are particularly interested in the students' ability to understand and apply core theoretical concepts. You know that the lecture and discussion materials you have for them in this area are complex and challenging, even for your strongest students. You want some quick way to assess students' ability to understand the theoretical concepts. There are several very simple and quick ways to gather data from students:

- *Minute paper* (also known as the "one-minute paper" or "half-sheet response"). Stop your class a few minutes early and have students respond to two questions: (1) What was the most important concept you learned during this class? (2) What important question remains unanswered for you?
- *Muddiest point.* At the end of class, have students write a brief response to the question, What was the muddiest point in this lecture today?
- *Modeling.* At any point in the class, have students draw a model that demonstrates the basic relationships among concepts. Have students discuss their models with each other and field their questions.
- *Metaphors.* Ask students to write a metaphor followed by a one- or two-sentence explanation. This is easily done as a fill-in-the-blank question. For example, the question is "Doing research is like _____." The answers—for example, "walking through molasses," "a puzzle," "going to the dentist," and "an adventure"—are very telling.
- *Defining features matrix.* The purpose of this exercise is to assess students' skills in categorizing information using a given set of critical defining features. Faculty can then do a quick check of how well students can distinguish between similar concepts and make critical distinctions. This assessment technique is particularly good for helping learners make critical distinctions between apparently similar concepts. Table 5–1 provides an example from a course on health education and an assessment of health behaviors.[10]
- *Documented problem solutions.* The aim of this assessment technique is to determine how students solve problems

TABLE 5–1 Defining Features Matrix: Example from a Course on Health Behavior

Features	Precede/ Proceed Model	Readiness for Change Model	Self- Efficacy Model
Precontemplation		X	
Predisposing factors	X		
Social assessment	X		
Maintenance		X	
Outcome expectation			X
Reinforcing factors	X		
Confidence			X
Relapse		X	
Enabling factors	X		
Self-confidence			X
Behavior and lifestyle	X		
Importance			X
Action		X	
Educational assessment	X		
Predisposing factors	X		
Contemplation		X	
Efficacy expectation			X

Adapted from Glanz K, Rimer B, Viswanath K (eds). Health Behavior and Health Education: Theory, Research and Practice, 4th ed. San Francisco: Jossey-Bass, 2008.

and how they understand and express their problem-solving strategies. This technique is particularly good in helping students to explicate their thought processes and approaches to solving problems. For example, in a biomechanics course, you could divide the class into groups and give each group a problem. Have the groups solve the problem and document each step of the problem-solving process. Then have the groups do a show-and-tell presentation on their problem solution approaches.

By collecting and reviewing these CATs, you will gain immediate insight into students' learning experiences, which will help direct your next class with them. Although CATs help teachers assess student learning problems, they also help enormously with actual student learning. That is, ongoing assessments of learning require that students stop and think about what they have learned and then synthesize and express in writing what they do and do not understand. Thus, CATs offset the global classroom problems of amnesia, fantasia, and inertia as well as individual learning problems, such as reluctance to ask for help.

CAT activities can be focused to meet a specific instructor need for feedback. A CAT, for example, can be used to determine whether students understand basic relationships among concepts. Students can be asked to perform many types of activities to demonstrate learning—be creative!

For example, have students express concepts by drawing, moving their bodies through space, or using Tinker toys (see the "modeling" description earlier).

You can also use CATs to assess attitudes and perceptions. The "metaphors" CAT described previously can be very helpful in identifying feeling states, often before the student is able to put feelings into words.

You might be wondering how your teaching goals apply to your selection of classroom assessment techniques. The link between the TGI and your CATs is that you should perform formative assessments on those targeted teaching goals that you value most. For example, many of us are interested in facilitating growth in students' critical thinking skills. How do we know that we are on the right track in our classroom experience with students? The "defining features matrix" CAT example given earlier, for instance, could be used to do a quick check on students' ability to distinguish core concepts. A quick scan of students' responses will help you identify ways in which students are confused.

Similar to other CATs, the "documented problem solutions" activity provides good information about students' problem-solving skills, but it is equally useful in helping students identify how they solve problems and in giving them ideas about other problem-solving approaches they might use.

For more examples of CATs, see Angelo and Cross's book, which remains the most widely used resource for classroom assessment techniques.[8]

Small Group Instructional Diagnosis

SGID[11,12] is a formative assessment that captures information from students, typically at about the midpoint in a course. The process takes about 15 to 30 minutes and entails five steps, as depicted in Figure 5–2. Two trained facilitators talk to the students while the instructor is not present. One facilitator introduces, explains, and facilitates the process. The other facilitator records the student groups' consensus and assists after the session with the students. A sheet with three questions is distributed to groups of three to seven students: (1) What is working well in the course? (2) What is not working well in the course? (3) What are your recommendations for change? Student groups discuss the questions and record their answers on the sheet. After about 7 minutes, the entire group of students is reconvened. Each question is posed to the class, and consensus is reached and recorded by the second facilitator. The sheets are then gathered for a postsession report. A report is generated by the facilitators of the results, and anonymity is preserved by giving typed reports. Because of the formative nature of an SGID, results are shared only with the instructor. The facilitators then meet with the instructor of record to review findings and offer any pertinent resources. The spirit of an SGID is twofold: (1) to improve one's teaching, and (2) to improve student learning. The last step in the SGID process is for the instructor to report back to students what was learned and to describe whether changes will be made and why some recommendations are not accepted. This report to students often gives them a greater sense of control over their learning and promotes a shared trust between students and instructor.

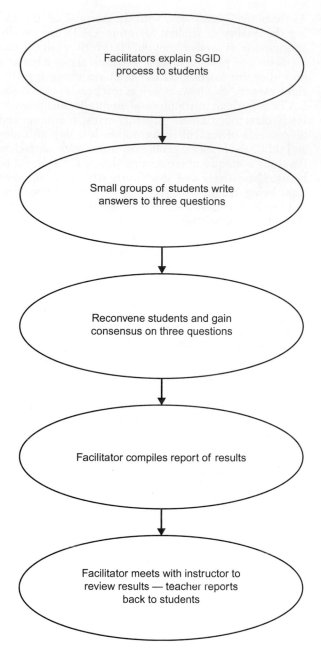

FIGURE 5–2 Steps in the small group instructional diagnosis process.

Quality Circles

Quality circles have long been used by Japanese companies as a way to get input from employees on how to improve production. Although this practice has been adopted by many American companies, it has not been used in education, primarily because ongoing formative assessment has only recently been accepted.[8,13]

To create a quality circle on the first day of the course, ask for a small group of three or four volunteers who would be willing to meet with you every few weeks for 15 or 20 minutes to give you feedback about how the course is going. Ask for a diverse group—that is, those who are particularly interested in the subject matter to be taught as well as those who are less interested. At the first meeting with students, ask them to be responsible for soliciting feedback from other students in the class and discuss with them how to give and receive feedback. That is, the quality circle will not be a "complaint session" but rather a discussion on what is going well in class and what might be improved in the course and how to improve it. The feedback is two-way: students give feedback to the instructor, and the instructor gives feedback to the students. The feedback is focused on anything that is happening in the classroom that facilitates or impedes student learning. Thus, discussions might include course assignments, classroom physical environment, use of cases and classroom exercises, communication between the instructor and the students, level of reading assignments, and evaluation and grading. The next time the whole class meets, members of the quality circle and the instructor make a brief report to the whole class on what can change and how, and on what can't be changed and why.[8]

Students take their quality circle roles seriously, and the discussions are thoughtful joint problem-solving ventures during which the instructor is allowed to grow, and students gain insight as to their own responsibilities for learning. For example, the instructor can ask the quality circle to suggest ways to increase class participation or why an assignment was generally poorly done. The atmosphere is collegial, and change is supported and applauded.

Peer Coaching

Peer coaching is often referred to as "peer review."[14] Both are professional strategies for instructors to consult and learn from one another through a series of meetings focused on discussions about shared teaching practices, observations in one another's classrooms or laboratories, and facilitation of collegiality and support. The intent is to help ensure quality teaching for students, resulting in good student learning experiences. Peer review is often routine in some programs to make decisions about hiring faculty and reviewing faculty for salary or merit decisions.[13]

Table 5–2 depicts the peer coaching process. In peer coaching, an experienced teacher is paired with a new teacher or with a veteran teacher who requests assistance. The two engage in conversations about teaching and reflect on and refine their practice. Their relationship is built on confidentiality and trust in a nonthreatening, secure environment in which they can learn and grow together. Peer coaching is generally conducted for formative (development) rather than summative (personnel decision) purposes. Formative evaluation activities provide instructors with information they can use to improve their teaching. It is intended for personal use rather than public inspection. All information gathered is private and confidential.

Components of the peer coaching process can include preobservation conferences, observation, and postobservation conferences. During preobservation conferences, the mentor and mentee can discuss any areas of concern or focus for the observation. Together, the pair can discuss the mentee's philosophy of teaching, review the course syllabus (e.g., learning objectives, course assessment methods, course schedule, and grading practices), discuss contextual issues of the course, and review the logistics of classroom observation.

A classroom or laboratory observation is scheduled in which the mentor takes descriptive notes and eventually identifies suggestions for improvement. The coach can

TABLE 5–2   Depiction of Peer Coaching Process

Step	Process
Step 1: Preobservation	Coach and instruct; meet and agree on the scope of the coaching process
	Discuss areas of concern or focus for the coaching
	Discuss instructor's philosophy of teaching
	Review the course syllabus, learning objectives, learning activities and grading, policies and procedures, course websites, course guides, etc.
	Discuss any contextual issues related to the course
	Schedule an observation of instructor's class and/or laboratory
	Review assignments and examples of completed student work
Step 2: Observation	Observe a class and/or laboratory session
	Coach takes descriptive notes during observation about:
	Teaching methods
	Multimedia use
	Content
	Effectiveness
	Student behaviors in session
	Consider videotaping the lesson or laboratory session
Step 3: Postobservation	Discussion about coach's descriptive notes: what went well and what didn't go so well
	Coach offers recommendations and resources
	Instructor can ask questions
	Additional follow-up meetings as mutually agreed on

Adapted from Chism NVN. Peer Review of Teaching, 2nd ed. Boston: Anker, 2007.

comment on the instructor's teaching methods, session content, and effectiveness. Videotaping one's teaching can also be done to serve as a visual point of reference for future discussions about the session.

A postobservation conference includes the discussion of notes, recommendations, and resources and answering any questions that emerge during the session. If videotaping was conducted, the mentee watches the video and takes notes about things that went well or did not go well. This can also provide an opportunity for the mentee to generate a list of questions or issues to discuss with the mentor. The mentor should also review the videotape with the mentee to point out strengths and weaknesses and may offer recommendations and resources for improvement. The postobservation conference is the time in which the mentor and mentee reach mutually agreed on micro and macro issues. Strategies are generated for each issue. Continued discussions can occur to conduct additional observations when the mentee has implemented strategies. The pair can continue to engage in conversations as desired.

End-of-Course Student Ratings

End-of-course evaluations, student rating forms, or student course evaluations are traditionally administered at the end of a term to collect students' evaluations of a course. Student feedback is a simple process and holds credibility for a number of reasons[15–17]: (1) the reliability is typically high because input is received from a number of student raters, (2) the ratings are made by those who have observed the teacher for many hours, and (3) there is high face validity in student ratings because the students have been personally affected by the teacher's performance.

Although student rating systems have credibility, they have important limitations: (1) Some of the student ratings are poorly constructed tools (e.g., double-barreled questions, asking about matters unrelated to student learning, use words that are unclear). (2) Occasionally, standardized procedures are not used. This leads to the inability to compare one faculty member against another. (3) Extraneous factors may not be taken into account that influence ratings (e.g., class size, student motivation, level of difficulty). (4) Interpretation can be difficult for tools that do not result in a statistical report. In some institutions, end-of-course evaluations from students are the primary or only data measure for teaching effectiveness. This is unfortunate because "writers on faculty evaluation are almost universal in recommending the use of *multiple* sources of data. No single source of data—including student rating data—provides sufficient information to make a valid judgment about overall teaching effectiveness."[16,17] Students are not qualified to judge many of the factors that characterize teaching effectiveness. Thus, students are not qualified to judge factors such as the appropriateness of course objectives, relevance of assigned readings, degree of currency of subject matter content, or the laxity or severity of grading standards.[15] These factors are best assessed by faculty colleagues.

PROGRAM ACCOUNTABILITY

Another major area of assessment in educational programs is the focus on ongoing and formal evaluation of all components of the educational program, including performance expectations and evidence of outcomes for students and faculty along with ongoing and formation evaluation of the clinical education program, professional curriculum, and evidence of graduate outcomes such as successful licensure and employment. Student learning and evidence of that learning in meeting performance expectations are a central component of accountability to all stakeholders.[3,4,18]

As physical therapy faculty, we must be accountable for what we say students will be able to know, do, and become as a result of completing their academic course of study. The course of study includes didactic and experiential components. Consequently, assessment of student learning is of concern at multiple levels within the educational institution, from courses to programs to school or college and institution.

University- or college-level outcomes must be explicated, and program-specific learning outcomes should link back or be *aligned* to the university or college student learning outcomes.[2,4,19] Mapping programmatic student learning outcomes to the university- or college-level student learning outcomes is helpful for several reasons. First, the documented link is an explication of the relationship between the two sets of student learning outcomes to faculty, administrators, students, and other pertinent stakeholders. Second, the alignment can serve as a resource when assessment reports are written. Third, the alignment is useful when revisions need to be made in a program based on previous assessment data (Table 5–3).

Programmatic student learning outcomes should be linked to course-level and co-curricular learning outcomes. Again, mappings of course and co-curricular outcomes should be documented to show their relationship to programmatic learning outcomes. A variety of measures should be used to report on student learning outcomes.

TABLE 5–3 Example of Aligning Assessment Goals across Levels: Clinical and Translational Science (CTS) Graduate Program

Component	Example Processes
University assessment goals	Undergraduate program assessment goals: Graduates will demonstrate disciplinary competence and/or professional proficiency. Graduate program assessment goals: Graduates will demonstrate the disciplinary competence and/or professional proficiency with a global perspective in service to others.
Program outcomes	Graduates will demonstrate working knowledge in core subject within the area of CTS. Graduates will effectively analyze, synthesize, and interpret biological data, including their own, and critically evaluate scientific information. Graduates will conduct research addressing specific scientific problems and be able to place their results in the context of previous knowledge. Graduates will formulate and execute a research plan to solve problems.
Assessment procedures and criteria	Biannual progress reports to the student's advisory committee before the student is allowed to register for the following term. Students will record minutes from each committee meeting for approval by the advisory committee. Qualifying exams (written and oral). Students will actively participate in discussions following seminars and presentations.
Assessment results	Progress and potential problems (either conceptual or technically) will be identified for the first cohort of graduates. Clarify and facilitate communication between the student and members of the committee. Pass or fail in qualifying examination. Grade in the seminar course (CTS791) will be based on the attendance, presentation, and active engagement in the discussion. Average grade point average 3.4 to 3.5 to enter program and 3.0 maintained throughout program.
Use of assessment results/ change	Potential problems (either conceptual or technically) are discussed and advice given by the committee. Use results of the progress reports and qualifying exams to re-evaluate entrance requirements for the program and basic course requirements. Courses or symposia will be developed and aimed at addressing weaknesses and trends seen in the progress of our students. Re-evaluate composition of graduate student advisory committees. Reassess content and goals of qualifying examination.

The terms *direct measures* and *indirect measures* are often used to categorize such assessment tools and efforts. Direct measures represent student performance that can be observed to assess how well students are achieving learning goals and objectives.[4,7] Examples of direct measures include examinations, papers, presentations, clinical evaluations, and certification examination scores. Indirect measures "capture students' perceptions of their learning and the educational environment that supports that learning."[7(p 88)] Examples of indirect measures include end-of-course student ratings, student satisfaction focus groups about the program, alumni and employers surveys, and self-assessments of clinical performance. The take-home message is that programs should use a variety of direct and indirect measures to report on program-level student learning outcomes (Figure 5–3).

Program- and course-level assessment should pose salient questions regarding student learning based on the

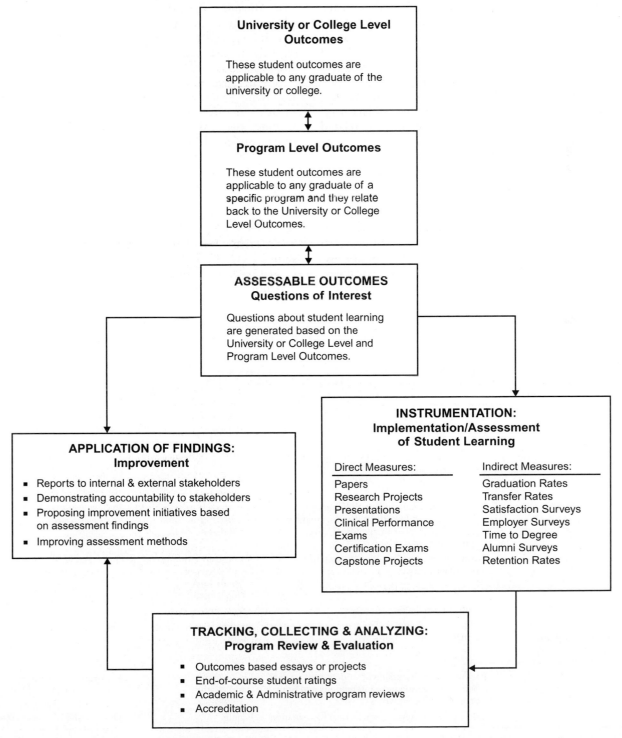

FIGURE 5–3 Overview of assessment of student learning process.

university- or college-level context. For example, a university-level learning outcome states that graduates will demonstrate professional competence and/or professional proficiency. The physical therapy faculty note a 3-year pattern of declining performance when students are in a pediatric clinical setting. This observation leads the faculty to ask, Why are our students performing poorly in pediatric clinical experiences? The faculty review the curriculum map to note where students learn about pediatric practice. Such courses and assignments are reviewed to ensure that necessary direct and indirect measures are used to assess student learning in pediatrics. When multiple data points are collected, the faculty review and evaluate the results. Once the faculty review the data, they make decisions on how to improve the student learning experience. For example, additional treatment plan assignments are developed and implemented within courses. After these improvements are implemented, the assessment cycle begins again, in that the data are collected and analyzed and further improvements are made. If the results are satisfactory, the faculty pose additional questions of interest related to student learning.

Remember that two of the "pillars of transformative assessment" include building a shared language and shared guidelines among program faculty. Accountability requirements for both specialized accreditation agencies (e.g., the Commission on Accreditation in Physical Therapy Education, or CAPTE[18]) as well as institutional accreditation agencies that accredit institutions of higher education all require assessment plans and ongoing evidence of how assessment data are used as a critical component of meeting expectations along with ongoing continuous quality improvement. Written assessment plans are now routine and must include evidence of the continuous implementation of assessment measures, analysis of that evidence, and actions taken to improve or address the problematic issue.

There are many tools and formats that can be used to implement and monitor the assessment process. A general framework of core categories (student, faculty, curriculum, environment, and graduate) can be used to frame a global program evaluation plan. Each of these dimensions is broken into very specific subcategories. Then, each subcategory is mapped out according to what assessment method will be used, who will implement the task, and when the task will be done. In Table 5–4, you see an example from the student dimension—that is, admissions. Note that the specificity of the subcategory makes it easier to identify an assessment method as well as to determine the *who* and *when*.[19]

Specific program assessment plans with evidence of improving student learning and student learning performance outcomes often use a similar column matrix that includes two critical accountability measures—summary of data collected (what was found in terms of student performance) and how the results are being used to change or modify the program, course, or curriculum (see Table 5–3). Program outcomes also identify and address the unique and innovative elements of the program and institution. These unique elements (e.g., producing graduates who will provide service to their community or an emphasis on rural health care) should be visible in mission and philosophy statements.

The crucial element in assessment is that a faculty "learning community" must be a real community that

TABLE 5–4 Example of the Student Component of Admissions for a Program Assessment Plan

Evaluation Component/ Tasks	Method	Who	When
Students: Admissions			
1. Prerequisite courses/student preparation for doctor of physical therapy program	Review of prerequisite courses to determine fit between student preparation and curricular demands	Department Admissions Committee	Done annually before preparation of admissions material
2. Characteristics of students fit with admissions criteria	Database profile for enrolled students by class that includes academic background and performance upon entry	Department Admissions Committee	Data prepared annually at beginning of academic year with assistance from School Admissions Office
3. Student recruitment strategies	Comparison of database with School of Pharmacy and Health Professions marketing plan (e.g., number of applicants, diversity of applicant pool)	School of Pharmacy and Health Professions Admissions Office	Performed at the beginning of each academic year
4. Application process	Feedback gathered by Admissions Chair from faculty	Admissions Committee Faculty/School Admissions Department	Immediately after admissions process each spring
	Applicant satisfaction surveys	Applicants	
5. Enrolled student review process by faculty for academic performance and professional behaviors	Academic performance: midterm and end-of-semester grade reports	Student faculty advisor	Ongoing—advisor follows up with students as needed
	Faculty group discussion of student professional behaviors from course interactions and other programmatic activities	Department Chair and faculty	Performed end of every semester/ongoing faculty meetings
	Clinical Competence Performance Examination	Faculty	Done at end of every semester

Adapted from Department of Physical Therapy, School of Pharmacy and Health Professions, Creighton University, Omaha, NE.

has shared motivation and trust. The assessment process is not the responsibility of one person, but rather of the entire faculty. The departmental assessment plan needs to be monitored and updated. It is an important accountability tool that needs to be a dynamic process for the program. Assessment committees need to be connected to the curriculum activities of the program. Finding ways to integrate the functions of curriculum and assessment can be a transformative process for the program. If you are in a school or college with several health professions, you may find it worthwhile to have an assessment task force across health professions that can be used for sharing resources and designing instruments that target issues of the institutional mission.

This chapter is about learning, assessment, and accountability. We began this chapter with a discussion of classroom assessment. We conclude the chapter by moving from a focus on classroom assessment to a discussion of the scholarship of teaching and learning. Here is where evidence of student learning that is a critical component of assessment can also be used to address important research questions about teaching and learning.

SCHOLARSHIP OF TEACHING

There continues to be interest in higher education about the meaning and scope of faculty scholarship and how the scholarly work of faculty is evaluated.[20–23] Boyer's classic book, *Scholarship Reconsidered*,[20] has had a profound effect on institutional discussions regarding standards for assessing faculty scholarship related to promotion and tenure. Boyer advocates that *scholarship* is a broader term than *research*. In addition to basic research, which he calls the "scholarship of discovery," he adds three additional forms of scholarship: the scholarships of integration, application, and teaching. The scholarship of integration is the need to make connections across the disciplines to a larger context, revealing the meaning of the data. The scholarship of application is asking how this knowledge can be "engaged" or applied to important real-world problems. The scholarship of teaching includes not only transmitting knowledge but also transforming and extending knowledge. Boyer's notion is that excellent teaching is visible through the same habits of mind that characterize scholarly work.

The scholarship of teaching includes a critical component of making the work visible or public (community property) of some or all of the act of teaching so that others can provide a constructive critique and evaluation and build on the work. The scholarship of teaching involves questioning, inquiry, and investigation, most often around issues of student learning. Although traditional research is driven by problems in need of investigation, when it comes to teaching, a "problem" is not something we want to have in our classrooms. Changing the status of the problem in teaching from terminal remediation to ongoing investigation is precisely what the movement for a scholarship of teaching is all about.[5,24]

The scholarship of teaching is about bringing the process of inquiry to the classroom. It has also been described as "going meta"—that is, having faculty frame and systematically investigate questions related to student learning.

What differentiates good teaching from scholarly teaching and scholarly teaching from the scholarship of teaching? The scholarship of teaching and learning provides a counterbalance to one of the liabilities of outcome assessment. In outcome assessment, the later we have the results, the later we have the knowledge of those results, which could be used to improve student learning and performance.

Case Example: Clinical Research Course—Reading the Literature

- *Good teaching approach:* The teacher gives a lecture on the core concepts for critical review of an article. Each step of the process is defined and discussed in class, with an exemplary article being used for application of each core concept. Students leave the class believing that they will be able to do an assigned article critique on their own.

  Working definition for good teaching: It is often described in terms of presentational and interpersonal skill based on student evaluations. Are the lectures enjoyable? Does the instructor care about the students? Are needed resources available?

- *Scholarly teaching approach:* The teacher brings a manuscript that he or she has submitted, having just received the review. After a brief review of concepts, the teacher guides the students through the review process of the manuscript. The teacher then shares the actual review he or she received and discusses with the students how the paper will need to be revised to move the paper toward publication.

  Working definition for scholarly teaching: The teacher brings the scholarship of discovery into class and works to connect current scholarship or knowledge development with the content of the course.

- *Scholarship of teaching and learning:* The teacher is interested in investigating what learning is taking place in small group work. Students are given a diagnostic quiz after an initial quick class review of core concepts in their assigned readings. In their assigned groups, they first exchange quizzes and correct the responses. Next, the group task is to critique an article that requires them to apply the concepts and supporting evidence for their judgment. Finally, they must go back to their initial quiz and do a self-assessment, answering these questions: (1) What were the most confusing concepts for you when you took the quiz? (2) What did you learn from your group? (3) What did you contribute to the group? (4) What would you do differently next time?

  Working definition for the scholarship of teaching: Teaching is examined from the perspective of the learner, examining student outcomes. What is the expected learning? The purpose is to improve the learning of students. Communication with one's peers is necessary in terms of making the work public for critical review and evaluation.

The issue of making the work public or community property is a critical issue for the scholarship of teaching.[22–24] Here, we discuss the application of two different types of assessment that lend themselves well to the scholarship of teaching: peer assessment and course portfolios.

PEER ASSESSMENT

Teaching is a complex activity that is often done individually, within the confines of the classroom. Most faculty would agree that some combination of evidence from the person who is teaching, the students who are learning, and professional colleagues who observe is useful in evaluation of teaching. As previously mentioned in the peer coaching process, peer review and assessment could be used for either formative or summative evaluation; we focus here on its use as formative assessment. This means our aim is on improvement of teaching, not on administrative decision making. Remember, the central focus in assessment is on *student learning*.[22–25]

Peer review of teaching responds to two current concerns with teaching in higher education: (1) the needs to make teaching more public and promote the idea of teaching as "community property" through peer collaboration and discussion, and (2) the need to make teaching a topic for public examination, debate, and engagement.

An argument made about teaching is that it is difficult to assess; therefore, it is not valued. Research on teaching, however, has demonstrated a great deal of consensus on what is effective teaching. Here are 10 strategies and characteristics of good practice, supported by research, that effective teachers use[25]:

- Have students write about and discuss what they are learning.
- Encourage faculty-student contact, in and out of class.
- Get students working on substantive tasks, in and out of class.
- Give prompt and frequent feedback to students about their progress.
- Communicate high expectations.
- Make standards and grading explicit.
- Help students achieve those expectations and meet those criteria.
- Respect diverse talents and ways of learning.
- Use problems, questions, or issues, not merely content coverage, as points of entry into a subject and as sources of motivation for sustained inquiry.
- Make courses assignment centered rather than text or lecture centered.

Course Portfolios

A second technique for assessment of teaching is a course portfolio. Portfolios can take many forms and have various purposes, from looking at a faculty member's teaching across courses to a student's account of her or his learning and professional development, or a practitioner's account of professional development and achievement.[26] Here, we focus on the use of a course portfolio as a tool for continuous improvement of teaching and learning. The course portfolio is different from a teaching portfolio in that it is a wide-angle lens that focuses on teacher performance *and* learner performance.[27]

We begin by outlining our working assumptions for creating a course portfolio.[5,27,28] A portfolio is a tool for self-directed reflective learning, not just an exposé of good work.

Portfolio development demands structure, yet allows for creativity, and provides a scaffold for reflective learning.

- A course portfolio should provide the teacher with a basis for improving teaching and student learning.
- Faculty will invest in this kind of assessment only to the extent that it connects goals, issues, and problems that really matter to them.
- Course portfolio assessment should be collaborative in that, just as a doctoral student works with a dissertation committee, following guidelines and seeking

consultation, portfolio assessment includes coaching, deliberation, and collegial exchange.[26]

So how does one go about designing a course portfolio? Hutchings proposes three core components in a course portfolio: design, enactment, and outcome.[5,27]

Design

A useful way to start is to think about what purpose the course portfolio will serve. For example, are you trying to examine how to become more interactive with students and do less lecturing in your course? Often a course portfolio begins with a teaching philosophy. This narrative will include a self-reflection on your beliefs and assumptions about teaching and learning, an explanation of your intended learning outcomes, the teaching practices you will use to reach those outcomes, and a rationale that connects the course goals to the teaching methods. It is this proposed relationship between your teaching methods and your learning outcomes that will serve as a framework for your analysis.

Enactment

Enactment is evidence or documentation of what happens in the class. This could take many forms, from the teacher's own self-reflections on the weekly progress of the course to the selection of class material samples that represent the connection between the course goals and the teaching strategies used to attain those goals. Following is a list of possibilities for documenting course enactment: videotapes, handouts, audiotapes of class interactions, hard copies of student-teacher online interactions, copies of lecture notes, examinations, readings, worksheets, and study guides. The important issue regarding evidence is not finding the evidence but rather selecting the evidence appropriate to your purpose.

Results/Outcome

The defining feature of the course portfolio is the focus on student learning. How do you decide what student work to include? Samples of good and poor work? All work? Here are some suggestions: (1) Examples of student work should demonstrate a good fit between assessment and course goals. (2) Use existing assessment data whenever possible. You probably have evidence of student learning outcomes that comes from activities that are part of your course. (3) Include a variety of sources of evidence—for example, examinations, projects, worksheets, and minute papers. (4) Select your evidence of student learning with purpose. You might want to randomly select a small cohort of students to track their outcomes over the course so that you have longitudinal data. Focus on key assignments that represent links with your course goals. The final component of the course portfolio is your reflective analysis and conclusions about your teaching and your students' learning— that is, a focus on lessons learned. As an example of the scholarship of teaching, the course portfolio should make a connection between the activity and the results.

SUMMARY

We have come full circle. We began the chapter by talking about student learning, classroom assessment, and the need to identify the teaching goals that we are working toward. We concluded the chapter by focusing on tools that teachers can use to examine their teaching in a way that will constantly advance their practice of teaching, improve student learning, and contribute to the scholarship of teaching.

THRESHOLD CONCEPTS

Threshold Concept #1: Understanding the central importance of student learning in the assessment process and the important interdependence of assessment and grading.

One of the challenges in higher education is the tendency to equate grades as the only measure of student learning and performance. Does this mean that grades do not matter? Of course not. Grades are important formative and summative indicators of student progression. The challenge is that grades are not sufficient when it comes to learning and understanding the complexities of student learning. It is important to appreciate the complexity of grading and use it as a tool for learning.[25] The more explicit we can be about the standards of performance that rest behind the grades, the better insight we will have that the grades do represent student learning and performance. Remember, if we want to know what may be problematic or why students may not be meeting the expectations or may be receiving good grades and yet not perform well in clinical or field experiences, that is where targeted investigation that looks in depth into student learning and performance can help us understand more fully what needs to be done to improve the learning.

Here are some of the practical and important uses of assessment[4]:

- Assessment activities can bring academic faculty and clinical faculty together to discuss and help better integrate the curriculum. *Students are having trouble with use and application of evidence across all years of the program.*
- Assessment can shine the light on areas that have been neglected for a long time. *What should we do about courses and performance expectations with modalities?*
- Assessment can be linked with scholarship of teaching and learning work and motivate collaboration across the faculty. *How can we improve students' development of clinical reasoning skills across the curriculum?*
- Assessment data can demonstrate excellent graduate outcomes that can be used in your recruitment of applicants.

Threshold Concept #2: Assessment is everyone's responsibility and is not just delegated to someone else (administrator, curriculum, or assessment committee).

Assessment is the responsibility of everyone. The misconception is that it is someone else's job to gather, analyze and report all of that data. This demonstrates a key misconception that assessment is about student learning and gathering evidence of student learning across all levels of education from classroom, laboratory, or program to school or institution. The other fallacy is that one must create special tools or use standardized tests for the assessment process. The reality is that there are many opportunities for assessment that are part of your ongoing teaching and learning activities.

An easy way to begin at the course level is to prepare an audit list of your course-embedded learning experiences, assignments, and tests. Then, identify what have been the major issues with which students struggle in your course (e.g., certain areas of knowledge, application of theory, skill performance). You may know this from past experience, or you may want to investigate a sample of student papers or tests to identify areas of weakness. Next, match the key learning or performance elements that are part of your assignments or tests with your desired course learning outcomes. Do they match? How do they fit with the learning and performance issues students may be having? This is an example of course assessment that can be easily undertaken in your regular teaching activities; in fact, it is likely to be something you are already doing informally.

ANNOTATED BIBLIOGRAPHY

Angelo TA, Cross KP. *Classroom Assessment Techniques: A Handbook for College Teachers.* 2nd ed. San Francisco: Jossey-Bass; 2004.

This is an outstanding resource for any academic department. The authors provide more than 50 examples of different classroom assessment techniques. The discussion of each technique includes an estimate of ease of use for the faculty, description of the technique, step-by-step procedures for adapting and administering the technique, practical advice, and pros and cons of the technique. The chapters focused on specific assessment techniques are grouped according to student learning goals (e.g., content knowledge, higher-order thinking skills, values, and attitudes).

Maki P. *Assessing for Learning: Building a Sustainable Commitment Across the Institution.* San Francisco: Jossey-Bass; 2004.

This book provides a good overview of both an institutional assessment process and program specific assessment. The book is loaded with good examples of charts, tables, and tools that can be used in designing and implementing an assessment process. There is an excellent section on sample criteria for standards of judgment.

Suskie L. *Assessing Student Learning: A Common Sense Guide.* 2nd ed. San Francisco: Jossey-Bass; 2009.

Suskie's book is a practical guide and excellent reference for planning and implementing assessment across all levels, courses, programs, and institutions, with the strongest emphasis on course and program assessment. Many practical examples and good ideas are shared in this text, including excellent recommendations for summarizing results to inform teaching, learning, planning, and decision making.

Van Note Chism N. *Peer Review of Teaching: A Sourcebook.* 2nd ed. Boston: Anker; 2007.

Written as a source book for administrators and faculty, this text is an outstanding resource for development of any peer review of the teaching process. The book is in two sections: the first provides a framework for designing and implementing peer review, and the second provides guidelines, protocols, and forms for each task in the process.

Walvoord B. *Assessment: Clear and Simple. A Practical Guide for Institutions, Departments, and General Education.* San Francisco: Jossey-Bass; 2004.

Walvoord's book is an outstanding simple and concise reference for anyone doing assessment. It is a step-by-step guide written so that all can understand the assessment process.

REFERENCES

1. Hatfield S. *Assessing your program level assessment plan.* IDEA Paper No. 45. Manhattan, KS: Kansas State University Center for Faculty Evaluation and Development; 2009. Available at: *http://www.theideacenter. org/sites/default/files/IDEA_Paper_45.pdf.* Accessed 15.07.11.
2. Mentkowski M, Rogers G, Doherty A, et al. *Learning That Lasts: Integrating Learning, Development, and Performance in College and Beyond.* San Francisco: Jossey-Bass; 2000:305, 359–405.

3. Huba M, Freed J. *Learner-Centered Assessment on College Campuses: Shifting the Focus from Teaching to Learning.* Needham Heights, MA: Pearson; 2000.
4. Suskie L. *Assessing Student Learning.* 2nd ed. San Francisco: Jossey-Bass; 2009.
5. Shulman L. *Teaching as Community Property: Essays on Higher Education.* San Francisco: Jossey-Bass; 2004.
6. Angelo TA. *Doing academic development as though we valued learning most: transformative guidelines from research and practice.* Available at: http://www.herdsa.org.au/wp-content/uploads/conference/1999/pdf/Angelo.PDF. Accessed 15.07.11.
7. Maki PL. *Assessing for Learning: Building a Sustainable Commitment Across the Institution.* Sterling, VA: Stylus; 2004.
8. Angelo TA, Cross KP. *Classroom Assessment Techniques: A Handbook for College Teachers.* 2nd ed. San Francisco: Jossey-Bass; 1993.
9. Priddy L. The view across: patterns of success in assessing and improving student learning. *On the Horizon.* 2007;15:58–79.
10. Glanz K, Rimer B, Viswanath K, eds. *Health Behavior and Health Education: Theory, Research and Practice.* 4th ed. Jossey-Bass: San Francisco; 2008.
11. Clark DJ, Redmond MK. *Small Group Instructional Diagnosis: Final Report.* Washington, DC: Fund for the Improvement of Postsecondary Education; 1982. ERIC ED 217 954.
12. Creed T. *A Model for Consulting with Faculty (Implementation of the SGID Process.).* Available at: http://www.ntlf.com/html/pi/9705/sgid.htm#sgid; May 1997. Vol 6 #4 National teaching and learning forum. Accessed 15.07.11.
13. Kogut LS. Quality circles: a Japanese management technique for the classroom. *Improving College and University Teaching.* 1984;32:123–127.
14. Chism NVN. *Peer Review of Teaching.* 2nd ed. Boston: Anker; 2007.
15. Hoyt DP, Pallette WH. *Appraising Teaching Effectiveness: Beyond Student Ratings.* IDEA Paper #36. Manhattan, KS: Kansas State University Center for Faculty Evaluation and Development; 1999. Available at: http://www.theideacenter.org/sites/default/files/Idea_Paper_36.pdf. Accessed 15.07.11.
16. Seldin P. *Evaluating Faculty Performance: A Practical Guide to Assessing Teaching, Research and Service.* San Francisco: Anker; 2006.
17. Cashin W. *Student Ratings of Teaching: The Research Revisited (IDEA Paper No. 32).* Manhattan, KS: Kansas State University Center for Faculty Evaluation and Development; 1995. Available at: http://www.theideacenter.org/sites/default/files/Idea_Paper_32.pdf. Accessed 15.07.11.
18. American Physical Therapy Association. *CAPTE Accreditation Handbook.* Available at: http://www.capteonline.org/AccreditationHandbook. Accessed 15.07.11.
19. Walvoord B. *Assessment Clear and Simple.* San Francisco: Jossey-Bass; 2004.
20. Boyer EL. *Scholarship Reconsidered: Priorities of the Professoriate.* Princeton, NJ: Carnegie Foundation for the Advancement of Teaching; 1990.
21. Glassick CE, Huber MT, Maeroff GL. *Scholarship Assessed: Evaluation of the Professoriate.* San Francisco: Jossey-Bass; 1997.
22. Hutchings P, Shulman LS. The scholarship of teaching. *Change.* 1999;31:11–15.
23. Hutchings P. *Making Teaching Community Property.* Washington, DC: American Association for Higher Education; 1996.
24. Bass R. The Scholarship of Teaching: What's the Problem? *Inventio* [serial online]. February 1999;1(1). Available at: http://www.doiiit.gmu.edu/Archives/feb98/randybass.htm. Accessed 15.07.11.
25. Walvoord B, Anderson V. *Effective Grading: A Tool for Learning and Assessment.* 2nd ed. San Francisco: Jossey-Bass; 2010.
26. Shulman L. Counting and recounting: assessment and the quest for accountability. *Change.* 2007;39:20–25.
27. Hutchings P. *The Course Portfolio.* Washington, DC: American Association for Higher Education; Sterling, VA: Stylus; 1998.
28. Hutchings P. *Opening Lines: Approaches to the Scholarship of Teaching and Learning.* Menlo Park, CA: Carnegie Foundation for the Advancement of Teaching; 2000.

APPENDIX 5-A TEACHING GOALS INVENTORY AND SELF-SCORABLE WORKSHEET

Teaching Goals Inventory

Please select ONE course you are currently teaching. Respond to each item on the inventory in relation to that particular course. (Your response might be quite different if you were asked about your overall teaching and learning goals, for example, or the appropriate instructional goals for your discipline.) Rate the importance of each goal to what you aim to have students accomplish in your course.

Please enter the name of the course you are rating:

_____

Please rate the importance of each of the 52 goals listed below to the specific course you have selected. Assess each goal's importance to what you deliberately aim to have your students accomplish, rather than the goal's general worthiness or overall importance to your institution's mission. There are no "right" or "wrong" answers, only personally more or less accurate ones. For each goal, choose only one response on the 1- to 5-point rating scale. You may want to read quickly through all 52 goals before rating their relative importance.

In relation to the course you are focusing on, indicate whether each goal you rate is:

(1) Not applicable	A goal you never try to achieve
(2) Unimportant	A goal you rarely try to achieve
(3) Important	A goal you sometimes try to achieve
(4) Very important	A goal you often try to achieve
(5) Essential	A goal you always/nearly always try to achieve

	1	2	3	4	5
1. Develop ability to apply principles and generalizations already learned to new problems and situations					
2. Develop analytic skills					
3. Develop problem-solving skills					
4. Develop ability to draw reasonable inferences from observations					
5. Develop ability to synthesize and integrate information and ideas					
6. Develop ability to think holistically: to see the whole as well as the parts					
7. Develop ability to think creatively					
8. Develop ability to distinguish between fact and opinion					
9. Improve skill of paying attention					
10. Develop ability to concentrate					
11. Improve memory skills					
12. Improve listening skills					
13. Improve speaking skills					
14. Improve reading skills					
15. Improve writing skills					
16. Develop appropriate study skills, strategies, and habits					
17. Improve mathematical skills					
18. Learn terms and facts of this subject					
19. Learn concepts and theories in this subject					
20. Develop skill in using materials, tools, and/or technology central to this subject					
21. Learn to understand perspectives and values of this subject					
22. Prepare for transfer or graduate study					
23. Learn techniques and methods used to gain new knowledge in this subject					
24. Learn to evaluate methods and materials in this subject					
25. Learn to appreciate important contributions to this subject					
26. Develop an appreciation of the liberal arts and sciences					
27. Develop an openness to new ideas					

Continued

	1	**2**	**3**	**4**	**5**

28. Develop an informed concern about contemporary social issues
29. Develop a commitment to exercise the rights and responsibilities of citizenship
30. Develop a lifelong love of learning
31. Develop aesthetic appreciation
32. Develop an informed historical perspective
33. Develop an informed understanding of the role of science and technology
34. Develop an informed appreciation of other cultures
35. Develop capacity to make informed ethical choices
36. Develop ability to work productively with others
37. Develop management skills
38. Develop leadership skills
39. Develop a commitment to accurate work
40. Improve ability to follow directions, instructions, and plans
41. Improve ability to organize and use time effectively
42. Develop a commitment to personal achievement
43. Develop ability to perform skillfully
44. Cultivate a sense of responsibility for one's own behavior
45. Improve self-esteem/self-confidence
46. Develop a commitment to one's own values
47. Develop respect for one's own values
48. Cultivate emotional health and well-being
49. Cultivate physical health and well-being
50. Cultivate an active commitment to honesty
51. Develop capacity to think for oneself
52. Develop capacity to make wise decisions
53. In general, how do you see your primary role as a teacher? (Although more than one statement may apply, please choose only one.)
    A) Teaching students facts and principles of the subject matter
    B) Providing a role model for students
    C) Helping students develop higher-order thinking skills
    D) Preparing students for jobs/careers
    E) Fostering student development and personal growth
    F) Helping students develop basic learning skills

Self-Scorable Worksheet

1. In all, how many of the 52 goals did you rate as "essential"?
2. How many "essential" goals did you have in each of the six clusters listed below?
3. Compute your cluster scores (average item ratings by cluster) using the following worksheet.

Cluster Number and Name	Goals Included in Cluster	Total Number of "Essential" Goals in Each Cluster	Clusters Ranked—from 1st to 6th—by Number of "Essential" Goals
I. Higher-Order Thinking Skills	1-8		
II. Basic Academic Success Skills	9-17		
III. Discipline-Specific Knowledge and Skills	18-25		
IV. Liberal Arts and Academic Values	26-35		
V. Work and Career Preparation	36-43		
VI. Personal Development	44-52		

A	B	C	D	E
Cluster Number and Name	**Goals Included**	**Sum of Ratings Given to Goals in that Cluster**	**Divide C by this Number**	**Your Cluster Scores**
I. Higher-Order Thinking Skills	1-8		8	
II. Basic Academic Success Skills	9-17		9	
III. Discipline-Specific Knowledge and Skills	18-25		8	
IV. Liberal Arts and Academic Values	26-35		10	
V. Work and Career Preparation	36-43		8	
VI. Personal Development	44-52		9	

From Angelo TA, Cross KP. Classroom Assessment Techniques: A Handbook for College Teachers, 2nd ed. San Francisco: Josey-Bass, 1993.
Web source: http://fm.iowa.uiowa.edu/fmi/xsl/tgi/data_entry.xsl?-db=tgi_data&-lay=Layout01&-view

6 AUTHENTIC ASSESSMENT: SIMULATION-BASED EDUCATION

Bradley Stockert ⊛ Debra Brady

How many times have you had a student demonstrate successfully their knowledge in the classroom on written examinations and with laboratory activities only to perform poorly in clinical situations? We recently had a student named Josh who performed well on written examinations that tested his knowledge base. He learned the information we requested, but he was unable to effectively apply that knowledge in patient care situations that required him to obtain, evaluate, and integrate new information from the patient in real time. The transformation of knowledge from classroom and laboratory activities to clinical situations can be problematic and overwhelming for many students. What Josh, and other students like him, really needed was time to practice patient care and receive constructive feedback about his performance in order to gain experience transforming and applying his knowledge and skills to clinical situations. Programmable patient simulators in a realistic environment offer one means to directly address the problem of creating a safe learning environment in which students can practice the application of their knowledge and skills in a clinical setting while receiving constructive feedback from faculty and other students that expands and transforms the clinical utility and application of their knowledge base and skills.

CREATING DIFFERENT LEARNING EXPERIENCES USING PROGRAMMABLE PATIENT SIMULATORS AS AN EDUCATIONAL TECHNIQUE

Simulation is a technique used in health care education to replicate the essential aspects of a clinical situation in an academic setting so that the participant can learn to

LEARNING GOALS

After completing this chapter, the reader will be able to:
1. Articulate the case for creating new and different learning experiences in health care education.
2. Distinguish the features of programmable patient simulators and high-fidelity simulation as an educational technique.
3. Explain the forms of immediate feedback (performance-based assessments) that are available with high-fidelity simulation, enumerating at least three approaches.
4. Analyze the term *frame of reference* as it relates to debriefing techniques following high-fidelity simulation.
5. Summarize reflective assessment techniques that can be incorporated into high-fidelity simulation, listing at least four approaches to assessment.
6. Discuss the benefits of using high-fidelity simulation to standardize student clinical experiences related to rare but critical events and interprofessional team training.

examine, assess, and manage the event more effectively when it occurs in clinical practice.[1,2] Although the use of patient simulators (e.g., role players and standardized patients) has been a long-standing practice in physical therapist education, the use of programmable patient simulators is relatively new. Programmable patient simulators are life-sized mannequins operated by sophisticated computer systems that control a variety of "patient" variables, such as vital signs, breath sounds, heart tones, and vocalizations. When programmable patient simulators are incorporated into a realistic setting (e.g., mock critical care unit with all of the lines, tubes, alarms, and monitors), the simulated environment and experience become *realistic, immersive, and uncertain* for the participant learning to work with complex patients or manage a clinical event.

INSTITUTE OF MEDICINE REPORT ON HEALTH CARE EDUCATION COMPETENCIES

The Institute of Medicine 2003 report,[3] *Health Professions Education: A Bridge to Quality*, challenges educators across all health care professions to redesign curriculum and restructure clinical learning experiences based on five competency areas: patient-centered care, interdisciplinary teams, evidence-based practice, quality improvement, and informatics. Competencies are defined in the report[3] as the "habitual and judicious use of communication, knowledge, technical skills, clinical reasoning, emotions, values and reflection in daily practice." Simulation using programmable patient simulators provides an opportunity to address, practice, and assess all five of these competency areas in the context of a realistic patient care setting. Articles in the nursing literature have shown that the use of programmable patient simulators had a positive impact on participant learning and improved performance on subsequent simulation experiences.[4–11] Studies with medical students have shown that there was significant improvement in critical assessment skills, performance, and retention of information when training included the use of programmable patient simulators.[12–15]

INTERPROFESSIONAL EDUCATION COLLABORATIVE EXPERT PANEL REPORT

The 2011 report from the expert panel of the Interprofessional Education Collaborative describes a series of core competencies for interprofessional collaborative practice.[16] This report envisioned interprofessional collaborative practice as "key to the safe, high quality, accessible, patient-centered care desired by all." The intent of the report was to define core competencies for interprofessional collaborative practice that build on each profession's disciplinary competencies. Four core competencies (domains) for interprofessional practice were identified[16]:

1. Values and ethics
2. Roles and responsibilities
3. Interprofessional communication
4. Teams and teamwork

The development and acquisition of interprofessional collaborative competencies will require health care education programs to move beyond profession-specific educational efforts to engage students from different health care professions in interactive learning with each other. Programmable patient simulation offers educators from all health care disciplines an opportunity to design interprofessional scenarios that address each of the core competencies (domains) noted in the report while engaging students in an interactive learning community with the common goal of building a safer and better patient-centered health care environment.

INSTITUTE FOR HEALTHCARE IMPROVEMENT REPORT TO IMPROVE PATIENT SAFETY

The Institute for Healthcare Improvement published a set of goals in 2006 designed to improve patient safety.[17] These goals set improved communication and teamwork among health care professionals during emergency situations as a priority. The Institute specifically focused on the use of programmable patient simulators as a means to improve communication and teamwork among health care professionals. Teamwork training is of particular importance because patient care has become more complicated and requires a multidisciplinary approach, yet education of health care professionals is still often provided in "silos" within each discipline.[18] Studies with Medical and Nursing students demonstrated improved emergency team performance when high-fidelity simulation was incorporated into their training.[19,20] There are a number of studies in the nursing and medical literature supporting the efficacy of programmable patient simulation for improving health care education outcomes and multidisciplinary team management of medical emergencies.[4,5,12,19,21–23]

FEATURES OF HIGH-FIDELITY SIMULATION AND PROGRAMMABLE PATIENT SIMULATORS

REALISM, IMMERSION, AND INTEGRATION

Fidelity is a term used to express the degree of realism present in the programmable patient simulator or the simulation. Programmable patient simulators have a variety of observable and clinical features available that add to the degree of realism present in the simulation. High-fidelity simulators have observable features that include the capacity for chest wall movements, pupils that are reactive to light, eyelids that blink, and the ability to converse and vocalize symptoms. Clinical features include breath sounds, heart tones, bowel sounds, and a library of normal and abnormal sounds for each. Simulators can be connected to a patient monitor that displays a variety of parameters in real time, such as electrocardiogram (ECG) data, blood pressure, and oxygen saturation among others. (Figure 6–1).

The features available in programmable patient simulators provide the operator with the ability to design scenarios that realistically replicate complex medical conditions and situations. For example, a "patient" can be stable when the simulation participant enters the room but develop chest pain and ECG changes associated with the onset of an acute myocardial infarction during the intervention. When the programmable patient simulator is incorporated into a high-fidelity setting with lines, tubes, alarms, and monitors, the simulated environment and experience becomes *realistic, immersive, and unpredictable* for the participant learning to work with complex patients or manage a clinical event. Simulation forces the participant to examine, assess, and integrate information in real time while witnessing the consequences of their decisions and actions.

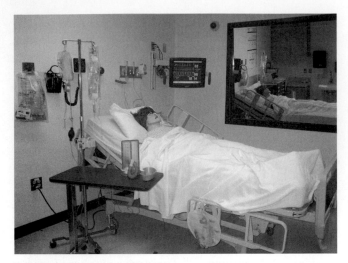

FIGURE 6–1 Example of a high-fidelity simulation environment. (Photo courtesy of Academic Technology and Creative Services, California State University, Sacramento, CA.)

TRANSFORMATIONAL LEARNING AND HIGH-FIDELITY SIMULATION

The goal of transformational learning is to develop learners with the ability to evaluate, interpret, and perform autonomous thinking, not simply memorize materials or assume the beliefs and judgments of an authority figure. Autonomous thinking is fundamental to professional practice in which each client presents with unique needs and requires creation of a plan of intervention developed in light of best practice guidelines (see Chapter 3 for additional information regarding metacognitive skills and reflective processes that facilitate autonomous thinking and transformational learning). Transformational learning affects the learner's *frame of reference*. Internal frames of reference are an adult learner's acquired "coherent body of experience—associations, concepts, values, feelings, conditioned responses" through which they interpret life experiences.[24] These frames of reference, based on knowledge, assumptions, and feeling, determine the actions people will take. The debriefing process is designed to uncover and analyze the participant's frames of reference that lead to the action taken (see later section, Debriefing Process). The discovery and analysis of a participant's frame of reference helps learners understand how their frame of reference was used to make a clinical decision as well as learn to scrutinize and transform that frame of reference in order to improve their professional performance on an ongoing basis.

Simulation has the potential to be a transformational learning experience that permanently changes the participant's view of the situation. Programmable patient simulation actively engages the participant in a student-centered learning environment. The simulation demands that they apply their subject mastery and clinical skills in the context of a realistic, unpredictable patient care situation. Learners "see" and "feel" the consequences of their actions, as well as their inactions, without compromising patient safety.

Simulation participants should go through a debriefing session following the simulation experience (see later section, Debriefing Process). The debriefing session challenges the learner to reflect on and explain their frame(s) of reference—that is, the assumptions and knowledge they used to reach their clinical decisions. A well-designed debriefing session fosters a discourse among participants regarding their frame of reference as well as how they could interpret the situation differently next time in order to improve their performance—that is, the debriefing session can transform the participants' frame of reference and their clinical behavior.

PERFORMANCE-BASED ASSESSMENTS WITH HIGH-FIDELITY SIMULATION
PREPARING THE LEARNER FOR THE SIMULATION EXPERIENCE

Effective high-fidelity simulation experiences that enable performance-based assessment of the specific knowledge, skills, and attitudes the learner is to achieve begin with development of targeted learning objectives and assignment of presimulation didactic content on which the simulation scenario is based. Ideally, simulation scenarios should be limited to three to four broad objectives, run 15 minutes or less, and include an immediate debriefing process that is equal to or double the time of the scenario.[21-25] More extensive objectives and longer simulations can overwhelm participants and lead to less focused debriefing discussions. Each objective can address several "essential or critical behaviors" the participant should perform. For example, Figure 6–2 illustrates a specific but broad objective for the participants. The critical behaviors listed in Figure 6–2 are what the participant is assessed on in the simulation to demonstrate understanding of the objective. Depending on the level of learner (novice, competent, expert), the facilitator may choose whether or not to provide the critical behaviors checklist as part of the simulation preparation. For members of the simulation group who are observing instead of participating at the bedside, the critical behaviors checklist can be an effective tool for helping formulate feedback and reinforcing the content of the objective.

Preparation for the simulation experience may take the form of readings, quizzes, concepts maps, video review of skills, laboratories, or practice on skill task trainers. This enables the participants to enter the simulation learning environment with the prerequisite knowledge and exposure to skills they are expected to synthesize in a patient-centered scenario.[26] In addition, participants need to be oriented to the simulator equipment so that lack of familiarity with the functions of the simulator does not affect their ability to perform.[27] Preparing students with the simulation objectives, didactic content, and prior practice with skills establishes a baseline for formative learning from which the student can demonstrate an ability to accomplish higher-order activities, such as application and integration of the material during the simulation experience. In addition, simulation enables the facilitator to immediately observe gaps in the ability of a student to apply and

Case Scenario: Mr. Jones is a 54 year old white male admitted to the ICU 48 hours ago with severe chest pain. He was subsequently determined to have suffered an acute myocardial infarction. Mr. Jones had frequent premature ventricular contractions and 2 runs of ventricular tachycardia initially, but no arrhythmias during the past 24 hours. He has an IV line, arterial line, pulmonary artery catheter, ECG, urinary catheter and he is on 2L oxygen via nasal cannula. *Student Role:* You are assuming Physical Therapy care for Mr. Jones. The patient was seen by another physical therapist for initial evaluation yesterday. You are to determine Mr. Jones' current status and if he is ready to begin cardiac rehabilitation.
Learning objective: During simulation the participants should demonstrate their ability to determine current patient status and assess the capacity of the patient to begin cardiac rehabilitation.

Critical behaviors that should be demonstrated	Met	Not Met	Comments
Patient examination			
Vital signs: current vs. past 24 hours			
Symptoms: monitored & aware of changes			
Ventilation: RR, % saturation & breath sounds			
Cardiovascular: BP, HR, circulation & heart tones			
Integument: integrity, irregularities			
Level of consciousness: impact on intervention plan			
Communication: calm, clear directions & explanations			
Patient mobility: ROM, strength & bed mobility			
Body mechanics: correctly used by PT and patient			
Lines & tubes: identified potential problems/limitations			
Pt modesty maintained: Pt appropriately covered			

FIGURE 6–2 Sample simulation case scenario, learning objective, and critical behaviors checklist.

integrate knowledge, skill, or convey appropriate attitudes during the simulation, which can then be addressed and clarified in the debriefing session. Subsequent simulation experiences that repeat the scenario or apply the same clinical concepts in a new scenario can form the basis for performance-based assessment using simulation.

SIMULATION LEARNING ENVIRONMENT

The tone the facilitator sets for the simulation experience and subsequent debriefing is pivotal to participant learning. Depending on the size of the learner group, participants may be divided into two groups of "active participants" and "observers." To enhance realism, the scenario should involve the number of active participants that would most closely mimic what is found in clinical practice, and the roles should be rotated in subsequent simulations.[21]

Performing in front of peers and a facilitator can be very stressful to participants.[21,25,28,29] Therefore, establishing a safe learning environment and a relationship of trust among the facilitator and participants is essential.[27,30] This involves understanding the ground rules for respectful communication and confidentiality. Maintaining confidentiality about

what happens in the simulation learning experience is an integral part of creating an environment of mutual respect. Addressing any use of video, audio, or written scenario summaries created during the simulation experience is part of this process. In fostering trust, the facilitator should explain how these materials will be stored, who will have access to them, and how and when they will be destroyed. This can be reinforced by having participants and facilitators sign a confidentiality and video/audio agreement, which is used in many simulation learning centers. Creating a psychologically safe and supportive environment where the students feel respected, valued, and free to explore questions, discuss mistakes, and reflect on how to improve practice is essential if the simulation experience and debriefing process are to be successful in creating transformational learning.[30,31]

In addition to establishing a safe learning environment, the authenticity of the simulation can affect participant performance. Ideally, participants should wear the professional attire they would expect to wear in the clinical situation being simulated. This enhances the fidelity of the scenario and expectation of professional demeanor. Care should be given to simulator moulage and props to create as close to a real-life situation as possible.[32] For example, if the participant is involved in working with a patient in the intensive care setting, then the appropriate monitoring equipment, audio alarms, invasive lines and tubes, and safety equipment should be in place (see Figure 6–1). As the "patient's" condition changes, the participant's recognition of or failure to respond to alarms and cues in the midst of other patient status changes can be explored in debriefing. Creating an atmosphere that mimics clinical reality allows the participant to suspend disbelief and encourages authentic engagement in the simulated experience to allow for deeper, more comprehensive performance assessment and discovery of the participant's frames of reference that are driving their clinical decision making.[30]

DEBRIEFING PROCESS

The cornerstone of simulation-based learning is the process of debriefing, or experience-analysis and feedback following the simulation experience during which the rationale for treatment choices is discussed and related to the learning situation the participant experienced.[25,29–31] There is general consensus in the literature and among simulation experts that optimal learning occurs when simulation is followed immediately by a verbal debriefing process rather than delayed.[26,28,33] Video of the simulation, debriefing logs generated by the simulator computer program, and behavior checklists can be used as objective tools to provide feedback and facilitate analysis. Skillfully led debriefing enables participants to express emotional states, explain their frame of reference, analyze their decisions, and synthesize information related to performance.[3]

One of the major benefits of the simulation experience is that performance data collected during the simulation can be used immediately by the participants and facilitator to provide objective feedback that helps with discovery of internal frames of reference that lead to appropriate or errant decision-making processes during a simulation. Debriefing facilitates the crucial step of reflection in the experiential learning process, which is essential for transformational learning. Structured time for reflection allows participants to develop insights into improving practice that can be applied in future situations.[30,34] A growing body of literature on simulation research in health care professions indicates that debriefing and this reflective process represent the most important aspect of the simulation-based learning experience.[4,5,21,25,26]

Role of the Facilitator in Debriefing and Performance Assessment

The role of the facilitator in debriefing is to first set a tone of mutual respect and open inquiry into the experience that generates group discussion following the simulation experience.[28–31] In contrast to the traditional lecture classroom setting where the instructor stands at the front of the classroom imparting knowledge, simulation debriefing is an active learner-centered event. A debriefing process when the facilitator speaks most of the time, reviews a checklists, or points out clinical problems on the simulation video is not considered best practice in debriefing and may be detrimental to the participant's self-esteem.[34] Effective debriefing is initiated by a facilitator that encourages and guides a

participant-led discussion, helps clarify clinical questions and practice standards as needed, and promotes reflection on the experience that enables the participant to discover the internal frames of reference on which their clinical reasoning is based.[25,29,33] The facilitators use of Socratic questions that incorporate why, how, and what encourages this type of dialogue. Depending on the level of the learner (novice, competent, or expert), the facilitator may need to do more coaching or clarifying in relationship to evaluation of skill performance and details of evidence-based practice guidelines.[30] For example, novice students will generally have a greater number of clarification questions than participants with more clinical experience. However, participant presimulation preparation and understanding of the learning objectives should enable the participants to engage in a deep analysis of their behaviors.[25,28]

The key in performance-based assessment using simulation learning is that the *participant is active* in the process and self-identifies areas in which performance meets expected professional standards and areas in which there is need for improvement. In the event the participants are not able to self-identify some problems in key aspects of the simulation experience, the role of the facilitator is to use objective data, clinical expertise, evidence-based practice resources, and a tone of respectful inquiry to guide discovery of internal frames of reference leading to errant behaviors. The discovery of the participant's internal frame of reference provides the learner the opportunity to analyze and incorporate new learning that will result in behavioral changes and ultimately improve clinical practice performance.[24,26,31]

Role of the Group in Debriefing and Performance Assessment

Debriefing with the observers and active participants following a clinical simulation disseminates the active learning experience to the entire group, and it creates a community for rigorous inquiry. Within the community of learners, participants become aware of their beliefs and assumptions so that they can redefine problems from another perspective. This discourse is a key aspect of transformational learning process.[24] Learners who are observing may do so behind one-way glass, through live video streaming, or off to the side in the simulation room. Observers might simply watch the scenario, take notes, or complete a critical behaviors checklist. (See Fig. 6–2.) A behaviors checklist provides observers who are watching the simulation a focus; facilitates addressing expected knowledge, skills, and attitudes related to each scenario; and provides a format for a constructive debriefing.

The benefit of the group approach in simulation learning is that observers provide different perspectives based on their prior experiences and internal frames. They can provide feedback on the application of knowledge, implementation of skills, or perceptions of attitudes conveyed that engage them in the learning experience, instead of depending on the facilitator to initiate all of the discussions or act as an authority figure. A checklist of critical behaviors based on the scenario objectives provides an excellent starting point for group discussions. Having students rotate the roles of participant and observer encourages sensitivity about how to provide respectful feedback and helps establish the professional norm for becoming a reflective practitioner.

Debriefing Techniques

Debriefing can take a variety of forms depending on the learning objectives for the simulation scenario and the level of the learner. The most frequent approach is facilitator-guided verbal debriefing, which may occur in an adjacent debriefing room or in the actual simulation area.[21,25,35] Video debriefing with the simulation group, individual simulation video debriefing, and written debriefing may be used in combination with verbal debriefing.

Four phases of the debriefing process are commonly discussed in the simulation literature and provide structure for the debriefing process: (1) describing the debrief process, (2) exploring participant response to the experience, (3) describing as well as analyzing the clinical scenario, and (4) integrating learning into future practice.[21,25,30,33] There are several models of a structured simulation debriefing in the literature.[25,31,34,36] Table 6–1 provides a succinct summary of the components of simulation and a structure for debriefing. The facilitator can implement the phases of the debriefing process to guide participants in discovering their internal frame of reference for clinical decision making and applying learned information in a new setting. The four phases of the debriefing process, which incorporate the categories of defusing, discovery, and deepening developed by Zigmont and colleagues,[26] are described in detail later.

Phase 1: Prebrief

Before beginning debriefing, the facilitator establishes the structure, goals, and time frame for the process. The facilitator is also responsible for establishing and modeling ground rules for the group regarding respectful tone of voice, confidentiality, and honest feedback that seeks to understand the thinking behind the behavior.

Phase 2: Defusing

The defusing phase enables the active participants to transition back into the group and move into analysis mode. Defusing follows a consistent pattern, with the facilitator first asking the participants how the experience was for them in order to address any emotional issues or concerns the participant may have because these issues may affect the ability to focus on key aspects of the simulation. Emotional responses can facilitate powerful learning experiences, but they can also impede reflection and assimilation of new perspectives if not addressed.[25,30,33] Initiating the debriefing process from the participant's perspective releases this emotion, gives the facilitator insight into the participant's perspective on the situation, and identifies areas that may require clarification. Encouraging participants to describe and recap the events chronologically is important in moving the group from "What happened?" to "Why did it happen?"[26] The facilitator prompts the participants by using opened-ended questions, such as, "How did this experience feel to you?" "From your perspective, what events lead to the patient's changing situation?"

Phase 3: Discovery

The goal in the discovery phase is to facilitate reflection among participants and observers about the simulation experience that encourages them to understand the internal frames of reference that prompted the behaviors and integrate new information that will improve performance and patient outcomes when a similar event occurs in clinical practice. During this phase, the facilitator and observers provide objective perspectives on the experience that enable the learner to recognize positive aspects of performance and areas for improvement. This phase involves

TABLE 6–1   Components of Simulation and Debriefing

Component	Activities
Creating a safe environment	Make learning group introductions Establish round rules and expectations Discuss confidentiality and sign forms Provide orientation to the simulation environment
Simulation experience	Define specific simulation objectives Enhance realism: mannequin moulage, lines/tube, drains, care environment Provide a challenging realistic scenario to invoke emotional response; scenario should be appropriate for level and area of clinical practice to be relevant, practical, useful to the participants
Debriefing phase 1: prebrief	Establish ground rules for respectful dialogue Clarify expectations on role of facilitator Explain format of facilitated debrief and participant/observer involvement
Debriefing phase 2: defusing[26]	Discuss emotions/feelings first Recap events (usually in chronologic order) Assess for issues that need clarification
Debriefing phase 3: discovery[26]	Promote reflection through objective observation, debriefing log, video review, observer feedback Discover internal frames of reference guiding behavior Discuss target internal frames of reference that should guide behavior Facilitate analogical reasoning
Debriefing phase 4: deepening[26]	Prompt individual to apply new information to practice setting and clinical events
Summary	Review the learning objectives discussed and lessons learned; consider using written reflection in addition to verbal Allow individuals to apply new information (repeat similar simulation exercise; clinical experience)

Data from references 25, 26, 33, and 34.

the community of learners in active dialogue regarding performance and practice standards. Objective data sources such as critical behaviors checklists, debriefing logs generated by the simulation program, and video of the experience can be used to encourage self-reflection.[37] Questions that encourage performance analysis might include, "What went well in the simulation?" "What would you want to do differently next time?" "Tell me a little about your thought process in making that decision?" Questions the facilitator can employ to engage the observers include, "How did the participant's actions reflect current practice guidelines for this situation?" "How have you handled a situation like this in the past?"

The participants may not be aware of the internal frames of reference that guide their behavior. A skilled facilitator, using a tone of respectful inquiry, engages the participants in conversations that probe at the rationale for behavior.[29,34,37] For example, the facilitator debriefing a simulation with physical therapy students might say, "I observed that when you were doing exercises with the patient in bed, the audio heart rate alarm went on indicating an accelerating heart rate. You paused, but did not stop the exercise. Can you tell us why you had the patient continue?" By phrasing the question with a tone of curiosity instead of judgment, the facilitator alerts the participant to the clinical concern but opens up dialogue about the rationale behind the behavior.[34] Once the participants explain their thought process, the facilitator can identify gaps in understanding and incorporate new information, as needed, that forms the basis for new learning. Prompting the learner group to make connections between past experiences that form their internal frames of reference and a new patient or clinical experience is the process of analogical reasoning.[26] Analogical reasoning involves expanding or changing the internal frame of reference to incorporate this new experience and attain the desired clinical performance.[24,26,31,34]

Phase 4: Deepening

Deepening is the phase in debriefing when members of the learning group are encouraged to make connections between the new frame of reference and clinical practice. The opportunity to immediately apply the new learning in another similar simulation or with a real patient is ideal in enabling the learner to test and embed the information for use in future practice situations.[21,33,34,38] If an immediate second simulation experience or clinical practice rotation is not possible, the facilitator can encourage deepening by asking reflective questions such as, "How could you use this new information in clinical practice?" "What did you learn here that you could implement to improve patient care?" The verbal debriefing process concludes with the facilitator providing a short summary of the topics addressed and the internal frames that were discovered, discussed, and modified as well as their potential impact on future clinical practice.[26]

Video-Assisted Debriefing

Video recordings of simulations can be used very effectively in meeting specific learning objectives.[25,38,39] During verbal debriefing, video clips can be shown during the discovery phase as an objective view that enables the participant to self-identify areas for improvement. The entire tape is not usually shown because this takes valuable time away from group discussion on analysis and integration of information into practice.[25] Instead, selected video clips are shown that center on specific learning objectives, skills, or crucial decision making points. Examples of reflective questions, the facilitator might ask the participants are, "What were your thought processes behind this decision?" "How did your actions reflect current practice guidelines for this situation?" "Would you do it the same way again?" "How would you do this differently?" To achieve deeper analysis, the facilitator can address questions to the participants and larger group such as, "How might you use this information in other similar clinical situations?" "What did you learn from this situation that changes how you will act in your future clinical practice?"

There may be instances when participants view the simulation video individually to facilitate private reflection.[40] For example, participants may be involved in a videotaped simulation with the learning objective of performing a specific clinical skill. During individual video review, they rate their performance based on a skills checklist, compare and contrast it to a model video of the skill, and submit their reflection to the faculty for discussion. Individual review could be especially effective when coupled with an opportunity to go back into simulation, experience the same or a very similar scenario in which the self-reflective learning could be actively applied, and then be debriefed in a facilitated group discussion.[30,34,38] The convenience of individual video review alone should not be substituted for the dynamic process of learner discourse that occurs during an interactive verbal debriefing session.

Written Debriefing

Another reflective technique to facilitate deepening of the learning experience is written debriefing. This is an experiential activity that occurs after verbal debriefing and provides opportunities for participants to reflect privately on their emotions, the events, their choices of behavior, and their internal frames of reference.[31,38] This process encourages the learner to synthesize the experience on a personal basis, connect new meanings to prior life experiences, and create mental models for how these new meanings can be applied in similar situations.[41] Written debriefing also gives the facilitator another format in which to connect with participants individually. This is especially important if there are members of the group that are intimidated in a group setting or uncomfortable speaking publicly. The facilitator might pose specific questions to prompt reflection such as, "What did you learn from this simulation that will affect your practice?" "How would you apply this learning differently or in another situation?" In addition to deepening the learning for the participant, written reflections provide the facilitator with another technique to assess individual performance.

Reflective Assessment Techniques

Several reflective assessment techniques can be used after initial simulation debriefing that can provide performance-based assessment of the experience and facilitate a transformational learning experience for the participant. In a designated time period (same day up to 1 week) after verbal debriefing, a group or individual assignment might include a second viewing of the simulation video recording and assigned questions that integrate research on current practice guidelines into analysis of performance and development of a treatment plans. Other activities could involve analyzing a written case study, or viewing a different simulation video and contrasting it to their simulation experience and best practice patterns. These various activities can be used to help the participants practice and develop their ability to evaluate, interpret, and perform autonomous thinking. In addition, these activities simultaneously provide the faculty and students with tools to assess how and to what degree the simulation and debriefing experience has transformed the participants' knowledge base, frame of reference, and clinical behaviors.

Reflective journaling is supported in the literature as an effective approach to facilitating integration of didactic content and clinical practice.[31,38,41] For example, reflective journal responses could be due weekly for a period of time after participants experience simulations and are involved in clinical rotations. Reflective questions might focus on analysis of the simulation experiences and instances in which scenario content was applied in clinical practice, or on ways in which evidence-based practice guidelines, discussed in simulation debriefing, were implemented by practitioners in the clinical setting.

STANDARDIZED STUDENT EXPERIENCES
STUDENT EXPERIENCES WITH RARE BUT CRITICAL EVENTS

Training students to manage complex patients and rare, but critical, clinical events challenges educators to provide opportunities for the participant to practice understanding and managing these events in an environment that does not compromise patient safety. Simulation is used in health care education to replicate the essential aspects of a clinical situation, so that the participant can learn to recognize and manage the event more effectively when it occurs in clinical practice.[1,2] Role players and standardized patients have been used to meet this end, but the use of programmable patient simulators allows the educator different options to develop more realistic and complex clinical situations. For example, during the course of therapy, a simulator can have a change in breath sounds, indicating a significant change in patient status. The change in patient status requires a response from the participant, whereas role players and standardized patients are unable to change their breath sounds or other clinical data in a realistic manner, reducing the fidelity and dampening the urgency of the situation for the participant.

The use of programmable patient simulators in a high-fidelity environment allows educators an opportunity to provide standardized experiences with complex patients and clinical situations before clinical internships. A variety of clinical conditions and situations, from simple to complex, can be standardized and provide each student an opportunity to practice and demonstrate competence with a variety of patient conditions as well as rare but critical events. Simulated clinical experiences replicate the essential aspects of the clinical situation and provide the participant an opportunity to demonstrate integrated subject mastery, clinical skills, competence, and autonomy for managing a number of clinical events before encountering these events with a real patient.

STUDENT EXPERIENCES WITH INTERDISCIPLINARY TEAMS

Programmable patient simulators in a high-fidelity environment give educators an opportunity to provide standardized experiences with complex patients and clinical situations for training interprofessional health care teams. Students from multiple health care disciplines, including nursing, medicine and physical therapy, can practice team communication and role clarification and other interprofessional core competencies[16] in a learning environment in which inexperience will not adversely affect patient safety and outcomes. Studies with medical students and nursing students have demonstrated improved emergency team performance when simulation was incorporated into their training.[19,20] In addition, simulation scenarios can be tailored to provide interprofessional team members an opportunity to practice the specific emergency protocols used in their particular clinical practice setting without compromising patient safety.

SUMMARY

The purpose of this chapter was to discuss the use of programmable patient simulators for creating new and different learning experiences that have the capacity to transform the learning and clinical behaviors of the participants. The features of high-fidelity simulators and the simulation environment were discussed. A variety of topics related to performance-based assessment were presented. The role and importance of the debriefing process, the components of the debriefing process, and the various ways in which debriefing can occur were presented in detail. A case was made for standardizing student clinical experiences with rare but critical events and for interdisciplinary health care team training through the use of programmable patient simulators.

THRESHOLD CONCEPTS

Threshold Concept #1: Preparing the learner for the simulation experience is essential.

Learners need to be prepared for the simulation experience. This may take several forms from readings, quizzes, concepts maps, video review of skills, laboratory sessions or skill task trainers.

Threshold Concept #2: Debriefing the learner provides a rich opportunity for reflection on the experience and continued learning.

Planning for the debriefing process following the performance-based experience is an important element in simulation-based education. The debriefing session provides an opportunity for experience-analysis and feedback. There is strong evidence supporting the value of immediate versus any time delay.

ANNOTATED BIBLIOGRAPHY

Fanning RM, Gaba DM. The role of debriefing in simulation-based learning. *Simul Healthcare*. 2007;2:115–125

This article provides a great deal of information regarding the process of debriefing. The authors include a description of several models of debriefing that can be used as well as describing the different roles a debriefing facilitator can used to improve the quality of the debriefing process. A list of organizations and institutions that offer formal training in the debriefing process is included.

Gaba D. The future vision of simulation in health care. *Quality Safety Health Care*. 2004;3:i2–i10

This article discusses the author's vision of how simulation can be used in the future to improve patient safety by having clinical personnel undergo systematic training, rehearsal, and performance assessments to refine their clinical practice. A significant portion of the article is devoted to a discussion of 11 identified attributes (dimensions) of simulation that can be used to address specific learning objectives for simulation.

Issenberg SB, McGaghie WC, Petrusa ER, et al. Features and uses of high-fidelity medical simulations that lead to effective learning: a BEME systematic review. *Med Teach*. 2005;27:10–28

The objective of this systematic review article was to evaluate the features and uses of high-fidelity medical simulation that lead to the most effective learning in simulation participants. The authors provide evidence that simulation-based learning allows participants to practice and acquire patient care skills in a controlled environment that, when combined with feedback (debriefing), boosts self-confidence and facilitates learning.

Weinschreider J, Dadiz R. Back to basics: creating a simulation program for patient safety. *J Healthcare Qual*. 2009;31:29–37

This article recommends and provides eight steps that can be used to develop and implement a simulation program. The process described is geared toward using simulation in healthcare as a process to promote patient safety and improve quality patient care.

Zigmont J, Kappus L, Sudkoff S. The 3D model of debriefing: defusing, discovery, and deepening. *Semin Perinatol*. 2011;35:52–58

This article describes the components of simulation and debriefing and provides a systematic approach to the debriefing process based on Kolb's Experiential Learning Theory, Adult Learning Theory, and the Learning Outcomes Model. The authors describe best practices in the debriefing process that lead to understanding of the rationale behind decision making and adaption of new learning to improve clinical performance.

REFERENCES

1. Gaba D. The future vision of simulation in health care. *Qual Saf Health Care*. 2004;3:i2–i10.
2. Morton P. Using a critical care simulation laboratory to teach students. *Crit Care Nurse*. 1997;17:66–69.
3. Greiner A, Knebel E, eds. for the Institute of Medicine *Health Professionals Education: A Bridge to Quality*. Washington, DC: National Academies Press; 2003.
4. Pauly-O'Neill S. Beyond the five rights: Improving patient safety in pediatric medication administration through simulation. *Clin Simul Nurs*. 2009;5:181–186.
5. Radhakrishnan K, Roche J, Cunningham H. Measuring clinical practice parameters with human patient simulation: a pilot study. *Int J Nurs Educ Scholarsh*. 2007;4:1–11.
6. Hennenman E, Cunningham H. Using clinical simulation to teach patient safety in an acute/critical care nursing course. *Nurse Educ*. 2005;30:172–177.
7. Medley C, Horne C. Educational innovations: using simulation technology for undergraduate nursing education. *J Nurs Educ*. 2005;44:31–34.
8. Rauen C. Using simulation to teach critical thinking skills. *Crit Care Nurs Clin North Am*. 2001;13:93–103.
9. Yaeger K, Halamek L, Coyle M, et al. High-fidelity simulation-based training in neonatal nursing. *Adv Neonatal Care*. 2004;4:326–331.
10. Shepherd I, Kelly C, Skene F, et al. Enhancing graduate nurses' health assessment knowledge and skills using low-fidelity adult simulation. *Simul Healthcare*. 2007;2:16–23.
11. Brannan J, White A, Bezanson J. Simulator effects on cognitive skills and confidence levels. *J Nurs Educ*. 2008;47:495–500.
12. Wayne D, Siddall V, Butter J, et al. A longitudinal study of internal medicine residents' retention of advanced cardiac life support skills. *Acad Med*. 2006;81:S9–S12.
13. Gordon J, Brown D, Armstrong E. Can a simulated critical care encounter accelerate basic science learning among preclinical medical students? A pilot study. *Simul Healthcare*. 2006;1:13–17.
14. Owen H, Mugford B, Follow V, et al. Comparison of three simulation-based training methods for management of medical emergencies. *Resuscitation*. 2006;71:204–211.
15. Steadman R, Coates W, Huang Y, et al. Simulation-based training is superior to problem-based learning for the acquisition of critical assessment and management skills. *Crit Care Med*. 2006;34:151–157.
16. Interprofessional Education Collaborative Expert Panel. *Core Competencies for Interprofessional Collaborative Practice: Report of an Expert Panel*. Washington, DC: Interprofessional Education Collaborative; 2011.
17. Botwinick L, Bisognano M, Haraden C. *Leadership Guide to Patient Safety. Institute for Healthcare Improvement Innovation Series White Paper*. Cambridge, MA: Institute for Healthcare Improvement; 2006.
18. Nishisaki A, Keren R, Nadkarni V. Does simulation improve patient safety? Self-efficacy, competence, operational performance, and patient safety. *Anesthesiol Clin*. 2007;25:225–236.
19. Devita M, Schaefer J. Improving medical emergency team (MET) performance using a novel curriculum and a computerized human patient simulator. *Qual Saf Health Care*. 2005;14:326–331.
20. Shapriro M, Morey J, Small S, et al. Simulation based teamwork training for emergency department staff: does it improve clinical team performance when added to an existing didactic teamwork curriculum? *Qual Saf Health Care*. 2004;13:417–421.
21. Jeffries P, Rizzolo M. Appendix A: final report on the NLN/Laerdal simulation study. In: Jeffries P, ed. *Simulation in Nursing Education*. New York: National League for Nursing; 2007.
22. Perkins G. *Simulation in resuscitation training. Resuscitation*. 2007;73:202–211.
23. Yee B, Naik V, Joo H, et al. Nontechnical skills in anesthesia crisis management with repeated exposure to simulation-based education. *Anesthesiology*. 2005;103:241–248.
24. Mezirow J. Transformative learning: theory to practice. *New Direct Adult Contin Educ*. 1997;74:5–12.
25. Dieckmann P, Reddersen S, Zieger J, et al. Video-assisted debriefing in simulation-based training of crisis resource management. In: Kyle R, Murray W, eds. *Clinical Simulation: Operations, Engineering, and Management*. Boston: Elsevier; 2008:667–676.
26. Zigmont J, Kappus L, Sudkoff S. The 3D model of debriefing: defusing, discovery, and deepening. *Semin Perinatol*. 2011;35:52–58.
27. Wickers P. Establishing the climate for a successful debriefing. *Clin Simul Nurs*. 2010;6:e85–e86.
28. Cantrell M. The importance of debriefing in clinical simulations. *Clin Simul Nurs*. 2008;4:e19–e23.
29. Rudolph J, Simon R, Dufrense R, et al. There's no such thing as "nonjudgmental" debriefing: a theory and method for debriefing with good judgment. *Simul Healthcare*. 2006;1:49–55.
30. Fanning R, Gaba D. The role of debriefing in simulation-based learning. *Simul Healthcare*. 2007;2:115–124.
31. Kuiper R, Heinrich C, Matthais A, et al. Debriefing with the OPT model of clinical reasoning during high fidelity patient simulation. *Int J Nurs Educ Scholarsh*. 2008;5:1–14.
32. Hwang J, Benchen B. Simulated realism: essential, desired, overkill. In: Kyle R, Murray W, eds. *Clinical Simulation: Operations, Engineering, and Management*. Boston: Elsevier; 2008:85–89.
33. Dreifuerst K. The essentials of debriefing in simulation learning: concept analysis. *Nurs Educ Perspect*. 2009;30:109–114.
34. Rudolph J, Simon R, Rivard P, et al. Debriefing with good judgment: combining rigorous feedback with genuine inquiry. *Anesthesiol Clin*. 2007;25:361–376.
35. Gurraja R, Yang T, Paige J. Examining the effectiveness of debriefing at the point of care in simulation-based operating room team training. (Volume 3: Performance Tools). In: Henricksen K, Battles J, Keyes M, eds. *Advances in Patient Safety: New Directions and Alternative Approaches*. Rockville, MD: Agency for Healthcare Research and Quality; 2008.

36. Owen H, Follows V. GREAT simulation debriefing. *Med Educ.* 2006;40:488–489.
37. Dieckmann P, Molin S, Lippert A, et al. The art and science of debriefing in simulation: ideal and practice. *Med Train.* 2009;31: e287–e294.
38. Ishoy B, Epps C, Packarnd A. "Do-overs" and double debriefing: a pilot study evaluating a different design for student simulation experiences. *Clin Simul Nurs.* 2010;6:e117.
39. Grant J, Moss J, Epps C, et al. Using video-facilitated feedback to improve student performance following high-fidelity simulation. *Clin Simul Nurs.* 2010;6:e177–e184.
40. Boet S, Bould D, Bruppacher H, et al. Looking in the mirror: self-debriefing versus instructor debriefing for simulated crisis. *Crit Care Med.* 2011;39:1–5.
41. Petranek C. Written debriefing: the next vital step in learning with simulations. *Simul Gam.* 2000;31:108–119.

STRATEGIES FOR PLANNING AND IMPLEMENTING INTERPROFESSIONAL EDUCATION

Teresa M. Cochran ☼ Brenda Coppard ☼ Gail M. Jensen

CHAPTER OUTLINE

Your Dean has just appointed you to the interprofessional education and practice task force for your institution. You are thrilled and anxious for creative planning and collaboration for the coming academic year. The initial meetings go well as the group brainstorms several possible activities and sets plans for a new interprofessional series of seminars and faculty development activities. You are in a group of early adopters and are so energized by the work. Now as you move toward implementation, each member must work with their discipline curriculum committee and program faculty to move forward with the plans. Suddenly you feel as if you are an outsider in your department. Although you anticipated some resistance from faculty because beginning this work will require some flexibility on the faculty's part, you are disappointed in the strength of the resistance. Now what?

LEARNING OBJECTIVES

After completing this chapter, the reader will be able to:
1. Justify the rationale in support of interprofessional education (IPE) learning experiences in health professions education.
2. Identify the key barriers for implementation and successful strategies to address these common challenges.
3. Identify core competencies for faculty development in interprofessional education.
4. Identify core competencies for student learning in interprofessional education.
5. Discuss the design and implementation of effective teaching-learning methods for facilitating effective IPE and team-based learning and practice.
6. Describe the strengths and weaknesses of common models for design and implementation of IPE programs.

WHY INTERPROFESSIONAL EDUCATION?

Does this sound like a familiar story? Discussions of how we can work across health professions to learn more about each other and how we can best collaborate to deliver efficient and effective patient care have been ongoing for several years, but the realities of health care reform and cost-effective care are upon all of us. Interprofessional collaborative practice is seen as the key to high-quality, accessible, patient-centered care. In order for students to be "workforce ready" to practice effective teamwork and team-based care, we must be intentional in the development and professional formation of our health professions students.

A cascade of federal reports have advocated during the past few decades for more interprofessional education and practice.[1-7] The 2011 report on Core Competencies for Interprofessional Collaborative Practice[7] is based on a core assumption that "... disciplinary competencies are taught within professions. The development of interprofessional collaborative competencies (interprofessional education), however, requires moving beyond these profession-specific educational efforts to engage students of different professions in interactive learning with each other. Being able to work effectively as members of clinical teams while students is a fundamental part of the learning."[7(p 1)]

All health professions share the responsibility for promoting good for their individual patients, but we also have a professional responsibility for promoting health as a public "good." Promoting the common good in health care requires health professionals to work together as stewards of scarce resources to deliver quality care and to take responsibility for shaping health policy that ensures access to care and promotes health. We need to remember that professional education is a powerful portal to professional life where students begin their formation of professional identity and "habits of mind."[8] We have an opportunity to build a strong foundation for interprofessional collaborative competencies through interprofessional education opportunities.

A good starting place for beginning to engage in interprofessional education is sorting out the operational definitions (Table 7–1).[7,9] Interprofessional education is defined quite simply as, "when students from two or more professions learn about, from and with each other to enable effective collaboration and improve health outcomes."[7] A key phrase in this definition is *learning about, from, and with each other.*[9] Interprofessional education is *not* sitting in the same classroom or sharing classes, nor is it engaging in a health screening for elders where the physical therapy student performs balance screening at a station and the occupational therapy students complete cognitive assessments at another station. What does it take to engage students in learning about, from, and with each other? Here is where we have the opportunity to help students grasp the critical importance of the underlying values and core components of professions' social contract. Here are key teaching and learning points to keep in mind:

TABLE 7–1 Definitions Used in Interprofessional Education and Practice

Concept	Operational Definition
Uni (disciplinary)	A health professional working independently to care for a patient
Interprofessional education	Students from two or more professions learn about, from, and with each other to enable effective collaboration and improve health outcomes.
Interprofessional collaborative practice	Multiple health workers from different professional backgrounds working together with patients, families, caregivers, and communities
Interprofessional teamwork	Levels of cooperation, coordination, and collaboration that are central to relationships between professions in patient-centered care
Interprofessional competencies in health care	Integrated enactment of knowledge, skills, and values/attitudes that define working together across professions, with other health care workers, with patients, families, and communities to improve health outcomes
Multiprofessional education	Various disciplines are brought together to understand a particular problem or experience and offer different perspectives on the problem. This is an additive approach, not an integrative approach.
Transdisciplinary	Health professional team members become familiar enough with the concepts and approaches of colleagues that they can "blur the lines" and the team can focus on collaborative analysis and decision making.

Data from Core Competencies for Interprofessional Collaborative Practice. Report of an Expert Panel. Interprofessional Education Collaborative, 2011; and Royeen CB, Jensen GM, Harvan R (eds): Leadership in Interprofessional Health Education and Practice. Sudbury, MA: Jones and Bartlett, 2009.

1. *Respect for human dignity as a moral compass.* Although students may readily grasp the meaning, behaviors, and actions that are consistent with demonstrating respect with their patients, they must begin to explore and experience how one builds mutual respect and trust when working with colleagues across professions.
2. *Understanding our collective interprofessional social contract.* Professions have an obligation to serve society and support the common good in health care. Real health improvement relies not only on direct care but also on addressing the environmental and social determinants of health, prevention, and health promotion.[7] Health care is a scarce resource that will continue to require health professionals working together with public health professionals in delivering care that is safe, efficient, and effective.
3. Moving beyond behavioral objectives to development of habits or dispositions. Although we continue to place much emphasis on professional core values and on abiding by codes of ethics, it is the professional formation and ways of "being" that are long-lasting. These elements of "who one becomes" are best facilitated through development of, not simple behaviors, but consistent patterns of behaviors that are habitual and predictable. Students' ability to engage in critical self-reflection in relation to professional identity and interprofessional professionalism is paramount.[9]

Interprofessional education has, as its centerpiece, teams working together in using the "distributed intelligence" of the team. The challenges in designing learning experiences that effectively build students' ability to be "collaboration ready" are important opportunities for educational innovation. This chapter provides a beginning blueprint for this work.

KEY STRATEGIES FOR ADDRESSING COMMON BARRIERS IN INTERPROFESSIONAL EDUCATION
IMPORTANCE OF ORGANIZATIONAL CAPACITY AND SUPPORT

As with any sustained organizational change, initiatives such as interprofessional education will require a mindset for producing change in the institutional culture, and a comprehensive, integrative approach is required to achieve successful outcomes.[10,11] It is critical to begin by knowing the culture in which your work will be situated. The extent to which programs are housed in public, private, or faith-based institutions and the institution's mission and available resources will drive the extent to which interprofessional initiatives will be developed. Regardless of institutional mission, one may argue that interprofessional care skills are consistent with the values of the health professions.[12(p 317)] As academic programs attempt to develop interprofessional education (IPE) and interprofessional practice (IPP) strategies for health care, few have effectively outlined the necessary components underlying a program's organizational context and culture that create the capacity for IPE. Greenfield has proposed the "interprofessional praxis audit framework" (IPAF) as a tool to identify the components of institutional capacity for IPE.[13]

The term *praxis* refers to the translation of theoretical knowledge into practice, and *audit* outlines the systematic process used to assess the concept of organizational culture for IPE. The IPAF is composed of five dimensions: context, culture, conduct, attitudes, and information. The model is helpful in considering the impact of the organization's shared values, beliefs, and behaviors, including its constraints, available resources, and the external policy and political milieu that will determine success for interprofessional initiatives.[13] Context is the key external environmental variable related to how interprofessional interactions are influenced by policies, guidelines, protocols, initiatives, and funding. Culture is designated as an internal variable that represents shared values and norms held by organizational staff.[13] Constructs, conduct, and information are the final audit variables described in the model that determine how individuals behave and communicate to enhance patient outcomes. The IPAF is a tool to help "map" the level of collaboration by facilitating a multidimensional and multi-level examination of the organization's level of capacity for and engagement with IPE.[13] When justification for interprofessional initiatives are clearly linked to mission, the mission becomes grounded in a manner that is difficult to deny. A clearly articulated mission statement should link societal needs and the social contract that health professionals should espouse to produce congruence and solid justification for IPE. This congruence should also be codified in the institution's strategic plan for the essential link to resource allocation as the activities are formalized.

Since interprofessional initiatives were introduced in the health professions nearly 45 years ago, a myriad of challenges beyond organizational culture have been identified. Many strategies are available to meet these challenges, but many problems may be resolved through the use of a few key strategies:

- Foster organic (or "grassroots") development of interprofessional interaction
- Foster connections between faculty and administration levels
- Build educational expectations for students
- Encourage wider faculty adoption of interprofessional interaction

Foster Organic Development

Begin where interprofessional interaction occurs naturally—allow and reinforce grassroots faculty efforts to develop in areas such as community-engaged learning in medically underserved communities where health-related concerns typically exceed the needs capacity of any single discipline to help, and the expertise of team is needed to extend scarce health resources. Other areas include educational initiatives that emphasize health promotion or disease prevention "cross-cutting" skills that are not discipline specific, yet are needed when promoting healthy lifestyle behaviors. Barr asserts that a fourth focus for IPE (in addition to preparing individuals for collaborative practice, teamwork,

and improvement of care processes) is to improve the quality of life in communities through academic-community partnerships and service learning experiences.[14,15] Geriatrics, management of chronic conditions, and rehabilitation are examples of other specific areas that are amenable to team functioning; consequently, physical therapists are frequently skilled at interprofessional collaboration because of the familiarity with interaction by virtue of their discipline-specific training.

Foster Connections

IPE is successful when coalitions are built at both grassroots faculty levels and across administrative stakeholders. Administrative authority is a critical factor for success, but it must include the right combination of faculty members capable of the grassroots collaboration fundamental to IPP and IPE. Just as the isolated effort of faculty collaboration is insufficient to lead to effective and lasting IPE, mandates by administrators in the absence of faculty buy-in and development are rarely sustainable.[11,16] Strategic implementation of initiatives led by early faculty "adopters" who are both competent and committed, within the culture of institutional support by leaders and administrators, has produced the most robust outcomes. It is important to recognize and reinforce early successes that have facilitated faculty interaction beyond individual course "boxes" or disciplinary silos.

Build Expectations

Build educational expectations for students linked to curricular and course-related outcomes, and include a visible reward structure such as certification programs or awards that reflect participation or mastery (Saint Louis University provides an excellent example).[12] Student leaders and champions must be developed, and recognition by some form of cross-professions leadership or honors programs are may be used as incentives (e.g., the University of Minnesota's "CHIP" program illustrates this important concept).[17]

Encourage Wider Faculty Adoption

Similar to development of student leaders, faculty development is a critical component. To change culture, faculty members beyond the "early adopters" must be allowed to develop the skills and attitudes needed for IPE. It is important to recognize that teams may function differently along the continuum of care (e.g., health professionals in an acute care environment may function very differently than practitioners coordinating patient care in rural home environments). Unfortunately, nuances for team function in various practice settings are frequently misunderstood by faculty members or administrators who have never practiced in the specific environment; therefore, it is essential for the right combination of expertise to be included as IPE initiatives are developed. The relationship and networks that are facilitated through faculty development opportunities enhance the collaborative foundation for the cultural shift and should not be underestimated. Reinforcing conditions for IPE should be reflected in the faculty role and reward structure, such as promotion and tenure documents, internal grant guidelines, and specific interprofessional awards not only to incentivize IPE but also to ensure that faculty members may successfully meet scholarship requirements within the academic enterprise.

FLEXIBLE CURRICULAR STRATEGIES TO ADDRESS BARRIERS IN INTERPROFESSIONAL EDUCATION

One of the most important concepts in designing interprofessional curricular activities is to realize that "one size does not fit all"—this is the reason why understanding the institution's culture is a prerequisite for curriculum development. Various approaches have been described, ranging from didactic mandatory and elective coursework, to practice-based simulations, to community-based health promotion activities. In a systematic review of formal IPE programs from 1966 to 2005 by the Best Evidence Medical Education (BEME) Collaboration of the United Kingdom, Hammick and colleagues[18] reviewed 399 studies, of which 107 met review criteria, and the 21 strongest evaluations of IPE were included in the analysis. Of the 21 programs, most of the studies were from the United States (54%) and United Kingdom (35%), with the majority of IP curricular learning experiences lasting longer than 2 days (54% lasting $\geq$7 days; 24% lasting 2 to 7 days), although curricular interventions ranged in duration from 1 to 2 hours to several months. IPE was equally distributed between hospital- and community-based environments (45% each).[18] The systematic review found that customization of curricular offerings and exposure of students to authentic environments were important mechanisms for positive outcomes of IPE. The authentic settings allowed participants to recognize their unique perspectives about themselves and others as they were forced to interact in a complex way within the IPE event. In addition, the strongest programs indicated that principles of adult learning for IPE are key factors for students to appreciate the outcomes of IPE. Hammick asserts that effective learning about being interprofessional occurs best in a context that reflects the students' current or future practice.[18] Some of the most effective IPE programs offer students a "menu" of learning opportunities, and examples of model programs are outlined in the concluding section of this chapter.

FACULTY DEVELOPMENT IN INTERPROFESSIONAL EDUCATION
HOW TO DEVELOP FACULTY: CORE COMPETENCIES AND TRAINING MODELS

Before interprofessional education initiation, "a systematic planning, development, and implementation process should be outlined including a plan for faculty and curricular development."[19(p 60)] Before faculty members move too quickly to adopt interprofessional educational experiences, they need to step back and think about developing the faculty! We cannot assume every faculty member has had positive interprofessional experiences in his or her clinical or academic work. Faculty development is an important step in shaping a collective vision among the faculty about interprofessional education. Purposes for faculty development

will need to be identified, and the faculty development model will need to be matched to the institutional context in order to align these elements for institutional success.

PURPOSE OF FACULTY DEVELOPMENT IN INTERPROFESSIONAL EDUCATION

IPE faculty development initiatives are necessary for educators and administrators[19]; Steinert proposed seven development approaches to promote IPE[20]:

1. Target change at the individual and organizational levels
2. Address the various stakeholders
3. Address major content areas (Table 7–2)
4. Include a variety of approaches (e.g., formal and informal, different settings)
5. During development activities, model the collaborative principles and practices of IPE
6. Weave principles of effective teaching and education design in IPE development
7. Attempt to disseminate the model for implementation

TABLE 7–2 Topical Areas Often Presented in Interprofessional Education Sessions for Educators

Area	Components
Interprofessional roles and responsibilities	Individual professional roles and responsibilities Limitations of respective professional role Group dynamics Professional role hierarchies
Professionalism	Educational requirements for each profession Consensus building within a team Conflict resolution and negotiation skills Interdependent relationships among professional members Valuing diversity
Communication	Effective verbal skills Active listening skills Communication barriers within teams Group facilitation techniques Ways to overcome miscommunication that frequently emerges from people holding differing perspectives
Pedagogy	Active learning techniques Ways to connect theory to practice Giving specific and sensitive feedback to students and partners Facilitation of critical reflection to recognize and implement change Passive role modeling Competency in using any technology used in interprofessional education activities Team teaching
Assessment	Selecting and administering targeted assessments related to learning objectives Identifying process improvements based on evidence

Data from references 19-22 and 24.

DEVELOPMENT MODELS

Faculty development models range from train-the-trainer sessions to self-study. Table 7–3 lists the various types of models that can be considered to develop faculty for interprofessional education. Regardless of the faculty

TABLE 7–3 Faculty Development Models, Definitions, and Considerations

Model	Definition and Considerations
Train-the-trainer	A trainer develops a cohort of faculty who become the trainers for select groups Who are the "trainer" and "trainers"? How are these people selected? How is the trainer viewed by those being taught?
Invited faculty development sessions	Select educators are invited to one or more sessions that addresses a particular topic How many sessions are needed to accomplish the objectives of the sessions? How are people selected and invited? Who will be the presenters for the sessions?
Voluntary faculty development sessions	Educators are invited as a whole to development sessions to address a particular topic How will the sessions address the potential participant learning needs? How are educators encouraged to attend?
Workshops with internal or external speakers	A workshop is held and facilitated by an "expert" Who are the experts in the topic to be presented? Does the facilitator request an honorarium to present the workshop?
Webinars	A webinar can be synchronous or asynchronous session that uses technology (Internet) to offer a development session Do the participants have access to the technology used in the webinar? Is the webinar interactive or not? Who is giving the presentation? Is it an internal expert or a vendor that provides faculty development?
Self-study; independent study processes	Materials are collected and offered to educators for study on an individual basis Who collects and determines appropriate resources? How will educators access such materials? How is success determined for self-study development activities?
Attendance at conferences	Educators choose professional conferences to attend that focus on interprofessional education How many people should attend the conference from a particular school, division, or program? How will conference attendees come back to their respective institution and share what they have learned with other faculty? Is there budget to send educators to attend the conference?

development model that is selected, there are a number of issues that must be addressed for such sessions:

- What are the goals for the faculty development sessions?
- What type of pedagogy is used for faculty development sessions?
- Who is the target audience and how will they be invited to development sessions?
- What are the indicators of success for accomplishing the faculty development sessions?

TOPICS FOR FACULTY DEVELOPMENT ON INTERPROFESSIONAL EDUCATION

Some consensus of topics exists according to developers who have a history in designing session on interprofessional education for faculty.[19,21-25] Such topics are listed in Table 7–2 and may include the following: purpose and goals for the interprofessional educational activities, ideal characteristics and attributes of educators and clinicians, and the competencies, components, and learning activities.[19] These topics must be addressed with all appropriate stakeholders involved in interprofessional education because many interprofessional experiences involve partnerships between academic institutions and health care or community sites.[21]

Stakeholders may include the didactic and clinical educators, teaching or graduate assistants, program directors, program curriculum committee members, program assessment committee members, and persons from clinical or community sites. Each interprofessional education cohort must identify appropriate stakeholders according to their specific context and interprofessional experiences.

STUDENT LEARNING AND PERFORMANCE EXPECTATIONS

The development of shared interprofessional core competencies for learners is an important foundational step in the implementation of any IPE program. Attempts to develop performance expectations or competencies for IPE have been in process for several years.

Although the United States' response to the Institute of Medicine's 2001 call for collaborative care has been somewhat slow (in comparison to similar core competencies have been developed in other countries since that time),[26] notable recent progress is evident. In 2009, with support by the Josiah Macy Jr, Robert Wood Johnson, and American Board of Internal Medicine Foundations, the Association of American Medical Colleges (AAMC), American Association of Colleges of Pharmacy (AACP), American Dental Education Association (ADEA), American Association of Colleges of Nursing (AACN), American Association of Colleges of Osteopathic Medicine (AACOM), and the Association of Schools of Public Health (ASPH) formed the Interprofessional Education Collaborative (IPEC), and a panel of experts was appointed by IPEC in 2010 to develop competencies to promote IPE and prepare clinicians for effective team-based care. Competencies across four domains were identified to ensure the foundation of knowledge, skills, and values for functioning as part of a team to provide effective patient-centered collaborative care. The core competencies, released in May 2011, include the following categories (Table 7–4)[7]:

- Values and ethics
- Roles and responsibilities

TABLE 7–4 Competencies for Interprofessional Collaborative Practice

General Competency	Examples of Specific Values and Competencies
Values and ethics for interprofessional practice: Work with individuals of other professions to maintain a climate of mutual respect and shared values	Place the interests of patients and populations at the center of interprofessional health care delivery Demonstrate respect, competence, cooperation, trust, and high standards of ethical conduct and integrity in relationships with patients, families, and other team members Ability is grounded in a sense of shared purpose to support the common good in health care and reflect a shared commitment to creating safer, more efficient, and more effective systems of care
Roles and responsibilities: Use the knowledge of one's own role and those of other professions to appropriately assess and address the health care needs of the patients and populations served	Recognize one's limits of professional expertise and role variance across specific care situations Recognize and communicate roles and responsibilities Engage resources when needed Practice at the "top" of one's scope of practice, or use the full scope of knowledge, skills, and abilities to optimize patient outcomes
Communication: Communicate with patients, families, communities, and other health professionals in a responsive and responsible manner that supports a team approach to the maintenance of health and the treatment of disease	Communicate in a firm but respectful manner when concerns about the quality or safety of care arise Select effective communication strategies Organize information Implement confident, respectful, and effective communication with patients, families, and health care teams, including listening, conflict resolution skills, and feedback
Teams and teamwork: Apply relationship-building values and the principles of team dynamics to perform effectively in different team roles to plan and deliver patient- and population-centered care that is safe, timely, efficient, effective, and equitable	Cooperate, problem-solve, and coordinate the patient-centered delivery of care, especially under conditions of uncertainty, to prevent gaps or errors in care Engage and integrate the skills of other health professionals in shared patient-centered problem-solving and care decisions Apply leadership practices, evidence, and accountability to perform effectively on teams and in different team roles in a variety of settings

Data from Core Competencies for Interprofessional Collaborative Practice. Report of an Expert Panel. Interprofessional Education Collaborative. 2011. Accessed August 3, 2011 from https://www.aamc.org/download/186750/data/core_competencies.pdf.

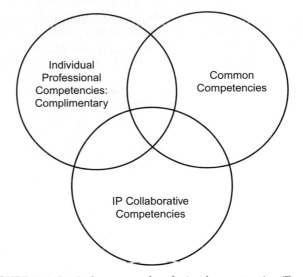

FIGURE 7–1 Barr's three types of professional competencies. (From Barr H, Koppel I, Reeves S, et al: Effective interprofessional education: Argument, assumption and evidence. Oxford: Blackwell, 2005.)

- Communication
- Teams and teamwork

To better understand the inter-relationships of these four domain of core competencies, it is helpful to consider Barr's model illustrating the "three types of professional competencies" (Figure 7–1), which include the following[7,27]:

1. Interprofessional collaborative competencies
2. Common competencies
3. Individual professional competencies: complementary

Barr describes *common competencies* as those expected of health professionals, and these are sometimes overlapping (e.g., application of various physical agent modalities or prescription of exercise regimens by physicians, physical therapists, occupational therapists, or nurses). Overlapping competencies may produce interprofessional tension at times because they are not identified as exclusive to a specific profession's scope of practice but may also be necessary to extend scarce health resources in medically underserved areas. *Complementary competencies* augment or improve the outcomes of other professions involved in providing care, such as a physical therapist improving the functional gains for patients who undergo total hip arthroplasty by the orthopedic surgeon. Although there will be some overlap related to pain management, as an example, the surgeon and physical therapist will provide mostly complementary expertise in managing the patient's condition. *Collaborative competencies* are skills that members of each profession need in order to function with others at a broader level, beyond interaction with other health care practitioners. Professionals must also function with patients and families, with nonprofessionals and volunteers, within and between organizations, within communities, and among policy makers.[27]

By establishing core competencies, it will not only be possible to coordinate the necessary curricular content, learning approaches, and assessment of outcomes across the health professions, it will also provide the foundation for a lifelong learning continuum for interprofessional competency as well as influence accreditation and licensure standards and evaluation research for interprofessional collaborative practice.[7] According to Aschenbrener, the health care we want to provide for the people we serve—safe, high-quality, accessible, person-centered—must be a team effort.[28] No single health profession can achieve this goal alone. These new competencies will build a path to a collaborative health care workforce and the improved care that we all desire.

Although the core competence consensus document provides a critical platform to advance IPE, it should be noted that the fundamental respect for professions is difficult to demonstrate when specific professions were not invited to be "around the collective" table for discussion. As Schmitt states: "A great deal of literature on IPE and practice is generated by and focuses on the TWO dominant health professions of medicine and nursing, whereas the health professions collectively encompass many more discrete fields of expertise, without which the quality of health care individuals and populations receive would be greatly compromised."[15]

It is clear that opportunity exists for the nonphysician health professions who are accustomed to practicing in settings that require team management of complex patient needs to provide modeling and leadership for team-based concepts in care.

ASSESSMENT TOOLS FOR INTERPROFESSIONAL EDUCATION

As the Core Competencies for Interprofessional Collaborative Practice are implemented into health professions' curricula, various instruments or methods for assessing student learning and performance related to IPE will be needed. According to a 2010 synthesis of six systematic review articles conducted by Reeves and associates, evaluation of IPE occurs with a variety of measures ranging from student satisfaction to patient care outcomes.[29] Within the academic setting, IPE outcomes typically involve formative assessments such as written assignments, reflective papers, and presentations. Learners' self-report of attitudes, perceptions, knowledge, and skills is typically assessed before, during (sometimes), and after learning experiences, and many programs collect two or more forms of data (i.e., survey and interviews).[29] Examples of three common assessment tools that have been validated in more than one study population and that can be administered to more than one group of learners are described later.[30]

The Readiness for Interprofessional Learning Scale (RIPLS), developed by Parsell and Bligh,[31] consists of 19 items anchored on a five-point Likert scale. It is designed to measure student attitudes toward and readiness for participating in interprofessional experiences, and it is composed of three subscales related to teamwork, professional identity, and roles and responsibilities. Although limitations existed because the original scale was validated in 120 undergraduate students, later validation involved administration of the questionnaire in a variety of populations, including both undergraduate and graduate students as well as practicing professionals.[32]

The Interdisciplinary Education Perception Scale (IEPS), developed by Luecht and colleagues,[33] is an 18-item self-report of attitudes toward interprofessional teamwork. Responses are recorded on a six-point Likert scale comprising four subscale measures related to competence and autonomy, perceived need for cooperation, actual cooperation, and understanding others' value. The instrument was validated with 143 subjects, representing the professions of medicine (including physician assistants), nursing, pharmacy, social work, occupational therapy, physical therapy, chiropractic, osteopathy, and podiatry.[34]

Attitudes Toward Health Care Teams Scale (developed by Heinemann and associates),[35] consists of 21 self-reported questions designed to compare attitudes of different members of health care teams. It can be divided into two subscales: the 14-item Quality of Care/Process subscale, measuring perceptions of the quality of care delivered by health care teams, and the six-item Physician Centrality subscale, designed to measure participant attitudes toward physicians' authority in teams and control over patient information. If IPE initiatives are successful, the scores for the Physician Centrality subscale should be expected to decrease over time and the Quality of Care/Process subscale measures should increase over time. The instrument was validated with national representation of 973 health care professionals practicing in geriatrics teams within the Veterans Administration health system.[35]

Finally, an emerging assessment option for IPE is based on the Objective Structured Clinical Examination (OSCE) used by medical schools to assess student performance patient evaluation and intervention. The Team Objective Structured Clinical Examination (TOSCE) has been developed, consisting of stations covering five common consultations in general medical practice,[36] and each station involves student completion of four tasks, including history, examination, diagnosis, and patient management plan. Teams of five students typically rotate through the five stations, allowing interaction and application of various roles in direct interaction with the simulated patient and the other health care professionals on the team. This technique is gaining some popularity for assessment of team function because study outcomes indicate the technique is relatively low-cost, students and raters have described the process as "fun," and the investment of time and labor by raters is not terribly burdensome. The utility of the TOSCE lies in its assessment of professional and interprofessional skills by learning through both self-reflection and peer feedback.[36]

Reeves' summary of current research literature about IPE reveals that most assessment data in IPE programs indicate positive changes in student perceptions, attitudes, knowledge, or skills related to IPE.[29] Although some studies failed to show change in attitudes over time, it is hypothesized that positive baseline attitudes toward collaboration were rated at a high level and remained high after completion.[37] According to Reeves' study, most students found value in IPE and reported favorable changes in their views toward collaboration with other professions. Knowledge and skills were also reportedly enhanced, especially related to role delineation, communication, and a better understanding of the specific nature of interprofessional collaboration.[29]

Figure 7–2 presents a comprehensive framework from the University of Toronto[37,38] that is useful for conceptualizing the complexity associated with assessing learner outcomes by illustrating the various levels of assessment as students progress from initial exposure and knowledge dimensions to application and competence of team-based practice.

Although there are difficulties in assessing IPE outcomes, such as the need for further development of research instruments to detect change and tendency for authors to interchangeably use terminology (e.g., *multiprofessional* or *collaborative training*), Reeves asserts that assessment of IPE initiatives has improved with clearly articulated definitions and methods and systematic use of specific assessment strategies.[29] There is a growing body of evidence that IPE may enhance practice and improve patient care,[29] but it is also recommended that more evaluations of IPE in simulated and authentic practice contexts are needed.[18]

TEACHING-LEARNING METHODS FOR INTERPROFESSIONAL EDUCATION

Although there is still much to understand about the most effective methods to foster student learning for interprofessional practice, many explicit methods have been employed with varying degrees of success. Research indicates that learning experiences based on characteristics of adult learners and involving elements of self-direction, choice, and active, practice-based learning in teams results in positive outcomes.[16,29] Cooke recommends that pedagogies involve clinical integration that allows progressive development of skills and attitudes.[39] Many interprofessional learning opportunities in community-based settings offer incredible complexity necessitating team skills, yet the interprofessional learning outcomes may not be explicitly stated. There exist many opportunities to build on or tweak existing learning experiences to

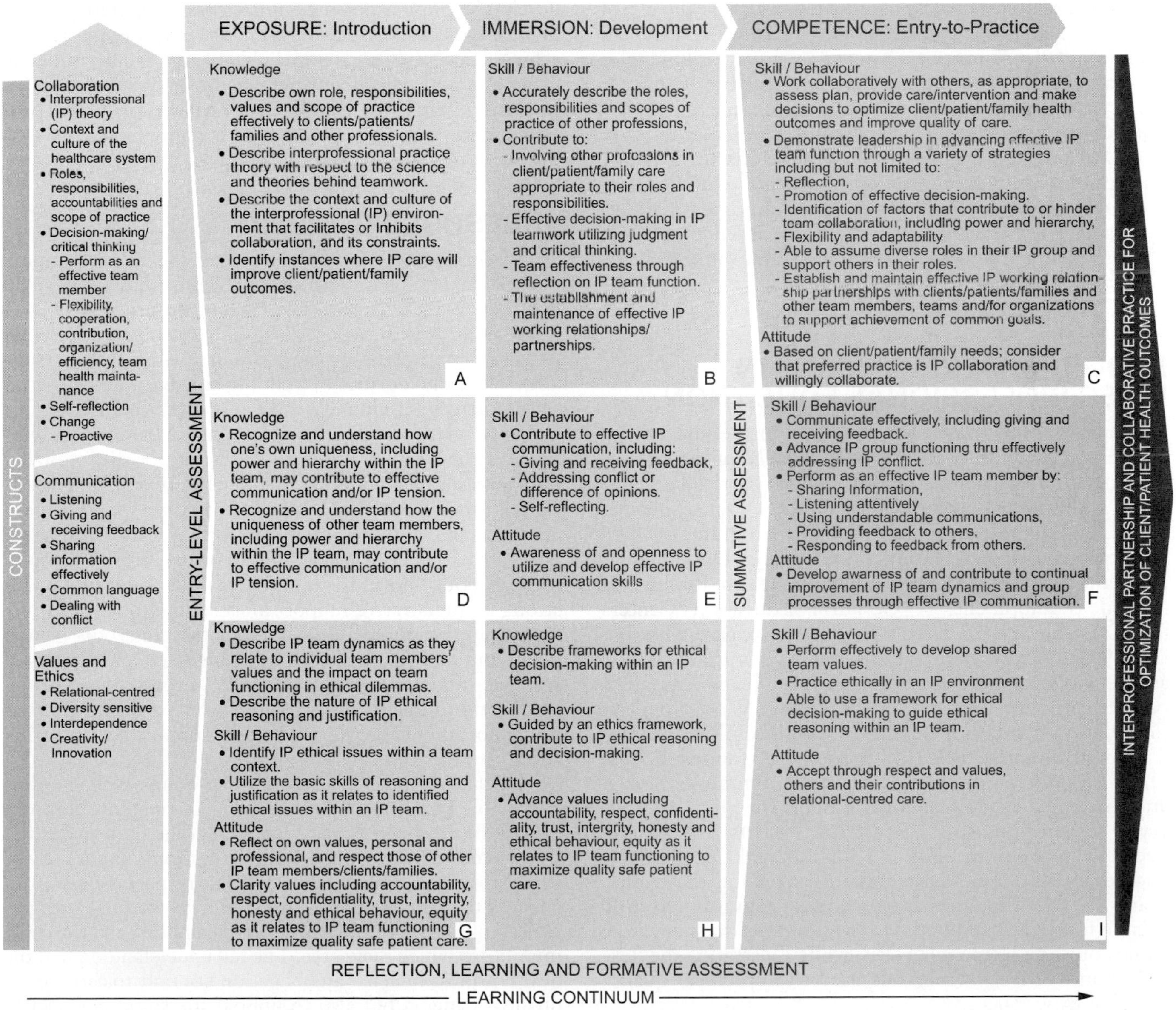

FIGURE 7–2 A Framework for the Development of Interprofessional Education Values and Core Competencies: Health Professional Programs, University of Toronto. From the University of Toronto, Centre for Interprofessional Education. Accessed February 2012.

provide an interprofessional focus. Faculty members must consider disciplinary preparation level of the learner (e.g., skill expectations at the end of the first semester versus end of third year of the professional curriculum) and whether learning experiences will be mandated or elective in nature.[7] In the absence of a systematic "menu" of multiple learning opportunities weaved throughout the curriculum, single elective experiences may send an implicit yet powerful message about the lack of importance of interprofessional culture. Finally, use of technology may facilitate IPE. Some programs have integrated simulations as a teaching modality for IPE; however, providing simulator activity for every student, and especially more than one student at a time, has been challenging.[40] Simulations appear to offer some promise for implementing feasible learning opportunities in an array of IPE activities.[40] Please refer to Chapter 6 for more detailed information on use of simulations.

In line with simulated patient management, a final consideration related to pedagogic issues in IPE is the use of distance technology and structuring learning experiences in online delivery formats. New educational technologies have allowed the educational environment to circumvent some of the traditional limitations of space and time.[41] Some practice settings, such as rural health delivery, do not have the luxury of multiple professions in the same physical proximity, yet effective patient care relies on effective communication skills. Distance technologies provide a mechanism for team interaction in the absence of direct physical contact, and the effectiveness and outcomes will need to be assessed.

PROGRAM DEVELOPMENT IN INTERPROFESSIONAL EDUCATION

Several programs have been described in the educational and research literature that serve as models for institutions that are interested in facilitating IPE. Historically, team-based training was attempted by the U.S. Department of Veterans' Affairs during the 1980s in programs such as the Interprofessional Team Training and Development program, and the federal Bureau of Health Professions funded development of Geriatric Education Centers (GECs), which also focused on collaborative care.[42] During the 1990s, private foundations financed initiatives such as the Collaborative Interprofessional Team Education (CITE) program (funded by the Robert Wood Johnson Foundation) and the Geriatrics Interdisciplinary Team Training Initiative (GITT) framework (funded by the Hartford Foundation). These types of programs developed and disseminated new national models for practice delivery.[30,42] Many notable and sustained efforts in IPE have been developed in the United Kingdom and Canada,[10,43,44] and several programs have gained traction in the United States.[16,45,46] Although many excellent programs currently exist, a few have been outlined in Table 7–5 to summarize some common elements of IPE, while illustrating the flexibility and variety of methods used to implement quality learning experiences.[10,46]

Programs vary by specific content offered, the combinations of participating professions, and the type and duration of learning experiences (see Table 7–5).[29] Reeves' synthesis of systematic reviews of IPE reveals that although programs varied, the following patterns were evident[29]:

- Various combinations of professions interact across the programs, yet medicine and nursing are the "core" professions represented.
- The most common combinations of learning experiences included didactic courses, seminar discussions, role-playing activities, and interactive cases or projects requiring group problem-solving strategies.
- Most learning experiences were elective or voluntary in nature.

There is little doubt that IPE will be necessary for developing the "collaborative-ready" health professionals needed in the challenging and changing health care environment.[6] This is a shared commitment that includes health professions education and clinical practice settings (Figure 7–3). Physical therapists may play an important role in modeling team-based competencies, and faculty members will need to develop learning experiences and assessment strategies that fit with their institution's mission and purposes in order to achieve success. "One size" will likely not "fit all" academic programs, and a flexible variety of opportunities grounded in clearly established competencies will be needed to promote successful interprofessional collaboration and ultimately improve patient care.

THRESHOLD CONCEPT

Threshold Concept #1: Understanding the critical importance of taking a strategic systems view of how to develop and implement interprofessional education.

Working within your discipline can be challenging enough, but negotiating the complexity of people, personalities, and the logistics of building collaboration and consensus across disciplines can seem overwhelming. The ability to "stand in the balcony" and take a broader, systems view can be very helpful in the IPE journey. Recognizing human resources and your personal networks and coalitions is critical, but organizational structures, policies, governance, and administrative support are also important factors to consider. Successful IPE work must be implemented both "bottom up and top down," meaning that strong administrative support must set the tone for expectations and resource allocation, but the grassroots faculty talent and leadership should be recognized and leveraged for role-modeling and sustainable success. The strong justification and guidelines offered by national and international documents provide additional support for garnering administrative resources.

The health professional's moral compass is a nonnegotiable component of educating competent, compassionate health professionals who are collaboration ready.

The centerpiece of the health professional's moral compass is respect for human dignity. This respect is a powerful concept that is fundamental for clinicians working with patients, colleagues within and across disciplines, and the communities in which they serve. The full understanding that the health professional has an obligation not only to care for individual patients but also to uphold the social contract in meeting societal needs and promoting the health of the nation is an essential cornerstone for interprofessional education.

TABLE 7-5 Examples of Model Programs for Interprofessional Education (IPE) in Canada and the United States

Program	Samples of IPE Learning Opportunities	Disciplines Involved
East Carolina University[46,47]	Stand-alone didactic courses sequenced to provide integration, case-based applications, and IPE service learning; rural immersion and workforce development projects	Medicine (including physician assistant), nursing, physical therapy, nutrition, psychology, health education, public health, child development and family relations, social work, health services management, health information systems
Medical University of South Carolina[16,46]	"C3 = Creating Collaborative Care" program: comprehensive, university-wide didactic coursework, IP electives, IP service learning in clinical rotations, national case competition, IPE social interactions	Medicine (including physician assistant), nursing, dentistry, pharmacy, physical therapy, occupational therapy, nurse anesthesia, cardiovascular perfusion, graduate biomedical sciences
Rosalind Franklin University of Medicine and Science[46,48,49]	Didactic coursework, service learning, culture focus, IP clinical experiences	Medicine (including physician assistant), podiatry, physical therapy, psychology, clinical laboratory sciences, medical radiation physics, nurse anesthesia
Saint Louis University[46,50]	Five designated IPE courses and service learning experiences culminating in Certificate in Interprofessional Practice on completion	Medicine, nursing, athletic training, clinical laboratory sciences, cytotechnology, nuclear medicine technology, nutrition, occupational therapy, physical therapy, radiation therapy
Thomas Jefferson University[37,46]	Health Mentor Program pairing students and adults with disabilities and chronic conditions, mandatory didactic coursework, experiential opportunities	Medicine, nursing, pharmacy, physical therapy, occupational therapy, couples and family therapy
University of Minnesota[46,51]	"1Health" program: mandatory didactic coursework and blended online modules, IP clinical experiences, national case competition, IPE social interactions formalized in "CHIP" program	Medicine, nursing, clinical laboratory sciences, occupational therapy, dentistry, pharmacy, veterinary medicine, public health
University of New England[46]	IP health education curriculum, simulation, cultural immersion project, research and clinical practice component	Osteopathy, nursing, pharmacy, occupational therapy, physical therapy, physician assistant, social work, nurse anesthesia, athletic training, exercise science
University of Pittsburgh[46,52]	Comprehensive incoming orientation coursework and case-based instruction with expert panels, interprofessional competition	Medicine, nursing, pharmacy, dentistry, public health, health and rehabilitation sciences
University of Washington[46,48,53]	Simulation-based team training; didactic learning experiences, web-based case scenarios, and team role modeling with standardized patients	Medicine (including physician assistant), nursing, pharmacy
Western University of Health Sciences[46,54]	Mandatory two semester didactic course for all first-year students, experiential courses, and clinical care	Osteopathy, nursing, podiatry, dentistry, veterinary medicine, physician assistant, physical therapy, optometry, pharmacy
Dalhousie University[10]	Mandatory program focusing on teamwork, professionalism, and specific topic areas through case-based discussions and interactions with expert panels	Medicine, nursing, physical therapy, occupational therapy, health and human performance, health service administration, pharmacy, dentistry
University of Alberta[10]	Mandatory 35-hour, case-based IPE course, including community-based group exercise	Medicine, nursing, physical therapy, occupational therapy, nutrition, and recreational therapy
University of British Columbia[10]	Multiple IPE electives and projects	Medicine, land, and food systems, applied sciences, arts, education, dentistry, and pharmaceutical sciences
University of Ottawa[10]	Rural Palliative Care Program focusing on IPP in palliative and end-of-life care in rural communities; involves continuing education opportunities	Medicine, nursing, social work, pharmacy, occupational therapy, physical therapy, dietetics, spiritual care providers
University of Toronto[10]	Core mandatory courses, IPE electives, case-based application for pain or palliative care, clinical component	Medicine (including physician assistant), nursing, dentistry, occupational therapy, physical therapy, social work, pharmacy, speech-language pathology, physical education and health, medical radiation sciences

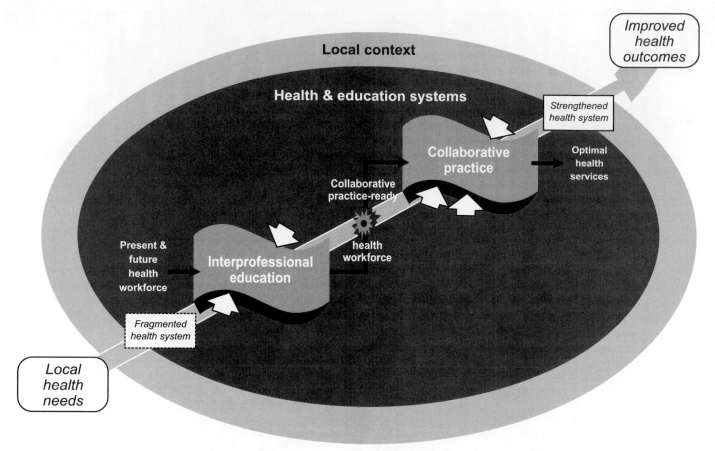

FIGURE 7–3 Framework for action on interprofessional education and collaborative practice. (From World Health Organization: Framework for Action on Interprofessional Education and Collaborative Practice. Geneva: World Health Organization, 2010.)

ANNOTATED BIBLIOGRAPHY

Barr H, Koppel I, Reeves S, et al. *Effective Interprofessional Education: Argument, Assumption and Evidence.* Malden, MA: Blackwell; 2005.

This books provides a systematic review of the effectiveness of interprofessional education in the health professions. There are chapters focused on conceptual models and potential theories that underlie interprofessional team work.

Core Competencies for Interprofessional Collaborative Practice. *Report of an Expert Panel. Interprofessional Education Collaborative.* https://www.aamc.org/download/186750/data/core_competencies.pdf; Accessed 03.08.11.

This document represents a critical point in health professions education in the United States as six health professions organizations came together to share ideas and generate a set of core team competencies. The core competencies represent a blueprint for all health professions. The document is a must read for all health professions educators.

Freeth D, Hammick M, Reeves S, et al. *Effective Interprofessional Education: Development, Delivery and Evaluation.* Malden, MA: Blackwell; 2005.

This is the first book on interprofessional education that provides examples of the development, delivery, and evaluation of interprofessional education. Interprofessional collaboration in education and practice settings in the United Kingdom, Canada, and Australia is far ahead of what has been accomplished in the United States given the structure of their national health systems.

Heinemann GD, Zeiss AM, eds. *Team Performance in Health Care: Assessment and Development.* New York: Kluwer Academic/Plenum; 2002.

This book describes the team functions and interaction in a variety of health care scenarios ranging from clinical practice to quality improvement committees. The strength of this book lies in its focus on evaluation of team function and its discussion of proven measurement instruments that capture the various dimensions of team performance. It is a good resource for faculty, students, clinicians, and health administrators who must facilitate effective teams.

Institute of Medicine. *Health Professions Education: A Bridge to Quality.* Washington, DC: National Academy Press; 2003.

The Institute of Medicine's 2003 report represents the second comprehensive report on interprofessional education (the first was *Crossing the Quality Chasm: A New Health System for the 21st Century*). This report develops a comprehensive new vision for clinical education in the health professions. These five core competencies for all health professionals were put forward: all health professionals should be educated to deliver patient-centered care as members of interdisciplinary teams, emphasizing evidence-based practice, quality improvement approaches, and informatics.

Royeen CB, Jensen GM, Harvan R, eds. *Leadership in Interprofessional Health Education and Practice.* Sudbury, MA: Jones and Bartlett; 2009.

This book on interprofessional health education and practice was the result of an interdisciplinary leadership conference focused on health care in rural and underserved settings. The book has six major sections covering topics such as strategies for promoting interdisciplinary education, leadership skills needed for interdisciplinary work, community development models, examples of collaborative teamwork, and a series of case studies on interprofessional health education and practice.

REFERENCES

1. Institute of Medicine. *Educating the Health Team.* Washington, DC: National Academy of Sciences; 1972.
2. O'Neil EH. *Recreating health professional practice for a new century.* San Francisco: Pew Health Professions Commission; 1998.
3. Institute of Medicine. *Health Professions Education: A Bridge to Quality.* Washington, DC: National Academy Press; 2003.
4. Institute of Medicine. *Priority Areas for National Action: Transforming Health Care Quality.* Washington, DC: National Academy Press; 2003.
5. Institute of Medicine. *Crossing the Quality Chasm: A New Health System for the 21st Century.* Washington, DC: National Academy Press; 2001.

6. World Health Organization (WHO). *Framework for Action on Interprofessional Education and Collaborative Practice.* Geneva: World Health Organization; 2010. *http://whqlibdoc.who.int/hq/2010/WHO_HRH_HPN_10.3_eng.pdf;* Accessed 10.06.11.
7. Core Competencies for Interprofessional Collaborative Practice. *Report of an Expert Panel.* Interprofessional Education Collaborative; 2011. *https://www.aamc.org/download/186750/data/core_competencies.pdf;* Accessed 03.08.11.
8. Sullivan W. *Work and Integrity: The Crisis and Promise of Professionalism in America.* 2nd ed. San Francisco: Jossey-Bass; 2005.
9. Royeen CB, Jensen GM, Harvan R, eds. *Leadership in Interprofessional Health Education and Practice.* Sudbury, MA: Jones and Bartlett; 2009.
10. Ho K, Jarvis-Selinger S, Borduas F, et al. Making interprofessional education work: the strategic roles of the academy. *Acad Med.* 2008;83:934–940.
11. Mitchell PH, Belza B, Schaad DC, et al. Working across the boundaries of health professions disciplines in education, research and service: the University of Washington experience. *Acad Med.* 2006;81:891–896.
12. Reubling I, Carlson JH, Cuvar K, et al. Interprofessional curriculum: preparing health professionals for collaborative teamwork in health care. In: Royeen CB, Jensen GM, Harvan R, eds. *Leadership in Interprofessional Health Education and Practice.* Sudbury, MA: Jones and Bartlett; 2009.
13. Greenfield D, Nugus P, Travaglia J, et al. Auditing an organization's interprofessional learning and interprofessional practice: the interprofessional praxis audit framework (IPAF). *J Interprof Care.* 2010;24:436–449.
14. Barr H. Interprofessional education: the fourth focus. *J Interprof Care.* 2007;21:40–50.
15. Barr H, Gilbert JHV, Schmitt MH. Interprofessional education and practice in health care: international perspectives. In: Harvan RA, Royeen CB, Jensen GM, eds. *Leadership in Rural Health Interprofessional Education and Practice.* Boston: Jones and Bartlett; 2009 Foreword.
16. Blue AV, Mitcham M, Smith T, et al. Changing the future of health professions: embedding interprofessional education within an academic health center. *Acad Med.* 2010;85:1290–1295.
17. University of Minnesota Center for Health Interprofessional Programs Student Center. Accessed 03.08.11 from http://www.chip.umn.edu/.
18. Hammick M, Freeth D, Koppel I, et al. A best evidence systematic review of interprofessional education. *Med Teach.* 2007;29:735–751.
19. Buring SM, Bhushan A, Brazeau G, et al. Keys to successful implementation of interprofessional education: learning location, faculty development and curricular themes. *Am J Pharm Educ.* 2009;73:60.
20. Steinert Y. Learning together to teach together: interprofessional education and faculty development. *J Interprof Care.* 2005;19:60–75.
21. Freeth D, Hammick M, Reeves S, et al. *Effective Interprofessional Education: Development, Delivery and Evaluation.* Oxford, UK: Blackwell; 2005.
22. Center for Health Science Interprofessional Education, Research, Practice. *Recent News.* May 31-June 3 University of Washington; 2011. *http://collaborate.uw.edu/about/news/recent-news.html* Interprofessional Training Accessed 19.07.11.
23. Interprofessional Education. *Our IPE Model.* Western University. http://www.westernu.edu/interprofessional-model; Accessed 19.07.11.
24. Faculty Development. *E-learning for clinical teachers. (2011). Background and policy context.* LondonDeanery. www.faculty.londondeanery.ac.uk/e-learning/interprofessional-education/background-and-policy-context; Accessed 19.07.11.
25. Center for Faculty Development. *University of Toronto at St. Michael's Hospital.* http://www.cfd.med.utoronto.ca/; Accessed 19.07.11.
26. Blue AV, Zoller J, Stratton TD, et al. Interprofessional education in U.S. medical schools. *J Interprof Care.* 2010;24:204–206.
27. Barr H. Competent to collaborate: towards a competency-based model for interprofessional education. *J Interprof Care.* 1998;12:181–187.
28. Aschenbrener CA. *Association of American Medical Colleges Press release: News Report Announce Competencies, Actions Strategies to Advance Interprofessional Education.* https://www.aamc.org/newsroom/newsreleases/2011/187630/110513.html; Accessed 28.12.11.
29. Reeves S, Goldman J, Burton A, et al. Synthesis of systematic review evidence of interprofessional education. *J Allied Health.* 2010;39:198–203.
30. Page RL, Hume AL, Trujillo JM, et al. AACP White Paper: Interprofessional education, principles and application: a framework for clinical pharmacy. *Pharmacotherapy.* 2009;29:145–164.
31. Parsell G, Bligh J. Shared learning between medical, dental, nursing, and therapy undergraduates. *Acad Med.* 1998;73:604–605.
32. Reid R, Bruce D, Allstaff K, et al. Validating the Readiness for Interprofessional Learning Scale (RIPLS) in the postgraduate context: are health care professionals ready for IPL? *Med Educ.* 2006;40:415–422.
33. Luecht RM, Madsen MK, Taugher MP, et al. Assessing professional perceptions: design and validation of an Interdisciplinary Education Perception Scale. *J Allied Health.* 1990;19:181–191.
34. Mu K, Chao CC, Jensen GM, et al. Effects of interprofessional rural training on students' perceptions of interprofessional health care services. *J Allied Health.* 2004;33:125–131.
35. Heinemann GD, Schmitt MH, Farrell MP, et al. Development of attitudes toward health care teams scale. *Eval Health Prof.* 1999;22:123–142.
36. Singleton A, Smith F, Harris T, et al. An evaluation of the team objective structured clinical examination (TOSCE). *Med Educ.* 1999;33:34–41.
37. Arenson C, Rose M, Lyons K. Model programs: Jefferson interprofessional education center, Thomas Jefferson University. *J Allied Health.* 2010;39:121–122.
38. University of Toronto. *Advancing the interprofessional education curriculum 2009. Curriculum overview. Competency framework.* Toronto: University of Toronto, Office of Interprofessional Education; 2008. *http://www.ipe.utoronto.ca/std/docs/IPE%20Curriculum%20Overview%20FINAL%20oct%2028.pdf* Accessed 20.07.11.
39. Cooke M, Irby DM, O'Brien BC. *Educating physicians: a call for reform of medical school and residency.* San Francisco: Jossey-Bass; 2010.
40. Shoemaker MJ, Riemersma L, Perkins R. Use of high fidelity human simulation to teach physical therapist decision-making skills for the intensive care setting. *J Cardiopulm Phys Ther.* 2009;20:13–18.
41. Weinstein RS, McNeely RA, Holcomb MJ, et al. Technologies for interprofessional education: e-classroom of the future. *J Allied Health.* 2010;39:238–245.
42. Heinemann GD. Teams in health care settings. In: Heinemann GD, Zeiss AM, eds. *Team Performance in Health Care: Assessment and Development.* New York: Kluwer Academic/Plenum; 2002.
43. *Center for the Advancement of Interprofessional Education Web site.* www.caipe.org.uk/about-us/defining-ipe; Accessed 06.07.11.
44. Gilbert JHV. Interprofessional learning and higher education structural barriers. *J Interprof Care.* 2005;19:87–106.
45. Lavin MA, Ruebling I, Banks R, et al. Interdisciplinary health professional education: a historical review. *Adv Health Sci Educ Theory Pract.* 2001;6:25–47.
46. Howell D. Interprofessional education programs today: surveying model programs in the U.S. *J Allied Health.* 2010;39:119.
47. Greer AG, Clay MC. Model programs: office of interdisciplinary health studies education, East Carolina University. *J Allied Health.* 2010;39:129–130.
48. Bridges DR, Davidson RA, Odegard PS, et al. Interprofessional collaboration: three best practice models of interprofessional education. *Med Educ Online.* 2011;16:1–10.
49. Rheault W, Stoecker J, Tappert S, et al. Model programs: Rosalind Franklin University of Medicine and Science. *J Allied Health.* 2010;39:125–126.
50. Ruebling I, Royeen CB. Model programs: Saint Louis university interprofessional education program. *J Allied Health.* 2010;39:123–124.
51. Brandt B, Buchanan J, Kostka S. Model programs: 1Health, the Center for Interprofessional Education, the University of Minnesota. *J Allied Health.* 2010;39:141–142.
52. Meyer SM. Model programs: interprofessional forum and competition, University of Pittsburgh. *J Allied Health.* 2010;39:139–140.
53. Zierler B, Ross B, Liner D. Model programs: the Macy interprofessional collaborative project, the University of Washington. *J Allied Health.* 2010;39:131–132.
54. Aston S, Mackintosh S, Orzoff J. Model programs: interprofessional education program, Western University of Health Sciences. *J Allied Health.* 2010;39:137–138.

PART II

EDUCATION IN PRACTICE ENVIRONMENTS

PREPARATION FOR TEACHING IN CLINICAL SETTINGS

Jody S. Frost

Teachers are those who use themselves as bridges, over which they invite their students to cross; then having facilitated their crossing, joyfully collapse, encouraging them to create bridges of their own.

      Nikos Kazantzakis in J. Canfield and M. V. Hansen's
      A 3rd Serving of Chicken Soup for the Soul.[1]

Case Situation 1

After earning a Doctor of Physical Therapy (DPT) degree and completing 6 months of clinical practice, I was informed that I would need to serve as a clinical instructor (CI) for a physical therapist assistant (PTA) student who would be arriving in 1 week! I was comfortable with managing a full patient caseload and all related activities, including using the patient management approach to care and evidence-based practice, applying concepts of defensible documentation in electronic health records, integrating the International Classification of Functional Disability and Health (ICF) in physical therapy and patient management, participating in case and family conferences, conducting quality assurance review, establishing and seeking positive interprofessional relationships, contributing to translating evidence into practice by participating in a journal club and weekly in-services, directing and supervising PTAs and other support personnel, and attending monthly professional meetings. Now, without more than a simple proclamation or an orientation,[2] I was to be assigned to a student for her first clinical education experience from a 2-year PTA program. Just when I was feeling like I finally had a handle on performing as a competent practitioner and meeting expectations, one more responsibility was "dumped" on me.

The center coordinator of clinical education (CCCE) hastily reviewed with me a copy of the academic program's curriculum and course learning objectives, dates of the 4-week clinical experience, name of the academic coordinator of clinical education (ACCE), and evaluation tool to be used to assess the student's performance for this first clinical experience. In addition, there was a brief student profile that provided her address, preferred learning style, and specific learning objectives for this experience. After this brief discussion, I was informed that the student would arrive at our clinical facility in 1 week and would need an orientation, "good" patients (excludes patients not covered by Medicare) with whom to practice her skills, and assurance that any patients selected would consent to care provided by a student under line-of-sight supervision. The CCCE asked me if I had any questions. After a brief pause, I quietly replied, "No." Not only did I not know where to begin to ask the first question, but also I was absolutely overwhelmed by the responsibility. I assumed that everyone who was assigned a student after 6 months of clinical practice must be capable of serving as a CI, and I did not want to respond any differently than my peers.

Afterward, I realized that in 1 week I would be responsible for this PTA student's clinical learning experience and had not a clue as to how to structure a planned experience. I was not completely familiar with the roles and responsibilities of a PTA student or the program's evaluation instrument because it was different than what I used as a DPT student. I had no experience providing a student orientation before and at best had only completed a new employee orientation. In reality, I knew very little about teaching students, let alone PTA students, in the clinic other than my recollections of being a student in the clinic and some classroom lectures on patient education and clinical education. For the next week I tried to informally question more experienced physical therapists and several PTAs about how they taught their students. I did not want them to know that I felt incompetent. I also tried to reflect on what my CIs did during my four clinical experiences by posing questions such as, How did they provide an orientation to the facility and the specific health care environment? What issues were discussed during the first few days of the experience? What were their expectations for my performance? Did I get a schedule on the first day and what was included on that schedule? What did they do to make me feel comfortable or uncomfortable? What did I remember most about my clinical educators that were positive or negative? Based on my limited discussions with others and my personal reflections, I developed a better, albeit limited, understanding of my perceived roles and responsibilities. All too soon it was time for me to teach my first student.

Case Situation 2

After 8 years of clinical practice in three different practice settings, including most recently a large teaching university hospital, and having earned both APTA Clinical Instructor and Advanced Clinical Instructor Credentials, I agreed to supervise two DPT students from the same program in a collaborative learning model on a 6-month internship. I was ready to try a new supervisory model of clinical education with two DPT students. This was their final 1-year internship of the program before graduation and eligibility to take the licensure examination. I had extended experience with managing, supervising, and evaluating students during their clinical education experiences, but this was my first opportunity to supervise two students in a collaborative learning model during an extended internship. My first concern was that I only possessed a Master of Physical Therapy (MPT) degree, with the addition of numerous continuing education courses provided by content experts and master clinicians in distance learning and face-to-face formats. I had been recently considering completing a postprofessional DPT degree; however, I had not made the commitment yet. Even with my years of clinical experience, earned American Physical Therapy Association (APTA) CI/Advanced CI Credentials, and additional training, I still had several pressing concerns. Was I adequately prepared to manage two DPT students in a long-term clinical experience and provide diverse and challenging learning experiences? Would the knowledge and skills that I possessed be adequate to keep pace with what they had learned in their program? What would I do with two students for 6 months because the longest clinical education experience that I had managed thus far was only 3 months? Was I well informed in how to apply the collaborative learning model? What if there was a significant disparity between the performances of these students? How would we address patient services provided by students where there are restrictions related to reimbursement and level of required supervision? What level of support was required of colleagues to manage two students during a 6-month internship?

In the past, I received excellent comments and feedback from students and academic programs regarding my performance as a CI, but those were different circumstances. Faced with the prospect of supervising two DPT students for a 6-month internship, I found myself questioning my ability and competence as a CI.

The first sketch is all too common in contemporary clinical education but illustrates a situation that can be prevented or eliminated given adequate training and resources. The second scenario is an emerging situation in physical therapy clinical education and describes new challenges confronting both experienced and novice clinical educators as a result of changes in doctoral professional education, lengthening[3] of clinical education experiences, exploration of different models of clinical supervision, and constraints related to patient reimbursement with students involved in the care. For both case situations, information provided in this chapter assists novice and experienced clinical educators with information and resources about the clinical education milieu; the roles and responsibilities of faculty, clinicians, and students involved in clinical education; preparation to be a successful clinical teacher; and alternative models and supervisory approaches for the delivery of clinical education.

LEARNING GOALS

After reading this chapter, the reader will be able to:
1. Understand the complexities of and relationships between different contextual frameworks in which students' academic and clinical learning occur.
2. Recognize the dynamic organizational structure of clinical education and the roles and responsibilities of persons functioning within this structure, including components of effective academic and clinical education partnerships.
3. Define the preferred attributes of clinical educators that contribute to enhanced student learning.
4. Identify hallmarks of quality clinical educator/preceptor/supervisor development training programs to facilitate planning, implementing, and evaluating clinical education programs and student learning.
5. Describe alternative clinical education models, supervisory approaches, and cooperative and collaborative approaches to providing student supervision and their relative strengths, considerations and limitations.

PHYSICAL THERAPY EDUCATION

Imagine education for physical therapists and PTAs occurring solely in an academic milieu or without any student clinical practice as an integral part of the educational process. Since the profession's inception, clinical practice as part of the curriculum has always been and continues to be of paramount importance and at the heart of students' educational experiences. Of significance is clinical practice's role in students' progression through the curriculum in preparation for entering practice. This is achieved by bridging the worlds of theory and practice, teaching in a real-world laboratory lessons that can only be learned through practice, introducing students to the peculiarities of the practice environment and the profession, and refining knowledge, psychomotor skills, and professional behaviors by managing patients with progressively more complex pathologies.[4] This aspect of the physical therapy professional curriculum is known as *clinical education*. On the one hand, clinical education is not currently constrained by type of practice setting or its geographical location, diversity of persons capable of serving as clinical educators, or the patient populations that clinical educators serve.[5–7] Strohschein and colleagues[8] believe, however, that the current climate of health care, with growing fiscal and time constraints, creates a growing tension between provision of appropriate patient care and provision of clinical education experiences for students. On the other hand, clinical educators are powerful role models for students during their professional education and significantly influence where, how, and with whom students choose to practice after graduation, and whether they choose to become future clinical educators.[9-11] Yet, in 2003 qualifications and credentials of supervising physical therapists in the United States were reported as quite varied, with the typical CI being female with a highest earned baccalaureate degree, more than 5 years of clinical practice, and 4 years of clinical teaching and has supervised two students in a 12-month period. Likewise, it was reported that the typical CI is not a member of the APTA and is neither APTA Credentialed nor a board-certified clinical specialist.[12] Thus, the outcome of physical therapy education is, in part, a reflection of the quality of clinical educators who help prepare graduates to deliver quality, cost-effective, and evidenced-based services to meet the needs and demands of society within an ever-changing health care environment.

DIFFERENCES BETWEEN ACADEMIC AND CLINICAL EDUCATION

The greatest fundamental difference between academic education and clinical education lies in their service orientations. Physical therapy academic education, situated within higher education, exists for the primary purpose of educating students to attain core knowledge, skills, and behaviors. In contrast, clinical education, situated within the practice environment, exists first and foremost to provide cost-effective and high-quality care and education for patients, clients, their families, and their caregivers. Academic faculties are remunerated for their teaching, scholarship, and community and professional services. Clinical educators are compensated for their services as practitioners by rendering patient and client care and related activities. In most cases, unless as a function of experience or as an employee of an academic institution, clinical educators receive little or no direct financial compensation for teaching students.[13] Physical therapy clinical educators are placed in a precarious position of trying to effectively balance and respond to two "masters." The first master, the practice setting, requires the practitioner to deliver evidenced-based, cost-effective, and high-quality patient services. The second master, higher education, wants the clinical educator to respond to the needs of the student learner and the educational outcomes of the academic program.

Other differences between physical therapy clinical education and academic education relate to the design of the learning experience. Educating students in higher education most often occurs in a predictable classroom environment that is characterized by a beginning and ending of the learning session and a method (written, oral, practical/simulated demonstration) of assessing the student's readiness for clinical practice. Student instruction can be provided in numerous formats with varying degrees of structure, including lecture augmented by the use of a variety of technologies, laboratory practice, discussion seminars, collaborative peer activities, tutorials, problem-based case discussions, computer-based instruction and patient simulations, and independent or group work practicums. With advancements in technology, including distance education,

hypermedia, virtual reality, and telehealth, contemporary teaching-learning archetype is being redesigned, and alternative structures and systems for classroom learning are clearly evolving.[14,15]

In contrast, the clinical classroom by its very nature is dynamic and flexible. It is an unpredictable learning laboratory that is constrained by time only as it relates to the length of a patient's visit or the workday schedule. Sometimes, to an observer, delivery of patient care and educating students in the practice environment may seem analogous in that they appear unstructured and even chaotic. Remarkably, student learning continues with or without patients and is not constrained by walls or by location (e.g., community-based services, service learning opportunities, international experiences, or home visits). Learning is not measured by written examination, but rather is assessed based on the quality, efficiency, cost-effectiveness, and outcomes of patient and client care provided by a student when measured against a standard of clinical performance.[15-17] Resources available to the clinical teacher may include many of those used by academic faculty, such as instruction using technology, practice on a fellow student or the clinical educator, online education or discussion, analysis of a journal article using principles of evidence-based practice,[18] or engaging in a teachable learning moment to enhance learning and foster intellectual curiosity.[19] Additional resources available to the clinical educator include collaborative and mentored student learning within and between professions, online libraries of patient cases, coaching strategies to more effectively manage clinical decisions, in-service education, grand rounds, surgery observation, special clinics and screenings (e.g., seating clinic, fitness screenings, community-based education to prevent common falls in the elderly population), presurgical examinations, on-site and online continuing education course offerings, interactions with other health professionals, and participation in clinical research. Rich learning opportunities are available in practice that complement, clarify, and augment much of what is provided in physical therapy academic education.[20]

Because learning occurs within the context of practice and patient care, the clinical teacher must be characterized as more of "a guide by the side" rather than the "sage on stage" that characterizes the classroom educator.[21] The clinical teacher, primarily through interactions, teaching, and handling of patients, assumes multiple roles, including facilitator, coach, supervisor, role model, mentor, and performance evaluator.[15] The clinical educator provides opportunities for students to experience safe practice. She or he asks strategically sequenced probing questions[22] that encourage learners to reflect, reinforces students' thinking and clinical decision making, fosters scholarly inquiry and sorting fact from fiction, and, by example, teaches and models for students how to manage ambiguities (e.g., balancing functional and psychosocial needs of the patient with available third-party payment for services).[21,23,24]

In summary, higher education and health care environments differ in relation to student learning because educators in each assume distinct roles and responsibilities that are circumscribed by the context in which learning occurs and the primary customer being served. Despite these differences, it is imperative that the two systems frequently communicate and interact with each other to fulfill the curricular outcomes of physical therapy programs and to ensure greater congruence between the theoretical, practical, and translational aspects of practice. In fact, academic and clinical educators, as partners in collaboration, must make concerted efforts to consciously bridge their differences given ongoing changes in health care and higher education that exist in different organizational structures. It is incumbent on the stakeholders in both communities to take the time to understand how these systems currently function and could function in the future. Thus, academic and clinical communities must explore new and innovative collaborative partnerships and organizational structures that enable quality learning experiences to continue in clinical practice in order to prepare safe, competent, and effective clinicians to meet the needs and demands of society.[8,25]

RELATIONSHIP BETWEEN CLINICAL AND ACADEMIC EDUCATION

The organization of clinical education is designed to provide a mechanism for academic faculty to share with clinical faculty their respective curricula and student expectations. In return, clinical faculty inform academic faculty of the relevance of the academic curriculum to entry-level practice and the ability of students to transform knowledge and theory into practice with patients as evidenced by their clinical performance.[26] Excluding students, the organizational system is often designed with persons providing three essential positions within clinical education. Persons assuming these roles must continually interact to ensure the provision of quality physical therapy education for students. These three roles are most commonly titled the Director of Clinical Education (DCE) or Academic Coordinator of Clinical Education (ACCE), the center coordinator of clinical education (CCCE), and the clinical instructor (CI). The DCE/ACCE is situated in the academy, whereas the CCCE and CI are based in clinical practice. Although, often not discussed as a part of the relationship between academic and clinical education, at the core of the clinical experience, first and foremost, is the patient (Figure 8–1).

Although the three primary players and the students largely manage physical therapy clinical education, it is important to remember that it is every physical therapist and PTA educator's responsibility to be vested in clinical education. Full-time clinical education represents a mean of 29.6% of the total curriculum[3] and is characterized as that part of the academic experience that allows students to apply theory and didactic knowledge to the real world of clinical practice.[3] As such, all academic faculty contribute to the effectiveness of the clinical learning experience because students' performance in the clinic is a direct reflection of how they were educated by faculty during the didactic portion of the curriculum. Faculty seek to understand how their classroom experiences relate to student performance in the clinic, and clinicians must comprehend how and what information presented in the classroom relates to the clinical education process and entry-level performance expectations. This is accomplished in a variety of ways, including faculty making clinical site visits and phone calls using established guidelines[27]; facilitating continuing education, external funding, and clinical research in

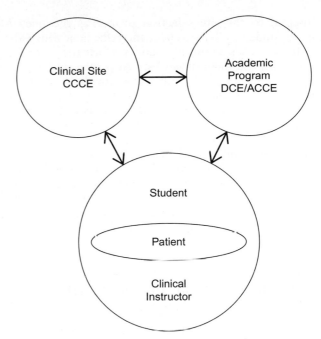

FIGURE 8–1 Relationship between clinical and academic education.

collaboration with clinicians; and serving as clinical educators in a self-contained model of clinical education.[28] Decisions about student clinical competence should not rest solely with the DCE/ACCE, but should reflect the collective wisdom of academic and clinical faculty assessments,[29,30] student self-assessments, consumers,[31] and employer assessments.[32] Additionally, the academic program has a responsibility to visibly demonstrate its commitment to clinical education by actively involving clinical educators in relevant aspects of curriculum design and development, including models of clinical education, implementation, and assessment of the physical therapy program.

CLINICAL EDUCATION ROLES AND RESPONSIBILITIES
ROLES AND RESPONSIBILITIES OF STUDENTS

The true messengers in clinical education are students. Students provide feedback to all stakeholders involved in the clinical education system. Given the various alternative models and supervisory approaches for providing clinical education, students bear a heavy burden because learning experiences are provided based on information received from academic programs that may be incomplete in relation to individual student learning needs. Only students can articulate their needs to the CI on a daily basis; therefore, they must take responsibility for their active learning if they wish to maximize their time in the practice setting.[33] Students must actively engage in the decision-making process of clinical site selection.[34,35] Interestingly, Gangaway and Stancanelli's 2007[36] study of students' perceptions of factors that were important for site selection determined that financial considerations, type of specialty offered by the facility, fulfilling program requirements, and reputation of the facility were found to be statistically more important than travel, proximity to school, and free or low-cost housing provided by the facility.

Integral to the site selection process is the need for ongoing student self-assessment and reflection, which identify the student's knowledge and performance strengths, deficiencies, and inconsistencies.[23] As part of this responsibility, students must feel comfortable providing constructive feedback to academic and clinical faculty. Faculty must remain open and flexible to student needs and be willing to modify the curriculum when revisions are shown to be necessary and feasible.

Self-accountability for behavior and actions is critically important for students as part of their learning contract. However, faculty should guide and model appropriate professional behavior and be willing to confront areas in which the students' professional values and behaviors are considered inappropriate or problematic.[37-39]

ROLES AND RESPONSIBILITIES OF THE DIRECTOR/ACADEMIC COORDINATOR OF CLINICAL EDUCATION

Since 1982, the roles, responsibilities, and career issues of the DCE/ACCE in physical therapy education have been investigated and discussed by several authors.[40-45] Although these studies span more than two decades, the essential responsibilities assumed by the DCE/ACCE have remained fairly consistent as related to administration and management, teaching, and service.[43,44] Additional skills that are incorporated in the role of the DCE/ACCE include increased use and application of technology for the purpose of communication, networking, and enhanced administrative efficiency and effectiveness, including the use of a clinical education consortia e-community, Web-based Clinical Site Information Form,[46] Web-based Physical Therapist Clinical Performance Instrument,[47] and Physical Therapist Assistant Clinical Performance Instrument,[48] use of more consistent student clinical performance assessment instruments that glean program and clinical education data[49] to manage and direct the clinical education program (including budget, personnel, affiliation agreements[50] and resources), assumption of leadership within clinical education, and other collaborative initiatives in working with program consortia, professional association groups, other health professions, and global clinical education opportunities including international clinical site placements.[51]

The DCE/ACCE functions in a pivotal faculty role in physical therapy education. She or he serves as the liaison between the didactic and clinical components of the program. In some programs, because of the number of students and the resultant number of clinical education sites required, more than one person has shared DCE/ACCE responsibilities (as co-ACCEs or as DCE/ACCE and assistant ACCE). The DCE/ACCE of a physical therapist program is a core faculty member and a licensed physical therapist with an understanding of contemporary physical therapist practice, quality clinical education, the clinical community, and the health care delivery system. Specific expectations of the DCE/ACCE based on their roles and responsibilities are articulated in the Evaluative Criteria for the Accreditation of Physical Therapist Programs.[6]

Additionally, the DCE/ACCE in a physical therapist program preferably has an earned DPT or doctoral degree or desire to pursue doctoral studies, has academic responsibilities including teaching, engages in scholarship, and provides community and professional service while balancing the many other unique administrative responsibilities associated with the position.[52] In 2010-2011, the highest degrees reported for DCEs/ACCEs were 12.8% PhD, 27.2% DPT degree, 34.3% postprofessional masters, and 11.6% bachelors.[3] The DCE/ACCE of a PTA program should be either a PTA or physical therapist with an earned bachelor degree or desire to pursue undergraduate studies. Additional preferred requirements include prior teaching experience; knowledge of education, management, and adult learning theories and principles; active involvement in clinical practice and professional activities at local, state, or national levels; and earned status as an APTA Credentialed Clinical Instructor.[53] The roles and associated responsibilities of a physical therapist program DCE/ACCE[43-45,52] are found in Table 8-1.

Additional activities that the DCE/ACCE should be involved with include the following[43-45,54]:

- Consortia activities (e.g., a group of regional academic programs and clinical educators that sponsor collaborative initiatives)
- Accreditation-related activities
- Program curriculum and university-based committee activities
- Clinical education research
- Management of budget related to clinical education
- Coordination of clinical education advisory committees
- State, regional, and national professional activities related to clinical education
- Leadership roles in bridging and strengthening academic-clinical partnerships in designing models for delivering clinical education
- Collaborating with others in managing clinical education

In some cases, DCEs/ACCEs have assumed a "broker" role in clinical education by linking clinical educators to facilitate clinical education research, arranging creative student clinical experiences (e.g., forming cooperative relationships for solo or rural practices), and forming collaborative working relationships with other academic institutions, faculty, or professions to increase access to clinical sites.

Given the unique responsibilities associated with this position in higher education and the ongoing need for clinical education program assessment, faculty performance assessment for the DCE/ACCE in support of this position is useful. There are several assessment tools available that define specific performance expectations for the DCE/ACCE. These tools are based on a 360-degree assessment of these performance expectations by program directors, academic faculty, students, CCCEs, CIs, and the DCE/ACCE. Assessments for the DCE/ACCE are beneficial to provide information about the DCE/ACCE's performance, describe workload responsibilities for those aspects associated with faculty and that are unique to this position, identify areas for professional growth and development, and provide constructive feedback about the clinical education program.[44,45,54]

TABLE 8-1   Roles and Responsibilities of the Director of Clinical Education/Academic Coordinator of Clinical Education

Primary Roles of the DCE/ACCE	Responsibilities Associated with Each Role
Communication between the academic institution and affiliated clinical education sites	Provide clinical sites with current program information (i.e., program philosophy, policy and procedures, clinical education agreements, clinical placement requests, student clinical assignments, required information for accreditation, performance assessments, and federal and state regulations that affect patient care provided by students). Foster ongoing and reciprocal communication between academic and clinical faculty and students through various mediums (e.g., phone, written, electronic and web-based correspondence, on-site visitations).
Clinical education program planning, implementation, and assessment	Perform academic and administrative responsibilities consistent with the Commission on Accreditation in Physical Therapy Education (CAPTE), federal and state regulations, institutional policy, and practice setting requirements. Coordinate and teach students about clinical education and related content, including the need to actively participate in the outcome of their clinical learning experiences. Remain current regarding issues in health care delivery and higher education that affect the provision of clinical education. Coordinate, monitor, and assess the clinical placement of students. Develop, maintain, and administer information and education technology systems that support clinical education and the curriculum. Coordinate, facilitate, and evaluate clinical education in the academic program, including instruments used for evaluation of the clinical education component of the curriculum for purposes of curricular assessment and revisions.[6,7,41-45,54] Review student clinical performance evaluations and provide feedback and interventions as required. Determine, in collaboration with program faculty, whether students have successfully met explicit learning objectives for the clinical experience to enable continued progression through the curriculum.
Clinical education site development	Develop criteria and procedures for maintaining quality clinical sites committed. Develop and maintain an adequate number of clinical education sites relative to quality, quantity, and diversity of learning experiences (e.g., continuum of care, life span, commonly seen patient diagnoses) to meet the educational needs of students and the academic program.
Clinical faculty development	Assess the faculty development needs of clinical educators. Develop, provide, and assess clinical faculty development programs that educate and empower clinical educators to effectively fulfill their roles as clinical teachers.[43-45,54]

Adapted from Department of Education. American Physical Therapy Association Model Position Description for the Academic Coordinator for Clinical Education/Director of Clinical Education. Alexandria, VA: American Physical Therapy Association, February 2011.

In 1988, Deusinger and Rose[55] challenged ACCEs to reexamine their role as part of physical therapy education by saying, "Like the dinosaur, the position of the ACCE is certain to become extinct in physical therapy education. The viability of this position is threatened because of the present preoccupation with administrative logistics and student counseling, a preoccupation that prohibits full participation as an academic physical therapist." They go on to suggest that "the role of the ACCE must be redefined for this faculty member to survive the demands of academia and serve the needs of the profession."[55] They expressed the hope that ACCEs would not become extinct in this position but instead would be transformed and emerge as an equal, valued, and respected member of the academic community. Twenty-three years later, the DCE/ACCE position still functions as a critical member of physical therapy core faculty with more well-defined roles and responsibilities that have expanded over the years. Today there are more doctoral-prepared DCEs/ACCEs with earned tenure (12.8%) or in tenure-eligible lines (14.3%). A majority hold the rank of assistant professor (50.6%), associate professor (18.1%), or full professor (1.6%). For those not with tenure, 40.3% of the DCEs/ACCEs are on a clinical track, and 32.6% are not eligible for tenure at their institution.[3]

ROLES AND RESPONSIBILITIES OF THE CENTER COORDINATOR OF CLINICAL EDUCATION

The CCCE's primary role is to serve as a liaison between the clinical site and the academic institutions. From the student's perspective, the CCCE serves in a unique but critical capacity. The CCCE is viewed as the neutral party at the clinical site who functions in the role of active listener, problem solver, conflict manager, and negotiator when differences occur between a student's perception of her or his performance and the CIs perception of the performance. In some situations, CCCEs function as mentors for individuals serving as CIs or those potentially interested in becoming CIs.[5]

Because of current pressure in health care settings to maximize human resources, it is as likely that the CCCE may be a physical therapist or PTA as it is that the individual may be a non–physical therapy professional (e.g., occupational therapist or speech therapist). In some professions, the use of a CCCE has facilitated the ability to assist in situations where there was an undersupply of clinical placements.[56] Whether the CCCE is a physical therapist or PTA or another health care professional, the following characteristics and qualities are considered universal to the role:

1. Interest in students and commitment to providing quality learning experiences
2. Experience in providing clinical education to students in the respective professions
3. Effective interpersonal communication and organizational skills
4. Knowledge of the clinical education site and its resources
5. Experience serving as a consultant in the evaluation process of students
6. Knowledge of professional ethics and legal behaviors
7. Knowledge of contemporary issues in clinical practice and the clinical education program, educational theory, and issues in health care delivery[5]

If the CCCE is a physical therapist or PTA, it is expected that he or she will possess attributes commensurate with that of CIs (see CCCE role responsibilities in the following list). CCCEs can assess their capabilities and competence by completing the APTA self-assessment for CCCEs.[5]

Responsibilities that are considered specific to the CCCE role associated with clinical site development include the following:

- Obtaining administrative support to develop a clinical education program by providing clinical education site administrators with sound rationale for development
- Determining clinical site readiness to accept students
- Contacting academic programs to determine whether the clinical site's clinical education philosophy and mission is congruent with that of the academic program
- Completing the necessary documentation to become an affiliated clinical education program (e.g., negotiated legal contracts that define the roles and responsibilities of the clinical site and the academic institution; clinical site information form [CSIF],[20] that documents essential information about the clinical site, personnel, and available student learning experiences made available in a web-based format in 2011[46,47]; policy and procedure manuals frequently available in an online format for ease of maintaining currency; and, in some cases, self-assessments for the clinical education site, the CI, and the CCCE[5]). The CCCE ensures that all required documentation is completed accurately and in a timely manner and is periodically updated as warranted by changes in personnel and the clinical site.[5] To assist the CCCE in managing his or her responsibilities, a *Reference Manual for Center Coordinators of Clinical Education*[57] was created that address administrative, managerial, supervisory, communication, and assessment components of this position.

Activities of the CCCE that are associated with preparing for and providing on-site student learning experiences include the following:

- Coordinating the CI student assignments and assessing the availability of learning experiences for students at the clinical site
- Responding to inquiries by academic program for available student placements and scheduling the number of students that can be reasonably accommodated by the clinical site on an annual basis
- Developing guidelines to determine when physical therapists and PTAs are competent to serve as CIs for students
- Providing mechanisms whereby CIs can receive the necessary orientation[2] and training to provide quality student clinical instruction
- Reviewing student clinical performance assessments to ensure their accuracy and timely completion
- Understanding legal risks,[58,59] including the Americans with Disabilities Act (ADA),[60,61] Family Education Rights and Privacy Act (FERPA),[62] and provisions associated with teaching and supervising students in the clinic

The role of the CCCE has changed over time given the milieu in which contemporary physical therapy clinical education occurs. Because of health care reform and resulting cost-containment measures that have occurred throughout the health care system, the CCCE may be a coordinator who manages administrative responsibilities associated with clinical education in large multicenter facilities, may be a physical therapist or PTA who can function as a mentor for new CIs, or may be a non–physical therapist or PTA who functions solely as an administrator without the expectations or necessary qualifications to mentor CIs or students, or the facility may not have a CCCE. It is critical that the profession continues to provide high-quality professional development programs that continue to educate the next generations of clinical teachers and mentors capable of ensuring the future quality and effectiveness of physical therapy services.[63]

ROLES AND RESPONSIBILITIES OF THE CLINICAL INSTRUCTOR

Example is not the main thing in influencing others. It is the only thing.
Albert Schweitzer. In Canfield J, Hansen MV, Rogerson M, et al (eds). Chicken Soup for the Soul at Work. Deerfield Beach, FL: Health Communications, 1996, p 125.

When asked if they can recall any of their CIs or preceptors, most health care professionals invariably answer "yes." Many say they remember not only the CIs who were exemplary role models but also those perceived to be poor role models. Likewise, they remember why a particular CI was remarkable or what they would have changed about their CI's performance. Impressions left by clinical educators are lifelong; a laudable tribute and commentary to the critical role that a CI plays in the life of every health profession student.

The CI is involved with the daily responsibility and direct provision of student clinical learning experiences. Central to every clinical learning experience is the student-CI-patient relationship. Often, students perceive that the success or failure of the clinical learning experience can be attributed solely to the CI. In reality, the quality of the learning experience is dependent on the interaction, management, and relationship of the learning triad of the CI, patient, and the student along with the community or environment in which learning occurs.[64] In physical therapy, the student supervisor is best known as the clinical instructor. Other synonyms for the CI include clinical tutor, clinical supervisor, clinical preceptor, clinical teacher, clinical mentor, and clinical educator. Each of these labels can be identified with one or more roles that this individual routinely performs. Much has been written in the health care literature about the CI's role, responsibilities, attributes of the CI that enhance student learning, and student and teacher perceptions of clinical instructor effectiveness.[12,37–39,65–72]

CIs significantly contribute to students' understanding of and competence in physical therapy clinical practice and serve as strong role models that guide students' visions of how they would like to practice in the future. Thus, the CI is responsible for providing an environment that fosters students' professionalism and encourages the development of an independent critical thinker and clinical decision maker through reflective practice to become a safe, competent, and effective entry-level practitioner.

Skills and Qualifications of a Successful Clinical Instructor

CIs' roles are multifaceted and encompass varied and diverse behaviors that include facilitating, supervising, coaching, guiding, consulting, teaching, evaluating, counseling, advising, career planning, role modeling, mentoring, and socializing. Before serving as a CI for students in physical therapy, competence should be demonstrated by the CI in several performance dimensions[5]:

- Clinical competence evidenced through the use of a systematic approach to care using the patient management model (i.e., examination, evaluation, diagnosis, prognosis, intervention, outcomes),[73–75] critical thinking skills, and effective time management skills
- Adherence to legal practice standards[58,59] and demonstration of ethical behavior[76–82] that meets or exceeds the expectations of members of the profession of physical therapy
- Effective communication skills, including the ability to provide feedback to students, demonstrate skill in active listening, and initiate communication that may be difficult or confrontational[67–70]
- Effective behavior, conduct, and interpersonal relationships with patients/clients, students, colleagues, and other health care providers[82,83]
- Effective instructional skills, including organizing, facilitating, implementing, and evaluating planned and unplanned learning experiences that take into consideration student learning needs, level of performance within the curriculum, goals of the clinical education experience, and the available facility resources
- Effective supervisory skills that include clarifying goals and student performance expectations, providing timely formal and informal feedback, making periodic adjustments to structured learning experiences, performing constructive and cumulative evaluations of student performance, and fostering reflective practice skills[84]
- Effective performance evaluation skills to determine professional competence,[38,39,71,85,86] ineffective or unsafe

practices,[83,84] constructive remedial activities to address specific performance deficits, challenging activities to engage exemplary performers, and the ability to engage students in ongoing self-assessment

Individuals can evaluate their readiness for or competence in serving as a CI by completing the self-assessment for CIs.[5] Higgs and McAlister[87] in their research identified six dimensions of a CI (Box 8–1). Different than competencies or a set of CI skills, these dimensions are oriented toward the CIs' socialization to their role and perception of themselves in the capacity of a CI.

In March 2010, a document entitled *Physical Therapist Clinical Education Principles*[88] was adopted by the APTA Board of Directors as a voluntary resource for physical therapist academic and clinical educators. Through a widespread consensus-based process and the involvement of multiple stakeholders, new graduate and CI performance outcomes were defined in this document. For the CI, 16 performance outcome categories were defined that increased the overall number and in some cases level of CI expected performance (Box 8–2).

When comparing the minimal qualifications for serving as a CI in 2000 with the expected qualifications for a CI in 2010, there is evidence that the expectations for the CI are

---

BOX 8–1   Six Dimensions of a Clinical Instructor

1. Having a sense of self
2. Having a sense of relationship with others as a central feature of clinical education
3. Having a sense of being a clinical educator
4. Having a sense of agency
5. Seeking dynamic self-congruence
6. Growth as a clinical educator

From Higgs J, McAllister L. Being a clinical educator. Adv Health Sci Educ Theory Pract 2007;12:187-200.

BOX 8–2   Categories Expected for Clinical Instructor Performance

- Teaching/instruction
- Planning and learning expectations
- Performance assessment and evaluation
- Self-assessment
- Practice management
- Communication
- Interpersonal skills
- Ethical and legal practice
- Professionalism
- Cultural competence
- Mentoring/coaching
- Supervision
- Modeling
- Professional development
- Level of practice performance/competence
- Qualifications

From APTA Physical Therapist Clinical Education Principles. Alexandria, VA, March 25, 2010. Accessed August 25, 2011: http://www.apta.org/uploadedFiles/APTAorg/Educators/Clinical_Development/Education_Resources/PTClinicalEducationPrinciples.pdf.

BOX 8–3 Comparison of Clinical Instructor (CI) Qualifications in 2000 and 2010

2000 CI Qualifications
- Minimum of 1 year clinical experience and the ability to perform CI responsibilities.
- Willingness to work with students by pursuing learning experiences in clinical teaching.
- Current state license, registration, or both (as required by specific state practice act), or certification or graduation from an accredited physical therapist assistant program.
- Positive representation of the profession by assuming responsibility for career and self-development and demonstrating this responsibility to students.
- Willingness to act as a professional role model and the ability to recognize the impact of this role on students.[63]

2010 Clinical Education Principles: CI Qualifications[88]
- Successfully complete APTA CI Credentialing[63] or equivalent training.
- Demonstrate a desire to educate students by pursuing learning experiences to develop knowledge and skill in clinical teaching.
- Be a licensed physical therapist when serving as the clinical instructor for the physical therapist student.
- Engage in ongoing self-assessment in the role and responsibilities of a CI.
- Maintain currency in professional policies, procedures, guidelines, code of ethics, and jurisdictional laws and regulations.
- Demonstrate effectiveness and proficiency in patient/client management.
- Determine the contributions of other health professionals to the student's learning experience.

BOX 8–4 Roles of the Practitioner and Clinical Instructor

Roles of the practitioner
- Patient referral and taking patient/client history
- Initial patient examination, evaluation, diagnosis, and problem identification
- Determining long-term functional goals mutually with the patient/client
- Defining short-term patient/client goals
- Clarifying patient/client plan of care
- Performing patient/client reexamination and assessing progression of care and interventions
- Assessing patient/client outcomes and readiness for physical therapy discharge

Roles of the clinical instructor
- Preplanning for the learning experience and providing an orientation to the clinical site
- Assessing students by identifying their strengths, learning needs, and previous experiences
- Setting overall student objectives and clarifying learning expectations with the assistance of students and the academic program
- Defining specific student behavioral and learning objectives
- Designing creative student learning experiences
- Providing formative student evaluations with modification of performance through feedback to achieve defined outcomes
- Providing summative student evaluations and assessing students' readiness for continued progress through the curriculum or entry into practice

Adapted from the American Physical Therapy Association Clinical Instructor Education and Credentialing Program, American Physical Therapy Association. The Clinician as Clinical Educator. Alexandria, VA: 2009; Section I, p 9.

---

different and elevated. Box 8–3 illustrates how these expectations have changed over a 10-year period. Of significance is a change from identifying a specific number of years of clinical experience to the successful completion of APTA CI credentialing or equivalent training. In addition, the more recent performance outcomes address issues of clinical practice in patient management, maintaining currency in professional policies, procedures, guidelines, and jurisdictional laws and regulations, and determining the contributions of other health professions to the learning experience.

Developing skills as a CI begins with an awareness of the parallels that exist between the roles of practitioner and CI. By recognizing these parallels, one can better understand how to transfer knowledge, skill, and behaviors used in delivering patient care to the task of designing a student clinical learning experience. Box 8–4 illustrates parallel relationships between practitioners and their patient management roles and CIs and their roles in coordination and implementation of student learning experiences.

Clinical Instructor Communication Skills

Several studies have focused on factors related to affective behaviors that are critical to effective learning experiences.[65,68,70,85,86] Affective characteristics of physical therapists found to contribute positively to patient and client care as well as effective clinical teaching include a positive attitude toward work, flexibility, compassion, sense of humor, openness to ideas and suggestions, friendliness, discipline and organization within the setting, and confidence in abilities and knowledge.[89] Students consistently rank communication, interpersonal relations, and teaching behaviors as the most valuable instructor behaviors in the clinical learning process. Interestingly, clinical nursing

faculty members were shown to possess four important qualities that collectively were important. These qualities were professional competence, interpersonal relationship, personality characteristics, and teaching ability.[39] When examining which of these qualities were shown to be most important, larger differences in scores were found between effective and ineffective teachers in the interpersonal relationship category, followed by the category of personality characteristics, with smaller differences in scores in the professional competence category and teaching ability category. The authors suggest that teachers' attitudes toward students, rather than their professional abilities, are the crucial difference between effective and ineffective teachers.[39] In a study by Young and Shaw, students rated university faculty as effective teachers for the majority of the rated items related to the affective domain.[90] Not surprisingly, the smallest differences found between "best" and "worst" clinical teachers were demonstrated in professional skills and knowledge.[65,91]

In a 1982 study by Emery, students ranked many of the behaviors identified to be necessary for effective clinical teaching as weak in their CIs.[65] APTA's CI Education and Credentialing Program (CIECP) was designed to provide an instructional program for CIs congruent with APTA's Guidelines for CIs. Because this program has been implemented in 1997, one might assume that behaviors required for effective clinical teaching are fully addressed through this professional development program. Recent studies demonstrate inconsistencies in the degree to which the APTA CIECP can be shown to produce a more effective CI. In a study by Morren and associates,[70] when examining the relationship between CI characteristics and student perceptions of clinical instructors, the authors found that students do not perceive the more qualified CI as being a more effective provider of clinical education based on the APTA Physical Therapist Student Evaluation: Clinical Experience and Clinical Instruction Survey (PTSE).[92] APTA CI Credentialing was shown to have a strong significant positive effect on four (provides timely feedback, clearly explains student responsibilities, integrates student learning styles, and provides constructive formal evaluation) of the 21 PTSE items measuring clinical instruction. In contrast, Housel and colleagues[93] found in their study using the New England Consortia–ACCE Student Evaluation that when the 27 CI-specific criteria were analyzed in summation, Credentialed CIs scored higher than non-Credentialed CIs, whereas when the 27 CI-specific criteria were analyzed individually, only 2 of these differences were statistically significant. Although APTA CIECP is one accessible professional development opportunity that provides CI training in physical therapy, it is not the sole determinant of CI effectiveness. Other mechanisms that support being a qualified CI include effective interprofessional and behavioral skills, instructional skills developed through other teaching and mentoring opportunities (e.g., classroom instruction, inservice programs, grand rounds), and performance evaluation assumed as a supervisor for other staff.

The area of student performance most frequently cited by CIs as lacking is also in the affective domain, specifically, interpersonal relations and communication.[94,95] DCEs/ACCEs previously reported that they are less comfortable failing students for solely affective problems unless they occur in conjunction with safety, psychomotor, or cognitive deficiencies.[96] In the past, physical therapy education did not have adequate mechanisms for clearly defining and assessing those professional, affective behaviors to which students should be held accountable in both classroom and clinic settings. However, instruments have been developed that can be used in the classroom (e.g., Professional Behaviors[97]) and the clinic[17,29,47–49,97,98] (e.g., physical therapist and PTA Clinical Performance Instruments, Clinical Internship Evaluation Tool, and Professional Behaviors) that clearly define performance expectations for student affective behaviors. Longitudinal studies should be conducted to determine whether the widespread use of these tools that clearly define expectations for acceptable professional behaviors translates into improved interpersonal relations and communication skills for both students and CIs.

Successful Clinical Instructors: Other Factors

Other factors that contribute to the success of clinical teaching and supervision are:

- The provision of student-centered teaching strategies that encourage activities such as reflection[21–24]
- Support for progressively increased student autonomy in approximating entry-level performance[99]
- Application of situational leadership theories applied in clinical learning that help students participate more responsibly in their learning experiences[100]
- Belief in a model of the best evidence-based clinical practices in physical therapy

- Explication of models of problem solving and decision making,[101–103] which can assist students in making better management decisions with sound clinical judgment, especially under ambiguous situations

Clinical teaching has also been shown to be more effective when systematic instructional strategies (e.g., preparation, briefing, planning, practice, debriefing) and repeated learning opportunities are available to students to reinforce learning.[100,104]

Enhancement of student learning occurs when the purpose of the learning experience is clearly defined, expectations for student and CI performance are clarified, the level of commitment is determined for all persons involved in the learning experience, and the timing, structure, frequency, and method of formative and summative evaluations are provided.[105] One of the greatest challenges for the CI is to find a balance for learners between nurturance and separateness. This is not unlike the delicate balance needed with patients and clients when providing physical therapy services. Specific techniques for teaching students in the clinical setting are discussed in Chapters 9 and 10.

PREPARATION FOR CLINICAL INSTRUCTION

To develop the requisite knowledge, skills, and behaviors needed to effectively perform their responsibilities as CIs, adequate formal preparation is strongly recommended in the areas of teaching, supervision, interpersonal relations, communication, evaluation, and professional skill competence.[106] Montgomery[107] believes that in addition to lack of formal training, many CIs also lack the "experience, maturity, and wisdom" to serve as mentors to physical therapy students. However, several studies describe CI characteristics as mature when most CIs are reported to have between 2 to 9 years of clinical practice experience and 5 or more years as CIs.[108,109]

Development and publication of voluntary *Guidelines and Self-Assessments in Clinical Education*[5] has significantly influenced clinical training courses and programs to use the six performance dimensions, described previously in this chapter under Skills and Qualifications of a Successful Clinical Instructor, as a basis for defining training objectives. In addition, many academic programs, clinical sites, and consortia provide training programs for CIs. In a 2006 study by Buccieri and associates,[108] CIs reported that they were effectively prepared and competent in their role. CI self-report was compared with the APTA's *Guidelines and Self-Assessments in Clinical Education*.[5] Positive relationships existed between CI self-report of effectiveness and the respondent's age, years in clinical practice, years as a CI, total number of students supervised, credentialing as a CI, and use of the *Guide to Physical Therapist Practice*.[73]

TRAINING PROGRAMS FOR CLINICAL INSTRUCTORS

Training programs for CIs should provide specific information about selecting appropriate, creative, and effective teaching methods that actively involve learners in both self-directed and guided experiences[110] Clinical teaching methods discussed might include demonstration-performance, teacher exposition, seminars, case analyses, case incident studies, role-playing and rehearsal, reflective diaries,[111,112] double-entry journal,[113] evidenced-based journal clubs,[114] clinical progression portfolio,[115] strengths-based teaching that emphasizes student empowerment, collaborative learning, and mutual growth,[116] conferences, brainstorming sessions, reflective discussions, and self-directed activities.[117]

Clinical training programs should also address the process of clinical evaluation. There are several key concepts in clinical evaluation:

- Feedback, summative, and formative evaluations
- Methods and techniques of evaluation such as competency-based, outcomes performance assessments, use of portfolios, and student self-assessment
- Problems in and legal aspects of clinical evaluation[50,58,59]
- A basic understanding of different evaluation instruments including how to critique their relative strengths and limitations and how to determine the most appropriate evaluation instruments for the specific clinical setting[17,29,30,49,118]

Development of effective communication and conflict management skills should be included in clinical training programs. Specific content to be addressed includes components of and barriers to communication; ways of improving interpersonal, professional, and organizational communication; sources of conflict in the clinical setting; and techniques for identifying, managing, and resolving conflict.[117,118]

Essential components of clinical educator training should include an understanding of the roles, characteristics, and responsibilities of the CI, organizational structure of the clinical education program, and management of students' experiences within the clinical environment.[5,13,119] Considerations in the management of the clinical environment include the following:

- Assessment of available learning resources
- Establishment of guidelines for a safe environment for patients/clients and students
- Understanding federal regulations related to the ADA,[60,61] FERPA,[62] and state regulations related to physical therapy practice
- Creation of an electronic filing system for confidential documents and other forms
- Development of a schedule for students
- Motivation of students to perform required tasks
- Development of a policy and procedure manual (printed or electronic) for students
- Selection of student orientation methods that are efficient and comprehensive (e.g., videotape of the clinical site, an established student orienting a new student)
- Understanding the management of patients/clients with diverse backgrounds
- Promotion of positive learning experiences through learning contracts or other approaches[63]

Frequently, as part of the tangible rewards of being a clinical educator, academic programs, clinical education consortia, or other clinical education special interest groups will sponsor continuing education programs for their clinical faculty at little to no cost.[11,120] Continuing education programs are generally identified as "basic or advanced courses" in clinical education. Training issues addressed in this chapter, in general, reflect content found in basic CI training courses with the exception of the Advanced CI Education and Credentialing Program. Regardless of the continuing education program, Notzer and Abramovitz[121] discovered in their research that long-term improvement of instructional skills continues after participation in even a brief workshop with a learner-centered approach that provides continuous feedback. Some training programs may offer state or regional credentialing or certificates and continuing education units (CEUs). However, most continuing education CI training programs do not have a mechanism for assessing the effectiveness of the training program in relation to knowledge, skills, and competence obtained by the learner.[122] Deusinger and colleagues[123] reported on a 1984-1985 pilot study, funded by APTA and directed by principal investigator Michael Emery in collaboration with Nancy Peatman and Lynn Foord in cooperation with the New England Consortium of ACCEs, Inc., which was conducted to develop a valid and reliable training and assessment system for credentialing clinical educators. A program was designed to ensure that clinical educators who complete the program are able to satisfactorily meet the APTA Guidelines for Clinical Instructors.

As a result of the successful pilot project, in 1997, APTA funded and developed a national voluntary CIECP[63] for physical therapist and PTA clinical educators to provide the essential knowledge and skills needed to plan, implement, and evaluate a quality clinical education program. This program is divided into two distinct parts: Part I, CI didactic curriculum through an interactive course format; and Part II, a credentialing process to assess participants' achievement of curricular outcomes through a six-station assessment center. Parts I and II are designed to be taught together to first provide and then assess the knowledge and skills identified as essential for physical therapist and PTA clinical educators. Part I is available to any health professional clinical educator with a minimum of 1 year of clinical experience or equivalency and interest in learning more about how to plan, implement, and evaluate a quality learning experience for students, whereas Part II is only available to physical therapists and physical therapist assistants who can earn the APTA Credential CI and CEUs (1.5). Completion of the didactic component of the program only for the non–physical therapy participant results in receiving CEUs (1.2). Today there are more than 34,500 physical therapists and PTAs that have become APTA Credentialed CIs.[124]

The didactic program addresses the following issues:

- Describing the parallels between the characteristics of the practitioner and clinical educator
- Planning and preparing for students during their clinical education experiences
- Identifying student learning needs
- Designing quality learning experiences
- Implementing clinical teaching methods and supervisory techniques that support ongoing learning
- Providing effective formative and summative evaluation
- Identifying legal and supervisory implications for clinical educators, including issues presented by ADA legislation, Medicare regulations, and the Patient's Bill of Rights
- Managing the student who is demonstrating problem performance or exceptional performance[125]

Only credentialed clinical trainers recognized by APTA can provide the CI Education and Credentialing program. To become a credentialed clinical trainer, U.S. and Canadian physical therapists/physiotherapists and PTAs must apply for the Train-the-Trainer course and meet established eligibility criteria to be invited to complete a 3-day intensive training program. By the end of the course, participants are expected to demonstrate mastery of the program content, an ability to manage and coordinate the assessment center, and an ability to competently teach, using active teaching strategies, selected content to audiences of different levels and disciplines. Credentialed clinical trainers are required to renew their credential every 3 years through a portfolio review process by the APTA Clinical Instructor Education Board. Typically there are between 150 and 185 active credentialed trainers available to teach the program throughout the United States and Canada.

In 2008, APTA launched a new voluntary Advanced Clinical Instructor Education and Credentialing Program (ACIECP)[126] to assist APTA Credentialed CIs, who were physical therapists, in integrating contemporary concepts provided to professional DPT students in the didactic component of the curriculum in clinical practice with patients. The ACIECP is also taught by Advanced Credentialed Trainers who have successfully met the competencies to teach this course. Topics address in the ACIECP include professionalism (includes the completion of three online modules before participating in the face-to-face course), clinical reasoning models, defensible documentation, evidence-based practice, *Guide to Physical Therapist Practice*, and Advanced Clinical Teaching concepts.[126] Today, more than 1000 physical therapist clinical educators have earned their APTA Advanced Credential CI.[124]

Finally, today we know more about what comprises the development of expertise as a CI. Thus, the process of learning to become an expert clinical teacher is a developmental experience[87] that in some ways mirrors what the CI strives to facilitate in their students. In Buccieri and associates' preliminary model, CI expertise was described as integration by the practitioner of professional development, teaching and learning, and relationships in a multidimensional process to acquire expertise in clinical instruction.[85] In Medicine, Graffam and colleagues[127] described a model of clinical instruction through observing clinician's teaching practices that consisted of seven interrelated behaviors labeled as engage, model, converse, measure, structure, conceptualize, and empower. They found that the degree to which clinicians shared their teaching philosophy generally correlated with the quality of their teaching. Not unlike the learning experiences designed for students, CIs require developmental opportunities to practice and reinforce knowledge and skills learned in clinical training programs, to learn from their mistakes,[128] and to apply this knowledge to real student situations, preferably with the guidance of a clinical teaching mentor.

Mastery of the subject matter related to providing effective clinical education, understanding the needs of learners and patients/clients to whom care is given, understanding the context in which clinical learning occurs, having competence and confidence in one's ability as a practitioner, and the ability to translate educational theory into the practice using sound principles of teaching and reflective practice as applied to the clinical setting all contribute to developing qualities of a master clinical teacher.[66,85,129]

MODELS OF CLINICAL EDUCATION

Although the most prevalent model of clinical education used in physical therapy is currently the integrated model,[3] the four models listed below can be found in selected physical therapist programs with new variations emerging in response to changing health care and higher education environments and cultures. These clinical education models are as follows[130]:

- Integrated model
- Independent and separate model
- Self-contained model
- Hybrid model

INTEGRATED MODEL

In the integrated model, the degree is conferred on completion of both didactic and clinical components with clinical education experiences interspersed throughout the curriculum and with shared responsibility between the academic program and clinical education sites. The clinical experiences may consist of both part-time (< 35 hours/week) exposures/experiences situated earlier in the program and longer clinical experiences (>35 hours/week) often in the final year. The full-time experiences may occur in two or three different clinic sites and health care systems representing different practice settings. This framework provides experiences addressing breadth and depth in patient management in preparing students for generalist practice competencies with a variety of patient populations in a variety of settings. Final clinical experiences may require a rehabilitation experience, acute or subacute care, and outpatient setting to address patients with simple and complex conditions across systems and the life span. These experiences are provided by clinical education faculty that are typically not paid by the academic institution. In addition, there are programs that use the integrated model and allow students who meet expected entry-level outcome competencies as a generalist practitioner to select an additional clinical internship in a more narrowed area of clinical practice.

INDEPENDENT AND SEPARATE MODEL

In the independent and separate model (e.g., medicine), the degree is conferred on completion of the didactic program, followed by a separate and independent clinical education experience, is frequently 1 year in length, with completion required to obtain a license to practice. Traditionally in medicine, the locus of control for the experience is the clinical education site and not the academic program, including readiness to progress through and exit the clinical experience and to be eligible to take the licensure examination. The student completes this experience in the clinical environment without oversight by the academic program, akin to a clinical residency in physical therapy. Representatives from the clinical agency interview the students for their placement, manage all aspects of the experience, and assess the performance of the students within the practice.

Within physical therapist education, a variation of this model (e.g., MGH Institute for the Health Professions[131]) exists whereby students complete a "shared internship model" to reflect the collaborative efforts of the academic program and clinical site. Students complete a final internship in which a portion (typically 2 to 4 months) of a 1-year internship is designed to complete entry-level program requirements to graduate and earn their DPT degree. Graduates are then eligible to sit for the licensure examination. Interns make a commitment to the clinical site for a full year, or 8 to 10 additional months following awarding of the degree. The licensed intern continues the remainder of the internship with the input and support of the academic program and clinical faculty, who provide ongoing mentoring and development of the intern in clinical practice. Interns are financially compensated throughout the yearlong internship.

SELF-CONTAINED MODEL

In the self-contained model (e.g., nursing and dentistry), the degree is conferred on completion of the didactic and faculty-supervised patient experiences. Nursing faculty serve as preceptors for students in groups supervised in clinical settings. Dentistry faculty serve as preceptors for dental students in a university-based dental clinic. Students complete supervised patient contact experiences with academic faculty members (salaries paid for by the academic institution) serving as advisors and clinical supervisors/mentors. In physical therapist education, the University of Pittsburgh[132] is involved as an academic-clinical partnership with the University of Pittsburgh Medical Center (UPMC), a large health care system where students can obtain nearly all of the necessary learning experiences within this system. For those experiences with limited exposures and availability (e.g., older adults, pediatrics) within UPMC, experiences are provided through non-UPMC affiliates. Students are required to complete a yearlong internship before graduation and to be eligible to sit for the licensure examination. Options are available for students to focus on one setting for the entire year; however, more often they request two different practice settings for a 6-month period. Supervision of students is provided by clinical educators that are employees of UPMC, where specific standards for clinical educators may be determined. In contrast, U.S. Army Baylor requires a full-time 12-month internship for students in a variety of clinical settings with emphasis on orthopaedics; however, they use only 13 clinical sites that are highly committed to clinical education and are contained within the military system.[133]

Another variation of the self-contained model was investigated by Nova Southeastern[134] as part of a contract awarded by APTA to study Alternative Models of Clinical Education based on a 2001 APTA House of Delegates motion (RC 36A/C-01). The purpose of this study was to investigate whether there was a difference in entry-level physical therapist skills between students clinically trained in a fully self-contained service-learning model and students trained in a combination model that consisted of first-level clinical experiences in a Self-Contained Model and final-level clinical experience in a traditional model. An additional purpose of the study was to determine whether there was a difference between the commitment and perception to underserved populations between students trained in the different two models. Based on statistical analysis, there was no difference in clinical skill level between students who received their clinical education in a hybrid model, including part-time collaborative self-contained service learning and traditional full-time 1:1 capstone clinical experiences, and those in the fully self-contained, service-learning collaborative model. The self-contained and the collaborative models were determined to be viable alternatives to the traditional 1:1 clinical education mode. Although the Self-Contained Model provided challenges, the overall benefits for students and faculty were reported to far outweigh the challenges.

HYBRID MODEL

In the hybrid model, clinical education experiences may occur in any combination of the previously mentioned models and may provide for simulated and real patient care in didactic and clinical environments.

MODEL SELECTION

There is no compelling evidence that directs physical therapy education to a preferred model of clinical education to which all involved stakeholders can agree.[135] As a part of the consensus-based discussion associated with the APTA Physical Therapist Clinical Education Principles,[88] a preferred model of clinical education was proposed as a springboard for further dialogue. One of the significant issues raised by the series of regional forums was the need for evidence in trying to change a model of clinical education for a profession. Given the paucity of research on the outcomes and effectiveness of various clinical education models, it is critical for the profession to investigate clinical education models with respect to student learning outcomes; cost-effectiveness to the clinic, student, academic program, and patients; patient outcomes; and feasibility of implementation and replication. In attempting to address the lack of evidence about the effectiveness of clinical education models, in 2011 APTA awarded a 2-year grant directed toward invesigation of "Innovation and Excellence in Academic and Clinical Education," to Jensen, Mostrom, Gwyer, Nordstrom, and Hack for their investigation of "Physical Therapist Education in the 21st Century." This is a critical study with potential findings to guide and shape the future of physical therapist DPT academic and clinical education.

Although the academic program, with consultation from the clinical education community, may elect to use any of the previously described models, that should not preclude the CI from using any of the alternative supervisory approaches discussed next when providing clinical education programs for students in practice.

ALTERNATIVE SUPERVISORY APPROACHES IN CLINICAL EDUCATION

To do justice to alternative supervisory approaches in clinical education would require space beyond that which can be allocated in this chapter. Therefore, only salient points are highlighted. Nevertheless, the reader is encouraged to explore references cited in this section and the subsequent summary table. Propelled by changes and constraints within health care delivery, federal and state policy issues, reimbursement, and the needs of CIs and learners, this topic continues to be an area of exploration and expansion in clinical education research in the health professions.

Although physical therapy clinical educators will comment that alternative approaches to student supervision were implemented in practice in the 1960s and 1970s, at that time little or no empirical evidence was reported that described these supervisory approaches, their benefits or limitations, or their outcome effectiveness. Since the 1990s and beyond, research describing the effectiveness of various approaches to student supervision has significantly increased investigating how best to provide student clinical education given limited personnel, financial, and space resources and the patients or clients involved. In a 2007 systematic review of the literature, Lekkas and colleagues[136] examined a variety of clinical supervisory approaches for physical therapist students (i.e., 1:1, 1:2, 2:1, 2:2, non-discipline-specific educator, and student as educator), and no single approach was found to be superior to another. Each model offered strengths and weaknesses, which were unique to the model. Although the purpose of many studies was to build placement capacity, most studies failed to identify the impact of the model on placement capacity. They concluded that there was no "gold standard" supervisory approach in clinical education.

Factors driving the use of different supervisory approaches in clinical education include preferences of the academic program and clinical facility, number of student placements accommodated by the facility at any one time and throughout the year, availability of qualified clinical educators, clinical educator schedules, requests from students, and the impact of federal and state regulations and payers. From 1990 to the present, pervasive changes have occurred in the configuration of practice and the delivery of physical therapy services; the breadth, depth, and design of physical therapist curricula in transitioning to the DPT degree to accommodate an expanding body of knowledge in physical therapy; the needs and changing values of students; the increasing numbers of students enrolled in physical therapy programs; increased length of full-time clinical education experiences in physical therapist programs[3]; increasing number of credentialed clinical residencies and fellowships; changes in the expected level of performance of clinical educators[88]; changes in payer regulations for students involved in patient-related services (i.e., Medicare Part-A and Part-B), and the level of experience of persons providing on-site student clinical supervision. Collectively, these changes have challenged the profession to rethink student-CI supervisory approaches and to consider and evaluate the use of other supervisory designs. Table 8–2 provides a reference and summary of varied clinical supervisory approaches, including their strengths, considerations, and limitations.[115,137–161]

COLLABORATIVE AND COOPERATIVE LEARNING

Collaborative and cooperative learning were originally developed for educating persons of different ages, experience, and levels of mastery of interdependence. Cooperative learning was principally designed for primary school education to assist children in becoming more efficient and effective in learning to work together successfully on substantive issues, to hold students accountable for learning collectively rather than in competition with one another, and to provide social integration regardless of issues of diversity. Collaborative learning is similar to cooperative learning in that the goal is to help students work together on substantive issues. However, collaborative learning was developed primarily to make students enrolled in higher education more efficient and effective in aspects of education that are not content driven, to shift the locus of classroom authority from the teacher to student groups, and to facilitate structural reform and conceptual rethinking of higher education.[162]

Although perceived by some to be synonymous and interchangeable terms, collaborative learning and cooperative learning within the context of small group learning are markedly dissimilar. Distinctions between collaborative and cooperative learning are generally drawn between the nature and authority of knowledge. The major disadvantage of collaborative learning is that, in attaining rewards of self-directed and peer learning, it sacrifices learner accountability.[162] Cooperative learning's major flaw is that by emphasizing accountability, it risks replicating within each small group the more traditional model of teacher autonomy.[163] These two approaches also differ in terms of style, function, and teacher involvement; the extent to which students need to be trained to work together in groups; different outcomes, such as mastery of facts, the development of judgment, and construction of knowledge; the importance of different aspects of personal, social, and cognitive growth among students; and implementation concerns (e.g., group formation, task construction, and grading procedures).[137,164]

Collaborative and cooperative learning, however, are based on the fundamental assumption that knowledge is a social construct, and open-ended tasks that facilitate collaboration and control by learners restructure the classroom environment.[162] The two philosophies also argue that learning in an active mode is more effective than passive reception—the teacher is a facilitator, coach, or "guide by the side," and teaching and learning are shared experiences between teachers and students, participating in small group activities to develop higher-order thinking skills and enhance abilities to use knowledge, accepting responsibility for learning as an individual and as a member of a group enhances intellectual development, articulating one's ideas in a small group setting enhances students' abilities to critically reflect on their thought processes and assumptions, belonging to a small group and supportive community increases student success and retention, and appreciating diversity is essential for the survival in a multicultural society.[163] Although there are distinctions between these two types of learning, for the purposes of exploring and implementing alternative supervisory designs in physical therapy clinical education, it is preferable to unite both learning approaches by drawing on each of their strengths to enhance the achievement of desired outcomes.

It is important to note that merely placing two or more students together during a clinical experience does not connote cooperative or collaborative learning. Specific

TABLE 8–2   Strengths, Considerations, and Limitations of Alternative Supervisory Approaches in Clinical Education

Design	Strengths	Considerations and limitations
One CI to one student (traditional design)	Allows the CI to maintain greater control of the learning experience Can easily monitor student performance Familiar student learning design Can easily provide line-of-sight supervision	Student less likely to learn from other clinicians Limited opportunities for collaborative learning Fosters student dependence on the CI
One CI to two or more students (collaborative-peer design)[115,137–146]	Fosters collaborative learning through peer interactions Enhances clinical competence related to clinical judgment Develops greater self-reliance, independence, and interdependence Teaches students to use and maximize limited resources Allows the CI to facilitate and guide the learning experience Fosters student problem-solving and critical thinking skills Makes orientation less costly and time-consuming Teaches students group presentation skills by providing collaborative projects or in-services Enhances service productivity in some settings (e.g., acute care)[140,141] Is useful for structured part-time group and early learning experiences	Initially requires more planning, effort, and organization time Requires that the total patient load is able to accommodate student needs Requires additional time to complete student performance evaluations Presents the possibility that too many patients will remain for the available clinicians after students have completed their training May be more likely used by an experienced CI Requires the CI to be highly flexible Can be problematic for CIs who wish to control learning experiences May be problematic for "needy" students or students requiring remedial work Is most successful when the CI carries a limited or no patient caseload
One PT and PTA/CI team to one PT and PTA student team (supervisor-director design)[147]	Enhances understanding and skills associated with direction and supervision Enhances understanding of the roles and responsibilities of the PTA Provides opportunities for PT students to learn appropriate use of the PTA through role modeling by the PT/PTA CI team Provides for collaboration and sharing of information between PT and PTA students Maximizes clinical site resources and minimizes competition for limited numbers of clinical sites when PT/PTA programs provide student clinical education concurrently	Assumes that a PTA is employed at the clinical site Requires that the PT/PTA/CI team clearly understands the appropriate direction, supervision, and use of the PTA, and role-models behaviors that demonstrate this understanding Assumes that the PTA and PT value and respect each other as coworkers Requires that the PT and PTA students are comfortable with their respective roles, strengths, and limitations so that they can learn from each other
One CI to two students paired from the same program at different clinical levels (student-peer mentor design)[137,142,148,149]	Same as one CI to two or more students design Allows the experienced student to develop supervisory skills Allows students to use each other as a resource and accept feedback more easily Allows the experienced student to orient the inexperienced student when beginning times are staggered Allows the experienced student to serve as the lead in situations in which the inexperienced student has not completed the didactic content Is useful in situations in which the inexperienced student has a shorter clinical experience	Same as one CI to two or more students design Can be problematic if students are not compatible in their learning styles or interpersonal interactions Requires alternative leadership design situations in which one student is the leader and the other is the aide, and vice versa
Two part-time CIs or two CIs on different rotations to one or more students[149]	Maximizes opportunities for part-time personnel to be involved as CIs (often experienced clinicians) Increases opportunities for clinical sites with part-time clinicians to participate in clinical education Exposes students to multiple approaches to care delivery Allows part-time and full-time CIs to show comparable abilities in providing learning experiences Permits students in the same setting to be exposed to different learning experiences with different CIs Allows a clinical site to accommodate more students by using multiple rotations within the same setting	Requires frequent and effective communication between CIs Can confuse students if expectations of the CIs differ Requires additional time for organization and planning Requires greater coordination between CIs in completing student performance evaluations Allows the possibility that students may compare CIs or CIs may compare students Can make it difficult for students to achieve their learning objectives Can decrease the variety and number patients/clients in the student caseload

TABLE 8-2 Strengths, Considerations, and Limitations of Alternative Supervisory Approaches in Clinical Education—cont'd

Design	Strengths	Considerations and limitations
Two part-ime CIs or two CIs on different rotations to one or more students (cont'd)	Allows for greater variability in length of the clinical experience Increases CI productivity in comparison with clinicians who are not involved Reduces supervisors' direct patient-related responsibilities Decreases the number of superficial questions posed by students	
Two CIs (one more experienced and one less experienced) to two or more students (teacher-mentor design or group supervision)[145,149]	Provides a mechanism to mentor and develop an inexperienced CI through role-modeling and teaching Allows students to learn to use parallel processes as inexperienced CIs Ensures that the experienced CI's knowledge is passed on to others Allows students to be part of a positive learning CI model that can be emulated	Requires an open and trusting relationship between CIs Requires that the inexperienced CI is comfortable knowing that he or she is inexperienced Confuses students as to which CI they are accountable Requires excellent communication and clarity of roles between CIs
Multiple rural or single practices offering collaborative clinical learning experiences (cooperative-network design)[150–152]	Permits solo practice settings to network with other sites to provide student clinical experiences Provides a support system for clinical teachers in rural settings Networking provides a mechanism to access clinical faculty training Enhances opportunities for students to be exposed to rural and solo practices Augments student learning experiences through interactions with multiple clinicians who provide care in different clinical settings Ensures that a mechanism is available for students to continue their learning experience uninterrupted in case of a CI's absence	Requires coordination and excellent communication between practice settings and CIs May be more difficult to implement because of different practice setting protocols and regulations Requires more complex coordination by the academic program with different legal contracts
One or more CIs from the same or different professions to one or more students from different professions (interprofessional cooperative design)[153 160]	Provides a learning model that teaches collaborative team learning among different professions Gives students a better understanding of the roles and relationships between different health care professions in clinical practice Teaches students team leadership and follower skills Models a learning environment to learn how to work more effectively together in an interprofessional setting Assists in minimizing "turf battles" that affect quality learning Teaches students consultative skills with other professions Supports Team-Based Competencies[161] to provide interprofessional and collaborative teamwork focused on patient-centered care	Applies only if different professions exist at the clinical site Requires excellent communication between and among the different disciplines Requires exceptional planning and organizational skills Requires that CIs trust, respect, and value each other's expertise and contributions to the learning process May cause problematic turf battles if interprofessional cooperation does not exist or where turf battles already exist Absence of role models demonstrating this model; resistance to change in using interprofessional team-based collaborative care

CI, *clinical instructor;* PT, *physical therapist;* PTA, *physical therapist assistant.*

components must be present for small group learning to be truly cooperative and collaborative. As Johnson and associates stated, "[a] group must have clear positive interdependence and members must promote each other's learning and success face to face, hold each other individually accountable to do his or her fair share of the work, appropriately use interpersonal and small group skills needed for cooperative efforts to be successful, and process as a group how effectively members are working together."[165]

Finally, assessment of any learning approach should be considered in light of several factors:

- The context in which learning must occur
- The academic program's expectations
- The available resources
- The availability of patients/clients
- The support of administration for clinical education specifically addressing productivity, cost-effectiveness, and reimbursement of care delivery
- The expertise, experience, and attributes of persons serving as clinical educators
- The relationship between all individuals involved in the teaching-learning process
- The characteristics of students

- Strengths, limitations, and considerations of a particular supervisory approach
- The time available for planning and evaluating the alternative supervisory approach
- The desired outcomes of the learning experience
- The strategies for ensuring successful implementation

SUMMARY

This chapter discusses topics perceived as most critical to understanding how to adequately prepare effective physical therapy teachers in clinical settings. It is understandable how situations like the two presented at the beginning of this chapter might readily occur. Today there are numerous resources and professional development opportunities for preparing future clinical educators and enhancing the knowledge and skills of experienced clinical educators. Many aspects of clinical teaching have been shown to be grounded in research that provides conceptual models and investigative studies that help to define components essential for quality education, expertise as a clinical instructor, and training programs for clinical teachers.

The reader is encouraged to explore references provided in the annotated bibliography at the end of this chapter to learn more about clinical instruction. As more clinical educators critically investigate the use of models of clinical education and alternative supervisory approaches, the profession will derive greater knowledge and understanding about the evidenced-based differences between these models and supervisory approaches and their resultant outcomes and effectiveness. Perhaps discussions espousing the benefit of one model design over another will be resolved based on empirical evidence rather than intuition, historical precedent, and personal anecdotes.[136]

It is my belief that implementing clinical teaching professional development programs is not sufficient. Ensuring the future long-term viability of physical therapy necessitates that the process of becoming a CI should begin when educating students during their professional studies.[165] Students should be oriented as part of their active participation in clinical education to understand the organizational structure and roles and responsibilities of the DCE/ACCE, CCCE, and CI as well as the rich learning experiences and gifts shared by patients who enable future generations to learn their craft. In addition, students should learn how to give and receive feedback, critically self-assess their learning experiences, and routinely perform self-assessments to monitor their growth and development throughout progressive learning experiences. They should begin to develop an understanding and appreciation for the analogous processes used in providing aspects of classroom teaching, clinical teaching, and physical therapy services. In this way, students will learn to translate the process of patient care delivery, which is the primary focus of their clinical education and initial practice, to teaching students in clinical settings, which is one of the first roles they will assume as practitioners.

Clinical educators must be held accountable for modeling those behaviors that they would like future practitioners to aspire to, and for demonstrating effective clinical teaching practices and evidence-based practice to ensure that students learn the knowledge, skills, and behaviors that are believed to be essential for entry into practice. Understanding one of the principles of pedagogy (i.e., that graduates will often teach in the clinical setting the way they were taught) means that CIs must critically examine their teaching and mentoring to determine whether their current approach is the legacy they wish to pass on. Andragogy, principles of adult learning, applies to physical therapy students and how they learn. Perhaps if CIs can recall their clinical education experiences as students, it will remind them of the pivotal role they play in the lives of all students. If CIs live by this rule, they can reshape clinical education. More important, individuals who serve to benefit most from these changes are the future graduates of physical therapist and PTA programs that will deliver quality, cost-effective, and evidence-based physical therapy care to patients and clients in an ever-changing health care environment.

THRESHOLD CONCEPTS

Threshold Concept #1. At the core of any clinical experience is the partnership and relationship between the CI, the student, and the patient.

Regardless of the practice setting, clinical environment, and academic institution, if the CI-student-patient relationship is compromised, then the overall learning experience may be jeopardized. As such, the interaction between clinical instructor, student, and patient is regarded as the strongest element in mentoring, modeling, and forming students' professional identity and in the development of expertise as a clinical instructor.[166]

TEACHING AND LEARNING ACTIVITY

- Design an activity that requires students to self-appraise and document how the management of different patients affects their development of knowledge, skills, and professional behaviors throughout the learning experience.
- Describe three learning experiences that could occur in clinical practice without patients and justify their relevance to patient management.
- Require that students keep a patient portfolio describing what they learned from each of their patient exposures and experiences to include personal reflections, lessons learned, and changes in their practice as a result of these patient episodes of care.

Threshold Concept #2. A strong collaborative partnership is required between the academic program and its affiliating clinical education sites to strengthen any model of clinical education within the curriculum.[131–133,160,167]

Clinical education is based on an infrastructure that requires strong partnerships between higher education and health care to address contemporary and future challenges and facilitate successful program outcomes. Individuals involved in clinical education are integral to the success of student clinical learning; however, without strong partnerships, they may not be able to function at an optimal capacity.

TEACHING AND LEARNING ACTIVITY

- Describe at least three ways in which academic and clinical partnerships could be strengthened in your organization.
- Define outcome measures that you would use to assess the strength of your current partnerships and any changes over time.
- Provide evidence for how your current partnerships facilitate or impede your relationships with students, clinical sites, and academic programs.

ANNOTATED BIBLIOGRAPHY

American Physical Therapy Association. *Guidelines and Self-Assessments for Clinical Education*. Alexandria, VA: American Physical Therapy Association; 2004.

This reference describes guidelines for clinical education sites, CIs, and CCCEs that were initially endorsed by the APTA House of Delegates in June 1993. These voluntary guidelines were designed to describe the fundamental and essential performance criteria that should guide the selection and development of clinical sites and individuals who serve as clinical educators. These guidelines are accompanied by three self-assessment documents that allow the clinical education site, CIs, and CCCEs to assess their performance as meeting the guideline, not meeting the guideline, or aspects of their performance being developed. Academic programs and clinical sites wanting to identify targeted areas for clinical faculty and clinical site development can use information gleaned from these self-assessments. Available at: http://www.apta.org/Educators/Clinical/SiteDevelopment/.

American Physical Therapy Association. *Physical Therapist Clinical Education Principles*. Alexandria, VA: American Physical Therapy Association; 2010.

A 2007 consensus conference on "Embracing Clinical Education Standards" was convened with critical stakeholders to systematically engage in a process of decision making about key components of physical therapist clinical education congruent with APTA's Vision 2020 and the DPT professional degree. Approximately 1000 persons were involved in the discussion of the draft principles across the United States during 15 regional forums. Agreement was reached on recommended performance expectations for new graduates and clinical instructors by more than 70% of the stakeholders (e.g., level of clinical competence, minimum required years of clinical experience, currency regarding professional policies, procedures, code of ethics, and jurisdictional law, training required for becoming a clinical teacher including APTA Credential CI or equivalency) and *preferred* clinical education infrastructure, organization and delivery that identified key components to enable clinical instructors to facilitate students' ability to achieve the new graduate performance expectations. APTA's Board of Directors adopted *Clinical Education Principles* for new graduate and clinical instructor performance as a resource for voluntary use by physical therapist academic and clinical educators. This resource document neither legislates nor dictates changes in clinical education, but rather provides for academic and clinical educators to use this document to inform their decision making and to stimulate further discussion among invested stakeholders about clinical education and explore future possibilities. Available at: http://www.apta.org/PTClinicalEducationPrinciples/.

Plack M, Driscoll M. *Teaching and Learning in Physical Therapy: From Classroom to Clinic*. Thorofare, NJ: Slack; 2011.

This text is an excellent resource for the health professional that models evidence-based principles by being grounded in strong theoretical and evidence-based approaches to teaching and adult learning within the context of health care. The framework for this text considers the capabilities, needs, and goals of learners, patients, and educators with ample opportunities for readers to integrate and reinforce learned concepts through personal reflection, thought-provoking questions, and real-world case situations. It is not often that a book models and practices what it espouses. Every teacher, clinician, and learner could benefit from this practical resource and should have this book in their office library to provide strategies to promote effective learning experiences for students and patients with application across health professions education and various practice settings.

Silberman M. *Active Training: A Handbook of Techniques, Designs, Case Examples, and Tips*. 3rd ed. San Francisco: Jossey-Bass/Pfeiffer; 2006.

This text is an excellent reference for academic and clinical teachers that provides active training approaches to engage audiences in the learning process. Silberman provides a systematic approach to active teaching that begins with the reflective planning process through design implementation and, finally, instructional and programmatic evaluation and active e-learning. Innovative strategies and case examples are provided to assist the instructor in developing variety in his or her teaching and for assessing which approaches may be best suited for different audiences. This reference is a must for anyone involved in teaching.

Watts N. *Handbook of Clinical Teaching*. New York: Churchill Livingstone; 1990.

This book provides a practical and user-friendly resource for health professionals to augment their knowledge and skills in providing clinical education for students. For illustrative and teaching purposes, Watts uses a multidisciplinary approach to understanding clinical teaching and encourages the completion of practice exercises in partnerships or collaborative interdisciplinary teams to reinforce learning. She facilitates learning through three essential teaching components: acquiring information, providing practice exercises, and giving immediate feedback. Some of the topics addressed include planning for student practice, performing a learning needs assessment, designing a learning contract, supervising practice of a complex skill, influencing student attitudes and values, giving effective feedback, and analyzing one's teaching style.

REFERENCES

1. Katzentzakis N. Canfield J, Hansen MV, eds. A 3rd Serving of Chicken Soup for the Soul. Deerfield Beach, FL: Health Communication; 1996:113.
2. McKinley MG. Go to the head of the class: clinical educator role transition. *AACN Adv Crit Care*. 2009;20:91–101.
3. Department of Accreditation. *Physical Therapist Program 2010-2011 Fact Sheet*. Alexandria, VA: American Physical Therapy Association; 2011.
4. Barnes MR. The twenty-sixth Mary McMillan lecture. *Phys Ther*. 1992;72:817.
5. American Physical Therapy Association. *Guidelines and Self-Assessments for Clinical Education*. Alexandria, VA: American Physical Therapy Association; 2004.
6. Commission on Accreditation in Physical Therapy Education. *Evaluative Criteria for Accreditation of Physical Therapist Programs: Accreditation Handbook*. Alexandria, VA: American Physical Therapy Association; 2011.
7. Commission on Accreditation in Physical Therapy Education. *Evaluative Criteria for Accreditation Physical Therapist Assistant Programs*. Alexandria, VA: American Physical Therapy Association; 2010.
8. Strohschein J, Hagler P, May L. Assessing the need for change in clinical education practices. *Phys Ther*. 2002;82:160–172.
9. Emery MJ, Gandy JS, Goldstein M. *Factors Influencing Career Selection of Students*. Presented at American Physical Therapy Association Combined Sections Meeting, Reno, NV.
10. Buchanan CI, Noonan AC, O'Brien ML. Factors influencing job selection of new physical therapy graduates. *J Phys Ther Educ*. 1994;8:39.
11. Gwyer J. Rewards of teaching physical therapy students: clinical instructor's perspective. *J Phys Ther Educ*. 1993;7:63.
12. Giles S, Wetherbee E, Johnson S. Qualifications and credentials of clinical instructors supervising physical therapist students. *J Phys Ther Educ*. 2003;17:50–55.
13. Gwyer J, Odom C, Gandy J. History of clinical education in physical therapy in the United States. *J Phys Ther Educ*. 2003;17:34–43.
14. Beckel C, Austin TM, Kettenbach G, et al. Computer and Internet Access for Physical Therapist Clinical Education. *J Phys Ther Educ*. 2008;22:19–23.
15. Sandroni S. Enhancing clinical teaching with information technologies: what can we do right now? *Acad Med*. 1997;72:770.
16. Scully RM, Shepard KF. Clinical teaching in physical therapy education: an ethnographic study. *Phys Ther*. 1983;63:349.
17. Roach KR, Gandy JS, Deusinger SS, et al. The Development and Testing of APTA Clinical Performance Instruments. *Phys Ther*. 2002;82(4):329–353.

18. Sabus C, Peck S, Lester J, Hinshaw G, et al. EBP partners: doctoral students and practicing clinicians bridging the theory-practice gap. *Crit Care Nurs Q*. 2009;32:99–105.

19. Rich VJ. Clinical instructors' and athletic training students' perceptions of teachable moments in an athletic training clinical education setting. *J Athl Train*. 2009;44:294–303.

20. Department of Education. *Clinical Site Information Form (CSIF)*. Alexandria, VA: American Physical Therapy Association; 2010.

21. Schön D. *Educating the Reflective Practitioner*. San Francisco: Jossey-Bass; 1987.

22. Barnum MG. Questioning skills demonstrated by approved clinical instructors during clinical field experiences. *J Athl Train*. 2008;43:284–292.

23. Jensen G, Denton B. Teaching physical therapy students to reflect: a suggestion for clinical education. *J Phys Ther Educ*. 1991;5:33.

24. Gandy JS, Jensen G. Groupwork and reflective practicums in physical therapy education: models for professional behavior development. *J Phys Ther Educ*. 1992;6:6.

25. Owen J, Grealish L. Clinical education delivery: a collaborative, shared governance model provides a framework for planning, implementation and evaluation. *Collegian*. 2006;13:15–21.

26. Peatman N, Albro R, DeMont M, et al. Survey of center clinical coordinators: format of clinical education and preferred methods of communication. *J Phys Ther Educ*. 1988;2:28.

27. Ebert MS. *Guide to Visiting Physical Therapist and Physical Therapist Assistant Students at Clinical Sites for Academic Coordinators of Clinical Education and Other Faculty*. New York: Columbia University; 1995.

28. May BJ, Smith HG, Dennis JK. Combined clinical site visits and regional continuing education for clinical instructors. *J Phys Ther Educ*. 1992;6:52.

29. Fitzgerald LM, Delitto A, Irrgang JJ. Validation of the clinical internship evaluation tool. *Phys Ther*. 2007;87:844–860.

30. American Physical Therapy Association. *Physical Therapist Student Clinical Performance Instrument*. Alexandria, VA: American Physical Therapy Association; 2006.

31. Dettman MA, Slaughter DS, Jensen RH. What consumers say about physical therapy program graduates. *J Phys Ther Educ*. 1995;9:7.

32. Mathwig K, Clarke F, Owens T, et al. Selection criteria for employment of entry-level physical therapists: a survey of New York State employers. *J Phys Ther Educ*. 2001;15:65.

33. Higgs J. Managing clinical education: the educator-manager and the self-directed learner. *Physiotherapy*. 1992;78:822.

34. Wojcik B, Rogers J. Enhancing clinical decision making through student self selection of clinical education experiences. *J Phys Ther Educ*. 1992;6:60.

35. Shoaf LD. Comparison of the student/site computer matching program and manual matching of physical therapy students in clinical education. *J Phys Ther Educ*. 1999;13:39.

36. Gangaway JM, Stancanelli J. Factors influencing student decision-making for clinical site selection. *J Allied Health*. 2007;36:124–141.

37. Ettinger ER. Role modeling for clinical educators. *J Optometr Educ* 1991;16–60.

38. Stenfors-Hayes T, Hult H, Dahlgren LO. What does it mean to be a good teacher and clinical supervisor in medical education? *Adv Health Sci Educ Theory Pract*. 2011;16:197–210.

39. Tang FI, Chou SM, Chiang HH. Students' perceptions of effective and ineffective clinical instructors. *J Nurs Educ*. 2005;44:187–192.

40. Harris MJ, Fogel M, Blacconiere M. Job satisfaction among academic coordinators of clinical education in physical therapy. *Phys Ther*. 1987;67:958.

41. Strickler EM. The academic coordinator of clinical education: current status, questions, and challenges for the 1990s and beyond. *J Phys Ther Educ*. 1991;5:3–9.

42. Clouten N. The academic coordinator of clinical education: career issues. *J Phys Ther Educ*. 1994;8:32.

43. Buccieri KM, Brown R. Evaluating the performance of the academic coordinator of clinical education in physical therapist education: determining appropriate criteria and assessors. *J Phys Ther Educ*. 2006;20:17–28.

44. Buccieri K, Brown R, Malta S, et al. Evaluating the performance of the academic coordinator/director of clinical education in physical therapist education: developing a tool to solicit input from center coordinators of clinical education and clinical instructors. *J Phys Ther Educ*. 2008;22:64–73.

45. Buccieri KM, Brown R, Malta S. Evaluating the performance of the academic coordinator/ director of clinical education: tools to solicit input from program directors, academic faculty, and students. *J Phys Ther Educ*. 2011;25:26–35.

46. American Physical Therapy Association. *Clinical Site Information Form Web*. Boston: Academic Software Plus; 2011.

47. American Physical Therapy Association. *PT CPI Web*. Boston: Academic Software Plus; 2008.

48. American Physical Therapy Association. *PTA CPI Web*. Boston: Academic Software Plus; 2010.

49. Proctor PL, Dal Bello-Haas VP, McQuarrie AM. Scoring of the Physical Therapist Clinical Performance Instrument (PT-CPI): analysis of 7 years of use. *Physiother Can* 2010;62:147–154.

50. Dye DC, Bender D. Duty and liability surrounding clinical internships: what every internship coordinator should know. *J Allied Health*. 2006;35:169–173.

51. Crawford E, Biggar JM, Leggett A, et al. Examining international clinical internships for Canadian physical therapy students from 1997 to 2007. *Physiother Can*. 2010;62:261–273.

52. American Physical Therapy Association. *Model Position Description for the Academic Coordinator/Director of Clinical Education: PT Program*. Alexandria, VA: American Physical Therapy Association; 2011.

53. American Physical Therapy Association. *Model Position Description for the Academic Coordinator/Director of Clinical Education: PTA Program*. Alexandria, VA: American Physical Therapy Association; 2011.

54. American Physical Therapy Association. *ACCE/DCE Performance Assessments*. Alexandria, VA: American Physical Therapy Association; 2010. *www.apta.org/Educators/Assessments/ACCE/DCE/* Accessed 25.08.11.

55. Deusinger SS, Rose SJ. Opinions and comments: the dinosaur of academic physical therapy. *Phys Ther*. 1988;68:412.

56. Rosenwax L, Gribble N, Margaria H. GRACE: an innovative program of clinical education in allied health. *J Allied Health*. 2010;39: e11–e16.

57. Trela P. *Reference Manual for Center Coordinators of Clinical Education*. Alexandria, VA: Clinical Education Special Interest Group; 2002. *http://www.apta.org/Educators/Clinical/EducatorDevelopment/*; Accessed 29.08.11.

58. Smith HG. Introduction to legal risks associated with clinical education. *J Phys Ther Educ*. 1994;8:67.

59. Fein BD. A review of the legal issues surrounding academic dismissal. *J Phys Ther Educ*. 2001;15:21.

60. Americans with Disabilities Act of 1990. PL No 101-336, 42 USC § 12101.103 (1990).

61. Ingram D. Essential functions required of physical therapist and physical therapist assistant students. *J Phys Ther Educ*. 1994;6:57.

62. Family Educational Rights and Privacy Act (FERPA). 20 U.S.C. § 1232g; 34 CFR Part 99.

63. American Physical Therapy Association. *Clinical Instructor Education and Credentialing Program and Manual*. Alexandria, VA: American Physical Therapy Association; 2009.

64. Plack MM. The learning triad: Potential barriers and supports to learning in the physical therapy clinical environment. *J Phys Ther Educ*. 2008;22:7–18.

65. Emery MJ. Effectiveness of the clinical instructor: students' perspective. *Phys Ther*. 1079;82:64.

66. Irby M. What clinical teachers in medicine need to know. *Acad Med*. 1994;69:333.

67. Dunlevy CL, Wolf KN. Perceived differences in the importance and frequency of clinical teaching behaviors. *J Allied Health*. 1992;21:175.

68. Emery MJ, Wilkinson CP. Perceived importance and frequency of clinical teaching behaviors: surveys of students, clinical instructors, and center coordinators of clinical education. *J Phys Ther Educ*. 1987;1:29.

69. Jarski RW, Kulig K, Olson RE. Clinical teaching in physical therapy: student and teacher perceptions. *Phys Ther*. 1990;70:173.

70. Morren KK, Gordon SP, Sawyer BA. The relationship between clinical instructor characteristics and student perceptions of clinical instructor effectiveness. *J Phys Ther Educ*. 2008;22:52–61.

71. Rogers JL, Lautar CJ, Dunn LR. Allied health students' perceptions of effective clinical instruction. *Health Care Manag (Frederick)*. 2010;29:63–67.

72. Ingrassia JM. Effective radiography clinical instructor characteristics. *Radiol Technol*. 2011;82:409–420.

73. American Physical Therapy Association. *Guide to Physical Therapist Practice*. revised 2nd Alexandria, VA: American Physical Therapy Association; 2003.
74. American Physical Therapy Association. *A Normative Model for Physical Therapist Professional Education, Version 2004*. Alexandria, VA: American Physical Therapy Association; 2004.
75. American Physical Therapy Association. *A Normative Model for Physical Therapist Assistant Education, Version 2007*. Alexandria, VA: American Physical Therapy Association; 2007.
76. American Physical Therapy Association. *Code of Ethics for the Physical Therapist*. (HOD S06-09-07-12). Revised 2009.
77. American Physical Therapy Association. *Standards of Practice for Physical Therapy (HOD S06-10-09-07)*. Revised 2010.
78. American Physical Therapy Association. *Guide for Professional Conduct*. Alexandria, VA: American Physical Therapy Association; 2010.
79. American Physical Therapy Association. *Professionalism in Physical Therapy: Core Values (HOD P05-07-19-19)*. June 2007.
80. American Physical Therapy Association. *Guide for Conduct of the Physical Therapist Assistant*. Alexandria, VA: American Physical Therapy Association; 2010.
81. American Physical Therapy Association. *Standards of Ethical Conduct for the Physical Therapist Assistant (HOD S06-09-20-18)*. November 2010.
82. American Physical Therapy Association. *Values-Based Behaviors for the PTA*. Alexandria, VA: American Physical Therapy Association; 2011.
83. Gleeson PB. Understanding generational competence related to professionalism: misunderstandings that lead to a perception of unprofessional behavior. *J Phys Ther Educ*. 2007;21:23–28.
84. Jette DU, Bertoni A, Coots R. Clinical instructor's perceptions of behaviors that compromise entry-level clinical performance in physical therapist students: a qualitative study. *Phys Ther* 2007;87:833–843.
85. Buccieri KM, Pivko SE, Olzenak DL. How does a physical therapist acquire the skills of an expert clinical instructor? *J Phys Ther Educ*. 2011;25:17–25.
86. Kelly SP. The exemplary clinical instructor: a qualitative case study. *J Phys Ther Educ*. 2007;21:63–69.
87. Higgs J, McAllister L. Being a clinical educator. *Adv Health Sci Educ Theory Pract*. 2007;12(2):187–200.
88. *APTA Physical Therapist Clinical Education Principles*. Alexandria, VA: American Physical Therapy Association; 2010. *http://www.apta.org/uploadedFiles/APTAorg/Educators/Clinical_Development/Education_Resources/PTClinicalEducationPrinciples.pdf*. Accessed 25.08.11.
89. Wojcik R. *Students' perceptions of the affective characteristics of physical therapists*. University of Illinois, Health Sciences Center: Master's thesis; 1984.
90. Young S, Shaw DG. Profiles of effective college and university teachers. *J Higher Educ*. 1999;70:670.
91. Irby DM, Ramsey PG, Gillmore GM, Schaad D. Characteristics of effective clinical teachers of ambulatory care medicine. *Acad Med*. 1991;6:54.
92. American Physical Therapy Association. *A Physical Therapist Student Evaluation: Clinical Experience and Clinical Instruction Survey*. Alexandria, VA: American Physical Therapy Association; 2010. *http://www.apta.org/Educators/Clinical/SiteDevelopment/*. Accessed 25.08.11.
93. Housel N, Gandy J, Edmondson D. Clinical instructor credentialing and student assessment of clinical instructor effectiveness. *J Phys Ther Educ*. 2010;24:26–34.
94. Foord L, DeMont M. Teaching students in the clinical setting: managing the problem situation. *J Phys Ther Educ*. 1990;4:61.
95. Ramsborg GC, Holloway R. Congruence of student, faculty, and graduate perceptions of positive and negative learning experiences. *J Am Assoc Nurse Anesth*. 1987;55:135.
96. Gandy JS. How academic coordinators of clinical education resolve student problems [abstract]. *Phys Ther*. 1985;65:695.
97. Warren M, Kontney L, Iglarsh ZA. *Professional Behaviors for the 21st Century*. http://www.marquette.edu/physical-therapy/documents/ProfessionalBehaviors.pdf; 2009–2010. Accessed 25.08.11..
98. Ullian JA, Blanc CJ, Simpson DE. An alternative approach to defining the role of the clinical teacher. *Acad Med*. 1994;69:832.
99. Kennedy TJ, Regehr G, Baker GR, Lingard LA. Progressive independence in clinical training: a tradition worth defending? *Acad Med*. 2005;80:S106–S111.
100. Keenan MJ, Hoover PS, Hoover R, et al. Leadership theory lets clinical instructors guide students toward autonomy. *Nurs Health Care*. 1988;9:82.
101. Denton B. Facilitating clinical judgment across the curriculum. *J Phys Ther Educ*. 1992;6:60.
102. Ajjawi R, Higgs J. Learning to reason: a journey of professional socialisation. *Adv Health Sci Educ Theory Pract*. 2008;13:133–150.
103. Slaughter DS, Brown DS, Gardner DL, et al. Improving physical therapy students' clinical problem-solving skills: an analytical questioning model. *Phys Ther*. 1989;69:441.
104. Allen SS, Bland CJ, Harris IB, et al. Structured clinical teaching strategy. *Med Teach*. 1991;13:177.
105. Anderson DC, Harris IB, Allen S, et al. Comparing students' feedback about clinical instruction with their performances. *Acad Med*. 1991;66:29.
106. Williams L, Irvine F. How can the clinical supervisor role be facilitated in nursing? A phenomenological exploration. *J Nurs Manag*. 2009;17:474–483.
107. Montgomery J. Clinical Faculty: Revitalization for 2001. In: *Section for Education and Department of Education, Pivotal Issues in Clinical Education Present Status/Future Needs*. Washington, DC: American Physical Therapy Association; 1988:7.
108. Buccieri KM, Schultze K, Dunget J, et al. Self-reported characteristics of physical therapy clinical instructors: a comparison to the American Physical Therapy Association's *Guidelines and Self-Assessments for Clinical Education*. *J Phys Ther Educ*. 2006;20:47–55.
109. Housel N, Gandy J. Clinical instructor credentialing and its effect on student clinical performance outcomes. *J Phys Ther Educ*. 2008;22:43–51.
110. Silberman M. *Active Training: A Handbook of Techniques, Designs, Case Examples, and Tips*. San Francisco: Jossey-Bass/Pfeiffer; 2006.
111. Mostrom E, Shepard KF. Teaching and learning about patient education in physical therapy professional preparation: academic and clinical considerations. *J Phys Ther Educ*. 1999;13:8.
112. Marland G, McSherry W. The reflective diary: an aid to practice-based learning. *Nurs Stand*. 1997;12:49.
113. Nolinske T, Millis B. Cooperative learning as an approach to pedagogy. *Am J Occup Ther*. 1999;53:31.
114. Elnicki DM, Halperin AK, Shockor WT, Aronoff SC. Multidisciplinary evidence-based medicine journal clubs: curriculum design and participants' reactions. *Am J Med Sci*. 1999;317:243.
115. Cooke M, Mitchell M, Moyle W, et al. Application and student evaluation of a Clinical Progression Portfolio: a pilot. *Nurse Educ Pract*. 2010;10:227–232.
116. Cederbaum J, Klusaritz HA. Clinical instruction: using the strengths-based approach with nursing students. *J Nurs Educ*. 2009;48:422–428.
117. Watts N. *Handbook of Clinical Teaching*. New York: Churchill Livingstone; 1990.
118. Hrachovy J, Clopton N, Baggett K, et al. Use of the Blue MACS: acceptance by clinical instructors and self-reports of adherence. *Phys Ther*. 2000;80:652.
119. Barr JS, Gwyer J, Talmor A. Evaluation of clinical centers in physical therapy. *Phys Ther*. 1982;62:850.
120. Department of Education/Clinical Instructor Education Board. *2000 Credentialed Clinical Instructor Survey*. Alexandria, VA: American Physical Therapy Association; 2000.
121. Notzer N, Abramovitz R. Can brief workshops improve clinical instruction? *Med Educ*. 2008;42:152–156.
122. Norcross JC, Stevenson JF. *Evaluating Clinical Training: Measurement and Utilization Implications from Three National Studies [abstract]*. Presented at the Annual Meeting of the Evaluation and Research Society, Toronto.
123. Deusinger S, Cornbleet SL, Stith JS. Using assessment centers to promote clinical faculty development. *J Phys Ther Educ*. 1991;5:14.
124. American Physical Therapy Association. *Clinical Instructor Education and Credentialing Program Databases*. Alexandria, VA: American Physical Therapy Association; 2011.
125. Emery MJ. The impact of the prospective payment system: perceived changes in the nature of practice and clinical education. *Phys Ther*. 1993;73:11.
126. American Physical Therapy Association. *Advanced Clinical Instructor Education and Credentialing Program and Manual*. Alexandria, VA: American Physical Therapy Association; 2008.

127. Graffam B, Bowers L, Keene KN. Using observations of clinicians' teaching practices to build a model of clinical instruction. *Acad Med.* 2008;83:768–774.

128. Pinsky LE, Irby DM. "If at first you don't succeed": using failure to improve teaching. *Acad Med.* 1997;72:973.

129. Grossman PL. *The Making of a Teacher: Teacher Knowledge and Teacher Education.* New York: Columbia University; 1990.

130. Education Division, American Physical Therapy Association. Clinical Education: Dare to Innovate. In: *A consensus conference on alternative models of clinical education.* Alexandria VA: American Physical Therapy Association; 1998:4.

131. Portney L, Knab MS, Applebaum DL. *Clinical Internship Resource Guide.* MGH Institute of Health Professions. Graduate Programs in Physical Therapy. Developed as part of a contract to study Alternative Models of Clinical Education: Implementation of a One-Year Clinical Internship in Physical Therapy Department of EducationAlexandria, VA: American Physical Therapy Association; 2004.

132. Kelly KK. *Clinical Education Principles and Economic Models: A Partnership in Action.* Presentation Combined Sections MeetingUniversity of Pittsburgh; 2010. *http://www.apta.org/Educators/Clinical/EducationResources/ModelsPrinciples/* Accessed 21.11.11.

133. Goffar SL. *U.S. Army-Baylor Clinical Internship Model: A Marriage Between Academia and Industry.* Presentation Combined Sections Meeting. http://www.apta.org/Educators/Clinical/EducationResources/ModelsPrinciples/; 2010 Accessed 29.08.11.

134. Gandy J. *Report to the 2004 House of Delegates. Investigation of Alternative Models of Physical Therapist Professional Clinical Education. (RC 36A/C-01).* Alexandria, VA: American Physical Therapy Association; 2004.

135. Martorello L. The optimal length of clinical internship experiences for entry-level physical therapist students as perceived by center coordinators of clinical education: a pilot study. *J Phys Ther Educ.* 2006;20:56–58.

136. Lekkas P, Larsen T, Kumar S, et al. No model of clinical education for physiotherapy students is superior to another: a systematic review. *Aust J Physiother.* 2007;53:19–28.

137. Secomb J. A systematic review of peer teaching and learning in clinical education. *J Clin Nurs.* 2008;17:703–716.

138. DeClute J, Ladyshewsky R. Enhancing clinical competence using a collaborative clinical education model. *Phys Ther.* 1993;73:683.

139. Nemshick MT, Shepard KF. Physical therapy clinical education in a 2:1 student-instructor education model. *Phys Ther.* 1996;76:968.

140. Ladyshewsky RK. Enhancing service productivity in acute care inpatient settings using a collaborative clinical education model. *Phys Ther.* 1995;75:503.

141. Ladyshewsky RK, Barrie SC, Drake VM. A comparison of productivity and learning outcome in individual and cooperative physical therapy clinical education models. *Phys Ther.* 1998;78:1288.

142. Chojecki P, Lamarre J, Buck M, et al. Perceptions of a peer learning approach to pediatric clinical education. *Int J Nurs Educ Scholarsh* 2010;7 Article 39.

143. Ladyshewsky R. Clinical teaching and the 2:1 student to clinical instructor ratio. *J Phys Ther Educ.* 1995;7:31.

144. Dupont L, Roy R, Gauthier-Gagnon C, Lamoureux M. Group supervision and productivity: from myth to reality. *J Phys Ther Educ.* 1997;11:31.

145. Holmlund K, Lindgren B, Athlin E. Group supervision for nursing students during their clinical placements: its content and meaning. *J Nurs Manag.* 2010;18:678–688.

146. Lindgren B, Brulin C, Holmlund K, Athlin E. Nursing students' perception of group supervision during clinical training. *J Clin Nurs.* 2005;14:822–829.

147. Jelley W, Larocque N, Patterson S. Intradisciplinary clinical education for physiotherapists and physiotherapist assistants: a pilot study. *Physiother Can.* 2010;62:75–80.

148. Escovitz ES. Using senior students as clinical skills teaching assistants. *Acad Med.* 1990;65:733.

149. Gerace L, Sibilano H. preparing students for peer collaboration: a clinical teaching model. *J Nurs Educ.* 1984;23:206.

150. Delehanty MJ. Recruitment and retention of physical therapists in rural areas: an interdisciplinary approach [abstract]. *Phys Ther.* 1993;73:70.

151. Clark SL, Schlachter S. Development of clinical education sites in an area health education system. *Phys Ther.* 1981;61:904.

152. Blakely RL, Jackson-Brownlow V. Interdisciplinary rural health education and training (IRHET) [abstract]. *Phys Ther.* 1993;73:66.

153. Russell L, Nyhof-Young J, Abosh B, Robinson S. An exploratory analysis of an interprofessional learning environment in two hospital clinical teaching units. *J Interprof Care.* 2006;20:29–39.

154. Anderson E, Manek N, Davidson A. Evaluation of a model for maximizing interprofessional education in an acute hospital. *J Interprof Care.* 2006;20:182–194.

155. Neill M, Hayward KS, Peterson T. Students' perceptions of the interprofessional team in practice through the application of servant leadership principles. *J Interprof Care.* 2007;21:425–432.

156. Bridges DR, Davidson RA, Odegard PS, et al. Interprofessional collaboration: three best practice models of interprofessional education. *Med Educ Online* 2011;16 doi:10.3402/meo.v16i0.6035.

157. Bowers HF. Designing quality course management systems that foster intra-professional education. *Nurse Educ Pract.* 2006;6:418–423.

158. Perkins J, Tryssenaar J. Making interdisciplinary education effective for rehabilitation students. *J Allied Health.* 1994;23:133.

159. Betz CL, Raynor O, Turman J. Use of an interdisciplinary team for clinical instruction. *Nurse Educ.* 1998;23:32.

160. Schilling D. *Interprofessional Clinical Education Model: Planning, Development, and Implementation.* Western University of the Health Sciences; 2010. Presentation Combined Sections Meeting*http://www.apta.org/Educators/Clinical/EducationResources/ModelsPrinciples/* Accessed 21.11.11.

161. Interprofessional Education Collaborative. Team-Based Competencies: Building a Shared Foundation for Education and Clinical Practice. Conference Proceedings. Supported by the Josiah-Macy Foundation, ABIM Foundation, and Robert Wood Johnson Foundation. Washington, DC, February 16-17, 2011. https://www.aamc.org/download/186752/data/team-based_competencies.pdf; Accessed 29.08.11.

162. Brufee KA. Sharing our toys: cooperative learning versus collaborative learning. *Change.* 1995;27:12.

163. Matthews RS, Cooper JL, Davidson N, et al. Building bridges between cooperative and collaborative learning. *Change.* 1995;27:35.

164. Gamson ZF. Collaborative learning comes of age. *Change.* 1994;26:44.

165. Johnson DW, Johnson RT, Smith KA. *Cooperative Learning: Increasing College Faculty and Instructional Productivity.* ASHE-ERIC Higher Education Report No. 4Washington, DC: George Washington University, School of Education and Human Development; 1991.

166. Laitinen-Väänänen S, Talvitie U, Luukka MR. Clinical supervision as an interaction between the clinical educator and the student. *Physiother Theory Pract.* 2007;23:95–103.

167. Tomlinson S. *Arcadia University Clinical Education Model.* Presentation Combined Sections Meeting. Philadelphia; 2010. http://www.apta.org/Educators/Clinical/EducationResources/ModelsPrinciples/; Accessed 21.11.11.

CHAPTER 9

TECHNIQUES FOR TEACHING STUDENTS IN CLINICAL SETTINGS

Karen A. Paschal

CHAPTER OUTLINE

Clinical education has long been recognized as a necessary part of physical therapy education. In 1968, Callahan and colleagues stated that the purpose of clinical education was "to assist the student to correlate clinical practices with basic sciences; to acquire new knowledge, attitudes and skill to develop ability to observe, to evaluate, to develop realistic goals and plan effective treatment programs; to accept professional responsibility; to maintain a spirit of inquiry and to develop a pattern for continuing education."[1] Despite major changes in health care delivery and physical therapy, this purpose reflects the present goal of physical therapy clinical education.

The importance of clinical education is expressed by students when they remind instructors that "real learning" in physical therapy occurs in the clinic. In fact, long after physical therapists forget what was taught in which course during academic preparation, they remember their clinical education experiences. Physical therapists remember not only specific experiences with patients but also their clinical teachers. It is not unusual to hear a clinical teacher say, "I remember when I was a student and my clinical instructor (CI) . . . ." Whether perceived as outstanding or mediocre, the clinical teacher has a profound effect on how students practice and how they want to teach the next generation of students. Much of what CIs know, do, and value in their positions was learned when they were students. However, as strong as those beliefs and ideas may be, the very personal ideas CIs have about clinical teaching may be perceived quite differently when enacted.

Consider these accounts of a clinical education experience described quite differently by a young CI and a student.

CLINICAL INSTRUCTOR: Jeff is a bright student. He's enthusiastic and eager to learn. I know this is only his second clinical affiliation and he hasn't had all of his classroom work yet, but he's on the right track. I've really tried to spend time teaching him. I wanted that when I was a student. My CI just let me go for it on my own. I mean, I learned, but I would have liked to have had someone there giving me feedback and teaching me more advanced skills. I think this approach has helped Jeff.

JEFF: This is different from my first affiliation. I'm really just watching my CI most of the time. Like with the new patient I saw this morning. I started the history, but she interrupted and just kept asking all the questions. Then, I started the examination, but I guess I wasn't doing something quite right, so she stepped in. It seems like she lectures to me all the time. I know I can't do everything perfectly, but I'd just like to try. I could think of most of the things she did with the patient, but all I got to do was watch her. That's not really true. She let me do the ultrasound.

This CI's intentions are good but are different when they translate into practice. In trying to improve on her experience as a student, the CI focuses on herself as the teacher rather than the student. How could she restructure her teaching to better facilitate learning? How could she teach and at the same time allow Jeff to learn by doing? This chapter focuses on pragmatic teaching techniques for use in the clinical setting. Avoiding highly specified, technical explanations of what clinical teachers do, this chapter uses an approach that recognizes the judgment of clinical teachers in the use of fundamental, practical, and realistic teaching techniques in typically unique and often ambiguous conditions that are the "real world" of physical therapy practice.

CONTEXT OF CLINICAL EDUCATION

Clinical learning is situated in the context of physical therapy practice. It occurs in real practice settings, with real patients, and with real physical therapists as clinical teachers. Figure 9–1 diagrams the essential elements in clinical education that provide context for the learning experience.

Historically, clinical education has occurred in settings in which administrators, directors, and, most important, physical therapy clinical teachers have been willing to provide it. As the treatment of patients with impairments and functional limitations related to human movement and movement dysfunction has moved from inpatient to outpatient settings, physical therapy clinical education has moved from hospitals to a variety of community-based centers, including outpatient health care facilities, schools, retirement centers, health promotion and wellness centers, and preschools. Changes in how and where health care is delivered have affected, for the most part positively, the traditional inpatient basis for students' clinical education. The modern teaching hospital has become a large intensive care unit, where physical therapy students have short-term access to critically ill patients who only represent a small and very ill portion of the total spectrum of physical therapy practice. Students get a fuller view of the quality of life of a patient when the patient is seen not only during acute illness requiring hospitalization, but also in outpatient clinics where patients are treated for movement-related disorders that affect everyday activities. The spectrum of clinical experiences that a student can have is tremendous.

Explicitly defining the desired outcome for each clinical experience dictates the appropriate timing in the curriculum, the duration of the experience, the type of setting, and the qualifications of the clinical teachers. Students' early experiences may be even more critical than experiences that occur after the completion of the didactic curriculum because they are generally short, and the impact of

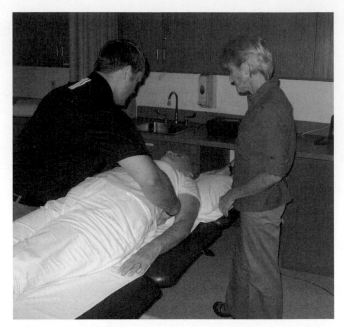

FIGURE 9–2 Patient, student, and clinical instructor co-participate in an early clinical learning experience.

the experience provides the framework for the student to develop patterns of lifelong clinical learning (Figure 9–2). The days of hands-off observation for students are over, although this may be the temptation in a busy clinical practice where productivity standards are high, and there is little time for teaching and practicing basic skills. Students must be ready to enter the clinic setting and interact with patients. They must know where to start. They must come with the expectation that they learn by thinking and doing with a patient.

What does a student need to know on day 1 of a clinical learning experience? What is best taught in the classroom or the laboratory? What is best learned during a clinical education experience? Basic knowledge and skills are prerequisites to clinical learning. Consider the example given in Table 9–1. Muscle performance examinations are routinely provided by physical therapists. Knowledge of these examinations, as well as rudimentary skill in performing them, is acquired in the classroom and laboratory. In the clinical setting, the student learns to use this knowledge and skill in clinical decision making and patient management.

ACADEMIC AND CLINICAL TEACHING: TWO DIFFERENT REALITIES

The primary difference between academic and clinical teaching is that control of academic teaching lies with the educational system, and control of clinical teaching lies with the health care system and, ultimately, the patient. This fundamental difference underlies all aspects of developing a clinical education program, and it must be recognized and accommodated in clinical education programs. The academic setting has been organized for the efficiency and convenience of the system, its administration and faculty, and technologies, whereas the clinical system is generally organized for the convenience of delivering health care to the patient. Most educational issues flow from this

Physical Therapy Practice Setting

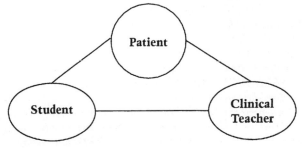

FIGURE 9–1 Fundamental elements of clinical education.

TABLE 9–1 Muscle Performance Examinations Provided by Physical Therapists

Learning Environment	Primary Learning Activity
Classroom	Acquisition of knowledge • Definition of muscle performance • Characteristics of performance • Mediators of performance • Reasons for examination • Selection of specific tests and measures • Expected examination outcomes
Laboratory	Acquisition of skill • Tests and measures for conducting a muscle performance examination, including generation of data
Clinic	Use of knowledge and skill for clinical decision making and patient management in • Evaluation • Diagnosis • Prognosis • Determination of appropriate intervention

Adapted from American Physical Therapy Association. Guide to Physical Therapist Practice, 2nd ed. Phys Ther 2001;81:9.

basic difference, including those of appropriate and attainable educational objectives, effective instruction and evaluation methods, effect of clinical education on the patient and patient care, and costs of teaching.

PREVAILING CONDITIONS IN THE CLINICAL ENVIRONMENT

The clinical setting is a unique and complex learning environment. Student performance is based on knowing and doing in a real situation with a real patient or client. The learning situation within the clinic is framed by several factors or ground rules.

Scully[2] suggests that there are three generic sources for the ground rules that frame the clinical learning environment: (1) those originating external to the clinical education facility, (2) those originating internal to the clinical education facility, and (3) those originating from within the clinical teacher. Table 9–2 gives examples of each. Although these delineations are helpful in understanding

TABLE 9–2 Ground Rules Framing the Context of the Clinical Education Experience

Sources	Examples
External	University mission and program objectives Assignment of students Time and length of assignment
Internal	Department policies and procedures Assignment of the clinical instructor Health requirements
Clinical teacher	Preparation and experience • Value judgments (i.e., patient primacy, professionalism)

Adapted from Scully RM. Clinical Teaching of Physical Therapy Students in Clinical Education. Ph.D. dissertation. New York: Columbia University, 1974.

the origin of factors influencing the context of the clinical experience, examples may not fit exclusively in one category.

Consider the examples of Natasha and Anne. Both are physical therapy students assigned to a pediatric clinical setting by their respective academic programs. Student assignment or placement is an academic prerogative, and the method used varies from program to program. The following descriptions of the placement procedures that affect Natasha and Anne provide an example of external factors that affect the clinical education experience.

NATASHA: A pediatrics rotation is important to me. I don't have much experience with children. But, I volunteered over the summer at a camp for kids with AIDS [acquired immunodeficiency syndrome], and I took the pediatric elective. It was tough, but I'm really excited about learning to do all we talked about. The student who was here last year said this was a great place!

ANNE: I'm not planning to get a job in pediatrics or anything. I just sort of got sent here—I was at the end of the lottery. I mean, I want to be well rounded and everything, but I don't want to work with kids. I just want to get the basics. You know, so if kids ever come into my office I'll know what to do with them.

On closer examination, however, the effect of this external factor, the placement procedures, may not be so clear cut. Consider values held by two physical therapists who could be assigned as Anne's CI:

CLINICAL INSTRUCTOR A: It's going to be a long 8 weeks. Anne doesn't want to be here. You can't just learn the basics and expect to be a good physical therapist. Where do I even begin with her?

CLINICAL INSTRUCTOR B: I appreciate Anne's honesty, and I hope I can work with her to become more diplomatic. I think there are many aspects of pediatric practice that apply to all patients. I think we can work together to create an excellent experience. I want to start by learning more about her interests.

The attitudes held by each of these therapists would greatly influence Anne's clinical education experience. Think of other external and internal constraints imposed on the clinical education process. In almost every case, the CI's knowledge, skill, values, and attitudes could reframe the learning context in a way that would dramatically change the outcome of the clinical experience.

Consider the demands imposed by the changing health care delivery system. Although addressed by academic programs in the curriculum, students often express the reality as follows:

ROBERTO: This hospital isn't a very good place right now. There's a lot of change going on. The patients are all seen in their rooms or in little satellite departments on the floors. It seems like all we do is get them out of bed. I don't have time for a complete examination before they're discharged. The biggest job the therapists have is deciding where to refer the patients when they're discharged from the hospital. I want to do real physical therapy.

The CI, Mariah, has the ability to reframe this response and challenge Roberto to make the most of his learning experience by expressing something like the following:

MARIAH: You're absolutely right. I think we sometimes get the notion that physical therapy means using our hands all the time. Sometimes, though, the emphasis is on using our heads to think and plan. We can learn about the patient's functional status before admission, we know what's happened here, and then it's our job to make the best possible guess about the future and make recommendations based on that. What a challenge! Discharge planning is a focus from the beginning, and even our treatments need to take that into consideration. What do you think about Mr. Baird, whom we saw this morning?

After the context of the clinical education experience is understood, physical therapists can develop ways to mold it as Clinical Instructor B and Mariah did. CIs can often reframe the circumstances if they view the ground rules as defining opportunities and challenges that allow them to better enable student clinical learning.

Prevailing conditions in the clinical environment provide additional opportunities and challenges for both the clinical teacher and the learner. The political climate of a given health care facility, reimbursement, interprofessional roles, productivity demands, and patient demographics represent just a few.[3] Given these prevailing conditions, it is important to ask the following: How do students learn in the clinic? What is helpful for clinical teachers to know and understand about the clinical learning process?

CLINICAL LEARNING

The purpose of this section is neither to review the work of learning theorists[4-9] nor to examine the literature related to student physical therapists' learning.[10-15] Rather, this section provides a contextual basis of clinical learning to use in the upcoming section, Roles of the Clinical Teacher: Diagnosing Readiness, Planning, Teaching, and Evaluating. John Dewey provided key descriptors of the clinical learning process when he stated, "education is not an affair of 'telling' and being told, but an active and constructive process."[16] Successful clinical learning requires the student to make meaning of knowledge in a clinical sense and then to enact that meaning when providing physical therapy services.

Clinical learning occurs in the context of the "whole" as opposed to isolated parts of physical therapy care. As students learn to practice and practice learning, they acknowledge that there are no simple patients. Holistic activities with concentrated work on the "hard parts" promote the acquisition of needed knowledge and skill with the opportunity to learn how to learn.[17]

STUDENT OWNERSHIP AND RESPONSIBILITY

The clinical education experience belongs to the student, despite the fact that it occurs in the CI's clinic. It involves patients to whom the CI has legal and ethical responsibilities. It requires the CI's time, energy, and creativity. It is imperative, however, that the student accepts ownership

TABLE 9–3 Principles that Dampen or Motivate Students to Enhance Competence and Encourage Self-Determination in Actions

	Dampeners	**Motivators**
Focus of goal orientation	Judgment	Development and learning
Performance expectations	Low	High
Learning opportunities	Governed by rules and regulations Prescriptive, mandatory experiences	Self-directed Multiple opportunities with recommendations
Instructional strategies	Routine Extrinsic rewards and incentives	Challenging Encourage deep and rich thinking processes
Feedback/ evaluation	Dominate and control behavior	Available but infrequent from external sources
Institutional/ personal premiums	Emphasize conformity	Emphasize creativity, innovation, and alternative perspectives

Adapted from Lewthwaite R, Burnfield JM, Tompson L, et al. Education and development principles. Presented at: Seventh National Physical Therapy Clinical Education Conference; April, 1995; Buffalo, NY.

and responsibility for the experience. Clinical education is not only an opportunity for a student to learn the knowledge, skills, values, and attitudes of the profession, but also is the first experience in a lifelong pattern of learning and continual development as a physical therapist. Table 9–3 summarizes principles that enhance competence and encourage self-determination in actions. It is important that students assume responsibility for learning what they need to know and how to go about learning it.

There are several learning experiences that can be used to encourage student ownership for clinical learning. The student should prepare for each experience by becoming familiar with the clinical site information form and any orientation materials sent before the student's arrival. Based on this information, the CI may wish to ask students to prepare specific personal goals and learning objectives they would like to meet during their time at the facility. This student-specific information provides an excellent basis for discussion during orientation, at which time the CI can affirm or revise student goals and plan relevant learning experiences. It is important to revisit these goals and objectives periodically. The CI can use them in weekly planning or as a part of the midterm evaluation by asking what the student has accomplished, what activities still need to be undertaken, or if further revisions or additions need to be made. Having the student develop objectives within the context of practice enables the student to further develop professional identity and mission as a physical therapist or physical therapist assistant. In doing so, the student acquires a framework for establishing lifelong learning habits.

PROCESS OF CLINICAL LEARNING

Clinical learning is a process of mutual inquiry conducted by the student and CI during the provision of patient care services. It is a process during which the student co-participates in clinical decision making with a skilled practitioner, the CI. As such, it is a situated learning experience in which teaching and learning occur around the patient in a series of complex interactions. Contrary to what CIs may think, *it doesn't just happen.* Consider Katie's experience as she and her CI described it to the Director of Clinical Education (DCE) for her academic program during his on-site visit:

CLINICAL INSTRUCTOR: She's doing fine. I don't have any complaints. You know, she's right where she should be. I don't mean that she's perfect, but time and more experience help. She just has the usual student problems. She asks questions. She fits in here, and she'll be a good physical therapist someday.

KATIE: I don't know. It's not bad, but I'm not sure that I'm learning. I mean, I know I'm learning, but I think I could be doing more. I sort of feel like a junior therapist. I come in, treat my patients with some help, and go home.

Katie is participating in the third of four clinical education experiences. She performs adequately but seems stuck. She thinks that she isn't learning as much as she is capable of, but she does not seem to know where to go from here. Consider steps the DCE might take, the CI's responsibilities, and what Katie needs to do to continue the learning process. The American Physical Therapy Association Clinical Instructor Education and Credentialing Program provides pragmatic instruction with case examples for facilitating learning in the clinical environment.[18]

Bridging Theory with Practice

A primary goal of clinical teaching is to enable the student to build bridges between theory and practice. Theoretical knowledge and fundamental skills taught in the physical therapy classroom and laboratory may be embedded in a patient problem orientation, but students rarely, if ever, learn in the clinical context until their first clinical education experience. The need for bridging theory and practice is made clear by example in this statement by Becky, a student in her first clinical education experience:

BECKY: I was doing okay until the patient threw me off track by giving the wrong answer to my question. I mean, she isn't supposed to have pain in her shoulder all night long, unless she has cancer or something bad like that. I was pretty sure she had a frozen shoulder.

Clinical practice is all about patient responses that don't fit with textbook diagnoses. There are no multiple choice patients for whom a circle around the best answer restores function. Academic knowledge needs to be reformatted in the contextual basis of patient care. Clinical wisdom is based on far more than building on the facts. It is a transformation of knowledge done by integrating reflective experience. This is illustrated in the following example:

STUDENT: My CI is so smart. How did she learn all she knows? Yesterday a patient tried to refuse treatment, but she just didn't take "no" for an answer. The patient ended up doing better during the treatment session than I had ever seen him do. Then, this morning, Mr. Jones said that he wasn't up to physical therapy.

She just said, "Okay, we'll check back later." An hour later, they called a code. I looked at his chart and everything. There was nothing to predict that. How did she know?

Physical therapists practice with a tacit knowledge not found in books and rarely described in the literature. Consider how this knowledge is conveyed to students.

The bridge between theory and practice is not a one-way street. Students often co-participate in practice and generate questions based on their experiences. These questions lead them back to the literature for increased knowledge and deeper understanding. Clinical education is all about transforming and putting knowledge to use. The role of the CI is to scaffold student performance to greater sophistication. Consider the learning experience Inara describes:

INARA: I evaluated my first patient yesterday. I had done parts of several exams with my CI, but this was the first in which I was responsible for the whole thing. My CI made suggestions, and I implemented them as I went along. It went pretty well. The patient will be back tomorrow, and I'm anxious to see how he's doing. After I finished the note (with revisions), I thought I was done. But my CI asked me to go home and compare what I had done with the *Guide to Physical Therapist Practice.* We'd used it at school, but I never thought about using it here in the clinic. Anyway, I had to find the practice pattern, and then I was surprised that it helped me think of things I hadn't thought of. With this CI, there's always more to learn . . . .

Inara's CI challenged her to move beyond "good enough." By suggesting a framework for reflecting on her actions, the CI fostered what Mentkowski and associates called "learning that lasts."[19]

Ability to Perform Effective Actions

Knowing is not enough. Students must learn to put their knowledge to work and, in doing so, practice and perform fundamental skills to enhance movement. Physical therapists examine, assess, evaluate, plan, and intervene. They palpate, stabilize, mobilize, facilitate, and inhibit. They teach, motivate, simplify, and modify. Skilled performance of these actions comes only with practice, development, and refinement. Lucía, a second-year student, describes her struggle with learning palpation:

LUCIA: I know anatomy, and I got 100% on the functional anatomy practical. But here I'm only positive that I differentiate skin and bone. There're layers of soft tissue in between! I touch every patient that comes in, and I still don't think I'm always feeling what my CI feels.

Lucía appears to be working hard to practice and develop her palpation skills. Consider what her CI's role is in helping her to perform effective actions.

Acculturation

Acculturation is the process by which a student is socialized into the profession of physical therapy. The socialization process is an account of how a new person is added to the group and becomes a member capable of meeting the traditional expectations of the profession. Physical therapy is a service-oriented profession. Clinical education occurs in settings where patients come to receive care. Patients are not exhibits who give time and money to come to a clinic to provide an example of a diagnosis for a student. They are real people with movement dysfunctions that limit their ability to live their lives the way they would choose. Students must learn what it means to provide service.

Most students use their own lives as the primary example for the way others live and may assume that their own beliefs, values, and socioeconomic status are those of the people whom they serve. Consider Cindy's comment. She is a 21-year-old student from a Midwestern farming community. She has been assigned to the liver transplant service of a metropolitan teaching hospital on the East Coast.

CINDY: Can you believe it? We are waiting to discharge this woman until her maid flies in from the Middle East. Her husband is too lazy to help her at the family house. I can't believe it. She doesn't even need that much help anymore.

Cindy's narrow norms of culture indicate a need for learning. Consider suggestions you could give her CI that would help Cindy enlarge her view.

Although most students have experienced physical therapy as a patient or have a friend or relative that has, they often fail to realize the broad scope of physical therapy practice, even after class work. Difficulties in learning within this very broad context of practice may not be evident until the clinical education experience. For example, consider the challenge Diego faced as you read about his experience, beginning with a phone call from his CI to the DCE in the third week of an 8-week affiliation on a trauma unit:

CLINICAL INSTRUCTOR: I'm sorry to bother you, but Diego's not back from lunch. I probably should have called about everything earlier, but things just kept getting worse slowly. Now I've had it! I don't even know where to begin. He's late all the time. He doesn't seem interested. I just can't engage him. It's almost as if he's avoiding the patients. He's smart enough and has good ideas about what to do, but I just can't get him to do anything. Sometimes up on the unit he just disappears. It's like he's hiding from me.

Diego's behavior was atypical in relation to his academic performance and previous clinical education experiences. During an on-site conference with the DCE the next morning, when Diego was asked how the affiliation was progressing, he focused exclusively on Jeff, a 24-year-old patient with a traumatic brain injury at Rancho Level I who had been injured in a motor vehicle accident when he was thrown from his car. He shared that Jeff's parents, siblings, and girlfriend were devastated, and Diego kept repeating, "Jeff is never going to be the same." As the conversation progressed, the DCE commented that Diego's CI had expressed her concern that Diego might be avoiding her. "What are you hiding from?" the DCE asked. He very honestly answered, "Life."

Experienced physical therapists may forget their initial reactions to the complexities of specialized practice settings, such as the trauma unit, skilled nursing facility, preschool program for children with developmental disabilities, athletic training room, neonatal intensive care unit, and hospice. Consider techniques a CI can use to explore personal feelings and reactions to difficult issues within professional practice and whether it is possible to validate a student's feelings while the student develops the ability to practice professionally in the challenging and sometimes overwhelming context of practice.

Critical Analysis of Clinical Competence

Accurate self-assessment is a critical ability for professional practice. Students acquire expectations about their own abilities from several sources. Successful experiences provide a foundation on which to build from observing role models or receiving verbal feedback provided by a clinical teacher or a patient.[20] Consider how a CI contributes to a student's ability to accurately self-assess performance and judge the outcome of professional actions, and how a student learns to evaluate his or her capabilities compared with entry-level competence or the performance of an expert clinician.[21]

OUTCOMES OF THE CLINICAL LEARNING PROCESS

The academic program formally defines the expected outcome for any clinical education experience. Ultimately, however, the goal of clinical learning is for the student to progress from other-assisted to self-assisted learning while developing patterns of learning that form the basis for a lifelong, reflective practice.[22,23]

Other-Assisted to Self-Assisted Learning

When students begin the clinical education process, their learning is directed by the academic faculty, CIs, and physical therapist role models. As they progress through their clinical learning experiences, however, each student assumes more responsibility for her or his learning. Selected statements from students at various stages in an academic program demonstrate this progress:

CLAUDIA: I wanted to show you this schedule that I received from my clinical site. Each of the 4 weeks has particular things I'm going to focus on. During the first week, I get an in-service on "overview of patient examination" and by the end, I'll do all of the peripheral joints.

Compare the assistance Claudia accepts from others with the initiative in self-assisted learning that Brad demonstrates:

BRAD: I kept thinking about this patient and his problem. I just had to devise a way to gain more mobility. I came up with a mobilization we hadn't learned in class and one that probably wouldn't even be possible on a normal elbow. I had the patient sit on a stool next to the treatment table and place his forearm on the table. I stood next to him and palpated for the displaced radial head. Then, I placed my thumbs on his head and directed a force caudally. At the beginning of treatment, only minimal displacement was possible. By the end, I believe 4 or 5 millimeters might have been possible. It was very interesting to think about this problem and satisfying to come up with a unique solution. I felt very good about being successful with it.

Consider how a CI interacts with each of these students to enable them to progress in self-assisted learning, and how the teacher knows when students are ready to assume more responsibility for their learning.

Lifelong, Reflective Practice

Lifelong, reflective practice is a hallmark of professional behavior. With so much to learn in the brief periods of clinical education, how does a student begin this endeavor? Students are often required to keep a journal or may be asked to present a case report as an in-service educational program during their clinical experiences. In addition to ongoing conversations with their CIs, these reflective activities encourage students to think about and question their actions. But these activities end at the conclusion of the clinical experience. Consider what might guarantee that the reflective process becomes lifelong, and what responsibility the clinical teacher assumes for this during the clinical education experience. One tool that is being used across disciplines is the portfolio.

The development of a portfolio offers an opportunity for students to reflect on their learning and professional development. By gathering and sorting examples of their professional work, defining moments of success and failure, and reflecting on the evidence they have presented, students are placed in a position of authority to assess and validate their personal development as professionals.[24] Portfolios should be structured and coached by the CI, academic faculty, or both for the purpose of guidance and feedback. They are often organized thematically. For example, a student might provide evidence of entry-level competence in the components of patient management. Beyond the selection of good examples of clinical work, the student must reflect on the content. If the student presented evidence of a patient examination, the student might ask herself or himself, "What is entry-level competence when performing this patient examination? What components are present or absent? How does my work differ from expert practice?"[21] By placing emphasis on judgment and meaning making, the student is encouraged to investigate her or his own learning experience. Consider Mark's example:

MARK: I needed to provide evidence that I could demonstrate mastery of entry-level professional clinical skills based on physical therapy examination, evaluation, diagnosis, prognosis, intervention, and appropriate health care use. I wrote a case study on a patient and included the literature I had used when I worked with the patient. I compared my patient care with the *Guide to Physical Therapist Practice*.[25] Then my CI and I discussed what I had discovered and the ideas I had to improve. He was especially helpful in prioritizing parts of the practice pattern to meet my patient's needs.

Writing the case study and comparing his practice to the *Guide* allowed Mark to reflect on his actions. His CI provided a further opportunity for learning by reflecting with Mark and offering his clinical wisdom. By including this example in his portfolio, Mark has provided evidence of his learning process, as well as created an opportunity for further reflection and learning in the future. The portfolio provides a vehicle for students to record and celebrate their professional growth and provides many opportunities for thoughtful deliberation and discourse. In addition, a portfolio may provide the student with a basis for planning in the crucial transition from student to new graduate.

ROLES OF THE CLINICAL TEACHER: DIAGNOSING READINESS, PLANNING, TEACHING, AND EVALUATING

Good clinical teachers enable student learning. They begin by inviting students to participate in the community of physical therapy practice, and then they plan, model, coach, question, encourage, instruct, supervise, and evaluate to optimize the learning experience. Box 9-1 highlights specific enabling acts used by good teachers. These are incorporated throughout this discussion.

Scully describes the role of the clinical teacher as "pacing the student to professional competency," which involves diagnosis of readiness, selection of clinical problems, supervision, and evaluation.[2] These categories, although not exhaustive or exclusive, provide an effective framework for considering the functions of the clinical teacher.[26]

DIAGNOSIS OF STUDENT READINESS

Traditionally, the clinical teacher has limited knowledge of a specific student's background before the student's arrival. It is incumbent on the academic institution to provide information about the educational program and the didactic curriculum for review. The clinical teacher needs to gain an understanding of the school's mission and the goals and objectives of the academic program because these frame the context in which the curriculum is presented. A list of completed classes and course descriptions provide the content to which a student has been exposed and suggest curricular themes around which the academic faculty have chosen to instruct. Recalling previous clinical education experiences of students from a particular program at your clinical practice may also be helpful.

Knowing the student's academic preparation to date, however, provides little information about the implicit curriculum; the personal context in which knowledge, skills, and values were learned and developed; or the clinical competency the student is able to demonstrate. Consider the cases of Natalie and Beth, classmates who are in the second week of their first clinical learning experience:

NATALIE'S CLINICAL INSTRUCTOR: Natalie has progressed much more quickly than most students during a first affiliation. Her 3 years of work as a physical therapist assistant are evident in her interaction with patients and other members of the health care team, as

BOX 9–1   Thirty-Five Enabling Acts for Clinical Teachers

1. Invite students to participate in a community of practice where good work has been done by former students.
2. Demonstrate the power truth telling exerts on learning.
3. Get students doing good work that counts for them and their patients.
4. Along with the students, start good work of your own.
5. Begin to know your students as people rather than as students.
6. Make it clear that you believe in the students' abilities to work at high levels of excellence.
7. Sit on the same physical level as your students when conversing with them, and speak in simple, clear language. Expect that they will do the same.
8. Avoid didactic monologues. Don't expect a given answer in discussions.
9. Encourage dialogues between the experiences and ideas of students and the experiences and ideas of experts.
10. Work from experience into theory and vice versa.
11. Move students from success to success, yet prepare them to accept occasional failure.
12. Help students view mistakes as opportunities.
13. Exercise imagination.
14. Capitalize on storytelling.
15. Provide opportunities for responsible decision making.
16. Enable students to think about learning as "finding" in addition to "receiving."
17. Enable understanding of the "whole" instead of "bits and pieces."
18. Become vulnerable to students by sharing feelings with them about the good work you are doing with and alongside them.
19. Arrange that students see, do, and remember in the context of practice.
20. Encourage humor and spontaneity.
21. Plan so that no learning experience is useless.
22. Enable students to own the knowledge, skills, and values of professional practice.
23. Cultivate rigor and joy in practice.
24. Help students refine their uses of emotion.
25. Make practice an act with meaning—always.
26. Avoid badgering and cruelty.
27. Avoid excessive praise of students' works.
28. Test the work of the student against work in the world outside.
29. Find ways of making public the good works of the students.
30. Show students that working habits taken on in the clinic will prove valuable in the future.
31. Provide evaluations of students' work when the evaluation least interferes with learning.
32. Give students ample time to complete their work.
33. Help students polish and refine work as they bring it to completion.
34. Sense the moments for letting go of students.
35. Never deny students their lives.

Adapted from Macrorie K. 20 Teachers. New York: Oxford University Press, 1984.

well as her fundamental handling skills. She observed me the first day, and then we began coevaluating and cotreating on day 2. We still work together, but she has assumed more and more responsibility for the patient. She is working hard to take our findings from the examination, make clinical judgments, and then work with the patient to set functional goals and think of creative ways to meet those goals. Because she's competent in so many of the "pieces," she's been able to focus on higher-level objectives.

BETH'S CLINICAL INSTRUCTOR: Beth was tentative the first week, and I felt I needed to push her to get involved. She was very apprehensive. She did say that this was really her first experience working with patients. They're never quite like your lab partner! She's doing well, though. After several days of observing, we're working with the patients together. She's participating in aspects of examination and intervention. This morning, for example, she re-evaluated the range of motion of a young man we're seeing following multiple fractures received in a motorcycle crash. She had planned a routine to minimize the need for the patient to change positions and practiced on her roommate last night. She's also going to be responsible for the subjective exam with an outpatient coming in today for the first time after a total knee replacement.

Life experiences, particularly those in health care, can alter a student's starting point in the clinic. Other, less definitive, factors can affect fundamental skills in communication, management, teaching, and a host of components of professional practice. Information specific to each student is essential to accurately diagnose readiness for learning experiences.

Pre-experience Planning for the Clinical Education Experience

Preparation for the clinical education experience is a key component that begins after a student is assigned to a CI. The CI should introduce herself or himself and begin to exchange information as soon as possible. The time and energy spent in this process allow the clinical teacher and the student to reap rich rewards during the experience. The instructor should communicate directly with the student. This can be done in person, by telephone, by mail, or by e-mail. See Figure 9–3 for a sample letter welcoming a student. This letter contains key elements important to any type of initial contact. It does the following:

- Welcomes
- Introduces the clinical teacher and facility
- Demonstrates *truth telling*, or telling the truth in a candid, forthright, honest, frank, and open manner
- Conveys expectations
- Encourages the student's active participation

The combination of information provided and requested allows the student and clinical teacher to begin thinking and planning.

Student Orientation to the Clinical Setting and the Clinical Education Program

The first day of any new experience can be overwhelming. A well-planned orientation session can handle administrative details, introduce the student to key members of the health care delivery team, and provide pragmatic information that the student needs. The fact that, for example, the hand-held dynamometers in the clinic are in the third drawer to the left of the hydrocollator packs between

Dear Student's First Name,

I was delighted to learn that you will be affiliating at ABCD Medical Center, in City, State. My name is Susannah Perez, and I will be your clinical instructor for the 16 weeks you are with us. I have been at ABCD Medical Center for 2 years; before that I worked for a private outpatient physical therapy practice here in the city. My primary responsibilities include patient care at a satellite clinic 4 miles west of the Medical Center where we see patients with a wide range of neuromusculoskeletal problems and management related to outpatient rehabilitation services at all of our sites. I also see patients in the osteoporosis clinic at the center one afternoon per week. My working hours are 7:00 a.m. to 3:30 p.m. I do work one weekend at the center every 6 to 8 weeks, and that's an opportunity you may want to consider.

This is an exciting time at the Medical Center. We recently consolidated with several other health care facilities and are in the process of restructuring the management of physical therapy services at all the sites. Although change can be a bit disconcerting at times, I think this will be a wonderful opportunity to experience first hand what changes in the health care delivery really mean! In addition, we'll work as a team with a physical therapist assistant, Ken, and another student who will be joining us for the last 6 weeks of your affiliation.

I enjoyed working with a student from your university 2 years ago, and I'm anxious to learn about any changes that have taken place since then. From looking at your curriculum, I know that you've had three short-term affiliations during your academic preparation and that this is your first of two affiliations before graduation. I'm enclosing a copy of our updated Clinical Center Information Form, a copy of brochures about the medical center and the city, and a list of additional clinical learning opportunities for students at our facility. I hope these will begin to answer some of the questions you may have and help you prepare for this affiliation.

I want to involve you in planning this experience so we can work together to meet your needs as well as the goals and objectives of your academic program. After you've had an opportunity to review the enclosed materials, please write down your goals and objectives for this experience. Please send them to me at least 2 weeks before you arrive. We'll devote 2 hours of your first morning to orientation, discussion, and planning for the 12 weeks, and getting you off to a good start.

In the meantime, if you have any questions or need additional information, please let me know. I can be reached at 123-456-7890 or by e-mail at sperez@medctr.org. If it's better to call you at home during the evening, just let me know. I look forward to meeting you in person!

Sincerely,

Susannah Perez, P.T., D.P.T., O.C.S.

FIGURE 9–3 Sample letter of welcome from a clinical instructor.

examination rooms three and four is probably not essential. These three questions may guide your planning: What does the student need to know before beginning to learn in the context of patient care? What can wait until later? What is best learned along the way?

Orientation is the time for the CI to begin assessing the student by verbal exchange. What can the student tell about herself or himself? Encourage the students to talk about physical therapy, and listen to what physical therapy means to them. Share experiences and describe your expectations and standards. If you are able to share less-than-perfect performances and what you learned from them, you give the student permission to take risks, make mistakes, and learn from them. Review the student's goals and objectives. They may not be realistic at this point, at your facility, or for a variety of reasons. Help students determine what they really want from this experience. Determine whether students' revised goals and objectives can be measured with the evaluation instrument required by the academic program. Review clinical education materials that the student may have from the academic program, and determine whether there are additional assignments for the student to complete.

Orientation is also the time to begin joint planning. Include in this planning expectations for yourself and the student. The verbal exchange and planning that occur during orientation set the tone for conversations and learning activities that continue throughout the clinical experience. It is essential for the instructor to convey the importance of open truth telling and create an environment that encourages it.

Student Self-Assessment versus Demonstrated Abilities

Self-insight and the ability to self-assess are skills based on knowledge and values. The student's self-assessment and the accuracy of that assessment are important components of the diagnosis of readiness. It is critical to evaluate whether a student's self-assessment matches the student's demonstrated abilities. The first days of any experience allow the instructor to assess the student's abilities. Ask yourself, "Is the information that has been shared congruent with what I'm seeing?"

Performance testing is an ongoing piece of clinical teaching that must be done in a manner that allows the student to focus on learning and development, rather than the adequacy of performance. Thad's CI did it in the following way:

THAD: At first, we talked about the patient before he came. If the patient had a preliminary diagnosis, I told Cassie, my CI, what I knew, and we figured out what I didn't know. Sometimes Cassie didn't know either, and then we looked it up. And then we planned where I'd start. I thought you started with the history, but you really start by watching the patient walk back from the waiting room. She helped me plan the history based on what we knew from the referral. I'd go in to the examination room with the patient and take the history. Cassie would knock and come in later, and I'd tell her what I knew, and we'd get the patient to chime in. Sometimes, Cassie asked questions if she didn't understand. That helped remind me of important things I might have forgotten to ask. Then it was up to me to tell the patient what I was going to do in the examination and do it. Cassie might say something like, "You might want to check _____ to see if _____," which would clue me in. Then I'd do it, and Cassie would help if I got stuck or seemed to be headed in the wrong way. It's hard to explain, but it's like the three of us are all working together to figure out the best way for the patient to get better. Now I do more on my own. I know Cassie won't let me really mess up, but I also know that I'm the one in charge, and she's not going to let me off the hook. I'm starting to feel like a real physical therapist!

TABLE 9–4   Questions to Enhance Clinical Learning

Types of Questions	Purpose
Knowledge	Recall facts or principles
Translation	Demonstrate understanding of knowledge
Excogitative	Challenge problem-solving and clinical decision-making skills
Evaluation	Require the student to make judgments about the value of ideas, solutions, and methods

Adapted from Abrams RG. Questioning in preclinical and clinical instruction. J Dent Educ 1983;47:599.

Cassie is able to determine Thad's performance capabilities by working and conversing with him over the patient right in the context of practice. She uses questioning to assist in assessing the congruency between self-assessment and demonstrated abilities. Abrams[27] describes four types of questions (Table 9–4):

1. Knowledge questions
2. Translation questions
3. Excogitative questions
4. Evaluation questions

Each can be an effective tool to gain understanding of the student's abilities, as well as an effective teaching tool.

Knowledge Questions

Knowledge questions are directed to guide the student to recall facts or principles. This information may have been learned in a classroom lecture, a text, or a previous clinical education experience. Never presume that a student has the prerequisite knowledge needed to examine or treat a patient with a particular disease, impairment, or disability, particularly during early clinical education experiences. Knowledge questions provide the clinical teacher with an understanding of the gaps in the essential knowledge of the student, confusions the student may have (i.e., the student has ideas that are fuzzy or not clearly differentiated), or errors in the student's perceptions. These questions should not be viewed as a test or an examination, but as a tool to aid in diagnosing a student's readiness for a particular learning experience. Knowledge questions need to be asked in a manner that encourages verbal exchange and provides the student with an opportunity to support and reinforce basic information or correct misconceptions. The following are examples of knowledge questions:

- Why does maintaining a moist wound bed facilitate re-epithelialization? (This question may lead to a discussion of wound dressings, their application, and the choice of dressing that a therapist might recommend for the patient being treated.)
- What motions are contraindicated for this patient immediately after a total hip replacement? (This question may serve to cue the student as he or she proceeds to the functional application of knowledge and begins to transfer the patient from a wheelchair to a mat table.)

Translation Questions

Translation questions require a student to demonstrate understanding of knowledge. They may require the student to perform a simple transformation (e.g., translating medical terminology to lay language for patient and family education) or to interpret the functional meaning of a laboratory test (e.g., the effect a low hematocrit may have on endurance). True learning in the clinical setting may not occur until the learner becomes the teacher—that is, until the student is able to translate her or his knowledge for a patient, a peer, the CI, or another health care practitioner. Translation questions enable the student to use knowledge. The following are examples of translation questions:

- How would you explain ultrasound to a 72-year-old patient? (This question provides an opportunity for the student to practice translating her or his classroom and laboratory knowledge into clear, concise, and understandable terms for a patient.)
- After observing the total knee arthroplasty in the operating room yesterday, what functional limitations might you expect this patient to have? (This question directs the student to consider the physical therapy meaning of a supplemental learning experience. The passive experience of observing a surgical procedure becomes active as the student is required to make meaning of it.)

Excogitative Questions

Excogitative questions challenge the student's problem-solving and clinical decision-making abilities. They require a student to reorganize knowledge, apply principles, and predict outcomes. These questions may be especially appropriate after a student has taken the patient's history and performed the objective examination. They may guide the development of goals as well as the treatment plan. The following are examples of excogitative questions:

- What is the patient's functional limitation? Based on your findings, what can you recommend to this patient? (These questions require that the student think about function related to the impairments found on examination. The student must then decide what can be done to improve function.)

Evaluation Questions

Evaluation questions "use all of the previous thought processes to judge the value of ideas, solutions, methods, or materials."[23] The process of self-assessment is a critical component of the lifelong learning process. Phrased properly, evaluation questions reinforce self-assisted learning and encourage critical analysis. The following are examples of evaluative questions:

- What criteria do you use to determine whether the patient is independent in transfers?
- How do you determine whether the patient is ready to return to work?
- After working with this patient for a week, how successful do you think the rehabilitation program will be?

(These questions, used within the context of patient examination, evaluation, and intervention, can enable a clinical teacher to gain a better understanding of what a student knows, what the student is doing, and why it is being done.)

Questioning can be used effectively to advance stronger critical thinking skills, reasoning, and clinical decision making. Refer to Chapters 3 and 11 for a more complete discussion of these topics. The need to maximize learning in smaller blocks of time with limited time for one-on-one teaching is a challenge in clinical education. Models have been developed to address this concern,[28,29] and the APTA Advanced Credentialed Clinical Instructor Program for the Physical Therapist provides additional instruction and practice for use.[30]

Ongoing Re-evaluation of Student Performance

Thad's depiction of his clinical learning experience, presented earlier, describes the opportunity his CI created for re-evaluating his performance on an ongoing basis. The context of patient care provides a unique environment in which the CI can evaluate student performance and teach, monitor and reinforce, and question and answer almost simultaneously. Ongoing re-evaluation is critical to ensure that selection of clinical learning experiences matches the student's readiness.

A note of caution: Accurate diagnosis of readiness can be a challenging endeavor. Just as in physical therapy patient care, assessment does not always lead to an accurate diagnosis. Consider the case of Daneen, a student in her first clinical experience, as she evaluated José, a 22-year-old man who was referred with shoulder pain:

DANEEN: José, I'm going to do your upper quarter screen. This is to rule out any problems with your cervical region, elbow, wrist, and hand so we can concentrate on your shoulder. Good. Now abduct your shoulder. That means bringing it out like this. That's to test your deltoid. It's innervated by the axillary nerve. That's C-5. Don't let me push it down. Good. Now I want you to …

Daneen's CI is concerned about her ability to provide patient education at an appropriate level for her patient. It could be argued that Daneen is not providing patient education at all. Rather, she is self-talking aloud. She is performing examination techniques that she has not mastered, and she needs to talk herself through the procedure, explaining to herself what she is doing and why. She has not yet reached a competency level that allows her to demonstrate proficiency in the skill while instructing the patient with appropriate patient-oriented language. An accurate diagnosis of readiness would lead the CI, in this case, to allow Daneen to practice the techniques until they were automatic; then, she would be able to orient her focus to the patient rather than use a scripted performance. Daneen needs to be able to perform an upper quarter screen without thinking about each step. This allows her to listen and talk with the patient.

SELECTION OF CLINICAL PROBLEMS

Clinical learning experiences or problems need to be selected based on the potential they provide for useful learning. The CI may be able to choose between patients, but this may not be possible in the real world of practice. More than likely, the CI needs to identify learning opportunities within the context of practice that day or even at that moment.

General guidelines for the selection of clinical learning experiences must acknowledge that students need to learn routines and standards before they develop creative alternatives. Students are searching for a right way to think and perform, and their tolerance for ambiguity, unexpected events, or variation is relatively low. Once confidence develops, students can discern when routine approaches fit and when they do not. Routines are rare when comparing patients, but there may be many similarities when considering "pieces" of physical therapy examination or intervention. For example, you may want to have the student work with patients with similar diagnoses to establish confidence in procedural reasoning and technical skills. Repeated actions over time enable students to look for patterns, develop hypotheses, and learn to respond to the unexpected. Once the pattern of learning is established, challenge the known and dare the student to stretch beyond his or her comfort zone.

Consider the following example: Mary has worked with Joe for the first 2 days of his first full-time experience after completion of the didactic curriculum in his educational program. So far he has been observing. He seems comfortable conversing with patients, asks appropriate questions, and demonstrates adequate fundamental handling skills when he participates in cotreating. Mary suggests the following:

MARY: Joe, you observed me evaluate Sam Jones, Dr. Stevenson's patient, who was 1-day post-op [postoperative] ACL [anterior cruciate ligament] reconstruction. It looks like Diane Reeves, a new patient coming in at 1:00 this afternoon, may have a similar diagnosis. I'd like you to see her. I'll be there if you have questions or need assistance, but I'd like you to take the lead. Why don't you take the next 20 minutes and outline how you would proceed? We can discuss your plans at 12:30, and then you'll be ready to go.

Mary selected this learning opportunity to extend Joe's experience from the previous day, when he had observed an examination of a patient with a similar diagnosis. This time, however, Mary can evaluate Joe's ability to plan the examination and his skill in performing it. By discussing his plans and participating in a supporting role during the examination, she can monitor his actions, protect the patient (if necessary), and instruct throughout the process as needed.

A student with more advanced knowledge and skills may be asked to focus on a different learning experience with the same patient, as in the following example:

CLINICAL INSTRUCTOR: I know that you've been working with several patients who have had ACL reconstructions. What would you think about treating them at the same time in more of a group approach? The staff has discussed this off and on. After an initial evaluation and setting up patients' treatment programs, could a group of five or six be scheduled at the same time? Are there activities they could do as a group? What effect would this have on outcomes? Could you help in developing a proposal for the staff meeting next month, considering this with factors such as time, cost, and outcome? Denise, our director, has gathered the data we have that might be relevant and suggested meeting with you tomorrow to share her ideas and begin discussing this project with you. Your knowledge and skills in working with patients with this diagnosis are good, beyond entry level, and I think you're ready to view the delivery of physical therapy service in a broader scope.

The selection of clinical problems and learning experiences progresses throughout the clinical experience with consideration of the student's readiness, types of patients, numbers of patients, and level of student responsibility. Choose clinical problems to challenge the student to learn. It is not so much a choice of patients, but what you choose to have the student do with them in the context of patient-centered service. Students should progress from self-centered to patient-centered learning in preparation for real-world practice. Specific clinical learning experiences are site dependent but should build on past experiences. *Clinical education is not intended to be a sampler in which each diagnosis is seen once and each technique is tried. There is no evidence that variety makes a better practitioner.* If a student can problem solve with a new patient of an unknown diagnosis and learn to improve the patient's function, the student should be able to use these problem-solving tools and generalize from one case to the next with improving skill.

SUPERVISION OF STUDENT PERFORMANCE

Supervision includes monitoring a student's performances, providing supportive guidance, and directing instruction. Refer again to Thad's description of his learning experience presented earlier. Cassie, Thad's CI, works alongside Thad and observes his performance on an ongoing basis. However, at a more advanced level, ongoing, direct observation may be less frequent, with information derived from written documentation or even patient outcomes. Most important, Cassie conveys to Thad her strong belief in his present and future clinical capabilities.

While providing supportive guidance to students, a clinical teacher must also provide targeted instruction. In the beginning of this chapter, Jeff's CI describes the instruction she provides to him. Her teaching is not focused and is perceived as a didactic monologue that got in the way of Jeff's learning. It is important to move beyond the book knowledge and laboratory skills a student brings to the clinic, but it is essential to listen to the student and teach in response to the student's questions—when asked or when you think the student should be asking. It is important to teach over the patient and enable the student to build the bridge between theory and practice. Make your reasoning process explicit while providing a safe environment for the student to develop an understanding of her

or his own reasoning process while working with you. Students should be encouraged to question their own practice, and they should be given permission to question the instructor's. The instructor should teach students to take effective actions.

Good clinical teachers do not have to know everything. One hopes that the student generates questions that the instructor can't answer. A vital component of clinical education is learning where to find those answers. The instructor should model and teach the student to use the resources available by looking in references, asking another therapist, asking the patient, or asking other health care practitioners.

Experienced clinical teachers admit that the most difficult part of working with students is giving up their own patients. Physical therapists value the relationships they develop with their patients and take pride in their ability to help them. Giving up ownership of that responsibility isn't easy for the therapist. Likewise, it is difficult to give up control of the student as the student moves from other-assisted to self-assisted learning. Supervision should focus on encouraging independence and professional initiative in the broadest sense of patient care while minimizing risk to the patient and student.

EVALUATION OF STUDENT PERFORMANCE

The purpose of evaluation is to measure performance, enhance attainment of goals, and minimize risk to patients. Evaluation begins in the pre-experience planning phase and continues throughout the clinical learning experience, concluding with a summative evaluation at the end of the experience. This summative evaluation incorporates multiple sources of information to make the decision about the student's readiness to practice by assessing the student's cognitive, psychomotor, and affective behaviors.[31] The evaluation is used by the academic institution to determine the success or failure of the student's clinical performance. Specific information and training regarding the use of the evaluation instrument used by a particular academic program are provided by the program. Summative evaluations are necessary to minimize risk to the consumer and determine entry-level competence. For the student, they represent an evaluation of his or her capabilities at a given moment and provide the opportunity for the clinical teacher to give input regarding the next phase of education or learning. Most important, they should encompass an element of self-assessment. Physical therapists occupy the role of clinical teachers and evaluators for only a brief period of time. It is imperative that the student learns to accurately self-assess his or her capabilities and areas that need improvement.

Formative evaluations need to occur throughout the learning experience as a continuous part of clinical teaching. Assess, with the student, where she or he is and where he or she is going. Students need to understand that clinical education is a learning experience. Yes, the student is expected to perform. But based on this performance, clinical problems are selected to provide opportunities for teaching and learning to enable the student to progress to competent professional practice. This is synonymous with the ongoing re-evaluation that occurs as a part of diagnosing a student's readiness.

Students often need assistance in distinguishing between their performance and their feelings about that performance. A student who lacks confidence may feel uncertain and judge his or her competencies to be lower than those observed by the clinical teacher. Another student, feeling satisfied with a patient's progress, might fail to consider aspects of his or her intervention in which improvement is needed. It is helpful for teachers to reflect on their own performance out loud. This includes acknowledgment of their limitations in knowledge and skill and errors in judgment, as well as their abilities to rethink and plan for improvement. Modeling is an effective teaching technique to encourage students to develop skill in accurate self-assessment. Students are able to self-assess based on their experiences. These experiences need to be designed to prepare them to self-assess objectively in the context of entry-level professional practice.

CIs rarely fail to identify significant problems that place a student at risk for not successfully completing a clinical education experience. Timing, however, is a key factor. If the instructor has concerns or suspects difficulty, it should be addressed immediately with the student. If the instructor is unable to resolve the problem, she or he should seek advice from the Center Coordinator of Clinical Education or the student's DCE. These are appropriate people from whom to seek information. Questions or concerns are best addressed before they become problems. Clinical educators at all levels are involved in the process of learning to provide better clinical education.

Often, a student is progressing satisfactorily, and then learning plateaus or stalls. In such a case, the instructor must give the student a jump start. If the student has been able to accomplish the program's goals and objectives and his or her personal goals, or is progressing toward that end, can the goals be extended or new goals set that move beyond entry-level competence to mastery? It is important for students to learn that professional development includes ongoing self-assessment and re-evaluation, followed by defining new goals targeted at enhancing knowledge and skills. Learning is a lifelong process that continues throughout clinical practice.

SUMMARY

This chapter attempts to deal simply with a complex subject. The answers to questions about clinical teaching are dependent on the context in which they are asked. Teaching techniques used by one CI must be molded and modified before they can be applied in another situation. Each topic addressed suggests many more questions. It is my hope that as we continue to plan, develop, and deliver clinical learning experiences that enable the transition from student to practitioner, the desires of physical therapists to continue learning will be reflected in self-directed efforts to know, understand, and become more able and skilled in the clinical education process.

THRESHOLD CONCEPTS

Threshold Concept #1: The integration of students' knowledge, skills and values and attitudes is an important outcome during clinical education experiences. They must combine what they know and practice what they can do in the context of patient care. Are there ways in which you can facilitate this integration? Let's look at an example.

A student is examining a patient who has sought physical therapy for shoulder pain. Following a brief history and systems review, the student begins gather data through the administration of a plethora of tests and measures. You are uncertain of the process he used to select the specific tests and measures and suspect that he is trying to do everything he learned in musculoskeletal class. What questions might you ask to facilitate thoughts about diagnostic hypotheses, evidence-based practice, and clinical decision-making?

Threshold Concept #2: Conceptual models for clinical teaching exist in the literature but are not often applied to the reality of teaching in day-to-day practice. Putting theory into practice is not an easy endeavor. Neher and colleagues described a five-step "microskills" model of clinical teaching that was used for clinical teaching of family practice residents.[28] This model, often referred to as the one-minute clinical instructor, may be especially helpful to maximize learning when you have limited blocks of time for one-on-one teaching.

Read the article. How does the model compare to your current clinical teaching methods focused on a student's decision-making processes? Give the five steps a try. What did you find most difficult in implementing the suggested strategies? Did you observe changes in student performance outcomes?

ANNOTATED BIBLIOGRAPHY

American Physical Therapy Association. *Credentialed Clinical Instructor Program.* Alexandria, VA: American Physical Therapy Association; 2009.

American Physical Therapy Association. Advanced Credentialed Clinical Instructor Program for the Physical Therapist. Alexandria, VA: American Physical Therapy Association, 2010. These two manuals provide comprehensive notes of the content presented in the two APTA education and credentialing programs. They are excellent resources for beginning as well as experienced clinical instructors.

Jensen GM, Gwyer J, Hack LM, Shepard KF. *Expertise in Physical Therapy Practice: Applications for Professional Development and Life Learning.* 2nd ed. Philadelphia: Saunders Publishing Company; 2007.

Based on observations and interviews with expert therapists, the authors describe a model of expertise in physical therapy practice and discuss how expert practitioners develop, think, reason, make decisions, and perform in practice. An excellent resource to compare with established performance behaviors expected for entry-level competence.

Lave J, Wenger E. *Situated Learning: Legitimate Peripheral Participation.* New York: Cambridge University Press; 1991.

Lave and Wenger locate learning in the processes of coparticipation and explore how practice grounds learning. They describe cases of Yucatec midwives, Vai and Gola tailors, naval quartermasters, meat cutters, and nondrinking alcoholics in which the learner participates in the actual practice of an expert to a limited degree and with limited responsibility for the product as a whole. This text is highly recommended to broaden the reader's perspective on situated learning beyond the realm of health care.

Lyons N, ed. *With Portfolio in Hand: Validating the New Teacher Professionalism.* New York: Teachers College; 1998

This book provides a rich description of the possibilities, potentials, and problems of portfolios in the practice and assessment of teaching. Helpful information is presented to guide the preparation of useful portfolios.

Mentkowski M, Associates. *Learning That Lasts: Integrating Learning, Development, and Performance in College and Beyond.* San Francisco: Jossey-Bass Publishers; 2000.

The authors define *learning that lasts* as the successful integration of learning, development, and performance. Based on work at Alverno

College, this text proposes a theory of learning with practical strategies for teaching.

Neher JO, Gordon KC, Meyer B, Stevens N. A five-step "microskills" model of clinical teaching. *J Am Board Fam Pract.* 1992;5:419–424

The need to maximize learning in smaller blocks of time with limited time for one-on-one teaching is a challenge in clinical education. The authors propose a five-step model focused on the student's decision-making process that includes getting a commitment, probing for supporting evidence, focusing on teaching, reinforcing what was performed correctly and correcting mistakes.

Perkins D. *Making Learning Whole: How Seven Principles of Teaching Can Transform Education.* San Francisco: Jossey-Bass Publishers; 2009.

This text introduces a practical, research-based framework for teaching using the metaphor of baseball. Learning in the context of the "whole game" is emphasized and the principles are well-suited to clinical teaching where learning is done in the context of patient-centered care.

Watts NT. *Handbook of Clinical Teaching.* New York: Churchill Livingstone; 1990.

Watts has contributed a practical handbook with sensible advice to enable clinical teachers to build bridges between the theory and practice of clinical teaching. Each chapter includes exercises and feedback that provide an opportunity for the reader to reflect on the information presented and begin to develop skill in application.

REFERENCES

1. Callahan M, Decker R, Hirt S, Tappan F. *Physical Therapy Education Theory and Practice.* New York: Council of Physical Therapy School Directors; 1968.
2. Scully RM. *Clinical Teaching of Physical Therapy Students in Clinical Education.* Ph.D. dissertation. New York: Columbia University; 1974.
3. American Physical Therapy Association. *Physical Therapist Clinical Education Principles.* Available at: http://www.apta.org/PTClinicalEducationPrinciples/; Accessed 15.08.11.
4. Skinner BF. *About Behaviorism.* New York: Knopf; 1974.
5. Bruner JS. *Beyond Information Given: Studies in the Psychology of Knowing.* New York: Norton; 1973.
6. Guba EG, Lincoln YS. *Fourth Generation Evaluation.* Newbury Park, CA: Sage; 1989.
7. Poplin MS. Holistic/constructivist principles of the teaching/learning process: implications for the field of learning disabilities. *J Learn Disab.* 1988;21:93.
8. Vygotsky LS. *Mind in Society.* Cambridge, MA: Harvard University Press; 1978.
9. Lave J, Wenger E. *Situated Learning: Legitimate Peripheral Participation.* New York: Cambridge University Press; 1991.
10. Van Langenberghe HVK. Evaluation of students' approaches to studying in a problem-based physical therapy curriculum. *Phys Ther.* 1988;68:522.
11. Graham CL. Conceptual learning processes in physical therapy students. *Phys Ther.* 1996;76:856.
12. Ladyshewsky RK, Barrie SC, Drake VM. A comparison of productivity and learning outcome in individual and cooperative physical therapy clinical education models. *Phys Ther.* 1998;78:1288.
13. Solomon PE, Binkley J, Stratford PW. A descriptive study of learning processes and outcomes in two problem-based curriculum designs. *J Phys Ther Educ.* 1996;10:72.
14. Hayward LM, Cairns MA. Physical therapist students' perceptions of and strategic approaches to case-based instruction: suggestions for curriculum design. *J Phys Ther Educ.* 1998;12:33.
15. Ladyshewsky RK. Peer-assisted learning in clinical education: a review of terms and learning principles. *J Phys Ther Educ.* 2000;14:15.
16. Dewey J. *Democracy and Education.* New York: Macmillan; 1916.
17. Perkins D. *Making Learning Whole.* San Francisco: Jossey-Bass; 2009.
18. American Physical Therapy Association. *Credentialed Clinical Instructor Program.* Alexandria, VA: American Physical Therapy Association; 2009.
19. Mentkowski M. Associates. *Learning that Lasts: Integrating Learning, Development, and Performance in College and Beyond.* San Francisco: Jossey-Bass; 2000.
20. Gagne RM, Driscoll MP. *Essentials of Learning for Instruction.* Englewood Cliffs, NJ: Prentice Hall; 1988.
21. Jensen GM, Gwyer J, Hack LM, Shepard KF. *Expertise in Physical Therapy Practice.* Boston: Butterworth-Heinemann; 1999.
22. Schon DA. *The Reflective Practitioner: How Professionals Think in Action.* New York: Basic Books; 1983.
23. Jensen GM, Paschal KA. Habits of mind: student transition toward virtuous practice. *J Phys Ther Educ.* 2000;14:42.
24. Lyons N, ed. *With Portfolio in Hand: Validating the New Teacher Professionalism.* New York: Teachers College; 1998.
25. American Physical Therapy Association. *Interactive Guide to Physical Therapist Practice.* Available at: http:www.apta.org/Guide; 2003. Accessed 15.08.11.
26. Houghland JE, Druck J. Effective clinical teaching by residents in emergency medicine. *Ann Emerg Med.* 2010;55:434–439.
27. Abrams RG. Questioning in preclinical and clinical instruction. *J Dent Educ.* 1983;47:599.
28. Neher JO, Gordon KC, Meyer B, Stevens N. A five-step "microskills" model of clinical teaching. *J Am Board Fam Pract.* 1992;5:419–424.
29. Ottolini MC, Ozuah PO, Mirza N, Greenberg LW. Student perceptions of effectiveness of the eight step preceptor (ESP) model in the ambulatory setting. *Teach Learn Med.* 2010;22:97–101.
30. American Physical Therapy Association. *Advanced Credentialed Clinical Instructor Program for the Physical Therapist.* Alexandria, VA: American Physical Therapy Association; 2010.
31. American Physical Therapy Association. *Physical Therapist Student Clinical Performance Instrument.* Alexandria, VA: American Physical Therapy Association; 2006.

WHAT MAKES A GOOD CLINICAL TEACHER?

Elizabeth Mostrom

CHAPTER OUTLINE

An exemplar *is a detailed description of a critical event, a defining or pivotal moment, or a turning point in one's professional or personal learning and development. The following narrative is a response from one outstanding clinical teacher when she was asked to describe an exemplar that shaped who she is and what she does as a clinical instructor (CI) for physical therapy students:*

[There are] two situations from my own clinical experience as a student: we had two clinical experiences back to back. [In] the first one I went to my clinical instructor was wonderful, top-notch; [in] the second one I did not enjoy [the] clinical instructor. I learned from both of them, things I want to do [as a CI] and things I try not to do.[1(p 5)]

Like many clinical teachers, this CI drew on memories of—and reflections on—her experiences as student physical therapist (an exemplar) to give context and shape to her beliefs about clinical teaching and learning. She also uses these memories to inform her everyday practice with her own students. Here are her reflections on her time with her "top-notch" instructor:

It wasn't necessarily her clinical skills that made me think she was such a good clinical instructor. I do think she had very good clinical skills but [they weren't] the key; it was more her personal skills. She treated me as a peer. She found learning opportunities for me, but she treated me as a peer in front of patients, in front of other staff members, in front of physicians, nurses, other team players. She gave me feedback and the confidence to continue with what I was doing [during an evaluation]. She had a lot of qualities . . . she was very thorough and she was very dedicated to her patients; she was a strong patient advocate. So some of those skills have affected me in positive ways as a clinician, but you also need those skills with a student. She was dedicated to my

learning and she was very thorough and thoughtful with my own learning.[1(p 6)]

That experience was in contrast to her less-positive memories of the second CI:

I felt like [he] did not treat me as a peer. He had an attitude that he was smarter and better, which he probably was, I'm sure, I mean I was a student and he's an instructor, but it was the attitude just of superiority; that we weren't on the same playing field. He didn't give me a lot of feedback, positive or negative, unless [I asked]. Again, it relates to confidence. He wasn't instilling confidence in me so I was second-guessing myself. In looking back, I think I just would have appreciated more feedback, positive or negative.[1(p 6)]

She also shared a particularly uncomfortable event that occurred when she was working with this CI:

We were in front of a patient, dealing with an upper extremity [problem] of some sort, and he asked me what I thought was a very strange question: "What is the key to the upper extremity?" And it was just a very strange question in my mind. I didn't know the answer so he said: "Well, you better go home and think about that." [It was] in front of the patient and [it] kind of made me feel like I don't know what I'm doing. The answer he was looking for was the clavicle because it's the only bony connection to the upper extremities, but it was just his choice of wording and [the fact that] he didn't rephrase the question. He didn't offer any additional information; he just kind of left it that vague. Again, in front of the patient.[1(p 7)]

Although the gifted clinical teacher whose voice you hear in this narrative was almost eight years removed from this distressing experience as a student, she still recalls it vividly and has committed to not having her students experience the same type of distancing and humiliation she felt during her time with the second CI.

This commitment is reflected in the first impressions of a student who was supervised by the exemplary clinical teacher whose words you have just read:

On my first day my CI welcomed me and gave me a very good impression. After having my last CI it made me appreciate it even more because it was completely opposite. She was just really—she made me feel relaxed right away. Then we started going over some things: the whole environment was completely foreign to me so I had no idea about anything. [She] helped me with that. She sat down with me and went through all that we needed to know in little bits and . . . let me know that I wasn't going to learn it all in one day, that it was going to take some time. She was a confidence booster right away. She's like "I know you're going to be great. I know you're going to be fine. So don't even worry about it." She had a really good attitude about everything and that just kind of set the theme for the rest of the clinical. Right away I felt comfortable with her. I knew I could ask questions, I knew she wasn't going to make me feel stupid or anything like that. [It] was really good from the start.[2](p 2)

Clearly this student is the beneficiary of the experiences in clinical teaching and learning borne of the CI's own experiences as a student. These are two of many other stories from and about exceptional clinical teachers that are shared in the pages to come. In this chapter, I present findings from a multiyear and multiphase qualitative investigation of CI mastery and student learning in physical therapist clinical education.

LEARNING GOALS

After completing this chapter, the reader will be able to:

1. Describe some characteristics and attributes of clinical instructors who have been identified as outstanding clinical teachers by their students and colleagues.
2. Discuss the relationships between a CI's teaching philosophy, teaching "style," and teaching behaviors and techniques.
3. Identify one exemplar that was a pivotal moment in the reader's own development as a CI or student and share the exemplar in a narrative form with a colleague.
4. Explore and clarify the reader's own beliefs about teaching and student learning in clinical environments; begin to articulate the reader's own clinical teaching philosophy based on those beliefs.
5. Craft a personal vision of what it means to be a good clinical teacher and develop a plan to assist the reader in achieving that vision.

INTRODUCTION

As the authors of several chapters in this handbook have clearly indicated, clinical education is a critical component of professional preparation and education for physical therapists at both the entry-level and postprofessional level (see Chapters 8, 9, 11, and 16). In the United States, the clinical education portion of the curriculum currently comprises more than 20% of the professional preparation program on average, and the trend has been toward increasing the length and amount of clinical education experience over the past few years.[3] Central to learning in clinical environments are the relationship and interaction between the student physical therapist or physical therapist assistant and the clinical instructor (CI) (or instructors) who provide supervision and guidance during clinical experiences. Although many studies[4-13] and several documents[14-16] have suggested desirable characteristics, attributes, professional behaviors, and teaching and clinical skills of physical therapy clinical instructors, only a handful have sought to describe expert or exemplary clinic instruction using qualitative approaches to inquiry[17-25] and exploring the perspectives and contextualized stories of *both* CIs and students.

In my own experience as a Director of Clinical Education for decades, there has been ample evidence of a wide variation in student experiences with clinical instructors; many students report tremendously positive experiences with CIs who facilitated their learning and development as future therapists, whereas others report experiences with CIs that were detrimental to their learning. Of greatest interest to me for the study I share in this chapter was the profound and positive impact on learning and development that students who have worked with exceptional CIs report. The landmark work of Jensen and colleagues[26-28] on expertise in physical therapy practice and some of my own inquiry into clinical mastery[29,30] spurred my interest in further exploring expertise in clinical instruction through the perspectives and voices of outstanding clinical instructors and physical therapist students with whom they have worked.

The broad purposes of the investigation were to undertake the following:

- Explore the professional learning and development of physical therapists who have been recognized as outstanding clinical teachers.
- Elucidate the nature and sources of their beliefs about teaching and learning in clinical settings.
- Describe the characteristics, attributes, and instructional practices of exceptional CIs from the perspective of those instructors and their students.
- Generate rich narrative descriptions of clinical teaching and learning to guide development of preliminary theory about expertise in clinical teaching and student learning in physical therapy clinical settings.

Some guiding questions for this investigation are shown in Box 10–1.

BOX 10–1 Guiding Questions for the Investigation of Good Clinical Teaching Practices

Clinical Instructors	Students
What makes a good clinical teacher in physical therapy?	What makes a good clinical teacher in the view of physical therapy students?
What can we learn from CIs who have been identified as excellent teachers?	What can we learn from students who have worked with exceptional CIs?
How can we best understand their own learning and development as a CI?	How do they describe the characteristics, attributes, and behaviors of those CIs?
What are their beliefs about clinical teaching and student learning?	How did their experience with the CI shape their learning and development as a student and future therapist?
What is their teaching philosophy?	What lessons were learned? How were they learned?
What teaching strategies or techniques do they employ?	

FINDINGS: THE VOICE OF OUTSTANDING CLINICAL INSTRUCTORS

The findings from phase 1 of the study (Figure 10–1) are discussed in the following section through the words and stories of these exemplary clinical teachers. (Please refer to Appendices 10–A to 10–C and Tables A2–1 and A2–2 for further detail about the study design, methods and participants.[31-38] The results have been broken down into two broad categories according to the type of data collection method involved:

1. Resume Sort
2. Clinical Instructor Interviews

RESUME SORT

Before the interviews, participants were asked to sort activities listed on their resumes and placed on note cards into piles of those activities they felt were "most," "somewhat," or "least" influential in their learning and development as a CI. There were six main categories of activities that appeared on resumes:

1. Formal educational preparation
2. Professional memberships and activities
3. Work experiences
4. Continuing education
5. Honors and awards
6. Community service

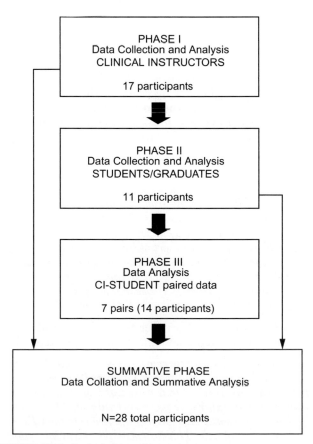

FIGURE 10–1 Study design and sequence.

During the interview, participants could then elaborate on the nature of the activities they felt were influential and how they contributed to their development as a clinician and clinical teacher. Not surprisingly, most saw their development as a clinician as tightly interwoven with their development as an instructor.

Most Influential Activities

Professional Memberships and Activities

These therapists highly valued their involvement in professional organizations and listed many of those activities as most influential in their development as a CI. All of them were members of the American Physical Therapy Association (APTA), and most were involved in various components of the organization at local, state, or national levels.

Several were members of other professional groups as well, such as the American Academy of Orthopedic Manual Physical Therapy, but they noted that there was some overlap between the categories of professional memberships/activity and continuing education because many of the continuing education activities they participated in were sponsored or supported by professional organizations. They valued offerings such as the Clinical Instructor Education and Credentialing Program (CIECP) and board certifications through the American Board of Physical Therapy Specialization (ABPTS). In addition to modeling involvement, many of these instructors engaged students during their internships in professional organizations and activities in an effort to encourage their future involvement.

One of the CIs described what he hoped to instill in his students:

> [T]hat it's not a matter of just coming to work and being a physical therapist, it's being involved in your Association and the importance [it] has on our profession. With respect to being a clinical instructor, it's trying to pass that on to students and helping them to value being a member, exposing them to different aspects of membership.[39(p 3)]

The CI went on to describe how he had traveled to a state legislative committee meeting the previous evening with one of his students so that they could "see the, not just social aspects of it, but the professional benefits too. Just getting everyone else's perspectives and things like that. I hope that what she saw there was how exciting it is to be able to network with people outside of your direct work environment."[39(p 3)]

Formal Educational Preparation

Most of the CIs felt that their formal educational preparation as a physical therapist or their postprofessional education was also very influential in shaping them as both clinician and CI. Interestingly, however, it was not the didactic curriculum per se that they saw as most important, rather it was academic and clinical faculty who they encountered along the way. Some of those faculty served as important mentors and models for whom they wanted to become; others served as reminders of whom or what they did not want to become as a therapist or clinical teacher. Although they saw their educational preparation as the "foundation" on which they built their practice as a CI, they recall it mostly as the source of their physical therapist student identity. This was an identity they frequently called on when describing exemplars (see the narrative at the beginning of this chapter) and when discussing their teaching philosophy, beliefs, and practices. One of the CIs in this study described the influence of his educational preparation this way:

> That was one of the most foundational points for me and I think it's a multi-faceted sort of reason for it. [That's] where I had my identity as a student. I remember working with both good CIs and CIs that I didn't think were so good.... I've never felt like I ever lost that feeling that I had the first time I went into a clinic.... I realize this is a real critical time in developing into a professional when you are a student. And I think it had lasting implications for me.[40(p 1)]

Work Experiences

The other frequently noted influential factor in the development of these CIs was their work experiences themselves. The CIs were constantly learning through doing in their everyday practice as therapists and teachers. The workplace environment was a critically important facilitator for these rich and meaningful experiences. These therapists had found their clinical practice "homes" in places that provided several supports for their ongoing learning and development. These included human resources, relationships and supports, and other administrative supports for their activities as a clinical teacher.

Two CIs explain how their professional work experiences helped them develop professionally:

> • I've had the pleasure of working with people that have had a significant amount of clinical experience and you can't help but absorb their most valuable types of treatments, their ways of educating patients, their ways of educating students. I think it's really accelerated my learning being around skilled clinicians.[41(p 2)]
> • The other thing that I thought was a significant ... piece of the puzzle is the environment that I work in because I get support from the manager and from the staff to implement [student] programs and to take time to do it. Without it I couldn't do what I do now with clinical education.[40(p 2)]

Somewhat Influential Activities
Continuing Education

The activities identified as "somewhat influential" were a variety of continuing education activities that most CIs saw as essential to keeping current for their practice but not as most influential in their learning and development as a CI. Thus, these CIs suggested that their knowledge of practice, what in the literature on knowledge in teaching might be called "subject matter or content knowledge,"[42] was important, but it was only one of several dimensions or domains of knowledge that contributed to good teaching.

Community Service and Honors and Awards

This "somewhat influential" category most often included the category of engagement in community service, viewed as important to their personal development and commitments; and honors or recognitions the CIs had received, most notably the recognition as a recipient of the Michigan Physical Therapy Association (MPTA) Outstanding Clinical Instructor Award. They described the award variously as an "honor," a "reinforcement," an "encouragement," and a "validation," although several pointed out that it did not or would not really change what they do as a CI:

> • You try to do the best job you can, but then when you get something like this, it's like WOW! I've been recognized for something you really like to do and that makes you strive to do even better.[43(p 2)]
> • It's the recognition.... I take away some sense of giving back and helping people through their education (by being a CI.) But ... it was nice to be recognized for my efforts being that I do care about these future PTs and the profession.[41(p 3)]

CLINICAL INSTRUCTOR INTERVIEWS
Exemplars

Description of exemplars as an interview strategy has been used in several studies of expertise.[26,28,31–33] The CIs in this study were asked to share one or two exemplars; they were urged to "tell me the story" or to "replay the video" of that event (see Appendix 10-B.). As forecast earlier, by far the most frequently shared exemplars were descriptions of experiences as physical therapy students working with CIs. In roughly half of the cases, the experiences were positive, and the CIs purposely sought to emulate the characteristics, commitments, and behaviors of that CI in their own clinical teaching. The negative experiences, which made up the other half of the experiences reported, defined what the CIs did not want to be (or become) for their students.

One example of both the positive and negative experiences of one of the CIs is provided in the narrative at the beginning of this chapter, but others had similar good and bad experiences:

> I had a situation when I was a student where this CI, I think, was on a mission to flunk me. It was strange I don't know where it was coming from.... She just wasn't open. If she had a concern it was all top secret you know. She wasn't really telling me what she was looking for or what the problems were. It was sort of like a CIA kind of thing. I never knew. I was always walking on eggshells and when you're a student your confidence is kind of flighty and she was harming that for sure. Maybe that was just her method, but I wasn't responding well to it. So I never forgot it.[44(p 9)]

This CI, however, also never forgot how another staff therapist and instructor saw the situation and stepped in:

> Luckily one of the other therapists there saved me. She saw what was happening and took me over and I never forgot that. She realized that what was happening was not kosher. So that experience has stayed with me.[44(p 9)]
> These experiences have been translated into the CI's current teaching style. This instructor felt it was important "to have it [expectations] all on the table. My goal is to be an

advocate and to create a great experience but also to meet expectations that are there from the school and from our facility ... but to be helpful and to gently pull people to a higher level.[44(p 9)]

A more positive experience with a CI was described by another participant:

It was my first rotation in my final year. My CI believed very heavily in education; [she] would take me aside and we would go through a lab in a sense—a practice lab—of what was coming up with the next patient. She was very, very energetic, a lot of fun, and I enjoyed [the labs] because it took the pressure off.... She was never condescending to me; it was always 'well, yeah, that will work [the way the student suggested], but maybe try this.' [She was] letting me choose and letting me make my mistakes without jumping on me.[45(p 5)]

The CI speaking here has purposefully attempted to emulate the enthusiasm for teaching, the respect for students, and the scaffolding for learning that was demonstrated by his memorable CI many years prior.

The other most frequent exemplars offered by CIs were stories of their learning through doing: learning through their own teaching experiences with students, through feedback from students, and, importantly, through reflection on those experiences. They asked themselves, What went well? What didn't go well? and Why? Often, such critical reflection was prompted by their work with difficult students, in some cases even those who didn't succeed. It is noteworthy that these CIs took seriously their responsibility to help students succeed and examined not only the performance of the learner but also their performance as a teacher in such cases.

In one instance, a CI described an experience with her most difficult student:

When I think about my whole career being a CI and having students, there's one student that comes to mind ... it was the most difficult student I had and one in which the student did not succeed. It was a real challenge for me ... But I was determined to make this work. As a CI I thought, I can do this. I have a challenging student and that's okay. And what do I need to do to make this work. And so for me it was a good experience.[46(p 5)]

For this CI, working with this student who didn't succeed was a "good experience" because she was forced to re-examine approaches to teaching and strategies that had previously worked for her with other students. She explored the student's learning needs and tried to adapt her teaching to best meet those needs. And, despite the fact that the student was not successful in the end, she felt the kind of deliberate reflection she engaged in about the student's learning and her teaching had transformed her as a teacher. She felt she had expanded the repertoire of approaches that she could employ for the variety of students she might encounter in her continued work as a CI.

The exemplars described by this sample of CIs are consistent with the findings of David Irby years ago in his studies of distinguished medical educators.[47,48] As Irby writes of his excellent clinical teachers: "They acquired their knowledge of teaching primarily from the experience of being a learner (the apprenticeship of observation of good and bad examples) and a teacher (reflecting on what worked and did

not work)."[49(p 339)] In a later study of clinical teachers in medicine, Pinsky and Irby[49] found that good teachers used the experience of failure to improve their teaching. They did so by using failure as a catalyst for several forms of reflection:

- *Reflection on action* involved assessing their teaching after a perceived failure.
- *Reflection for action* (anticipatory reflection) involved planning for future teaching in light of past experience.
- *Reflection in action* involved assessing and trying to adapt teaching in the moment in the context of a teaching/learning activity that did not seem to be going well.

Similar forms of reflection were also reported by Buccieri and associates[18] based on a study with a small sample of expert physical therapist clinical instructors. These findings also resonate with a large body of research on teacher thinking summarized by Clark and Peterson[50] and Clark.[51] The experienced teachers those authors describe engage in intentional, interactive, improvisational and reflective thinking about their teaching: "They reflect on and analyze the apparent effects of their own teaching and apply the results of these reflections to their future plans and actions. In short, they have become researchers on their own teaching effectiveness."[50(p 292)]

Influential People

In a follow-up question to the resume sort activity and the description of exemplars, CIs were asked to identify people (vs. events or activities) who influenced their learning and development as a CI and to describe how these individuals influenced them. Some of the findings presented elsewhere in the chapter overlap with responses to this question. In fact, it's worth noting how many of the descriptions of events or activities were infused with vivid memories of the people who were characters in those narrative accounts of events. Responses to this question were categorized as the following influential people:

- Teachers or professional colleagues
- Students
- Patients

Teachers and Professional Colleagues

In the category of teachers, 11 participants identified academic faculty members who served as professional role models for them as both clinicians and clinical educators. These academic faculty members were almost universally described, as shown in Box 10–2.

One CI described how an academic faculty member influenced his approaches to clinical teaching:

He influenced ... how I think, how I critically analyze. If I go to a course, I'm not going to believe it just because they tell me [it is correct]. Same thing with a research article ... just because it's there, I'm going to look for the flaws in it and how that might influence whether I can use that [information] clinically or not. He modeled evidence-based practice long before it became cliche.[52(p 7)]

Thus, the CI today reports a commitment to assisting his students to incorporate this type of critical analysis into

---

BOX 10–2 **Characteristics, Attributes, and Behaviors of Individuals with Positive Influence**

Academic Faculty Role Models and Mentors
- Very involved in professional organizations, physical therapy education, and clinical practice
- Dedicated to the field and to their students
- Knowledgeable and up to date
- Encouraged students to think critically, to ask why
- Modeled evidence-based practice
- Positive and respectful interactions with students; made students feel recognized and unique as a person in their encounters

Clinical Instructors
- Very involved in professional organizations and activities
- Respectful and supportive of students and professional colleagues
- Dedicated to their patients; being a patient advocate
- Open, clear, and honest in their communication; made expectations clear and provided regular feedback
- Patient; made student feel comfortable and welcome
- Treated student as a member of the team
- Committed to assisting student learning and development; let me "try my wings"
- Well-rounded

Professional Colleagues and Mentors
- Very involved in professional organizations and activities; encouraged professional engagement
- Knowledgeable and current in their areas of practice
- Creative; "think outside of the box"
- Supportive of the CI as a clinician and clinical teacher; "took me under their wing"
- Modeled professional behaviors; respectful of patients and colleagues
- Collaborator; team player
- Dedicated to their work and patients

---

their learning experience with him: "I want them to know why they are doing a particular technique, not just [do it] because it was shown to them."[52(p 8)]

As discussed earlier, other teachers who were very influential in the learning and development of these CIs were clinical faculty members: their CIs when they were students. The characteristics, attributes, and behaviors of CIs that were viewed as positive influences for the CIs who participated in the study are shown in Box 10–2. Most of the CIs indicated that they seek to emulate many of these attributes and behaviors in their work with students.

Alternatively, negative characteristics and behaviors by their previous CIs usually revolved around these factors:

- CIs not sharing or making expectations clear
- Supervision at the shoulder during the entire experience
- A lack of regular feedback
- A disrespectful or condescending attitude toward the student
- Public humiliation of the student (in front of patients caregivers or colleagues)
- Outright unethical behavior

Some of these negative experiences were described earlier in this chapter. The following describes the experience of one of the CIs with a clinical supervisor who taught her how she did not want to be with her own students:

> *I had an instructor who would not leave me ever, ever, to the point where they would sit right next to me and write things down as I was doing things. I even had to say once, 'Do you have to be right there?' 'Well, yeah.' And so I said I would never make my students that uncomfortable.... I said that I would never, ever be that way with my students.[43(p 4)]*

Eleven of the 17 CIs also identified professional colleagues as powerful role models and mentors for them as both clinicians and CIs in their respective communities of practice.[20,53,54] As you might expect, and as has been borne out by these findings, the professional identities of "clinician" and "clinical educator" are interwoven in the view of the CIs in this sample. The most frequently described characteristics, attributes, and behaviors of these professional colleagues and mentors are listed in Box 10–2 and mimic those in the previous two categories of clinicians.

One CI describing two colleagues who had been mentors to her put it this way: "They showed me that you didn't have to be an 8 to 5 PT. There was much more to it than managing your caseload. There is that personal side. That's how I practice. I don't practice by the numbers and things like that; I practice by the people."[43(p 5)]

Students

The students themselves were influential for the CIs involved in the study. All of the CIs reported that they learned something from every student they had worked with, from excellent students to very challenging students. The common refrain was "the experience works both ways" or "it's just a great two way street."[55(p 8)] Here is one description from a CI who has worked with numerous students for more than 12 years: "Every student is a teacher. I learn something from every student that I have. It sort of all molds together ... the more students I have, the more I learn about them and teaching.[40(p 8)] This same CI went on to report that the students he learns most from are those that provide him with honest feedback on his performance as a CI, which he genuinely appreciated. He also remarked on how the wide spectrum and diversity of students he has worked with require him to constantly "reconfigure my (his) approach" according to the student's learning needs.

In all cases, these CIs viewed the student-CI relationship as one of reciprocal teaching and learning, and they valued lessons learned from students about learners, learning, and their own teaching. Often these CIs made their beliefs about this reciprocal relationship explicit to the students early in their experience with them. This is the way one CI put it:

> *I think a lot of my students bring as much to the clinical as what I can give back to them ... and I always make it a point to say that to them. 'Don't be afraid to express or inform us of those things that you've learned along the way because I feel the clinical education experience works both ways. You don't come here and I just give you all this knowledge and then you leave. I like to see the interaction back and forth because there are always things that you can teach me. I'm not the all-knowing wise one here. I know what I know, but you also know what you know, so it works both ways.[56(p 8)]*

Sharing this viewpoint early in the experience with the student goes a long way in diminishing the socially conferred status differential between teacher and learner by explicitly valuing their knowledge and respecting what they can uniquely bring to the learning experience.

Patients

Finally, influential people for these CIs included the patients they have worked with throughout their careers. They saw their relationship with patients as similar to that with students in some ways; that is, the relationship is one that involves reciprocal teaching and learning, partnering, mutual respect, and mutual responsibility. As one CI stated: "As therapists we are teachers ... and healing and learning are joint efforts."[45(p 8)] The CIs reported that they translate the lessons learned from their patients over the years into their encounters and teaching with students. Such lessons included the importance of respectful interaction, using people first language, treating the patient as a person as a whole versus a body part, obtaining informed consent, being an active listener, and being patient: "I want the student to be respectful to every patient they see and know that they are not a body part or a problem; they're a person. I want them to evaluate the whole body, the whole person, not just a knee."[52(p 9)]

One CI learned about using patient-first language from one of his patients; it is a lesson he passes on to his students:

I treated an English professor years ago. He kept overhearing PTs refer to their patients as the 'shoulder lady' or the 'guy with the knee.' He was recovering from a tibial fracture and wanted to be referred to as the 'guy who will ski again' rather than a 'tibial fracture.' What this taught me is that how we label patients could have a substantial effect on their view of themselves, how we treat them, and perhaps their outcomes.[57(p11)]

Beliefs about Student Learning and Clinical Teaching

When asked about how they felt students learn best, the CI's responses merged with another question about the type of environment that enhances learning. The recurring themes in response to these questions are shown in Box 10–3.

One quote from a CI captures many of the facilitative elements mentioned in Box 10–3:

I think the best environment for a student is one where they are kept busy but not overly busy ... where they have that hands-on experience but with support. Where they have an opportunity and a comfort zone to talk to the CI frequently if need be and not feel like they are left out on a limb to struggle.... I don't want to come across as a know-it-all because I'm not. I want to make them feel like it's okay for them to come and talk to me—that it's not a bother for me. That's why I'm there working with them.[45(p 10)]

As you might expect, when CIs were asked to share their beliefs about what factors might impede or constrain student learning, their descriptions tended to be on the opposite end of the continuum from those factors identified earlier in this section. Impediments or barriers to learning included, first and foremost, student fear and discomfort in the view of these CIs. The sources of fear and discomfort

---

BOX 10–3 Facilitators and Impediments to Student Learning from Clinical Instructors' Perspective

Facilitators of Student Learning	Impediments to Student Learning
• An environment and CI that make the student feel welcome, comfortable, supported, not threatened	• Today's health care environment—productivity demands and restrictions on what students can and cannot do in clinical settings
• CI who is accessible and approachable	• CI not available, approachable
• CI who wants to teach and cares about student learning	• Lack of clinical instructor feedback; constructive criticism (or destructive criticism) not balanced with positive feedback, affirmation
• CI who provides honest and constructive feedback	
• CI who is not "all knowing"	
• CI who uses questioning as a tool for fostering insight and learning versus as a practical examination	• Not sharing expectations openly with students— "cards under the table"; not being honest and up front with students
• CI who invites the student to be a partner in the design and decisions about the experience and providing multiple opportunities for learning	• Public questioning of students or questioning in ways that could be embarrassing or humiliating
• CI who provides hands-on experience at the right time and place—sequencing and pacing the learning activities and experiences according to student readiness and needs	• Too much to do, too fast for student; not sequencing and pacing activities
	• Too little or too much supervision or guidance (in some cases trying to create a "clone" of the CI)
• CI who grades the level and amount of supervision according to where students are at the moment with attention to where they need to go	• Student perfectionism
	• Student passivity; not actively engaging and taking responsibility for one's own learning

---

could be from the environment itself (the demands of today's health care system), the CI, other staff, or the student (see Box 10–3). Note how they contrast with perceived facilitators of student learning.

These CIs did suggest that the fear of being wrong was a constraint on learning. They felt such fear could be engendered by the demands of the environment or the behaviors of the CI, or be related to factors intrinsic to the student. For example, public questioning by the CI could cause the student to be fearful of being wrong and potentially damage their confidence and/or the trust of the patient in their care. Alternatively, if the student never wanted to be wrong (often linked to perfectionism or a passive approach to learning), such fear limited golden opportunities to learn through their mistakes.

Many of the CIs discussed how they negotiated the way that questioning would be used early in clinical experiences with students. In the quote that follows, one CI describes how she adapts her approach to questioning according to student responses. In the case described here, she and the student had already agreed that the student wanted to have the CI give feedback and ask questions as he worked with patients because he felt that was the way he learned best; that is, by getting immediate feedback.

I will ask questions of the student, but if they don't look like they are on the same page, I'll hold most of our discussion until we are in a private setting.... I'm not a drill sergeant-type of clinical instructor. If they are right on with their responses, then the questions will continue. And if they're drawing a blank, I'll bring them out of the treatment setting and we'll talk about it.... I won't continue to grill them if they're just not there. Maybe change the direction of the questioning, but definitely not continue to fluster them. You hate to have them come up with the wrong answers in front of the patient. That just isn't good for either party.[58(pp 7, 9)]

Teaching Philosophy and Teaching Style

When asked about their clinical teaching philosophy or principles that guide their approaches toward students, several interrelated themes emerged. The three most frequent and consistent responses across these CIs are shown in Table 10–1. For these CIs, their teaching philosophy translated into what they often referred to as their teaching style; their philosophy reflected their core beliefs and commitments and was a driver for their actions as a clinical educator. When they discussed their teaching style, they were often describing what might be viewed as enactment strategies based on their foundational philosophy. The

TABLE 10–1 Key Themes for Clinical Instructors: Philosophy of Teaching and Philosophy in Action.

Philosophy of Clinical Teaching	Characteristics of Philosophy	Philosophy in Action (Enactment Strategies)
Clinical teacher as guide, facilitator of learning and student advocate	• "Meet the student where they are" • "Help them reach their potential"	• Welcoming activities, establish "comfort zone" early on • "Find out where they are"- diagnosis of readiness* – dynamic assessment of learner • Provide opportunities to prepare for anticipated learning experiences – take potential for anxiety "down a notch"
Clinical teacher and students are partners in learning	• Students are "part of the team" • Student as colleague	• Mutual goal setting, activity planning, and pacing of the experience • "Let the student be in the driver's seat" some of the time
Teaching is not telling	• Not "spoon feeding" • Encourage discovery learning • Encourage critical self-reflection • "Plant the seeds" for lifelong learning	• Not telling – rather, asking the right questions and the right time and place • Negotiate the ground rules and "set the stage for questions" – why, when, how • Help the student "find the answer within"

"Diagnosis of readiness" was a term used by Scully and Shepard (1983) in an early ethnographic study of clinical teaching in physical therapy. They referred to diagnosis of readiness as a tool used by clinical teachers for pacing of the clinical experience in accordance with student learning needs.

linkages between the CIs teaching philosophy and that "philosophy in action" are also shown in Table 10–1.

Over and over again, the CIs described their role as a teacher as that of guide, facilitator, and advocate for the student. They all viewed a commitment to "meet the student where they are" and then "going from there" as a starting point for fulfilling this role: "I think the overall philosophy is to reach the student at the level they're at—find out what that is first. Meet them where they are and then get the most out of them so they can reach their potential. My favorite (moment) is when you see their potential is beyond what they see as their potential."[40(p 9)]

This CI went on to say that this vision of student potential is powerful motivation for his continued involvement in clinical education. Another CI describes this commitment to meeting the student where they are as

first getting a feel for what they're (the student) bringing to the table, to see where they are and what they are comfortable with ... and then picking up on what we need to augment.... It's trying to tailor each experience to that particular student's needs.[44(p 8)]

Another core philosophical commitment articulated by these CIs was to viewing clinical teaching and learning as a partnership. Students were viewed as "part of the team" and colleagues in this educative endeavor. Finally, all of the CIs expressed their belief that "teaching is not telling" or "spoon feeding." Rather, their aims were to create an environment and teacher-learner relationship that was conducive to discovery learning and fostered critical self-reflection through thoughtful questions and support of the student. As one CI put it, they wanted to "plant the seeds" for lifelong learning. In short, these instructors saw themselves as primarily walking side by side with the student in this journey—occasionally pulling them along to new insights and at other times giving a gentle nudge toward self-revelation of those insights.

It is important to note that the CIs in this sample were *able* to articulate a clinical teaching philosophy. Although many physical therapists may readily be able to articulate their philosophy of patient care or physical therapy clinical practice, I suspect far fewer are able to clearly articulate a philosophy of clinical teaching. But like the sample of expert clinicians studied by Jensen and colleagues,[26-28] the practice of these outstanding clinical instructors with students was infused with and shaped by their clinical teaching philosophy. In a recent observational study of clinical teachers in medicine, Graffam and colleagues[59] found that those teachers who had what they called "conceptualizations" of teaching (a teaching philosophy) were the most effective teachers. They were more learner centered, more intentional in their teaching toward desired purposes and aims, and most likely to empower their students as learners and future practitioners.

Ideal Student versus Challenging Student

When I asked CIs to provide descriptions of an "ideal student" and of the "most challenging student" there was virtually full consensus regarding the characteristics, attributes, and behaviors that emerged. Like the descriptions of facilitators and impediments to learning discussed earlier

TABLE 10–2 Clinical Instructor Descriptions of the Ideal Student and the Most Challenging Student

The Ideal Student	The Most Challenging Student
Is enthusiastic, energetic, willing to learn, willing to do, and open-minded	Lacks commitment to learning, is close minded, a "know-it-all"
Takes initiative, self-motivated, and self-directed	Does not put effort into learning; "you teach me;" "an 8-4 job"
Assumes responsibility, is accountable, follows through, takes advantage of learning opportunities	Passive learner, limited evidence of receptivity and follow-through; doesn't seek out or take advantage of learning opportunities available
Has passion and is committed to the patients and the profession; is bright and responsive	Seems disengaged with the learning process, "going through the motions"
Is socially capable, has people skills—respectful interaction, professional	Has poor interaction skills—insensitive or inappropriate exchanges with CI, patients, or others
Is self-aware, accurate self-assessment	Has limited self-awareness, poor self-assessment
Adequate academic preparation	Lacks requisite foundational knowledge or skills

in this chapter, these descriptions tended to represent two ends of a continuum in several domains, as illustrated in Table 10–2.

Ideal students, like these CIs, are enthusiastic, willing, and open-minded learners who take initiative, assume responsibility, learn from their mistakes, and are self-aware and motivated to advance their development. They are described as socially capable and respectful in their interactions with patients, caregivers, and other staff. Finally, they take a genuine interest in their patients, have passion for what they do, and are committed to the profession.

The most challenging and difficult students were those with poor interactional skills, especially as conveyed by insensitive or inappropriate remarks to or about others, and those who felt they knew it all, were close minded, or were perceived to be just going through the motions. Such attitudes often translated into a perceived lack of commitment to learning on the part of the student that was detrimental to the goal expressed by CIs for the establishment of a teacher-learner partnership. Lack of self-awareness, poor self-assessment, and unprofessional behaviors were often part of the constellation of concerns presented by challenging students in the view of these CIs. These descriptions resonate with findings from other studies of physical therapy clinical educators by Hayes and associates[60] and later Wolff-Burke[61] who called such behaviors "generic inabilities."

Ethical Distress in Clinical Education

Therapists often encounter moments of ethical distress, discomfort, or dilemmas in their everyday clinical work. I was interested in exploring the types of ethical distress that clinical instructors were encountering during their work with students. In response to a question about

moments of ethical distress, these CIs described situations that fell into four primary categories:

1. Reimbursement, resource allocation, and productivity issues
2. Struggles between patient autonomy and the therapist's duty of beneficence
3. Observations of disrespectful interactions, mistreatment, suspected negligence, or abuse
4. Inappropriate use of support staff

Detailed descriptions of some of the therapists' stories about these distress points and their responses to them can be found elsewhere,[62] but I will briefly provide a few examples of encounters that fell into each of these categories.

In the reimbursement, resource allocation, and productivity category, examples were concerns about denial of services believed needed for patients, or considerations around billing for student time and services when their efficiency or skills were not equal to the CI. Struggles between the patient's right to autonomy and the therapist's duties of beneficence and nonmaleficence often centered around discharge planning and decision making. In these cases, the therapist and students wanted to allow patients and families to make decisions for themselves, but sometimes the desires of the patient were not viewed as in the best overall interest of the patient in the eyes of the health care team, or there was concern that the patient's decision may even cause harm. In these instances, the balancing of the sometimes competing principles of autonomy and beneficence is challenging at best. What was important for the CIs who encountered these struggles with their students is that they became important teaching/learning moments—moments that encouraged reflection, dialogue, and exploration of the values and beliefs of both CI and student.

Unfortunately, some CIs and their students had encountered several situations involving observations of disrespectful interactions with patients, caregivers, or staff and, at the extreme, suspected or actual negligence or abuse. In the latter case, one situation was in a pediatric clinic where the welfare of a child became a concern and required action. In another case, the CI and student encountered a dying patient who had sustained an injury from a bed rail but had not been attended to by a nurse for a long period of time because "she's going to die anyway." The CI went on to describe his and the student's feelings and response to the situation this way:

When we were in there trying to untangle this patient, you could see that both of us felt so bad, we were ready to cry, we felt so bad for this person. They couldn't do anything for themselves really and then to hear the comment that we did. It was very hard…. It was not patient care, it was patient abuse. And so the student and I talked a lot about what is considered quality care with somebody and what do you do when you run into a situation like this and what are the levels (through which you need to proceed). Obviously, we have to go farther than just talking to her (the nurse) because somebody else needed to know this had occurred. So that was a learning experience for both (of us) because that was the first time I had ever really run into that.[45(p 14)]

In this heart-wrenching and unfortunate case, the student traveled the path of patient advocacy with the CI in territory where he had never been before, including joint discussions with the nurse, supervisors, and other appropriate personnel.

The last category of ethical distress identified revolved around observations of inappropriate use or overuse of support staff. Again, as before, when detected and questioned, the CI and student discussed the concerns and jointly engaged in actions to try to change the practice in accordance with appropriate standards of care. In fact, in all cases of ethical concern described, these CIs spent time with their students discussing feelings and necessary actions associated with the situation and most often had them travel the path of altruism, advocacy, integrity, and professional duty with them in response.

Take-Home Message for Learners

To conclude the interviews, the CIs were asked two culminating questions. The first of these was about what they hoped the "take-home message" or lesson learned would be for the students with whom they worked. The universal refrain was "Never quit learning, ever! Every day be open to new learning. Be aggressive in obtaining (new knowledge and skills) because in our profession there is so much to know and learn."[44(p 12)] Several of the CIs added that this engagement in the process of lifelong learning was not just for the purpose of the student or therapist's own development but for the higher aims of "bettering the care we provide for our patients" and advancing the profession of physical therapy. Several of them referred to this as "passing on" their learning, knowledge, and skills to students and professional alike:

- *Your profession is lifelong learning and you have a responsibility to continue your growth after your graduation and pass that on.*[40(p 14)]
- *When you feel you're ready, start taking students and teach them what you know.... If you are really good at what you do and you believe in what you do, you should want to share that. So just don't break the chain. Keep on learning and teach someone else.*[56(p 12)]

These take-home messages were intertwined with several others focused on being an advocate for the patient and treating every patient as a unique human being and a teacher, taking the most from each patient encounter, and loving your work.

- *Every patient is unique and every patient is a little case report with a lesson in discovery waiting to be had.*[57(p 18)]
- *...be the best that you can be, always give it as much as you have. Every day is not the same for you or your patient— everyday is new. Keep things in perspective and love what you are doing. Always, always learn because there are always opportunities to get better at what you do.*[63(p 6)]

Advice for Novice Clinical Instructors

When asked about their advice for novice CIs, there were several recurrent themes that emerged (Box 10–4).

BOX 10–4   Advice for New Clinical Instructors

- Remember what it's like to be a student; remember how it was when you were in your students' shoes, go back and reflect on those experiences.
- Don't try to know it all! You don't need to know everything. If you don't know something, admit that to the students and learn with them.
- See each student as a unique individual—"You can't make them mini-me's"; build on each student's strength and help the weak areas strengthen.
- Be self-aware and true to yourself; know your own strengths and weaknesses.
- You're not alone; use all of the resources around you to assist you in becoming a CI—training courses, reference materials, and other clinical and academic faculty

---

A few final quotes from CIs capture these points well:

- *The clinical instructor can learn as much from the student, I know I do, as I hope I am giving to them. I learn by sharing my knowledge base with them and they are also challenging me ... so I have to be extremely prepared too. I just can't wing it ... Everybody I've found here (at this clinic) is the same way. They are fired up and excited about having a student and they want it to be the best experience ever for them.*[58(p 13)]
- *You're going to know things that they (the students) don't know and vice versa.... Don't even worry about that. You're not a CI because you know everything. You are a CI because you want to be. I really do enjoy having the students here. It keeps me fresh, it keeps me alive, ever searching the literature, going to continuing education. It just keeps me going.*

In conclusion, all of these exceptional CIs are dedicated to their work as clinicians and clinical educators. They are invested in their students' learning and development and also have served as models and mentors for therapists preparing for or assuming new roles as CIs. They love what they do and see their work with students as personally fulfilling, as a learning and developmental experience for them, and as a way of "giving back" to the profession. Indeed these intrinsic rewards and benefits of clinical teaching were front and center for this sample of gifted CIs in their conversations with me; this finding is consistent with those of others who have investigated the perceptions of physical therapists regarding their role as clinical instructors.[64,65]

FINDINGS: THE VOICE OF STUDENTS

So what do students who have worked with exceptional CIs have to say about their learning during those clinical experiences? I turn now to findings from Phase 2 and share the words and stories of 11 students who worked with outstanding CIs (Figure 10–1; see also Appendix 10-C and Tables A2–1 and A2–2).

DESCRIPTION OF EXEMPLAR

In this sample of students, when asked for a description of an exemplar, all 11 participants felt that there was not one single event that met our definition of an exemplar. An exemplar was defined for these participants as "a personal and narrative account of an event or experience that you feel contributed in a significant way to your learning and development as a physical therapy student and future professional." Instead, the students felt it was an accumulation of numerous "little things" across the course of their experience that contributed most to their learning.

- *It wasn't one experience that changed everything. It was all the little things that you got right from the start.*[66(p 8)]
- *The thing that stands out to me, which is ironic about this question, is that with (my CI) it wasn't one big event. It was the everyday routine that really contributed to my learning.*[67(p 10)]

Examples of those "little things" were further described by the students when we asked additional questions about their CI's teaching style and the strategies they employed to foster the student's learning. These "little things" will be discussed in more detail in the next sections of this chapter. They included, but were not limited to, the positive and nonthreatening use of questioning, mutual brainstorming, and exchange of ideas for patient care; acceptance and support of students' ideas and "ways of doing" while also offering alternatives; adapting the amount and type of supervision provided according to the learner's needs; the CIs serving as a guide to resources for addressing questions that arose; the CIs modeling professional engagement and enthusiasm for their work with patients and students; and the CIs modeling patience and caring as they interacted with patients and their students.

TEACHING PHILOSOPHY AND TEACHING STYLE

Three primary themes emerged as students described the teaching philosophy and style of their CIs (Figure 10–2). All participants felt that their CI's teaching philosophy was one that involved the fostering of discovery learning by asking questions of the student as opposed to teaching through telling. As one student stated, "He would quiz me on ways that I might progress a patient without giving me the answers."[68(p2)] Another participant reported that "She pushed me to figure it out for myself . . . she always made me come up with the answer first . . . and then she would

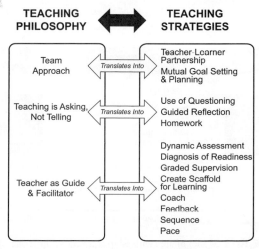

FIGURE 10–2 Student descriptions of the teaching philosophies and teaching strategies of the outstanding clinical instructors with whom they worked.

kind of direct me."[66(p1)] Part of the discovery learning process for these students and CIs involved holding the student accountable for seeking out answers to questions and following through on assignments or "homework." Likewise, CIs also sought out answers to questions they had and assisted students by identifying possible resources that could aid their investigations into clinical questions. In this way, both student and CI were involved in discovery learning, evidence-based practice, and exploration of clinical reasoning—and mutual sharing of new learning and findings: "It was always about discussion and investigating and we never could take anything at face value.... There always had to be a rationale, a reason (for what you are doing) and your thought process."[67(p4)]

It is important to note that none of the students reported feeling threatened by the use of questioning as a pedagogical tool by their CIs. As we all know, the form, function, timing, and linguistic and paralinguistic features of questions can dramatically change our emotional and cognitive responses to them. In medical education, in fact, the pervasive use of some forms of questioning has come to be known as "pimping" and is accepted as a pedagogical tool that is clearly hierarchical in its nature; at its worst, it is referred to as "malignant pimping" and can result in the humiliation of learners.[69] In contrast, these students felt empowered by their CI's questions; they were often viewed as a way of inviting student opinions, valuing their knowledge, and refining their clinical reasoning skills.

The second teaching philosophy identified by the students was one we labeled as a "team approach" to learning. In this approach the students felt like a partner in learning and were treated as respected colleagues. One student put it as follows: "I didn't feel like I was really, truly a student. She treated me as more of an equal . . . she was kind of like a co-worker."[70(p 5)] Another student reported, "She would ask for my opinion and get me involved in the conversation and that would make me feel really good too, because somebody was asking for my opinion. It made me feel like I knew something."[71(p1)]

This team approach included establishing mutual goals and objectives for the clinical experience both formally and informally. In some cases, the goal setting, revision, and refinement happened on a daily basis as indicated; in others, there were more structured weekly meetings to reflect on the learning and growth that occurred in the past week and anticipate the next week of the clinical experience.

Finally, the third philosophy identified by most of the students was one in which the CIs served as a guide for the students and tailored their teaching and the clinical experience to the needs and level of the students. To do this, CIs inquired about the learning styles, needs, and hopes of the students early on and also engaged in ongoing dynamic assessment of the students' learning needs and progress as the experience unfolded. One student explained how their CI did this at the start of and throughout the clinical internship: "(He worked at) . . . first establishing where I am at, then figuring out where I need to be, and then exploring how to get there."[72(p3)] Another student stated: "We kind of prioritized what I wanted to learn from my clinical right from the start."[66(p2)]

Such assessments served as a tool for "diagnosis of readiness,"[17] determination about the level of supervision and guidance needed for the student, and the scaffolding of the experience that permitted the student to move gradually toward more independence in increasingly complex clinical encounters:

(As the internship progressed) . . . if we had time we would go over anything I felt I needed to work on. So he kind of tailored his teaching to what kinds of needs I had. He would ask me what I'd like to work on.... It was pretty much tailored to what I needed.[73(p 2)]

It is important to note that the three teaching philosophies of CIs described by this sample of students—teaching as asking versus telling, a team approach to teaching-learning, and teacher as guide and facilitator—are in total agreement with the teaching philosophies that our sample of CIs articulated (see Table 10–1).

TEACHING STRATEGIES OR TECHNIQUES

Not surprisingly, the teaching philosophies of CIs translated into specific teaching strategies or techniques that the CIs used when working with their students. The descriptions of the most frequent teaching strategies employed by the students' CIs and their CIs' teaching philosophy is summarized in Figure 10–2. All students indicated that they felt like a partner in the learning experience, that is, a respected member of the "team," and engaged with their CI in mutual goal setting and planning of the experience. This process often involved a collaborative "replay" of the past week, reflection on prior learning and experience, and anticipation or forecasting of future learning needs with an eye toward the overall goals for the clinical experience.

All students reported the use of questioning by their CIs as a strategy that facilitated their learning by encouraging them to seek resources and answers to clinical questions independently ("doing homework"), reflecting on the meaning and relevance of past experiences to current situations or encounters, and inviting them to share their findings and insights to inform CI-student team clinical decision making.

One student described how her CI would set her on the search for answers to questions:

(The CI would say) 'We have resources in our library. Why don't you go up there and see what you can come up with?' So it was like she wasn't giving me the answers, but she would always point out things in a non-threatening way that I did appreciate.... When you learn things on your own, it does make it stick with you a little bit more.[70(p 6)]

Like the student quoted here, these students consistently reported being challenged by the questions their supervisors asked but not threatened. As one student put it, "She would ask me questions but it would be more like a conversation back and forth."[71(p 1)]

Finally, the students felt their learning and development as a therapist was assisted by the CI's ability to assess their need for guidance and supervision from moment to moment, day to day, and week to week and adjust the amount, type, and level of supervision and guidance provided to the needs of the student. They identified this grading of supervision and as a teaching strategy that enhanced their "learning through doing." Most described this

grading as "coaching" that began with an assessment of where the student was, followed in sequence by CI modeling and demonstration, student observation, informal and formal instruction, practice sessions, and finally "doing" with patients paired with formative feedback. In addition, the students' level of independence in their work with patients was characterized by a gradual movement from direct supervision of the CI, to indirect supervision, to relative independence.

- *(My CI) was understanding as to where each person is in their development. She asked what I wanted and needed at the beginning and then she was able to grade accordingly.*[74(p 6)]
- *At the beginning, (my CI) was always there. Like at first I just watched her . . . the first couple of days, kind of got the feel for things. And then I'd treat patients and she'd be in the room, especially for evals.... She would just kind of sit and let me do the eval and if there was anything to discuss, we would do it either during or afterwards. Gradually, she'd be around less and less and in the end sometimes she wasn't even there.*[2(p 5)]

This student went on to point out, however, that even when she was given independence, her CI was always accessible and available as a support and resource when needed.

All of these teaching techniques and strategies combined to create a "scaffold" for learning for these students during clinical internships. A model of the many activities that comprised this scaffold is shown in Figure 10–3 and will be discussed further in relation to several theoretical constructs at the conclusion of the chapter.

CHARACTERISTICS, ATTRIBUTES, AND BEHAVIORS OF CLINICAL INSTRUCTORS

When we asked the students in our sample to describe some of the personal and professional characteristics, attributes, and behaviors and of their CIs, the findings were categorized as descriptions of the CIs' "ways of being" and their "ways of doing," as shown in Table 10–3. As is evident

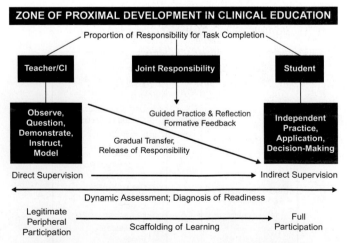

FIGURE 10–3 Model of apprenticeship learning in the Zone of Proximal Development in clinical education. The model incorporates several key concepts from social constructivist theories of learning and development.

TABLE 10–3 Student Descriptions of the Characteristics, Attributes, and Behaviors of Outstanding Clinical Instructors Illustrating the Relationship between "Ways of Being" and "Ways of Doing"

Personal and Professional Characteristics and Attributes: "Ways of Being"	Personal and Professional Behaviors: "Ways of Doing"
Respectful and nonjudgmental of students, patients, colleagues, and others	Treated student as a colleague; each learner and patient as unique "She never once made it seem that I wasn't important."
Accessible and approachable; personable	Available when needed; invited questions and asked about learner's needs and goals
Open and receptive to student ideas and the ideas of others	Asked for and valued students' opinions and ideas and those of others
Positive professional role model; an advocate for the patients and the profession	Engaged in professional organizations and activities; served as an advocate for patients
Knowledgeable and committed to continued advancement of knowledge and skills; respected by colleagues	Sought evidence to support the practice; participated in continuing education and shared learning with others
Caring and compassionate; patient	Attentive and responsive listener; was patient and caring in interactions with students, their patients, and caregivers

barriers to communication with patients, (2) multilayered psychosocial issues that arose in the context of patient care, and (3) situations that had legal or ethical implications. The communication category included students' work with patients with language, hearing, or speech impairments, those with cognitive impairments, or those who did not speak English. In the psychosocial category, the most frequent challenges centered around work with patients with unusual and sometimes unexplained symptoms that did not appear to be all of somatic origin, those with extremely complicated social circumstances or concurrent psychiatric diagnoses, and those with behavioral issues such as aggression. Some of the legal and ethical issues revolved around the suspicion of potential neglect or abuse at the extreme or questions about appropriate use of support personnel or students in the provision of and reimbursement for clinical services.

In response to these challenges, virtually all of the students reported initially feeling "overwhelmed" and not adequately equipped to manage the situation. But in all cases, they said that their CIs were an invaluable resource in trying to understand the situation, explore their feelings around it, and determining an appropriate course of action. Furthermore, all students reported that there were memorable lessons learned as a result of these challenging situations and that they carried those lessons forward into their future practice as therapists.

in the table, there is a clear relationship between these ways of being and doing, and they were intertwined in student descriptions of their CIs. The following quotes from three students capture many of the characteristics, attributes, and behaviors of CIs listed in Table 10–3.

- *She was respectful to everybody ... respecting the things we wanted to get out of the internship, respecting our thoughts and feedback and everything. She was very knowledgeable as a therapist, which was important.... She was an excellent role model in a lot of ways.... Just having high standards for herself and her students and supporting the profession too.*[67(p 6)]
- *He was real receptive to my ideas and receptive to any other knowledge I could give him. He was really interested in what else I could bring in. He was interested in learning from me ... we tried to see each other more as co-workers. But of course I was a student and I still asked questions. He really respected my opinions and treated me more like a therapist than a student.*[73(p 4)]
- *She was just awesome when it came to communicating with patients. She answered all their questions, took her time. It never felt like she was in a rush to leave to get to the next person.*[70(p 10)]

MOST CHALLENGING EXPERIENCES

When asked about their most challenging moments when working with their CIs, the students in this sample described three primary categories of experiences that were difficult during their internships. These were (1) various

TAKE-HOME MESSAGE AND LESSONS LEARNED

In the same way we asked CIs about their intended "take-home messages" for students, we asked students what they viewed as the primary take-home message or lesson learned from their work with an exceptional CI. Interestingly, these were all closely aligned with the messages our sample of CIs reported.

The loudest and clearest message for all students was to be inquisitive, to "never stop learning," and to continuously seek to advance their knowledge and skills.

- *Keep asking yourself questions.... Always ask why, why, why, and have a rationale for what you're doing.*[67(p 14)]
- *Always further your knowledge ... try to know more and do more.*[74(p 11)]

The second primary lesson learned for these students focused on the importance of adopting a patient-centered approach to care that was caring, compassionate, and holistic.

- *Be honest about the patient's progress, but hopeful.... Always be respectful to the patients and their families and caregivers ... be supportive and an advocate.*[2(p 6)]
- *She taught me to view the patient as a whole and not just the diagnosis they came in for.*[66(p 6)]

The final key take-home message was to be professionally involved and to take pride in their work and profession.

- *Professionalism, professionalism ... become involved in other aspects of physical therapy (beyond direct patient care).*[75(p 5)]
- *Be proud of what you do and have pride in your good work.*[76(p 9)]

FINDINGS: PAIRED CLINICAL INSTRUCTOR AND STUDENT DATA

As mentioned earlier, our two samples of CI and student data yielded a subsample of seven sets of data in which outstanding CIs could be paired with the students with whom they worked. Further examination of these pairs of data did not reveal any new findings that were not described earlier in this chapter, except that there were very clear matches between what the therapists had hoped to impart and achieve as a clinical teacher and what their students learned and took from their experiences.

In my view, this additional finding speaks to the powerful positive influence exceptional CIs can have on shaping their students, future professionals, and thus, the future of the profession in many ways. All of the students who worked with these excellent teachers indicated that they have sought to emulate and embody some of the characteristics, attributes, commitments, and behaviors of their CIs both in their work as physical therapists and as current or future CIs.

CONCLUDING THOUGHTS: MAKING SENSE AND CREATING MEANING

What I have attempted to do in this chapter is provide the reader with a personal and contextualized view of good clinical teaching in physical therapy by sharing the stories and voices of exceptional clinical instructors and the students who had the opportunity to work with them. As indicated in the chapter objectives, my hope is that clinical instructors will use these stories as a catalyst for reflection and will now be inspired to engage in thoughtful reflection on their own experiences as a CI—to identify and share an exemplar with another colleague, to clarify their beliefs about clinical teaching and learning, to articulate their philosophy of clinical teaching, and finally, to craft a personal vision of who and what they want to be as a CI and set a course to accomplish that vision.

There is much to be learned from the clinical instructors and students whose voices you have heard here, and it is, indeed, good news! These CIs truly enjoy their work with students, and their engagement in clinical education is a powerful stimulus for their own ongoing learning and development. They espouse, live, and model many of the core values described in the APTA's professionalism document[77] and are true examples of what it means to be a reflective practitioner.[78,79] They share the qualities of expert clinicians described in the landmark work of Jensen and colleagues.[26–28] These CIs are both patient centered and learner centered and are committed to delivering high-quality patient care and learning experiences for students at the same time. Their teaching is intentional, guided by their teaching philosophies, but it is also individualized and improvisational according the unique level and needs of the student as they enter and move through clinical experiences. Furthermore, these CIs are engaged in regular reflection on and inquiry into their own teaching and effectiveness as clinician and clinical educator; they are constantly "remaking" themselves as clinical teachers through their enlarging repertoire of experiences working with students. The other good news is that their students want to emulate the characteristics, attributes, and behaviors of these CIs in their own clinical practice and teaching. So the admonitions from CIs to "pass it on" and "don't break the chain" have been heard and carry with them great promise for future students and developing professionals.

Many of the findings reported here connect with existing and expanding literature on the characteristics, attributes, and behaviors of good clinical teachers in physical therapy[4,5,8,18,20–22,80] and medicine.[49–51,61,81–84] My goal, however, was not to move from description to a universal prescription for good teaching in physical therapy clinical education. Although models of clinical instruction can be very useful, they also can easily become devoid of context and oversimplify very complicated phenomena. Clinical education is extremely complex and is situationally and relationally negotiated moment to moment in the constantly shifting environment of health care today.

What I do leave the reader with as further "food for thought" is a model of apprenticeship learning in clinical education that tries to capture the multiple layers, dimensions, and complexity of good clinical teaching (see Figure 10–3). This model draws heavily on social constructivist theories and views of learning that emphasize the situated and social nature of learning and the importance of authentic activity and experience for facilitating human learning and development. Such views have a long history dating back to the early 20th century when some of the theoretical underpinnings of social constructivism were formulated by educational philosopher John Dewey[85,86] and Russian psychologist Lev Vygotsky.[87–89] More recently, the term *cognitive apprenticeship* has been proposed and widely adopted as a description of the learning and cognitive development that takes place when novices and experts interact in authentic practice environments around genuine tasks.[90–93] The importance of the embedded, situated, and social nature of such learning in communities of practice has been further emphasized and elaborated on by Jean Lave and Etienne Wenger.[53,54,94] All of these authors draw on a key assertion put forth by Vygotsky[87] that cognitive development is inevitably social and that mind, or higher intellectual or mental processes, is socially co-constructed. Vygotsky developed the concept of the zone of proximal development (ZPD) to describe the socially mediated interpersonal space where learning and development occur as a result of interaction between learner and more capable others. Vygotsky defined this boundary zone as:

> *The distance between the actual developmental level as determined by independent problem solving and the level of potential development as determined through problem solving under adult guidance or in collaboration with more capable peers.*[87(p 86)]

In the model I share in Figure 10–3, I suggest that the gifted clinical teachers described in this chapter are in fact constantly assessing and operating in the learner's ZPD. The ability to accurately gauge what a student knows and is capable of doing at the start of a clinical experience and to anticipate what the student may be capable of doing while proceeding through the experience is essential to movement through the ZPD and the accomplishment of new ways of knowing, thinking, feeling, and doing for the student. This ability is based on ongoing dynamic assessment of the learner across the experience that permits diagnosis of learner readiness for various clinical situations and encounters.

Dynamic assessment also permits the CI to make informed determinations about the amount and level of supervision necessary for students and to scaffold experiences in a way that supports and advances their learning and development. Scaffolding is a metaphor used in education meant to evoke the vision of a scaffold built alongside a building while it is in construction and later removed piece-by-piece when it is no longer needed.[91] It is important to note that scaffolding is not a singular concept; it involves many of the behaviors and strategies suggested in the figure: questioning, instruction, demonstration, modeling, guided practice, guided reflection, reciprocal teaching and learning, the provision of formative feedback, and gradual transfer of responsibility for task completion from the teacher to the learner. Finally, as the instructor assists the learner through the ZPD and then "fades" as director of learning, the student is able to move from what at first was legitimate peripheral participation in the physical therapy community of practice to full participation in that community.[53]

Among the numerous activities that make up scaffolding, feedback is especially important in clinical teaching and learning. For a detailed review of numerous forms, functions, and aspects of formative feedback, I refer readers to an excellent article by Shute[95] (see Annotated Bibliography). Shute also offers another metaphor for scaffolding that may be helpful to readers and applicable to the clinical teaching and learning I have described in this chapter. Shute evokes the vision of teaching a child to ride a bicycle. We start the process with a child on a bicycle with training wheels and over time we remove the training wheels, then run along side the child, arms stretched toward them ready to react and catch them when at risk, finally standing back and observing as they cycle away independently and gradually round a corner to disappear from view.

I offer one more observation on the notion of the ZPD as an organizing framework for understanding the many activities that contribute to optimal teaching, learning, and development in clinical environments. As originally described and envisioned by Vygotsky,[87] the ZPD and cognitive development is not just about intellectual growth—it is inherently relational and intersubjective, grounded in interpersonal interactions between teacher and learner and others in the sociocultural milieu that surrounds them. As such, Goldstein,[96] drawing on the early work of Noddings,[97] reminds us that the ZPD is a "relational zone" and that caring relationships are critically important in the co-construction of mind. I draw attention to this point because the students described in this chapter repeatedly shared the fact that they felt respected and cared for by their CIs. Thus, the importance of creating a teaching-learning relationship in which students feel nurtured, supported, and safe in this "construction zone" cannot be overstated.

Acknowledgments

I would like to recognize and thank several of my graduate students who assisted with data collection and analysis during phase 2 of this study that spanned several years: Tammy Baldwin, DPT, Brandi Barriger, DPT, Tina Cook, DPT, Heather Couillard, DPT, Shannon Erdody, DPT, Onya Glenn, DPT, Jordan Hogan, DPT, and Erica Monroe Hemerline, DPT. Their insights into the experiences of students during clinical experiences and their contributions to the investigation were invaluable.

THRESHOLD CONCEPTS

Threshold Concept #1: A philosophy of clinical teaching serves as both a foundation and framework for excellent clinical instructors in physical therapy.

This philosophy is grounded in beliefs about student learning and clinical teaching that often emerge out of one's own experiences as a student and clinical teacher. The philosophy of many good clinical teachers is both patient centered and learner centered.

Learning activity: Reflect on your past experiences as a student completing clinical internships and also your experience as a CI if applicable. Can you identify some critical moments in those experiences (exemplars) that were turning points for you in your own learning and development as either a student or an instructor? What were they? Describe them in a narrative form and share them orally or in writing with another colleague to further explore the meaning of those experiences. Then begin to think across all your experiences and what you know about clinical education to develop a vision of yourself as an excellent clinical teacher. Now, craft a paragraph that describes your personal philosophy of clinical teaching.

Threshold Concept #2: Ongoing dynamic assessment of student learning, understandings, clinical reasoning, performance, and behaviors is essential to the process of scaffolding learning and grading/fading of supervision during clinical learning experiences.

Learning activity: If you are a CI, identify and describe three strategies you could use or have used to assess student learning (or to "diagnose their readiness" for a clinical encounter) during clinical education experiences. How would you translate the assessment information gained into a new learning experience or teaching approach for a student? If you are a student, identify and describe three ways that you could use or have used to make your level of learning, understanding, knowledge, or skills visible to your CI.

Threshold Concept #3: Good clinical teachers are investigators of their own teaching and their student's learning. They learn from failures as well as teaching-learning successes.

Learning activity: Think back over some memorable clinical education experiences you have had. Identify one time when you experienced "failure" or when things didn't go as anticipated (went wrong) and another time when you experienced "success" (things went very well!). Describe what, exactly, went wrong and what went well in each situation. Why do you think things went as they did? What "lesson learned" do you take from the experiences? Is there anything you will do differently if you encounter a similar situation in the future?

ANNOTATED BIBLIOGRAPHY

Clark CM. *Thoughtful Teaching*. New York: Teachers College Press; 1995.
One volume in an international series of books on teacher development. Clark artfully brings together findings from research on teaching with stories of teaching and learning that exemplify "thoughtful teaching." Divided into four parts—Reflections on Thoughtful Teaching, Research on Thoughtful Teaching, Portraits of Thoughtful Teaching, and Cultivating Thoughtful Teaching—this volume is a must read and inspiration for those who wish to truly be "thoughtful teachers."

Ende J, ed. *Theory and Practice of Teaching Medicine*. Philadelphia: American College of Physicians Press; 2010
The first in a series of six volumes in a "Teaching Medicine" series published by the American College of Physicians. Ende and his contributors bring together theory, research, experience, stories, and practical suggestions into an accessible volume that has numerous lessons for those that want to improve their clinical teaching and advance student learning and development.

Dennen VP. Cognitive apprenticeship in educational practice: research on scaffolding, modeling, mentoring, and coaching as instructional strategies. In: Jonassen DH, ed. *Handbook of Research on Educational Communications and Technology*. 2nd ed. Mahwah, NJ: Lawrence Erlbaum Associates; 1999:813–828.
An excellent review of the literature on cognitive apprenticeship (CA) with descriptions of many of the concepts and strategies that comprise the larger concept of CA, including, but not limited to, scaffolding, the zone of proximal development, intersubjectivity, fading, modeling, pacing, mentoring, and coaching.

Shute VJ. Focus on formative feedback. *Rev Educ Res*. 2008;78:153–189.
A comprehensive review of the literature on formative feedback defined as "information communicated to the learner that is intended to modify his or her thinking or behavior to improve learning." The review discusses multiple forms of feedback and variables that interact with feedback that can influence whether or not feedback is, in fact, successful at promoting learning. The review concludes with several useful summary tables that provide guidance on "things to do" and "things to avoid" when providing feedback. The review should be a thought-provoking and useful tool for clinical teachers.

Sutkin G, Wagner E, Harris I, Schiffer R. What makes a good teacher in medicine? A review of the literature. *Acad Med*. 2008;83:452–466.
These authors conducted a systematic review of the literature published between 1909 and 2006 addressing the question of "What makes a good clinical teacher in medicine?" The review points to the multifactorial nature of excellent clinical teaching and highlights the importance of noncognitive attributes in addition to teaching knowledge and skills. The article concludes with a multipage appendix that summarizes all studies evaluated and provides descriptions of the many characteristics of good clinical teachers in medicine.

Weise J, ed. *Teaching in the Hospital*. Philadelphia: American College of Physicians Press; 2010.
The fourth of six volumes in the "Teaching Medicine Series" published by the American College of Physicians. The focus in this volume is on the unique demands and requirements for teaching and facilitating learning in inpatient hospital settings. The chapters on teaching clinical reasoning, nonclinical skills, and the use of "teaching scripts" in inpatient environments may be very helpful for therapists working with students in those settings.

Wenger E. *Communities of Practice: Learning, Meaning, and Identity*. New York: Cambridge University Press; 1998.
This book provides a thorough description of a social constructivist theory of learning that starts with the assumption that "engagement in social practice is the fundamental process by which we learn and so become who we are." The concept and meaning of communities of practice is clearly articulated and how individuals learn, negotiate shared understandings, and develop identities within those communities is explored.

REFERENCES

1. CI-1 (Clinical Instructor 1 – see Table A2–1).
2. S-1 (Student 1 – see Table A2–2).
3. Commission on Accreditation in Physical Therapy Education. *Physical Therapist Education Programs 2010-2011 Fact. Sheet*. Alexandria, VA: American Physical Therapy Association; August 16, 2011.
4. Emery MJ. Effectiveness of the clinical instructor: students' perspective. *Phys Ther*. 1984;64:1079–1083.
5. Emery MJ, Wilkinson CP. Perceived importance and frequency of clinical teaching behaviors: surveys of students, clinical instructors, and center coordinators of clinical education. *J Phys Ther Educ*. 1987;1:29–32.
6. Jarski RW, Kulig K, Olson RE. Allied health perceptions of effective clinical instruction. *J Allied Health*. 1989;18:469–478.
7. Jarski RW, Kulig K, Olson RE. Clinical teaching in physical therapy: student and teacher perceptions. *Phys Ther*. 1990;70:173–178.
8. Buccieri KM, Schultze K, Dungey J, et al. Self-reported characteristics of physical therapy clinical instructors: a comparison to the American Physical Therapy Association's Guidelines and Self-Assessments for Clinical Education. *J Phys Ther Educ*. 2006;20:47–55.
9. Morren KK, Gordon SP, Sawyer BA. The relationship between clinical instructor characteristics and student perceptions of clinical instructor effectiveness. *J Phys Ther Educ*. 2008;22:52–63.
10. Weatherbee E, Nordrum JT, Giles S. Effective teaching behaviors of APTA credentialed versus noncredentialed clinical instructors. *J Phys Ther Educ*. 2008;22:65–74.
11. Housel N, Gandy J. Clinical instructor credentialing and its effect on student clinical performance outcomes. *J Phys Ther Educ*. 2008;22:43–51.
12. Giles S, Weatherbee E, Johnson S. Qualifications and credentials of clinical instructors supervising physical therapist students. *J Phys Ther Educ*. 2003;17:50–55.
13. Page CG, Ross IA. Instructional strategies utilized by physical therapist clinical instructors: an exploratory study. *J Phys Ther Educ*. 2004;18:43–49.
14. American Physical Therapy Association. *Guidelines and Self-Assessments for Clinical Education*. Alexandria, VA: American Physical Therapy Association; 2004.
15. American Physical Therapy Association Department of Education. *APTA Physical Therapist Clinical Education Principles*. Alexandria, VA: American Physical Therapy Association; March 25,2010. Available at: http://www.apta.org/PTClinicalEducationPrinciples/; Accessed 26.09.2011.
16. American Physical Therapy Association. *Clinical Instructor Education and Credentialing Program and Manual*. Alexandria, VA: American Physical Therapy Association; 2009.
17. Scully RM, Shepard KF. Clinical teaching in physical therapy education: an ethnographic study. *Phys Ther*. 1983;63:349–358.
18. Buccieri KM, Pivko SE, Olzenak DL. How does a physical therapist acquire the skills of an expert clinical instructor? *J Phys Ther Educ*. 2011;25:17–25.
19. Kelly SP. The exemplary clinical instructor: a qualitative case study. *J Phys Ther Educ*. 2007;21:63–69.
20. Plack MM. The development of communication skills, interpersonal skills, and a professional identity within a community of practice. *J Phys Ther Educ*. 2006;20:37–46.
21. Plack MM. The learning triad: potential barriers and supports to learning in the physical therapy clinical environment. *J Phys Ther Educ*. 2008;22:7–18.
22. Healey WE. Physical therapist student approaches to learning during clinical education experiences: a qualitative study. *J Phys Ther Educ*. 2008;22:49–57.
23. Laitinen-Vaananen S, Talvitie U, Luukka MR. Clinical supervision as an interaction between the clinical educator and the student. *Physiother Theory Pract*. 2007;23:95–103.
24. Laitinen-Vaananen S, Luukka MR, Talvitie U. Physiotherapy under discussion: a discourse analytic study of physiotherapy students' clinical education. *Adv Physiother*. 2008;10:2–8.
25. Weatherbee E, Peatman N, Kennedy D, et al. Standards for clinical education: a qualitative study. *J Phys Ther Educ*. 2010;24:35–43.
26. Jensen GM, Gwyer J, Hack LM, et al. *Expertise in Physical Therapy Practice*. Newton, MA: Butterworth-Heinemann; 1999.
27. Jensen GM, Gwyer J, Shepard KF, et al. Expert practice in physical therapy. *Phys Ther*. 2000;80:28–43.
28. Jensen GM, Gwyer J, Hack LM, et al. *Expertise in Physical Therapy Practice*. 2nd ed. St. Louis: Butterworth-Heinemann; 2007.
29. Mostrom E. Wisdom of practice in a transdisciplinary rehabilitation clinic: situated expertise and client centering. In: Jensen GM, Gwyer J, Hack LM, et al. *Expertise in Physical Therapy Practice*. Newton, MA: Butterworth-Heinemann; 1999:207–230.
30. Mostrom E. Situated expertise: the wisdom of practice in a transdisciplinary rehabilitation clinic. In: GM Jensen, Gwyer J, Hack LM,

et al. *Expertise in Physical Therapy Practice.* 2nd ed St. Louis: Butter-worth-Heinemann; 2007:214 239.

31. Benner P. *From Novice to Expert: Excellence and Power in Clinical Nursing Practice.* Menlo Park, CA: Addison-Wesley; 1982.

32. Martin C, Siosteen A, Shepard KF. The professional development of expert physical therapists in four areas of clinical practice. *Nordic Physiother.* 1995;1:4–11.

33. Benner P, Tanner CA, Chesla CA. *Expertise in Nursing Practice: Caring, Clinical Judgment, and Ethics.* New York: Springer; 1996.

34. Maykut P, Morehouse R. *Beginning Qualitative Research: A Philosophic and Practical Guide.* Bristol, PA: Falmer Press; 1994.

35. Thomas DR. *A general inductive approach for qualitative data analysis.* School of Population Health, University of Auckland; [serial on internet]; August, 2003. Available at: http://www.fmhs.auckland.ac.nz/soph/centres/hrmas/_docs/Inductive2003.pdf; Accessed 15.10.03.

36. Thomas DR. A general inductive approach for analyzing qualitative evaluation data. *Am J Eval.* 2006;27:237–246.

37. Miles MB, Huberman AM. *Qualitative Data Analysis: An Expanded Sourcebook.* Thousand Oaks, CA: Sage; 1994.

38. Lincoln YS, Guba EG. *Naturalistic Inquiry.* Beverly Hills, CA: Sage Publications; 1985.

39. CI-2 (Clinical Instructor 2 – see Table A2–1).

40. CI-14 (Clinical Instructor 14 – see Table A2–1).

41. CI-3 (Clinical Instructor 3 – see Table A2–1).

42. Shulman LS. Knowledge and teaching: foundations of the new reform. *Harvard Educ Rev.* 1987;57:1–22.

43. CI-15 (Clinical Instructor 15 – see Table A2–1).

44. CI-11 (Clinical Instructor 11 – see Table A2–1).

45. CI-5 (Clinical Instructor 5 – see Table A2–1).

46. CI-7 (Clinical Instructor 7 – see Table A2–1).

47. Irby DM, Ramsey PG, Gillmore GM, et al. Characteristics of effective clinical teachers of ambulatory care medicine. *Acad Med.* 1991;66:54–55.

48. Irby DM. What clinical teachers in medicine need to know. *Acad Med.* 1994;69:333–342.

49. Pinsky LE, Irby DM. "If at first you don't succeed": using failure to improve teaching. *Acad Med.* 1997;72:973–976.

50. Clark CM, Peterson PL. Teachers thought processes. In: Wittrock M, ed. *Handbook of Research on Teaching.* 3rd ed. New York: Macmillan; 1986:255–296.

51. Clark CM. *Thoughtful Teaching.* New York: Teachers College Press; 1995.

52. CI-17 (Clinical Instructor 17 – see Table A2–1).

53. Lave J, Wenger E. *Situated Learning: Legitimate Peripheral Participation.* Cambridge, UK: Cambridge University Press; 1991.

54. Wenger E. *Communities of Practice: Learning, Meaning, and Identity.* Cambridge, UK: Cambridge University Press; 1998.

55. CI-12 (Clinical Instructor 12 – see Table A2–1).

56. CI-8 (Clinical Instructor 8 – see Table A2–1).

57. CI-10 (Clinical Instructor 10 – see Table A2–1).

58. CI-4 (Clinical Instructor 4 – see Table A2–1).

59. Graffam B, Bowers L, Keene KN. Using observations of clinicians' teaching practices to build a model of clinical instruction. *Acad Med.* 2008;83:768–774.

60. Hayes KW, Huber G, Rogers J, et al. Behaviors that cause clinical instructors to question the clinical competence of physical therapy students. *Phys Ther.* 1999;79:653–671.

61. Wolff-Burke M. Clinical instructors' descriptions of physical therapist student professional behaviors. *J Phys Ther Educ.* 2005;19: 67–76.

62. Mostrom E. Teaching and learning about the ethical and human dimensions of care in clinical education: exploring student and clinical instructor experiences in physical therapy. In: Purtilo R, Jensen GM, Royeen CB, eds. *Educating for Moral Action: A Sourcebook in Health and Rehabilitation Ethics.* Philadelphia: FA Davis; 2005: 265–283.

63. CI-13 (Clinical Instructor 13 – see Table A2–1).

64. Gwyer J. Rewards of teaching physical therapy students: clinical instructor's perspective. *J Phys Ther Educ.* 1993;7:63–66.

65. Davies R, Hanna E, Cott C. "They put you on your toes": physical therapists' perceived benefits from and barriers to supervising students in the clinical setting. *Physiother Can.* 2011: preprint. doi:10.3138/ptc.2010-07.

66. S-6 (Student 6 – see Table A2–2).

67. S-11 (Student 11 – see Table A2–2).

68. S-2 (Student 2 – see Table A2–2).

69. Wear D, Kokinova M, Keck-McNulty C, et al. Pimping: perspectives of 4th year medical students. *Teach Learn Med.* 2005;17:184–191.

70. S-10 (Student 10 – see Table A2–2).

71. S-8 (Student 8 – see Table A2–2).

72. S-9 (Student 9 – see Table A2–2).

73. S-5 (Student 5 – see Table A2–2).

74. S-4 (Student 4 – see Table A2–2).

75. S-7 (Student 7 – see Table A2–2).

76. S-3 (Student 3 – see Table A2–2).

77. American Physical Therapy Association. *Professionalism in Physical Therapy: Core Values.* Alexandria, VA: American Physical Therapy Association. Available at: http://www.apta.org/Professionalism/; Accessed 4.10.2011.

78. Schon DA. *The Reflective Practitioner: How Professionals Think in Action.* New York: Basic Books; 1983.

79. Schon DA. *Educating the Reflective Practitioner.* San Francisco: Jossey-Bass; 1987.

80. Morren KK, Gordon SP, Sawyer BA. The relationship between clinical instructor characteristics and student perceptions of clinical instructor effectiveness. *J Phys Ther Educ.* 2008;22:52–63.

81. Crandall S. How expert clinical educators teach what they know. *J Cont Educ Health Prof.* 1993;13:85–98.

82. Sutkin G, Wagner E, Harris I, et al. What makes a good clinical teacher in medicine? A review of the literature. *Acad Med.* 2008;83:452–466.

83. Ende J, ed. *Theory and Practice of Teaching Medicine.* Philadelphia: American College of Physicians Press; 2010.

84. Skeff KM, Stratos GA. *Methods for Teaching Medicine.* Philadelphia: American College of Physicians Press; 2010.

85. Dewey J. *How We Think: A Restatement of the Relation of Reflective Thinking to the Educative Process.* Lexington, MA: DC Health; 1933.

86. Dewey J. *Experience and Education.* New York: Macmillan; 1938.

87. Vygotsky LS. *Mind in Society: The Development of Higher Psychological Functions.* Cambridge, MA: Harvard University Press; 1978.

88. Vygotsky LS. The genesis of higher mental functions. In: Wertsch JV, ed. *The Concept of Activity in Soviet Psychology.* New York: Sharpe; 1981:144–188.

89. Vygotsky LS. Thinking and speech. In: Reiber RW, Carton AS, eds; Minick N (transl). *The Collected Works of L. S. Vygotsky.* New York: Plenum; 1987.

90. Brown JS, Collins A, Duguid P. Situated cognition and the culture of learning. *Ed Res.* 1989;18:32–42.

91. Collins A, Brown JS, Newman SE. Cognitive apprenticeship: Teaching the craft of reading, writing, and mathematics. In: Resnick LB, ed. *Knowing, Learning, and Instruction: Essays in Honor of Robert Glaser.* Hillsdale, NJ: Lawrence Erlbaum; 1989:453–494.

92. Rogoff B. *Apprenticeship in Thinking: Cognitive Development in Social Context.* New York: Oxford University Press; 1990.

93. Dennen VP. Cognitive apprenticeship in educational practice: research on scaffolding, modeling, mentoring, and coaching as instructional strategies. In: Jonassen DH, ed. *Handbook of Research on Educational Communications and Technology.* 2nd ed. Mahwah, NJ: Lawrence Erlbaum Associates; 1999:813–828.

94. Lave J. *Cognition in Practice: Mind, Mathematics and Culture in Everyday Life.* Cambridge, UK: Cambridge University Press; 1988.

95. Shute VJ. Focus on formative feedback. *Rev Educ Res.* 2008;78: 153–189.

96. Goldstein LS. The relational zone: the role of caring relationships in the co-construction of mind. *Am Educ Res J.* 1999;36:647–673.

97. Noddings N. *Caring.* Berkeley, CA: University of California Press; 1984.

APPENDIX 10-A STUDY DESIGN AND METHODS

The overall study design and chronology are shown in Figure 10–1. The study was a multiphase and multiyear investigation employing ethnographic methods in a multiple-case design that allowed for across-case and within-case analysis. The study spanned more than 5 years of data collection and analysis from outstanding clinical instructors (CIs) and former students of exceptional CIs. Instruments and methods included demographic questionnaires, a resume sort activity[26,31,32] completed by CIs before and during an interview, reviews of clinical teaching/learning artifacts, and semistructured interviews that included a detailed description of an exemplar.[31,33] The interview guide for CIs is provided in Appendix 10-B. The interview guide for students is provided in Appendix 10-C. All interviews of CIs were conducted by this author (EM). Student interviews were conducted by some of my graduate physical therapist (PT) students (see Acknowledgments at the end of this chapter), and data were analyzed in collaboration with EM.

Each interview lasted about 45 to 75 minutes. Interviews were audiotaped and transcribed verbatim. Transcripts of interviews were returned to participants for review to confirm the accuracy of the transcript and to provide the participants the opportunity to add or correct information if desired. This review served as one strategy—a member check—to enhance dependability and credibility of the data. Interview transcripts were analyzed using a constant-comparative method[34] and a general inductive approach as described by Thomas.[35,36] Several strategies were employed to establish the trustworthiness of the data and analysis following recommendations by Miles and Huberman[37] and Lincoln and Guba.[38] To triangulate data, several sources and methods for data collection were used as described previously. For the student data, multiple investigators allowed for independent open coding of data initially with subsequent group analysis and coding to achieve consensus on codes, categories, and themes. Finally, an audit trail was created consisting of questionnaires, resume sort cards (for CIs), interview transcripts, investigator field notes, coding drafts, and final reports.

The first phase of the study focused on collection and analysis of data from CIs (see Figure 10–1). The initial sampling frame for the study was a group of individuals who were recipients of an Outstanding Clinical Instructor Award given on an annual basis by the Special Interest Group for Clinical Education (SIGCE) of the Michigan Physical Therapy Association (MPTA). Candidates for the award are nominated by PT or physical therapist assistant (PTA) students during or immediately following the final year of their educational program. The nomination process requires that students complete a nomination form, developed based on studies of clinical teacher effectiveness conducted by Emery,[4,5] and provide narrative data

in support of their nominee. A committee established by the SIGCE comprising academic and clinical faculty invites nominations from students or recent graduates from all PT or PTA educational programs in Michigan annually. The committee reviews nominations, seeks additional supporting information from the CI and professional colleagues, and then selects one or more recipients each year. Awardees and nominees are recognized at an MPTA annual conference and through chapter newsletters. A record of nominees and nominators is maintained by the SIGCE and recorded in committee minutes and files.

The second sampling frame for the study was individuals who had nominated one of the recipients of the Outstanding Clinical Instructor Award. These potential participants were former students of the CIs and were now graduates and practicing PTs at the time phase 2 of the study commenced (see Figure 10–1). Further description of participant recruitment and selection is provided below.

Participants

Once the sampling frame for CIs was established, a purposive sample of those outstanding CIs who met additional inclusion criteria was sought, and these CIs were invited to participate in phase 1 of the study. Additional inclusion criteria were that the potential participant had continued his or her involvement in clinical education as a CI and/or a Center Coordinator of Clinical Education (CCCE) during the past 5 years and had consented to participate. A final sample of 17 CIs was included in this phase of the study, at which point the data were saturated and no further interviews were conducted.

Demographic data on the CI participants is provided in Table A2–1. As can be seen in this table, overall this was an experienced group of therapists and CIs, although 2 of the 17 therapists had less than 5 years of experience. Collectively, these CIs had worked with a large number of students during the 5 years before their entry into the study, and all indicated that they enjoyed being a CI. Furthermore, all were committed to their own ongoing learning and development, and many had advanced their credentials by completing the Clinical Instructor Education and Credentialing Program (CIECP)[16] or a postprofessional degree, or had obtained certification as a clinical specialist.

For phase 2 of the study, we sought former students who had nominated their CIs for the MPTA Outstanding CI Award. Additional inclusion criteria for this purposive sample were simply that the potential participant was currently practicing as a PT and consented to participate. This group of individuals was more difficult to locate and recruit, and it took 3 years to gather data from 11 participants, at which point we felt confident that those data were saturated. Demographic data on student/graduate participants is shown in Table A2–2. Most of these participants were still novice PTs, with 9 of the 11 having 2 years or less experience. The 2 more experienced therapists had both served as CIs themselves, but the less experienced therapists had not yet assumed that role.

Phase 3 of the study consisted of further examination of seven pairs of CI and student data (see Figure 10–1). This represents a subsample of the CI and student data sets in which the Outstanding Clinical Instructor Award recipient and the student who nominated the person for the award were examined side by side. The parallel construction of several of the interview questions for participants provided fertile ground for this additional comparative analysis. (See Appendices 10-B and 10-C.) In Tables A2–1 and A2–2, these seven pairs are identified as CIs 1 through 7 and student/graduates 1 through 7.

TABLE A2–1 Clinical Instructor Demographics at the Time of Entry into the Study*

Participant Identifier	Entry-Level Degree	Gender	Age (yr)	No. of Years as PT	No. of Years as CI	No. of Students Past 5 Years	APTA CI Credential	Postprofessional Degree	Clinical Specialization
1	MSPT	F	31	7	6	6	Y	N	N (planned)
2	DPT	M	28	3	2	4	Y	N (planned)	Y (GCS)
3	MSPT	M	30	4	4	4	N (planned)	Y (in process)	N
4	BSPT	F	39	15	15	5	N	Y	Y (OMPT, OCS)
5	MSPT	M	37	10	8	14	Y	N	N
6	MSPT	F	33	7	6	7	Y	N	N (planned)
7	BSPT	F	39	17	16	6	Y	Y	N
8	BSPT	M	46	22	20	20	N (planned)	N	N
9	BSPT	F	51	30	20	12	Y	Y	N (planned)
10	BSPT	M	43	21	11	11	N	Y	Y (OCS, FAAOMPT)
11	BSPT	M	43	18	7	7	N	Y	Y (OCS)
12	MPT	F	33	8	8	20	Y	N	N
13	BSPT	F	54	32	28	15	N	Y	N
14	BSPT	M	36	13	12	15	Y	Y	Y (OCS)
15	MSPT	F	31	9	5	6	N	N	N
16	BSPT	F	47	25	20	5	N	N	N
17	MSPT	M	40	17	16	3	N	N (planned)	Y (OCS)
N = 17	BSPT = 9 MSPT = 7 DPT = 1	F = 9 M = 8	Range: 28-54 Mean: 39	Range: 3-32 Mean: 15	Range: 2-28 Mean: 12	Range: 3-20 Mean: 9.4	Y = 8 N = 9 (2 planned)	Y = 8 N = 9 (1 planned)	Y = 6 N = 11 (3 planned)

DPT, *Doctor of Physical Therapy*; F, *female*; FAAOMPT, *Fellow of the American Academy of Orthopedic Manual Physical Therapy*; GCS, *Geriatric Clinical Specialist*; M, *male*; MSPT, *Master of Science in Physical Therapy*; N, *no*; OCS, *Orthopedic Clinical Specialist*; *planned, plan to seek credential, certification, or degree in near future*; Y, *yes*.
*Numbers for demographic variables are rounded to the closest whole value.

TABLE A2-2 Student or Graduate Demographics at Time of Entry into the Study

Participant Identifier	Entry-level Degree	Gender	Age (yr)*	No of Months or Years as PT*	No. of Weeks with Nominated CI*	Setting of Clinical Experience with CI	Primary Patient Population(s) Seen
1	DPT	F	25	6 mo	14	Inpatient subacute rehabilitation unit	Neurology, medical-surgical; adults and geriatrics
2	MSPT	F	26	2 yr	14	Inpatient subacute rehabilitation unit	Neurology, medical-surgical; adults and geriatrics
3	MSPT	M	27	10 mo	9	Private practice outpatient clinic	Musculoskeletal disorders; adolescents and adults
4	MSPT	M	27	1 yr	14	Private practice outpatient clinic	Musculoskeletal disorders, chronic pain; adolescents and adults
5	MSPT	F	30	4 yr	14	Hospital-affiliated outpatient clinic	Musculoskeletal disorders, neurology; adults
6	MSPT	F	27	1 yr	7	Hospital-based outpatient clinic	Neurology, oncology, burns; adults
7	MSPT	F	33	8 yr	8	Hospital-affiliated outpatient clinic	Musculoskeletal, neurology; adult and pediatric
8	MSPT	F	25	1 yr	8	Hospital-based outpatient clinic	Musculoskeletal disorders; adults
9	DPT	M	25	1 yr	14	Private practice outpatient clinic	Musculoskeletal disorders; adults
10	DPT	F	27	1 yr	8	Inpatient acute care and long-term care hospital	Musculoskeletal Disorders, neurology, cardiopulmonary; adults and geriatrics
11	DPT	F	33	1 yr	12	Hospital-affiliated outpatient clinic	Musculoskeletal disorders; pediatrics to adults
N = 11	MSPT = 7 DPT = 4	F = 8 M = 3	Range: 25-33 Mean: 27	Range: 6 mo to 8 yr; 8, <2 yr	Range: 7-14 wk Mean: 11 wk		

DPT, *Doctor of Physical Therapy*; F, *female*; M, *male*; MSPT, *Master of Science in Physical Therapy*.
Numbers for age and years as a physical therapist (PT) are rounded to the closest whole value.

APPENDIX 10-B CLINICAL INSTRUCTOR INTERVIEW GUIDE

Note: Probes or additional cues in italics—use as necessary.

A. Introductions, Consent Review, and Equipment Check

B. Review of Resume Sort Activity

In preparation for this interview, I asked you to complete a resume sort activity. To start the interview, I would like to review and discuss that activity with you. As you recall, I asked you to sort pieces of your resume that I had placed onto note cards into three categories: (1) those events or activities that you considered MOST important or influential in your development as an outstanding clinical instructor (CI)/educator; (2) those that were SOMEWHAT influential; and (3) those that were LEAST important.

Let's start with those events or activities that you felt were **MOST** important or influential:

- How did this event/activity influence your thinking and practice in clinical education?

  - What was most meaningful about this experience? (people, event, course...)
  - In what way exactly did it affect you?
  - How did you begin to think differently about clinical education?
  - Did you begin to practice differently? In what way?
  - Would you consider it a positive experience that changed you or a negative one?

Now lets discuss those that were **SOMEWHAT** important or influential:

- How did this event/activity influence your thinking and practice in clinical education?

  - What was most meaningful about this experience? (people, event, course...)
  - In what way exactly did it affect you?
  - How did you begin to think differently about clinical education?
  - Did you begin to practice differently? In what way?
  - Would you consider it a positive experience that changed you or a negative one?

Finally, lets review activities or events that were **LEAST** important in your development as a CI:

- Why do you think this activity was *not* important in shaping your thinking or practice as a CI?
- **Summary** of resume sort activity:

  - Do you notice any similarities between activities in each of these three categories? That is, are there any similarities in items/events that you felt were most important? Somewhat important? And least important in your growth as a CI?
  - *For example, do the majority fall into continuing education activities? Or clinical practice experiences? Or any particular category?*

C. Reporting of Exemplar

In preparation for this interview, I also asked you to identify and reflect on an experience that you felt was a critical event or turning point in your professional development as a clinical educator. I would like to give you the opportunity now to **describe that experience in detail**. You can think of it as telling a story ... or playing back a videotape for me. ...

(Probes as indicated in follow-up—include questions about further detailed description of the experience AND thoughts, feelings, and insights related to the experience.)

D. Additional Professional Development and Practice Questions

Thus far, we have talked primarily about events, activities, and experiences that you feel contributed to your development as a CI. Now I'd like to take a closer look at **PEOPLE** who you feel influenced your growth as a CI.

- Are there any teachers or professional colleagues who have been especially influential in your development as a CI? (Mentors, academic or clinical faculty, clinicians)
- Why do you feel they were so influential?
- How were you changed as a result of their influence?
- Are there any students who were especially influential?
- Why do you feel they were so influential?
- How were you changed as a result of their influence?
- Are there any patients who were especially influential?
- Why do you feel they were so influential?
- How were you changed as a result of his or her influence?
- Anyone else? (Including people outside of your professional life...)

(Beliefs about clinical teaching ... clinical practice)

- If you had to describe your overall "philosophy" of teaching and teaching "style" for student physical therapists, what would that be?
- How has this changed over the time you have been working with students? (Or has it?)
- What do you believe accounts for this change? Does this philosophy/style translate into your work with patients? How?

(Beliefs about student learning...)

- How do you feel students learn best in clinical settings?
- What kind of environment do you feel creates opportunities for learning?
- What impedes or constrains student learning in the clinic?

(Practice in clinical instruction...)

- What do you actually DO when working with students to try and facilitate their learning?
- What do you DO to try and overcome impediments/constraints to student learning in the clinic?
- Can you describe an **ideal student** to work with in the clinic? Please be specific. Feel free to provide an example of a student who was "ideal," just don't tell me his or her real name...
- *(What are their characteristics, attributes, behaviors, background, etc.?)*
- Can you describe the **most challenging situation or student** you have worked with in the clinic?
- Why was this situation or person so difficult?
- How did you deal with the situation?
- What was the outcome?

In the course of clinical experiences, many CIs and students encounter everyday **ethical distress or dilemmas**. Can you identify some times in your experience working with students like this? *(For example, observing treatment of a patient that one feels is not caring, or discharging of patients before recommended timelines...)*

- How do you approach such situations when working with students?
- What are you trying to teach in these situations?
- What institutional/professional barriers or facilitators are factors?
- If you had one **"take-home" message or lesson** that you want students to take from their work with you as an instructor, what would that be?
- What **advice** or suggestions would you give to novice CIs who want to develop expertise in clinical instruction/education?
- Is there anything else you want to share with me about your learning, development, and practice as a CI?

E. Conclude Interview/Final Notes

APPENDIX 10-C STUDENT NOMINATOR INTERVIEW GUIDE

Note: Probes or additional cues in italics—use as necessary.

A. Introductions, Consent Review, and Equipment Check
B. Initiate Interview

To "set the stage" for the rest of the interview, can you tell me about the environment at the clinic where you were working with the clinical instructor (CI) you nominated for an Outstanding Clinical Instructor Award?

- Type of clinical setting?
- Types of patients you were working with?
- Number of staff members?
- Nature of interactions among PT staff and other professionals?
- Types of learning experiences outside of direct patient care available?
- *(Others? Follow-up as indicated.)*

How did these environmental factors influence, enhance, or detract from your learning and development while there?

Reporting of Exemplar

In our project consent form, we talked about having you provide us with an exemplar. An exemplar is a personal and narrative account of an event or experience that you feel contributed in a significant way to your learning and development as a physical therapy student and future professional. In this case, we are interested in an event or experience that occurred while you were working with the CI that you nominated for the Outstanding Clinical Instructor Award. I would like to give you the opportunity now to **describe that experience or event in detail**. You can think of it as telling a story or playing back a videotape for me.

(Probes as indicated in follow-up to exemplar—include questions about further detailed description of the experience AND thoughts, feelings, and insights related to the experience.)

We'd like you to tell us more about your CI now.

- How would you describe your CI's "teaching style" in general?
- Did your CI seem to have an overall "philosophy" of teaching students in the clinic? If so, what was it? And how did you learn about it?

(Explicit discussion of this? Or implicit learning about it?)

- What were some of the specific teaching/instructional strategies or techniques your CI used that helped you learn?

(Seek specific and detailed examples of the use of these techniques.)

- Can you describe the type and level (or amount) of supervision you received from your CI during the course of your clinical experience? How was this graded over time?
- Tell us about some of the personal characteristics or attributes of your CI that you feel enhanced your learning in the clinic. Why or how did these help you learn?
- Were there any characteristics, attributes, or behaviors of your CI that interfered with your learning? How?

(For example, one student reported that the CI was so knowledgeable that the student at first felt a bit intimidated. Another student wanted a bit more independence toward the end of the clinical experience.)

- So far, we've been talking about your CI primarily. In clinical education, however, it is rarely just the CI and student involved in teaching and learning. There are patients, their family members and caregivers, and other health care personnel. Please describe the nature of your CI's interaction with:
  - Patients
  - Family members/caregivers
  - Other health care personnel
- What was your most challenging or difficult experience during this clinical affiliation? Please describe it in detail. How did your CI assist you (or not) in dealing with this situation? What was the final outcome?

(Note: If the participant does not describe a situation that entails ethical distress or dilemmas, then ask specifically: Did you encounter any situations that caused you ethical distress or discomfort during the experience? How did you and your CI handle this situation? Probe for thoughts and feelings about the situation.... What did the student take from that experience?)

- Based on your work with this CI, what were the primary "take-home messages" or "lessons learned" from your CI?
- How has your experience with this CI changed or shaped your practice as a physical therapist?

Questions Regarding Participant's Role as CI

- Have you served as a CI for other students?

If YES:

- How has your experience with an outstanding CI shaped *your* practice as a CI?
  - What things do you do that are similar to your former CI?

181

- What things do you do that are different?
- How do you try to create an environment that facilitates learning?

If <u>NO</u>:

- How do you feel your experience with an outstanding CI may influence your future practice as a CI?
  - What things will you try to do like your CI?
  - What things will you do differently? Why?

- How will you try to create an environment that facilitates learning?
- Is there anything else you would like share with us about your experience with this CI?

C. Conclude Interview; Record Final Notes to Self

CHAPTER 11

FACILITATING THE TEACHING AND LEARNING OF CLINICAL REASONING

Nicole Christensen ⊙ Terry Nordstrom

First off, we weren't really told anything about clinical reasoning to start, and then it sort of, that word or phrase or whatever, just sort of infiltrated the system but nobody discussed what it was. It just was.

I think that with the terms used in different classes, applying to different examples of situations, and so maybe we have formed our own idea of what clinical reasoning is. I don't know if we've ever heard it actually being defined ... to me it sounds more like a mathematical process or ... scientific method to apply ... if you have a hypothesis and you narrow it down to maybe a few options?

When I heard the words "clinical reasoning" I didn't know what it was. I still don't know what it is, I think ... to me it's like logic, like you have explanations of the things that you do. Why you're doing the things that you do, and then we use our tools, coming from knowledge, coming from your head. It comes from the school, what we learn ... encounters from the past. But I don't really know what is "clinical reasoning," and I don't think it's straightforward ... and I don't know what it is.

These are excerpts from three separate focus group discussions, held with students from three different physical therapist educational programs, where they were discussing their current understandings of and their learning of clinical reasoning.[1] Each of the three students quoted above was close to completion of their entry-level education, and each was expressing a degree of uncertainty in their descriptions of clinical reasoning, relating this to not having ever heard clinical reasoning overtly defined or discussed as part of their professional educations, in either the academic or clinical education settings. Each had been listening to fellow students discuss their ideas, and each was attempting to provide an explanation for the brief, superficial, and sometimes contradictory

descriptions the group had been able to generate in their discussions so far.

What can and what should student physical therapists understand about clinical reasoning? How can their learning be facilitated during this time of professional formation? In this chapter we discuss how research-derived descriptions of the skillful clinical reasoning of expert clinicians, as well as insights gained from research describing student physical therapists' understanding of clinical reasoning, can guide the focus of explicit teaching strategies for the learning of clinical reasoning, including ethical reasoning, during professional education.

LEARNING GOALS

After completing this chapter, the reader will be able to:

1. Recognize current research-derived models of clinical reasoning in the physical therapy literature and how this knowledge enhances the teaching and the learning of clinical reasoning in practice.
2. Recognize characteristics of the clinical reasoning of expert physical therapists and how these can be used to guide students' learning of clinical reasoning.
3. Discuss the interdependence of deductive and inductive reasoning in adopting a biopsychosocial approach to patient care.
4. Discuss implications of recent research on the clinical reasoning of student physical therapists for professional education, including the need to link clinical reasoning to professional formation and the need for explicit links between the academic and clinical educational settings.
5. Describe elements of a clinical reasoning capability model and discuss this as a framework within which to develop strategies for facilitating the learning of clinical reasoning.
6. Develop teaching and learning opportunities for facilitating clinical reasoning in the academic setting.
7. Implement strategies for facilitation of clinical reasoning in the clinical education setting.

WHAT IS CLINICAL REASONING?

Clinical reasoning is a term that is used with different meaning in a variety of health care professions and contexts, and it is understood differently even among various members of the physical therapy profession. To most effectively situate this chapter's discussion of teaching and learning of clinical reasoning, it therefore becomes necessary to first establish a common and current understanding of this concept.

The term *clinical reasoning*, in the context of allied health professional literature, is most commonly understood to represent the thinking and associated decision making of the clinician in practice. During the past three decades, this simple description of clinical reasoning has been significantly expanded and transformed by developments within the allied health professions literature. Seminal research into expert practice in nursing,[2,3] clinical reasoning of experienced occupational therapists,[4] and clinical reasoning attributes of expert physical therapists,[5,6] as well as theoretical literature concerned with the nature and scope of clinical reasoning,[7,8] all contributed to a shift in the original conception of clinical reasoning in medical literature: an individual process of diagnosis occurring inside of the clinician's head. This more recent allied health literature characterized the reasoning process in an expanded way—involving the patient, occurring during the initial diagnostic encounter, and evolving throughout the subsequent interaction and management over the entire course of a patient's care.

A recent description of clinical reasoning, applicable to the practice of multiple health care team members (medical doctors, nurses, physical therapists, and occupational therapists), was proposed to be "a process of reflective inquiry, in collaboration with a patient or family (as appropriate), which seeks to promote a deep and contextually relevant understanding of the clinical problem, in order to provide a sound basis for clinical intervention."[9] This definition represents a step in the right direction toward achieving a common understanding of clinical reasoning, but even this description can be considered incomplete in that it does not explicitly encompass the clinical reasoning involved with clinical tasks beyond diagnosis and choice of intervention (e.g., those related to decisions about how to interact with patients, how to teach and facilitate learning in patients, how to determine a prognosis, and how to act when faced with ethical dilemmas).[6]

Today, our research-derived understanding of skillful clinical reasoning in physical therapy has evolved to include the following aspects[10]:

- Clinical reasoning involves the interaction of individuals in a collaborative exchange to achieve a mutual understanding of the problem and to negotiate an agreed-on plan for addressing that problem.[11,12]
- Clinical reasoning is patient centered and situated within a biopsychosocial model of health.[5,6]
- Clinical reasoning involves both deductive and inductive reasoning.[6,11]
- Clinical reasoning is complex, nonlinear, and cyclical in nature.[11,13]

- Clinical reasoning plays a critical role in reflective learning from practice experiences and in the development of clinical expertise.[7,11]

WHAT CAN WE LEARN FROM THE CLINICAL REASONING OF EXPERT PHYSICAL THERAPISTS THAT CAN INFORM OUR TEACHING?

A common finding across research that distinguishes characteristics of expert physical therapists' practice is their ability to create a collaboratively oriented clinical reasoning exchange with their patients, caregivers, and other members of the health care team.[5,11,14–16] These types of exchanges are built into the structure of physical therapy practice. Jensen and colleagues[5] characterized expert practice as consisting of several interrelated dimensions, each influencing and influenced by the other (Figure 11–1):

- A dynamic, multidimensional base of knowledge
- A central focus on assessment of movement as linked to functional deficits
- Consistent virtues seen in caring and commitment to patients
- A clinical reasoning process wherein patients were interacted with as people

Each of these dimensions also contributed to, and was influenced by, the experts' philosophy of practice.

Clinical reasoning, as practiced by the experienced physical therapists participating in the study, was collaborative and patient centered in nature: the physical therapists' focus was on patient function and expectation rather than a medical diagnosis.[5] Further, the physical therapists' practice was focused on understanding a patient's story, and they used clinical reasoning as a tool to fit the patient story within their clinical and experiential knowledge. These practice methods served to facilitate the collaboration that the expert practitioners valued in clinical practice.

Although the experienced therapists studied by Jensen and colleagues[5] were not selected as participants based

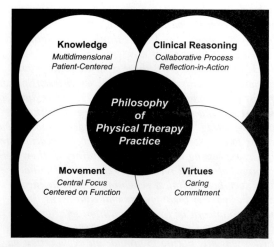

FIGURE 11–1 Dimensions of expert physical therapists' practice. (From Jensen GM, Gwyer J, Shepard KF. Expert practice in physical therapy. Phys Ther 2000;80:28-43; discussion, 44-52.)

on objective criteria related to their clinical outcomes, subsequent research[16] linked the expert clinician characteristics identified by Jensen and colleagues[5] to superior measurable clinical outcomes, providing validity to the characterization of the clinical reasoning of experts as being associated with effective, efficient patient care, as well as being collaborative and patient centered.

The clinical reasoning of novices, in contrast, has been characterized as more therapist centered, lacking in collaboration, with less focus on understanding of the patient as a person in favor of a more narrow focus on only the physical aspects of a patient's presentation.[14–16] These differences between the clinical reasoning characteristics of novice and experienced therapists can be attributed at least in some part to the very different stages of professional practice development they represent.[2] Although it is clear that novice clinicians cannot be "experts" at time of entry to practice, they can be explicitly educated to recognize aspects of clinical reasoning that align with more skillful practice and how they influence outcomes. Novices can be provided strategies to promote their own clinical reasoning development within the context of an explicitly biopsychosocially oriented, patient centered, collaborative approach to physical therapist practice.

CLINICAL REASONING STRATEGIES MODEL

Edwards and colleagues[6,11] explored the nature of expert clinical reasoning with their research-derived model of clinical reasoning strategies. These researchers studied the clinical reasoning of expert physical therapists in multiple practice contexts (orthopaedic, neurologic, and home health settings) and proposed a model to depict and make explicit the different types, and broad scope, of reasoning "activities" associated with all areas of clinical practice. The eight strategies composing the model (Table 11–1) were further subdivided into three broad categories[6,17]:

- Strategies used for diagnosing the patient
  - Diagnostic reasoning
  - Narrative reasoning
- Strategies used throughout the management components of patient care
  - Procedural reasoning
  - Interactive reasoning
  - Collaborative reasoning
  - Reasoning about teaching
  - Predictive reasoning
- The ethical reasoning strategy used to drive ethical problem solving as it arises in the diagnostic and management phases of patient care
  - Ethical reasoning

These strategies were employed by the therapists in a dynamic manner, resulting in a cue-based decision-making interplay, in which different forms of reasoning were used when judged appropriate to further the mutual inquiry process by therapist with patient (Figure 11–2).[6] In other words, these skilled clinical reasoners were able to respond to the emerging data and cues they perceived in a very fluid and individualized manner, most appropriate for an individual patient as he or she presents in a particular moment in time.

As noted in Table 11–1, there are different forms of reasoning employed within the whole of the model. Deductive reasoning, for example, employs development and systematic testing of hypotheses to establish a cause-and-effect relationship between variables.

Conversely, inductive reasoning does not involve the development or testing of hypotheses, but rather it proceeds from a thorough understanding of the particulars of the case, including the context in which the physical therapist interacts with the patient. As applied to this situation, inductive reasoning can be defined as the eliciting of data directly from patients, from their perspective, in order to understand that individual's own perspective or story. In the case of narrative reasoning, a similar goal of understanding cannot be achieved by making assumptions about how one might feel if in a similar circumstance: what characterizes narrative reasoning is the focus on achieving an understanding of the person's situation and having this validated by the patient, thereby minimizing the influence of a clinician's bias or faulty assumptions on the reasoning process (Box 11–1). The focus of inductive reasoning is on the particulars of the case and making decisions about these.

The fluid shifts between inductive and deductive reasoning are a key finding in the research done by Edwards and colleagues.[6] This shifting occurred within the therapist's diagnostic process and throughout the patient's continuing management. How these shifts occurred has important implications for teaching and practice: not only, then, should the therapist consider the specific findings from the patient interview and examination to come to a diagnosis, but the therapist also needs to come to a confirmed understanding of the person's beliefs, culture, values, and experiences (i.e., all of the factors that contribute to the context in which physical therapy occurs) to fully understand how to be most effective with this particular person.

When the therapist and patient discuss the nature of the problem that brought the patient to physical therapy and how the course of physical therapy will be constructed, the discussion includes results of both the deductive (diagnostic) and inductive (narrative) reasoning processes. Thus, clinical reasoning is characterized by a dialectic, in which the therapist thinks about and integrates findings from these distinctly different thinking processes. The dialectical nature of clinical reasoning and how it can be reinforced in learning are taken up later in this chapter.

A similar dialectic occurs in ethical reasoning, the third main category of clinical reasoning in this framework.[18] Deductive reasoning in ethics involves consideration of the norms of ethics, primarily bioethical principles, a profession's code of ethics, and the accepted values of a profession. To engage in ethical reasoning from these norms alone would neglect critically important factors such as the patient's and caregiver's beliefs, relationships, culture, and values.[19] The particular therapist's narrative, which incorporates the therapist's values, beliefs, and experiences, is an integral part of inductive reasoning.[18] The conscious integration of the therapist's personal narrative in ethical reasoning requires a critically self-reflective practitioner; that critical self-reflection provides the foundation for the therapist's continued moral development.[18,19]

TABLE 11-1 Clinical Reasoning Strategies Model

Reasoning Strategy	Description	Example
Diagnostic reasoning	Strategy that requires knowledge of: • What information is needed • How that information is interpreted Necessary information and interpretation strategies must be implemented for data from both the patient interview/interaction and the physical examination. Diagnostic reasoning is a deductive strategy.	Using a diagnostic reasoning strategy to create initial diagnostic hypotheses based on interpreted data from the patient interview and examination. The hypothesis includes the identification and validation of: • Activity/participation restrictions • Physical impairments • Pathology of body structures • Pain mechanisms • The broad scope of relevant contributing factors (e.g., physical, environmental, psychosocial, emotional, behavioral) Multiple hypotheses are formulated, related to particular impairments that could be contributing to the activity or participation restrictions experienced by the patient. Hypotheses are tested via systematic questioning and physical examination testing, in order to narrow the possibilities and settle on a likely cause-and-effect relationship between impairment(s) and restricted activities
Narrative reasoning	Strategy that requires the establishment of and understanding of the "person" inside the patient. This strategy involves an understanding of the patient's: • Story • Illness experience • Context • Beliefs • Culture Validation of these elements is equally important; the therapist should reflect the therapist's understanding back to the patient for confirmation of understanding. The elements that make up the patient's life experience should be explicitly integrated into the clinical reasoning and decision process. Narrative reasoning is an inductive strategy.	Using open-ended questions to ask a patient about her beliefs concerning her potential for a full recovery. The therapist then repeats those beliefs back to the patient as he has understood them to confirm she has been correctly understood. The therapist explains that he will keep these beliefs in mind as he conducts the examination, and overtly includes discussion of his findings related to his prognosis for full recovery in comparison to the patient's beliefs. Any discrepancy is discussed further, and the plan of care reflects this discussion
Procedural reasoning	Strategy that requires choice in administration of interventions. This strategy uses re-examination to help determine progress and outcomes. Procedural reasoning can be both a deductive and an inductive strategy.	Therapist formulates several hypotheses about interventions likely to benefit her current patient. She selects one, asks for and receives consent from her patient to trial the intervention, and chooses impairment(s) and relevant related activity restriction(s) to re-examine upon completion of the intervention (following the session, at the end of the week, etc.) Therapist decides to continue with the chosen intervention based on results of re-examination, indicating progress toward achieving anticipated outcomes
Interactive reasoning	Strategy that requires a means of approach and interaction with the patient; the goal in this interaction is the establishment of rapport. Interactive reasoning can be both a deductive and an inductive strategy.	Therapist notices his patient responds more positively to a quiet, calm tone of voice (assessed by nonverbal communication cues and improved ability to focus on motor control retraining tasks) compared with her performance while he had been joking with her earlier on in the visit. Therapist modulates his communication and consciously maintains a quiet, calm tone throughout the rest of the session, despite his own preference for establishing rapport through joking and laughing with his patients.
Collaborative reasoning	Strategy that requires a working relationship with the patient. The relationship will include a distribution of power in the decision-making process. Collaborative reasoning fosters a consensual approach in: • Interpretation of examination data • Setting and prioritization of intervention goals • Choice of intervention approach	Therapist asks her patient what her goals are for physical therapy. Patient states she has two "less important" goals, and those mirror the therapist's hypotheses for appropriate goals. However, the goal she indicates as "most important" is one that the therapist hadn't considered, and while it is still appropriate, feels is much less important to focus on. Therapist and patient discuss these differences explicitly and come to an agreement for a plan of care wherein the patient's wishes for prioritization of her main goal are honored, and the other goals are also integrated simultaneously.

	Collaborative reasoning can be both a deductive and an inductive strategy.	The patient and therapist agree that this is reasonable, and although the therapist feels the patient may not achieve the goals that the therapist thinks are most important as quickly, as a result of spending some of the time in therapy focused on the goal the patient values most, both agree that the mutually derived plan of care is acceptable.
Reasoning about teaching	Strategy that requires approaches and strategies for educating patients. Like narrative reasoning, this strategy requires the therapist to verify that new information has been understood by the patient. The reasoning about teaching strategy can be both a deductive and an inductive strategy.	A patient returns for a follow-up session and reports that he has not performed the home exercise program prescribed at the last session. The therapist hypothesizes that the patient may not have remembered how to do the exercises and/or may not have remembered to do them during his busy work day. The therapist, however, also invites the patient to offer more of his perspective by asking, "Can you tell me more about why you didn't perform the home program?" before beginning to reinstruct the patient or problem-solve about ways to fit the exercises into the work day. The patient indicates that he didn't really see the relevance of those particular exercises to his particular participation restrictions and so chose not to do them. The therapist then initiates a discussion of his perception, and they come to a mutual understanding of an exercise program that is perceived as relevant to the patient and appropriate to the therapist.
Predictive reasoning	Strategy that requires focus on the process of developing a prognosis. Choices about management and the implications of those choices should be explored and considered (e.g., what factors influence development of the worst-case scenario vs. best-case scenario). Predictive reasoning can be both a deductive and an inductive strategy.	The patient is a woman with three very young children, all of whom require lifting for sleep, changing, and eating throughout the day. She presents to the physical therapist with a recent onset of severe lower back pain. Upon completion of the examination, the therapist discusses her prognosis for recovery from her acute back. He explains what he would predict her course of recovery could be if she could get assistance with her children and avoid lifting for a period of time, and explains how the time would likely be longer to achieve the same degree of recovery should she be unable to get help with the lifting of her children in the short term. The therapist and patient discuss her situation in light of these two possible outcomes and develop the plan of care and goals with timeframes accordingly.
Ethical reasoning	Strategy that requires the awareness and resolution of both ethical and pragmatic dilemmas in patient practice. The end result should be "doing the right thing" as dictated by all of the situational variables and constraints. Ethical reasoning can be both a deductive and an inductive strategy.	A physical therapist working in a for-profit private clinic has received a continuation of therapy referral from a physician for a patient with Medicare insurance who she recommended should be discharged to a home program. This therapist's manager suggests she should continue to see the patient "to make the physician happy" because the patient has available benefits remaining. The therapist must come to a decision about continuing or not continuing care for this patient, while weighing factors related to her responsibilities to her patient, her employer, and her relationship with the referring physician. The therapist uses deductive (principle-based) and narrative reasoning to come to a context-appropriate decision.

Data from Edwards I, Jones M, Carr J, et al. Clinical reasoning strategies in physical therapy. Phys Ther 2004;84:312-335.

Thus, inductive reasoning in ethics provides the means through which the patient's, the caregiver's, and the therapist's voices counterbalance the deductive reasoning process. Just as with clinical reasoning, expert physical therapists engage in a fluid back-and-forth between deductive and inductive when considering the ethical dimensions of their work with patients and caregivers. Each side of the dialectic informs the other, with neither alone sufficient. Expert physical therapists' ethical reasoning is also characterized by their recognition of patterns among the different ethical situations they have encountered through their careers.[18,19]

This case-based reasoning, or *casuistry* (in which previous reasoning patterns are used to determine current action),

is the means through which experienced physical therapists link their narrative and principle-based reasoning strategies. Edwards and Delany[19] use the metaphor of an ethical reasoning bridge (Figure 11–3), with one pylon being the ethical principles applicable to the case and the other pylon the particulars of the case gained through narrative. The therapist uses the patterns from familiar, exemplar cases to connect the two pylons and thereby arrive at a deeper understanding of the ethical dimensions of the case, further developing their clinical expertise.

As mentioned previously, novices (and one might argue some less skillful experienced clinicians) have been shown to reason clinically with a focus mainly on a patient's physical presentation,[14-16] as opposed to a more holistic focus

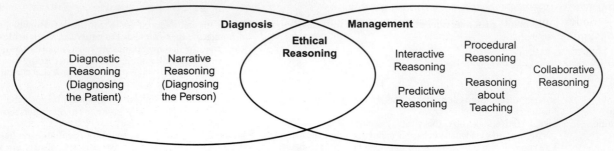

FIGURE 11–2 Clinical reasoning strategies in diagnosis and management.

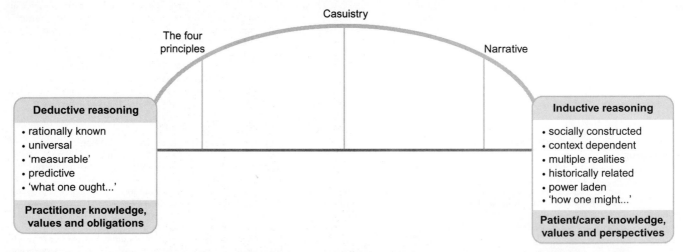

FIGURE 11–3 The ethical reasoning bridge. (Modified from Edwards I, Delany C. Ethical reasoning. In Higgs J, Jones M, Loftus S, Christensen N [eds]. Clinical Reasoning in the Health Professions, 3 rd ed. Amsterdam: Elsevier, 2008.)

BOX 11–1   Example of Narrative Reasoning Dialogue

- Dialogue:
  - Therapist: "How do you feel your life has been affected by your condition?"
  - Patient: "I feel I am not being a good father because I can't play soccer with my kids after work like I used to."
  - Therapist: "What I hear you saying is that you feel your back pain is keeping you from playing soccer with your kids, and that is important to you as a father."
  - Patient: "Yes, that's right."
  - Therapist: "Let's make sure to prioritize that in our plan for physical therapy then; we will work on ways you can build back up to being able to safely play soccer with your kids again."
  - Patient: "That would be great".
- Outcome of dialogue: achievement of understanding by therapist that this patient's experience has been one of not only being limited from playing soccer with his kids, but also a feeling of losing his ability to participate in this particular way with his children as he would like to as their father.
  - This understanding then is explicitly carried into developing the plan of care, which will include prioritization of interventions that will enable the patient to return to safely playing soccer with his children.

on both the physical and psychosocial aspects of the patient.[1,20] It is proposed that explicit education about and practice in application of the breadth of clinical reasoning strategies, including ethical reasoning, that are used by skilled clinical reasoners (experts) can be a part of the clinical reasoning education of novices.[20,21]

STUDENT PHYSICAL THERAPISTS' UNDERSTANDING OF CLINICAL REASONING

We have discussed the ways in which current research-derived models of expert physical therapists' practice describe their clinical reasoning. Rather than a therapist-centered, stepped, and linear process of problem solving, this research supports a more complex interactive, cue-based, and non-linear process involving multiple forms and foci of reasoning. Implications from this research have been used to inform suggestions for physical therapy educational curricula; we also will use these models to inform the educational suggestions we propose in this chapter.

Instruction in clinical and ethical reasoning as part of a physical therapy curriculum is commonplace, but it is only recently that researchers have begun to focus on the outcome of that instruction, particularly concerning students transitioning to professional practice.

Recent research by Christensen[1] explored what a group of student physical therapists understood about clinical reasoning, how they developed this understanding, and what factors influenced their learning of clinical reasoning. This qualitative research employed a hermeneutic approach, wherein texts were analyzed in an iterative manner, themes identified, and answers to the research questions interpreted. Methods of data collection included focus group and individual interview discussions, including postclinical observation interviews. A model of students' existing understanding of clinical reasoning was constructed, and key factors perceived as influencing their learning were identified.

The research revealed that the student participants understood clinical reasoning to be a sequential, linear process of deductive problem solving, and variably understood related aspects such as types of knowledge used, the roles of physical therapist and client in clinical reasoning, and how to evaluate the quality of their clinical reasoning. Students demonstrated a lack of awareness of the role of collaboration in the clinical reasoning process. Their understanding was characterized by not fully comprehending the importance of the inter-relationships among the different types of clinical reasoning and how reasoning is integrated into thinking in practice. Finally, these student participants demonstrated an absence of understanding of how to use critical reflection as an experiential learning tool. Factors identified as influential in their learning included variable, largely implicit academic and clinical education curricula and inconsistent opportunities to work with clinical educators skilled in facilitation of clinical reasoning.[1,21,22]

Research by Nordstrom[20] examined the role of physical therapy students as moral agents while on final clinical experiences. This research specifically asked what types of ethical issues these students encountered, how the students reasoned through those ethical issues, and how they negotiated action with their clinical instructors (CIs) and patients in their role as moral agents. Data were collected from physical therapy students and their CIs through journals, multiple interviews with each participant distributed throughout the clinical experience, and focus groups (separated by participant type: student or instructor) at the end of the clinical experiences.

The ethical issues encountered by the students were similar to those seen in other studies of physical therapists and students, including the importance of caring.[23-32] These ethical issues were considered in a clinical context as opposed to in isolation as "ethical problems."

The students' reasoning was characterized by several different strategies:

- Deductive reasoning strategies, in which they considered the ethical principles and norms of the profession at issue in the situation; clinical and lay language was used rather than the specific language of bioethics.
- Inductive reasoning strategies, where the students' personal narratives were evident, and formed primarily by the students' past histories and their interpretations of their roles as both students and future physical therapists.

The students also described inductive reasoning processes that involved understanding of the patients' narratives, as described in journals and interviews. The students did exhibit dialectic thinking between deductive and inductive reasoning, but unlike the study of expert physical therapists,[18] casuistry was not evident. The students' actions occurred along a continuum from choosing not to act to telling the patient what the student had decided and letting the patient decide by negotiating a mutually agreed-on action with the patient.

Throughout the students' self-reflection on their personal narrative and what they were learning from the patient, the CIs and other physical therapists were important. The CIs preferred to act as role models and to provide support, guidance, and background explanations rather than tell the student what to do or step in and act on behalf of the student.

The student-CI interactions were more explicitly about the clinical aspects of the case rather than the ethical implications, except if there were significant ethical issues (e.g., whether something should be brought to the ethics committee). One participant consulted with her CI and other supervisors about what to do when she discovered that a patient, who was a Christian Scientist, was being given medication against her will, and whose capacity for medical decision making was being questioned but had not yet been determined. In another example, a CI discovered that a student was disclosing a patient's personal health information in the clinic's waiting area. The CI talked to the student about the legal and ethical implications of that behavior.

There are several important implications of clinical reasoning in the clinical and academic aspects of entry-level physical therapy education from these two studies.

The World Health Organization's International Classification of Functioning (ICF),[33] now the profession's standard as the model underlying physical therapy practice, has as a central feature a holistic view of the patient in a biopsychosocially oriented manner. In Christensen's study,[1] the students did not see the connection between collaboration, communication, and clinical reasoning. These students took a limited view of the areas on which they focused in their reasoning processes rather than considering the areas' full scope. That view was often narrowly focused on the clinical aspects of the case with little understanding of the relationship between their role and the patient's role in clinical reasoning. This more clinician-centered focus is inconsistent with the ICF's biopsychosocial model. In the specific case of ethical reasoning,[20] when the concerns were focused on the moral implications of the situation and the effects on the patient as a person, there was more variability among the students: some students did not consistently describe a collaborative process with patients and how they sought to gain an understanding of the patient's narrative, whereas other students more frequently engaged in this collaborative and narrative reasoning.

A goal of entry-level education is to prepare clinicians who can practice effectively and also have the ability to learn and grow as professionals throughout a career. Christensen's research[1] showed that participants were unaware of the potential for, and therefore unprepared to actively, systematically, and optimally utilize, critical reflection of the clinical reasoning process as a vehicle for learning from their own practice. A potential for developing conscious critical self-reflection as a means to professional development was seen in Nordstrom's ethical reasoning study[20] when, during the post-hoc discussion of ethical issues in the interviews, some students reflected on how their actions were influenced by their biases and judgments. Both the Christensen[1] and Nordstrom[20] studies, however, illuminated a disconnect in student learning between the academic and clinical environments.

Christensen[1] described a disconnect between academic and clinical settings for the learning and practice of clinical reasoning. As illustrated by the quotes from student participants in this research, included in the introduction to this chapter, students experienced curricula that address clinical reasoning in the academic setting in a mostly implicit way. These findings suggest that explicit attention to—and practice with—clinical reasoning and associated thinking and learning skills, in addition to technical and other professional "doing" skills, is key to development of proficient clinical reasoning capability in new graduates.[21] Physical therapist education programs are required to address ethics,[34] and there is explicit ethical content within these programs, although we do not have a current understanding of how programs approach the ethics curriculum and instruction.[35]

Nordstrom's student participants, however, did not discuss how they used classroom learning about ethics in their ethical reasoning and did not rely on consultation with academic faculty during their clinical experiences, and the CIs' influence was more implicit than explicit.[20] Therefore, it appears that there is also a disconnect in the realm of ethical reasoning between the academic and clinical environments, with a more implicit approach to ethical reasoning in the clinical environment and perhaps the need for a more clinically focused approach to ethics in the academic environment (Box 11–2).

ROLE OF PROFESSIONAL FORMATION IN LEARNING CLINICAL REASONING

Professional formation is a critical aspect of the education of professionals.[36-40] Not only are students learning to "do" physical therapy, they are learning to "be" a physical therapist. Professional formation implies the creation of an identity as a physical therapist and adopting the spirit and ethos of the profession.[41] Professional formation involves the transformation of a layperson into a health care practitioner who is able to respond with skilled know-how and respect for patients as people who have significant concerns about their health within that profession's community.[36,37] When one becomes a member of a professional community of practice, not only does it affect what the practitioner does, but it also affects that person's identity and interpretation of the world.[42] Within the context of physical therapy, that identity also involves the therapist's conception of personal beliefs about the relationship a health care provider has with patients,[43] the moral role of physical therapists,[44] and how they should interact with other health care providers within an interprofessional team. Who they are and how they should present themselves as a professional includes how they frame the situation, how they identify problems, how they think through those problems, and how they act in practice—all of which are consistent with and embedded in clinical and ethical reasoning.

Part of developing one's professional identity includes developing a philosophy of practice, as seen among expert physical therapists. Curricular design features, such as a portfolio, that include the development of a philosophy of practice, moral development, and the development of clinical reasoning, can make explicit what is often implicit

BOX 11–2   Educational Implications: Suggested Strategies to Address Students' Disconnects in Understanding of Clinical Reasoning

Students construct narrowly focused, shallow understandings of clinical reasoning from an implicit curriculum in both academic and clinical education settings	Explicit teaching of clinical reasoning theory, models, and research in the academic setting, with opportunities for application, practice, assessment, and feedback on performance in simulated clinical contexts threaded throughout appropriate patient/client management courses in the curriculum
Students are unaware of the links between clinical reasoning and collaboration, patient centeredness, and/or communication	
Students are unaware of the links between critical self-reflection on their own clinical reasoning and the development of clinical practice expertise over time	Explicit teaching about, opportunities for application and assessment of, and feedback on performance of critical self-reflection on clinical reasoning (including ethical reasoning) during simulated clinical performances (e.g., practical exams, standardized patient experiences)
	Explicit facilitation of students' awareness of the learning skills they are developing, how they relate to clinical reasoning, and how they link to development of self-directed, lifelong learning skills to development of clinical expertise
Students experience inconsistent opportunities to work with educators in both academic and clinical settings who provide skillful facilitation and mentoring of students' clinical reasoning skills This includes development of awareness of the ethical reasoning interwoven throughout diagnostic and management decision making	Explicit focus on development of clinical reasoning skills (including both thinking and experiential learning skills) in the clinical education setting
	Provision of experiences to discuss and reflect on, and development of goals and assessment of progress specifically oriented around clinical reasoning skills performance
	Explicit training for both academic and clinical educators to develop their own teaching (facilitation/mentoring) and assessment skills related to the development of the broad range of clinical reasoning strategies (for diagnosis and management, and ethical problem solving) and critically reflective learning skills of students

in entry-level education. Adoption of the ICF and a biopsychosocial approach as a foundation of the entry-level curriculum can be an important step in developing professional identity. That step can only be effective in identity formation if those approaches are clearly reinforced through all of the courses in the curriculum, the assessment methodologies within those courses, and as part of the assessment of the overall curricular outcomes (Table 11–2). In this way students and faculty are held accountable for achieving learning outcomes that provide evidence that graduates practice with skilled know-how and respect for the people who are their patients.

Research findings[1,20] suggest there is a need for stronger connections between the academic and clinical education contexts in physical therapy education as it is related to clinical and ethical reasoning. Several means to strengthen those connections that merit consideration include the following:

TABLE 11-2   Curricular, Co-Curricular, Classroom, and Clinical Strategies to Address Professional Formation as Part of Clinical Reasoning

Curricular	• Adoption of a specific philosophy for the approach to patients integrated through all applicable courses in the curriculum • A biopsychosocial approach, e.g., ICF model

Co-curricular	• Portfolio that includes development of a philosophy of practice through the course of matriculation in the program
	  • The student's personal beliefs about the relationship a physical therapist has with patients
	  • The student's beliefs about the moral role of physical therapists
	• Opportunities for interprofessional collaboration
	  • Community service volunteer activities with students from other professions
	  • Interprofessional practice opportunities in "mock" clinic or community-based clinic

Classroom	• Standardized patients for practical exams • Rubrics that include students' use of clinical reasoning strategies • Student's written critical self-reflection on the clinical reasoning strategies in standardized patient encounters
Clinical	• Clinical faculty development workshops mentoring students' clinical reasoning capability • Use rubrics on clinical reasoning from standardized patient encounters in the academic setting for feedback and mentoring during clinical experiences • Ask for student's critical self-reflection on their clinical reasoning strategies following patient visits • Clinical faculty development workshops mentoring students' clinical reasoning capability • Rubrics on clinical reasoning from standardized patient encounters in the academic setting used for feedback and mentoring during clinical experiences • Students' critical self-reflection on their clinical reasoning strategies following patient visits

1. Clinical faculty development focused on mentoring students in the development of clinical reasoning capability through continuing education workshops[45]
2. Preparing students for clinical practice through the use of authentic, holistic assessment methods such as standardized patients in which the rubrics focus on the students' ability to use clinical reasoning strategies and sharing those rubrics with clinical faculty
3. Asking students to use clinical cases, including ethical cases, in classroom learning and assessment and including clinical faculty in the development, supervision, and/or assessment of those learning activities[46]

HOW CAN THE TEACHING AND LEARNING OF CLINICAL REASONING BE FACILITATED IN PROFESSIONAL EDUCATION?

To facilitate the learning of clinical reasoning in professional education most effectively, the associated teaching must be explicit and interwoven throughout contextually relevant content matter as a theme that is applied and experienced, or practiced, across the entire academic and clinical education curricula. We present here several suggestions based on research findings presented earlier[1,10,21,22] for how the learning of clinical reasoning (including ethical reasoning) can be facilitated. These include considerations of teaching that is situated in the context of developing capability in specific thinking and experiential learning skills associated with skillful clinical reasoning; inclusion of specific models and research-derived evidence about skillful clinical reasoning in the academic curriculum (e.g., the Clinical Reasoning Strategies Model[6] presented earlier); and application of, feedback on, and the skillful facilitation of critical self-reflection on clinical reasoning experiences in the clinical education setting.

DEVELOPING CLINICAL REASONING CAPABILITY

The model of clinical reasoning capability was developed as one of the main outcomes of the research, conducted by Christensen and colleagues,[1,21,22] describing student physical therapists' understanding and experiences of learning clinical reasoning. This model was grounded in descriptions of capability in the higher education literature,[47] in which the term *capability* has been operationally defined as "the justified confidence and ability to interact effectively with other people and tasks in unknown contexts of the future as well as known contexts of today." Specifically, capability is observed in the following ways:

- Confident, effective decision making and associated actions in practice
- Confidence in the development of a rationale for decisions made
- Confidence in working effectively with others
- Confidence in the ability to navigate unfamiliar circumstances and learn from the experience

Capable individuals are motivated to develop their knowledge intentionally, through application and processing of their knowledge by reflective learning from practice.[48]

Clinical reasoning capability, then, has been described as the integration and effective application of thinking and learning skills to make sense of and learn collaboratively from clinical experiences (Figure 11–4).[22] This model proposes four key dimensions of clinical reasoning capability, which are congruent with the descriptions of thinking and learning skills inherent in the clinical reasoning of expert physical therapists.[5,11] These skills are linked to the development of excellence as both a clinical reasoner and an experiential learner:

1. Reflective thinking
2. Critical thinking
3. Complexity thinking
4. Dialectical thinking[1,21,22]

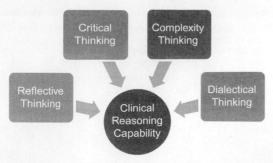

FIGURE 11–4 Dimensions of clinical reasoning capability. (Data from Christensen N, Jones MA, Higgs J, Edwards I. Dimensions of clinical reasoning capability. In Higgs J, Jones MA, Loftus S, Christensen N [eds]. Clinical Reasoning in the Health Professions, 3rd ed. Amsterdam: Elsevier, 2008, pp 101-110.)

Reflective thinking is the ability to think about a situation at various moments in time, in order to make sense of and evaluate it. Schön[49] described three occasions when reflection is necessary in practice:

1. *Reflection on action* is described as occurring after the clinical action has stopped and is a way of cognitively organizing experiences or making sense of things.
2. *Reflection in action* occurs in the midst of action and allows for modification of the situation as new information emerges. Another way of conceptualizing reflection in action is "thinking on your feet."
3. *Reflection for action* involves planning for future encounters by thinking back on past experiences and making links between past and anticipated future events.

Wainwright and colleagues[50] recently described how reflection is used in practice by novice and experienced physical therapists. Their findings included the observation that reflection in action was less commonly used by the novice clinicians and focused mainly on the patient's performance. In contrast, more experienced clinicians were able to think on their feet more often and were focused not only on the patient's performance but also on monitoring their own thinking (reasoning) and actions. These findings highlight the ability to think about one's thinking (meta-cognition) while in action as being a differentiating factor between novice and more experienced clinicians and suggest that this would be an important area of focus for optimizing the facilitation of learning from clinical reasoning.

Critical thinking is intimately linked to reflective thinking but involves an active process of not only analyzing and evaluating information but also questioning assumptions.[51] In the context of clinical reasoning, critical thinking applies both to the examination and evaluation of a particular clinical presentation and to the critical evaluation of one's own thinking or reasoning.[22] "The outcome of thinking critically in practice is the achievement of a coherence of understanding. This can be defined as an awareness of assumptions, and how these assumptions connect to the reasoning used within the context of a situation to create new knowledge and generate an appropriate new action."[52(p 1)] Underlying assumptions are explored and

their adequacy and appropriateness evaluated, and therefore it becomes possible to bring to light blind spots or gaps in knowledge that may be adversely affecting a clinician's clinical reasoning through a given situation.

Complexity thinking is a way of thinking that allows for recognition of the dynamic and interdependent relationships between the many elements and players influencing a given situation.[53,54] Complexity thinking allows a clinician to effectively recognize and consider the relative weighting of all relevant internal (within the person) and external (the context in which the person is functioning) factors acting to produce a given clinical presentation.[13,22,55] Effective clinical reasoning within each of the reasoning strategies also requires an awareness and understanding of how each aspect affects the others, in the context of the complex human being who is the patient.[6,10]

Dialectical thinking is used here specifically to refer to the way in which expert physical therapists were observed to demonstrate a fluidity of reasoning between both deductive and inductive thinking styles within the various clinical reasoning strategies.[6,11] This thinking ability is proposed to be necessary for clinicians to develop a holistic understanding of the person who is the patient and their clinical presentation,[6,21] consistent with a biopsychosocial approach to health care practice that is in accordance with the ICF model.[33]

The intent of facilitation of the thinking and learning skills evident in the clinical reasoning of capable (expert) physical therapists in the novices who are our entry-level student physical therapists is not that these students can or will graduate as "experts" in clinical practice. Rather, by empowering students with these thinking and learning skills, the goal is to graduate students who are confident and able to take responsibility for their own continued personal and professional development.[19,56] Given the current lack of coordination and lack of quality control experienced by many students between the academic and clinical education setting components of their professional education, the facilitation of the development of capability in clinical reasoning can be considered one step educators can take toward equipping novice clinicians to direct their own learning and development even in less than optimal clinical situations.[1,10,21]

EXPLICIT TEACHING AND LEARNING STRATEGIES FOR THE ACADEMIC SETTING

Wenger[42] describes one characteristic of communities of practice, such as the physical therapy profession, as the utilization of a process by which that community gives form to concepts and experiences central to practice in order to facilitate the shaping of experience by members of a practice community; it results in "focusing our attention in a particular way and enabling new kinds of understanding."[33(p 60)] Likewise, it has been proposed that clinical reasoning—a complex, abstract practice phenomenon—is a key component of practice that can and should be given form, or made visible, in the academic classroom setting.[1] Figure 11–5 illustrates ways in which clinical reasoning can be made explicit and woven through a curriculum.

Definitions and models of clinical reasoning, such as the Clinical Reasoning Strategies Model[6] discussed earlier, can

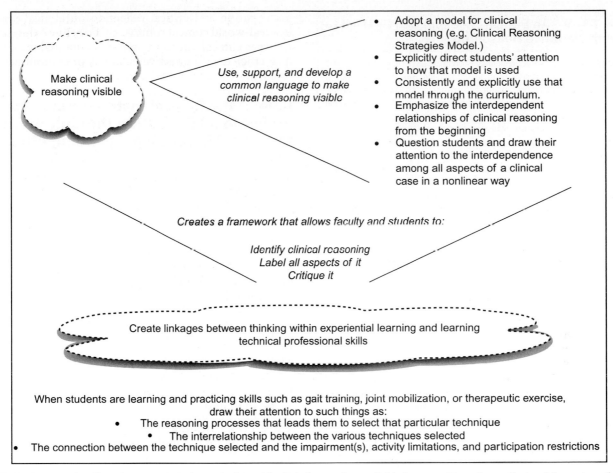

FIGURE 11–5 Example of key characteristics of a curriculum with clinical reasoning explicitly integrated into the professional formation of students.

assist this process. By fostering students' awareness of all components involved in a particular clinical reasoning process (e.g., participants, various areas that are a focus of attention and reasoning), the interactions between these components, and the various thinking skills inherent in a dialectical model of clinical reasoning, educators can reinforce a complex understanding and encourage complexity thinking about interdependent relationships between aspects of a patient case. The explicit exploration of the ways in which clinical reasoning is described in theoretical and research-derived models can allow educators to "create points of focus around which the negotiation of meaning becomes organized."[42(p 58)]

The importance of learning a common language through which students and their faculty can describe, reflect on, and learn from reasoning experiences (their own or those of others) presented in a simulated clinical context within the academic setting has been well argued in the literature[57,58] and is strongly supported by implications from our own research.[1,20] This is consistent with the perspectives of educators designing curricula to promote capability, who emphasized that "it is important to make ways of seeing visible to students."[59(p 40)]

Once a model has been adopted as a framework within which faculty and students can identify clinical reasoning, label it, and critique it, the teaching and learning of more technical professional skills (e.g., therapeutic exercise, gait training, joint mobilization) can be embedded or situated

within the context of clinical reasoning. This then facilitates the building of explicit links in students' knowledge between the "doing" of physical therapy practice and the thinking and experiential learning processes within which the doing takes place.

Curricular Design that Integrates Ethical and Clinical Reasoning

Although there is literature that addresses the ethics curriculum in physical therapy education,[60–63] and Jensen and Paschal[46] discussed means to develop the necessary skills and habits of mind for professional practice, there is no literature available that specifically addresses curricular design to integrate ethical and clinical reasoning. There are elements of curricular design that can support the integration of ethical and clinical reasoning. First, and as was mentioned previously, building a curriculum on a biopsychosocial approach to clinical practice and using the ICF model in all courses where it is directly applicable provides the foundation for an approach to clinical reasoning consistent with the literature. Course sequencing can also play a role in regard to integrating both types of reasoning. Given the importance of narrative reasoning in both and the parallels between hypothetical-deductive reasoning in clinical reasoning and principle-based reasoning in ethical reasoning,[64] a curriculum can be designed to introduce these concepts

BOX 11-3   An Ethical Case that Can Be Used to Develop Narrative Reasoning

Glen is a physical therapist at Community Hospital. Glen is seeing Ms. Williams 3 days after an arthroscopic surgery on her left shoulder. Ms. Williams arrives at the clinic wearing a sling for her left arm. The referral states, "PT s/p arthroscopic subacromial decompression surgery." The referring physician, Dr. Blanding, is the orthopedist who does the highest volume of orthopedic surgery at Community Hospital. During the history, Ms. Williams states that she tore her rotator cuff when she fell while walking her dog and that the surgeon told her he was "going to clean out her shoulder joint." She describes it as a "straightforward" thing, and she expects to be able to use her shoulder again in the next couple of weeks. Ms. Williams tells Glen that the surgeon told her to wear her sling for a week, when she is scheduled to see Dr. Blanding again. Glen finishes the patient interview and lets Ms. Williams know that he needs the operative report from the physician so that he is clear as to what procedure was done. Because it is late in the day, he reschedules Ms. Williams for the next day and makes an effort to obtain the operative report. Glen receives the operative report via fax 5 minutes before Ms. Williams' appointment, and it indicates that a torn supraspinatus tendon was observed. The report states the tendon was surgically repaired using sutures. Glen is now ready to see Ms. Williams and know if he delays the visit any further, he will get behind for the rest of the day. He walks into the room and Ms. Williams asks, "What did the operative report say?"

in close proximity to one another in the curriculum and then reinforce these parallel concepts among the courses. As an example, students can be introduced to narrative reasoning in an ethical context very early in the curriculum through the use of ethical cases (Box 11–3) and role playing, and then, when the concept is later incorporated in clinical reasoning, students bring a familiarity with it at both a conceptual and practical level. By distributing courses that focus on ethics and professional development through the curriculum, one has the opportunity to make further linkages between clinical and ethical reasoning and to use actual cases from the students' preceding clinical experiences that can be used to further develop students' ethical and clinical reasoning capability. An explicit norm among the faculty that establishes the importance of collaboration when developing course learning objectives, approaches to teaching clinical reasoning, and the rubrics faculty use to assess student learning can further integrate clinical reasoning in a consistent manner through the curriculum. As related to clinical reasoning, if those rubrics include criteria that require evidence of ethical reasoning as part of the overall assessment, such as with a standardized patient examination, then students appreciate the inseparability of these forms of reasoning.

Explicit Facilitation of Learning through Clinical Reasoning in Practice Settings

Within clinical education, it has been proposed that clinical reasoning capability can be facilitated through interaction with skilled clinical educators who are aware of, and able to facilitate application of, clinical reasoning models and language that students have been exposed to and practiced in the academic setting.[1] In addition, for true capability in clinical reasoning to be developed, these clinical educators must also be skillful in guiding students toward a personal understanding of clinical reasoning through

participation and critical reflection on clinical reasoning in a real-world clinical context.[1,21] To achieve this, it is critical that clinical and academic classroom educators organize efficient and effective channels of communication in order to coordinate their efforts.

Role of the Clinical Instructor in Fostering Professional Formation through Attention to Clinical Reasoning, Including Ethical Reasoning

The clinical environment, with its frequent demand for clinical and ethical reasoning strategies, provides an ideal avenue for critical self-reflection to foster professional formation. Clinical educators can continue the work begun in the academic setting by continuing to have students write journals on their reasoning processes that build on the four key dimensions of clinical reasoning capability.[41,65] These journals can be guided by specific questions that accomplish the following:

- Reveal the students' meta-cognitive processes (reflective thinking)
- Question their assumptions (critical thinking)
- Examine their relationships with patients and caregivers (complexity thinking)
- Evaluate their deductive and inductive thinking (dialectic thinking)

Table 11–3 provides examples of the types of guided questions one might use in the clinic to develop ethical reasoning skills. Furthermore, given the importance of social processes[66,67] involved in the formation of professional identity, bringing forth the student's beliefs and opinions about clinical and ethical reasoning through dialogue can help students further develop professional identity[68]; this dialogue can occur with either the CI or other physical therapists. A dialogue with a student could use a combination of recent patient encounters and the reflective journals to explore the student's thinking. Because clinical reasoning has multiple possible perspectives, and because the CI and student wish to respect each other's point of view while the CI seeks to develop the student's confidence, that dialogue could take the form of a conversation as opposed to a more directed inquiry.[68] While CIs intentionally model the behaviors they wish to see in students, it is important to make that modeling explicit. Conversations about the student's observations and analysis of the CI's behaviors that exhibit caring, clinical reasoning strategies, and moral approach to patients would bring those modeled behaviors alive in the student's mind.

Central to professional formation is the integration of the moral role of the professional into a student's way of being. The moral role of physical therapists is founded on the trust the patient has placed in the physical therapist to act in the patient's best interest over all others,[45] and with that moral role comes the responsibility to act as a moral agent.[69] Clinical experiences provide an ideal setting to direct specific attention to how students act as moral agents. Students notice the moral aspects of clinical care they observe from CIs and integrate that into their conception of their identity as a physical therapist.[20,68] The student and the CI can each raise questions and explore their ability

TABLE 11-3 Guided Questions to Develop Capability in Ethical Reasoning

Dimension of Clinical Reasoning Capability	Example of a Guiding Question for Journals Using Ethical Reasoning
Reflective thinking	• Write about what you considered as you reasoned through and made a decision that involved ethical considerations. Think about what you included in your reasoning and what you might have omitted.
Critical thinking	• Think about a patient you found difficult to work with. What made the person difficult for you? What role do you think your approach or attitude might have had in making that person difficult to work with?
Complexity thinking	• Write about a time that you found a patient and/or caregiver a challenge for you to deal with. As you think about that challenge, reflect on all the factors you considered in the interaction, including your thinking and feeling. How did those various factors come together to influence the outcome?
Dialectic thinking	• Think about a time that presented an ethical problem for you. For example, you were blocked from doing what you knew was "right," or there were at least two choices of what the right thing to do was, but there was no best thing to. • To what extent did you think of ethical principles, rules, or "everyone who is a physical therapist ought to do this"? • What did you know about the personal story of the other key people involved? What were their motivations? What were their beliefs? How did their past experience influence their thinking, behavior, or emotion? How well did you explore this with these people versus come to conclusions from assumptions?

to act as moral agents when they are thwarted by constraints, such as payment policy or the action of other health care practitioners. To leave this learning at an implicit level would be a disservice to the student and not give adequate recognition to the complexities of the physical therapist's moral role.

Facilitating Critical Self-Reflection about Clinical Reasoning

The facilitation of experiential learning is in itself a skill that requires practice to develop. This type of facilitation can, to a limited extent, take place during practice encounters (e.g., when a CI is observing a student working with a patient) and can be more extensively engaged when done retrospectively, involving the facilitation of critical reflection on a student's past clinical encounters. Ideally these encounters will have been witnessed by the CI, but it is possible (although less ideal) to facilitate a student's critical self-reflection even when the clinical encounter was not witnessed by the CI (e.g., the CI reviews documentation or is presented with a summary of the patient encounter by the student).

Facilitation of critical reflection involves dialogue and questioning. The intent is to help the student to realize what she or he knows and to identify any gaps in knowledge that can direct new learning. By engaging students with strategic questions (rather than "telling" students what they need to know) and probing for blind spots, a CI can lead a student to construct a new understanding. When engaging with students with the intent of facilitating self-reflection on their clinical reasoning, it is important to remember that the focus of the discussion should be just that: What they were thinking? Why they were thinking it? How do they judge the quality of that clinical thinking? The following conceptual framework has been proposed as a useful tool for structuring the breadth and focus of the facilitation and is based on four types of reflection[10]:

Reflective attention is focused on four distinct areas to facilitate critical self-reflection in all relevant aspects of clinical reasoning and experiential learning[70]:

• Content reflection
• Process reflection
• Premise reflection
• Reflection on learning

Content reflection involves critical examination of how a clinician has decided to describe the patient presentation—what it "consists of." Examples of questions that could be posed to a clinician to facilitate this type of critical reflection include, "What do you think are the cause-and-effect relationships underlying the presentation?" and "What is your understanding of the patient's perspectives on his problem?"

Process reflection involves critical examination of the problem-solving (reasoning) strategies being used. Examples of questions that could be posed for this area include, "How did you empirically validate (hypothesis testing) any cause-and-effect relationships you have recognized?" and "How did you determine that you understood your patient's perspectives or story?"

Premise reflection involves questioning the validity of the underlying assumptions that may have guided thinking or actions. Examples of questions to facilitate premise reflection include, "What do you think your assumptions are about the way this type of patient problem usually presents in clinic?" "Do you have any assumptions or biases about the 'type' of patient or person this is?" and "How do you know your assumptions are valid or invalid?"

Finally, reflection on learning involves drawing the students attention to what they feel they have learned through the process of critical self-reflection. Questions that can facilitate this type of synthesis for the learner include, "What have you learned from questioning your assumptions?" "Should you or should you not revise your own perspectives?" and "Will you think or do anything differently in the future based on this experience?"

Our research and teaching experiences strengthen our support for the proposal that active facilitation of the various thinking and learning skills required for both clinical reasoning and reflective learning are critically important for the development of capability in clinical reasoning.[1,21] It has been suggested that facilitation of these thinking and learning skills to enhance continual learning from clinical experiences is beneficial to clinicians of all levels of practice experience[10] and therefore can be viewed as building foundational skills that will continue to enhance lifelong learning and contribute to clinical reasoning capability growth throughout a practitioner's career.

SUMMARY

The clinical reasoning capability of student physical therapists at the time of graduation is arguably the most critical indicator of how well equipped these new graduates are to become increasingly skillful clinicians through critically reflective processing of clinical practice experiences. The intentional provision and facilitation of learning opportunities that guide students toward the development of capability in clinical reasoning, therefore, are an important way in which educators can contribute to improving professional entry educational outcomes. This explicit intention toward development of thinking and learning skills inherent in the practice of skilled clinical reasoners might best be viewed as the development of "ever more sophisticated ways of interpreting experience. So understood, the most critical aspect of a teacher's role is not provision of information, but participation with learners in the development of strategies to interpret that information."[54(p 131)]

THRESHOLD CONCEPTS

Threshold Concept #1: Understanding clinical reasoning

This activity is appropriate for learners at multiple levels of professional education (e.g., entry level, residency, fellowship, transitional Doctor of Physical Therapy); however, the example here is provided from experiences teaching at the entry level.

As discussed in the body of this chapter, an important finding from recent research exploring the understanding and capability in clinical reasoning of student physical therapists[1] was that their understanding of clinical reasoning was limited in breadth and depth and was generally inconsistent with current research-derived models of skilled clinical reasoning and a patient-centered, collaborative approach to practice. The importance of facilitating students' understanding of clinical reasoning was also discussed previously. Therefore, the first threshold concept we have chosen to illustrate with an example of an associated teaching/learning activity is understanding clinical reasoning, consistent with current research-derived models.

In this example, students engage in this small group exercise before receiving any formal curricular content on clinical reasoning definitions, theory, or research-derived models. Students are asked to create a concept map representing their answer to the question "What is clinical reasoning?" To begin, they are instructed to brainstorm onto a large piece of paper anything they can think of that is related to clinical reasoning. Once the group has exhausted their ideas and all are listed on the paper, they are then asked to group these ideas into related categories, name the categories, and determine relationships between the categories. Finally, they are asked to draw a representation of the group's answer on another large piece of paper. This drawing can take any form from a flow chart with arrows to a metaphoric story representing the concepts the group has generated by their brainstorming session (e.g., a tree with roots and branches representing the way disparate concepts function together [see Figure 11–6, A]). Each group then presents their ideas to the larger group, and a discussion is facilitated by the instructor about similarities and differences among the different groups' concept maps. The students sign the back of their map, and the instructor stores these away.

Sometime later, after students have had academic exposure to explicit clinical reasoning content, and after they have had some clinical education exposure, they are asked to repeat this exercise, ideally in the same small groups. The procedure is the same, and the maps are presented to the larger group. The instructor then reveals to each group their first map (or, if done yearly over a 3-year curriculum, their first two maps) and has each group of students reflect on ways in which they feel their current concept map differs from their original map (Figure 11–6). They then present again to the larger group their self-assessment of their own learning over the curriculum, related to clinical reasoning. Integration of a more collaborative, patient-centered approach to clinical reasoning can be seen when contrasting the first drawing (see Figure 11–6, A), with its absence of explicit involvement of the patient, to the second (see Figure 11–6, B), in which the patient and the physical therapist are equal "ingredients" in the cocktail recipe. These types of observations are made by the students themselves as they critically examine their maps, and faculty facilitate the drawing out of other such comparisons in discussion with the larger group.

This educational activity is designed to facilitate the instructor's understanding of where the students are in terms of breadth, depth, and complexity of their understanding of the "whole" of clinical reasoning (e.g., as represented in the Clinical Reasoning Strategies Model[6]). The second time the students generate this map, the instructor is facilitated in understanding what students have learned, and students are facilitated in self-reflection on their understanding and their learning.

Threshold Concept #2: How to teach/facilitate movement between deductive and inductive reasoning within the clinical reasoning strategies

The second threshold concept discussed here is learning dialectic thinking within ethical reasoning. Although the example is focused on ethical reasoning, the approaches to this concept could be used in clinical reasoning in general.

The curriculum at Samuel Merritt University includes two courses on ethics and professionalism, one in the first semester and one in the final semester. The first-semester course (Box 11–4) occurs in the semester before students begin in-depth study of clinical reasoning. Students have two 8-week, full-time clinical experiences before the final course (Box 11–5), and they have a subsequent 6-month internship.

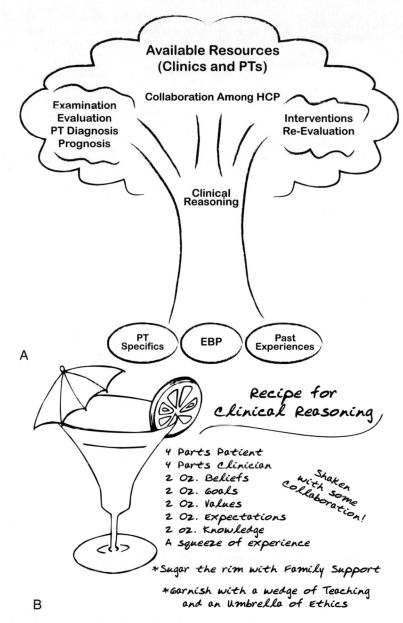

FIGURE 11–6 Clinical reasoning concept maps from **(A)** early in the program, and **(B)** later in the program.

BOX 11–4   Approaches to Teaching and Learning in Professional Issues I Oriented Toward Dialectic Thinking

The model of dialectic thinking in ethical reasoning based on Edwards and Delany's work[19] is introduced conceptually as a whole, and then the deductive and inductive elements are introduced and explored in depth.

Throughout this unit, an ethical case based on a patient with an unclear medical and surgical history who has arrived at the clinic expecting to receive physical therapy that day is used. This case has to be constructed such that the clinical aspects of the case are easily understood, and it was intentionally structured such that the ethical issues at question were embedded in the common occurrences in the everyday practice of physical therapy. The back stories of the people in the case, including the patient, a physical therapist, the clinic manager, and a physician, are purposely left out. The students work in small groups immediately after the discussion of each topic as described below. The case mentioned previously and included in Box 11–3 is an example of the case used for this purpose.

Deductive thinking is introduced through a personal and a professional values sort exercise, which is followed by the introduction of the American Physical Therapy Association (APTA) Core Values.[71] The four ethical principles and ethical rules[72] are introduced, and then the APTA Code of Ethics is introduced and discussed.

The students analyze the case in light of each of these aspects of deductive thinking.

Narrative reasoning is used to begin a discussion of inductive thinking. After a lecture that includes first-person narratives of illness from the literature, students work in small groups, and each student constructs the narrative of one character in the ethics case. The students role-play the case in which they are asked to discover the narrative of the character involved. One group performs the role-play in front of the entire class; this is followed by a large group discussion of the narratives of the case and how those influence ethical decisions. Finally, the students are asked to come to a resolution of the case that requires them to consider both deductive and inductive thinking as they have discussed it in their groups.

The final examination in the course includes an ethical case in which the students must address the key ethical principles involved in the case, distinguish the pertinent principles from the APTA Code of Ethics, and identify questions they would use to discover the narratives of the patient and her caregiver that are at the center of the case. They must come to a resolution that incorporates both elements of the dialectic.

BOX 11–5   Approaches to Teaching and Learning in Professional Issues II Oriented Toward Dialectic Thinking

In this course, the students bring a case that presented ethical problems for them from their just completed clinical experience. That case then provides the basis for further discussion during the semester. There is a review and discussion of the ethical reasoning model presented in the first course. The students then write a guided critical self-reflection that asks them to address their deductive thinking that occurred in the clinic while they experienced the case, what their thinking is in that regard in retrospect, and what their narrative reasoning was in the moment and in retrospect. This critical self-reflection is reviewed by the instructor and, with their written case, serves as the basis for a series of discussions with groups of 4 to 6 students, 8 to 12 students, and 18 to 20 students. The latter two groups are facilitated by the instructor, whereas the smallest group discussion is not. The instructor directs the discussion toward aspects of deductive or inductive reasoning that may have not been given due consideration and the possible implications arising from that lack of consideration, including how a better understanding of the ethical reasoning might have resulted in a different outcome.

The students then write a critical analysis and self-reflection of their case in which they must discuss their deductive and inductive reasoning, including the importance of the absence or too little attention to either element of the dialectic played in their ethical reasoning. They also address how biases, assumptions, and judgments affected their reasoning and how they addressed any residuals from the case.[73] They conclude the paper with a reflection in which they think forward to their roles as a physical therapy intern, a physical therapist, and a CI as related to ethical reasoning and teaching ethical reasoning to future students. The grading rubric for the paper aligns with all of these required elements.

ANNOTATED BIBLIOGRAPHY

Edwards I, Delany C. Ethical reasoning. In: Higgs J, Jones M, Loftus S, Christensen N, eds. *Clinical Reasoning in the Health Professions*. 3rd ed. Amsterdam: Elsevier; 2008

This chapter places the empirical research that Edwards and colleagues did on clinical reasoning and ethical reasoning in the broader context of ethics. It provides a foundation for dialectic thinking in ethical reasoning as well as models that can be used for teaching ethical reasoning that are easily understood. The model of ethical reasoning can serve as a foundation to build inductive and deductive thinking when considering ethical reasoning. The authors provide both a solid grounding in ethical theory and practical application in education and practice.

Edwards I, Jones M. Clinical reasoning and expertise. In: Jensen GM, Gwyer J, Hack LM, Shepard KF, eds. *Expertise in Physical Therapy Practice*. 2nd ed. Boston: Elsevier; 2007:192–213

In this chapter, Edwards and Jones present the full dialectical clinical reasoning model with explanatory text. The model is represented graphically, and the explanation of this qualitative research-derived description of expert clinical reasoning is layered in easily digested pieces, effectively facilitating the reader's understanding of how the clinical reasoning strategies are situated within this larger context of dialectical reasoning, comprising deductive and inductive components.

Purtilo RB, Jensen GM, Brasic Royeen C. *Educating for Moral Action: A Sourcebook in Health and Rehabilitation Ethics*. Philadelphia: FA Davis; 2005.

This sourcebook provides a series of writings that meet the editors' intended goal of challenging common thinking about ethics and how it is taught in the rehabilitation professions. Each chapter is written by a leading scholar in the field and addresses relevant and diverse topics as stigma, social responsibility, and spirituality. Of particular note for the content in this text are chapters by Swisher on the professional ethics curriculum and Mostrom on clinically based learning about the ethical basis of care.

REFERENCES

1. Christensen N. *Development of clinical reasoning capability in student physical therapists*. Doctor of Philosophy Thesis. Adelaide, South Australia, Australia: University of South Australia; 2009. Available at *http://arrow.unisa.edu.au:8081/1959.8/77781*.
2. Benner P. *From Novice to Expert: Excellence and Power in Clinical Nursing Practice*. Menlo Park: Addison-Wesley; 1984.
3. Benner P, Tanner C, Chesla C. *Expertise in Nursing Practice: Caring, Clinical Judgment, and Ethics*. New York: Springer; 1996.
4. Mattingly C, Fleming MH. *Clinical Reasoning: Forms of Inquiry in a Therapeutic Practice*. Philadelphia: FA Davis; 1994.
5. Jensen GM, Gwyer J, Shepard KF, Hack LM. Expert practice in physical therapy. *Phys Ther*. 2000;80:28–43.
6. Edwards I, Jones M, Carr J, et al. Clinical reasoning strategies in physical therapy. *Phys Ther*. 2004;84:312–335.
7. Higgs J, Jones MA. Clinical decision making and multiple problem spaces. In: Higgs J, Jones MA, Loftus S, Christensen N, eds. *Clinical Reasoning in the Health Professions*. 3rd ed. Amsterdam: Butterworth Heinemann Elsevier; 2008:3–18.
8. Jones MA, Jensen G, Edwards I. Clinical reasoning in physiotherapy. In: Higgs J, Jones MA, Loftus S, Christensen N, eds. *Clinical Reasoning in the Health Professions*. 3rd ed. Amsterdam: Elsevier; 2008:245–256.
9. Nikopoulou-Smyrni P, Nikopoulos C. A new integrated model of clinical reasoning: development, description and preliminary assessment in patients with stroke. *Disabil Rehabil*. 2007;29:1129–1138.
10. Christensen N, Jones MA, Edwards I. *Clinical reasoning and evidence-based practice. Independent Study Course 21.2.2: Current Concepts of Orthopaedic Physical Therapy*. 3rd ed La Crosse, WI: Orthopaedic Section, APTA; 2011.
11. Edwards I, Jones M. Clinical reasoning and expertise. In: Jensen GM, Gwyer J, Hack LM, Shepard KF, eds. *Expertise in Physical Therapy Practice*. 2nd ed. Boston: Elsevier; 2007:192–213.
12. Edwards I, Jones M, Higgs J, Trede F, Jensen G. What is collaborative reasoning? *Adv Physiother*. 2004;6:70–83.
13. Stephenson RC. Using a complexity model of human behaviour to help interprofessional clinical reasoning. *Int J Ther Rehabil*. 2004;11:168–175.
14. Jensen GM, Shepard KF, Gwyer J, Hack LM. Attribute dimensions that distinguish master and novice physical therapy clinicians in orthopedic settings. *Phys Ther*. 1992;72:711–722.
15. Jensen G, Shepard KF, Hack LM. The novice versus the experienced clinician: insights into the work of the physical therapist. *Phys Ther*. 1990;70:314–323.
16. Resnik L, Jensen GM. Using clinical outcomes to explore the theory of expert practice in physical therapy. *Phys Ther*. 2003;83:1090–1106.
17. Jensen G, Gwyer J, Hack LM, Shepard KF. *Expertise in Physical Therapy Practice*. 2nd ed. St. Louis: Saunders Elsevier; 2007.
18. Edwards I, Braunack-Mayer A, Jones M. Ethical reasoning as a clinical-reasoning strategy in physiotherapy. *Physiotherapy*. 2005;91: 229–236.
19. Edwards I, Delany C. Ethical reasoning. In: Higgs J, Jones MA, Loftus S, Christensen N, eds. *Clinical Reasoning in the Health Professions*. 3rd ed. Amsterdam: Butterworth Heinemann Elsevier; 2008:279–290.
20. Nordstrom T. *Physical therapist students as moral agents during clinical experiences [EdD Dissertation]*. Available through Dissertation Abstracts International 69(06) 2008A. UMI Number ATT 3317689. San Francisco: University of San Francisco Press; 2008.
21. Christensen N, Jones MA, Edwards I, Higgs J. Helping physiotherapy students develop clinical reasoning capability. In: Higgs J, Jones MA, Loftus S, Christensen N, eds. *Clinical Reasoning in the Health Professions*. 3rd ed. Amsterdam: Elsevier; 2008:389–396.
22. Christensen N, Jones MA, Higgs J, Edwards I. Dimensions of clinical reasoning capability. In: Higgs J, Jones MA, Loftus S, Christensen N, eds. *Clinical Reasoning in the Health Professions*. 3rd ed. Amsterdam: Elsevier; 2008:101–110.
23. Barnitt R, Partridge C. Ethical reasoning in physical therapy and occupational therapy. *Physiother Res Int*. 1997;2:178–194.
24. Barnitt R. Ethical dilemmas in occupational therapy and physical therapy: a survey of practitioners in the UK National Health Service. *J Med Ethics*. 1998;24:193–199.
25. Barnitt R. Truth telling in occupational therapy and physiotherapy. *Br J Occup Ther*. 1994;57:334–340.
26. Carpenter C. Dilemmas of practice as experienced by physical therapists in rehabilitation settings. *Physiother Can*. 2005;57:63–76.
27. Geddes EL, Wessel J, Williams RM. Ethical issues identified by physical therapy students during clinical placements. *Physiother Theory Pract*. 2004;20:17–29.
28. Greenfield B. The meaning of caring in five experienced physical therapists. *Physiother Theory Pract*. 2006;22:175–187.
29. Greenfield BH, Anderson A, Cox B, Tanner MC. Meaning of caring to 7 novice physical therapists during their first year of clinical practice. *Phys Ther*. 2008;88:1154–1166.

30. McGee BJ, Ogger J. *Journaling of ethical considerations during the clinical internship year.* [Masters Thesis] Mt. Pleasant: Program in Physical Therapy, Central Michigan University; 2000.

31. Stiller C. Exploring the ethos of the physical therapy profession in the United States: social, cultural, and historical influences and their relationship to education. *J Phys Ther Educ.* 2000;14:7–15.

32. Triezenberg HL. The identification of ethical issues in physical therapy practice. *Phys Ther* 1996;76:1097–1107; discussion, 1107–1108.

33. World Health Organization. *International Classification of Functioning, Disability and Health.* Geneva: World Health Organization; 2001.

34. American Physical Therapy Association. *Evaluative criteria for accreditation of education programs for the preparation of physical therapists.* Alexandria, VA: American Physical Therapy Association; 2005.

35. Finley C, Goldstein M. Curriculum survey: ethical and legal instruction—a report from the APTA Department of Education and the APTA Judicial Committee. *J Phys Ther Educ.* 1991;5:60–64.

36. Benner P, Sutphen M, Leonard V, Day L. *Educating Nurses: A Call for Radical Transformation.* San Francisco: Jossey-Bass; 2010.

37. Cook M, Irby D, O'Brien B. *Educating Physicians: A Call for Reform of Medical School and Residency.* San Francisco: Jossey-Bass; 2010.

38. Foster C, Dahill L, Golemon L, Tolentino B. *Educating Clergy: Teaching Practices and Pastoral Imagination.* San Francisco: Jossey-Bass; 2006.

39. Sullivan W. *Work and Integrity: The Crisis and Promise of Professionalism in America.* 2nd ed. San Francisco: Jossey-Bass; 2005.

40. Sullivan W, Colby A, Wegner J, Bond L, Shulman W. *Educating Lawyers: Preparation for the Profession of Law.* San Francisco: Jossey-Bass; 2007.

41. Sullivan W. Can Professionalism Still be a Viable Ethic? *Good Society.* 2004;13:15–20.

42. Wenger E. *Communities of Practice: Learning, Meaning, and Identity.* Cambridge, UK: Cambridge University Press; 1998.

43. Jensen GM, Gwyer J, Shepard KF. Expert practice in physical therapy. *Phys Ther* 2000;80:28–43; discussion, 44–52.

44. Triezenberg HL. Examining the moral role of physical therapists. In: Purtilo R, Jensen G, Brassic Royeen C, eds. *Educating for Moral Action: A Sourcebook in Health and Rehabilitation Ethics.* Philadelphia: FA Davis; 2005:85–97.

45. American Physical Therapy Association. *Advanced Credentialed Clinical Instructor Program for the Physical Therapist.* Alexandria, VA: American Physical Therapy Association; 2007.

46. Jensen GM, Paschal KA. Habits of mind: student transition toward virtuous practice. *J Phys Ther Educ.* 2000;14:42–47.

47. Stephenson J. The concept of capability and its importance in higher education. In: Stephenson J, Yorke M, eds. *Capability and Quality in Higher Education.* London: Kogan Page; 1998:1–13.

48. Doncaster K, Lester S. Capability and its development: experiences from a work-based doctorate. *Studies Higher Educ.* 2002;27:91–101.

49. Schön D. *Educating the Reflective Practitioner: Toward a New Design for Teaching and Learning in the Professions.* San Francisco: Jossey-Bass; 1987.

50. Wainwright S, Shepard K, Harman L, Stephens J. Novice and experienced physical therapist clinicians: a comparison of how reflection is used to inform the clinical decision making process. *Phys Ther.* 2010;90:75–88.

51. Scriven M, Paul R. *Defining critical thinking.* Available at: http://www.criticalthinking.org/aboutCT/definingCT.shtml; Accessed 28.07.06.

52. Forneris SG. Exploring the attributes of critical thinking: a conceptual basis. *Int J Nurs Scholar* 2004;1: Article 9.

53. Plsek PE, Greenhalgh T. Complexity science: the challenge of complexity in health care. *Br Med J.* 2001;323:625–628.

54. Davis B, Sumara D, Luce-Kapler R. *Engaging Minds: Learning and Teaching in a Complex World.* Mahwah, NJ: Lawrence Erlbaum Associates; 2000.

55. Stephenson R. The complexity of pain: Part 2. Pain as a complex adaptive system. Phys Ther Rev. 1999;4:183–194.

56. Jones MA, Rivett DA. Introduction to clinical reasoning. In: Jones MA, Rivett DA, eds. *Clinical Reasoning for Manual Therapists.* Edinburgh: Butterworth Heinemann, 2004:3–24.

57. Loftus S, Higgs J. Learning the language of clinical reasoning. In: Higgs J, Jones MA, Loftus S, Christensen N, eds. *Clinical Reasoning in the Health Professions.* 3rd ed. Amsterdam: Butterworth Heinemann Elsevier; 2008:339–348.

58. Ajjawi R, Higgs J. Learning to communicate clinical reasoning. In: Higgs J, Jones MA, Loftus S, Christensen N, eds. *Clinical Reasoning in the Health Professions.* 3rd ed. Amsterdam: Butterworth Heinemann Elsevier; 2008:331–338.

59. Bowden J, Marton F. *The University of Learning: Beyond Quality and Competence.* London: RoutledgeFalmer; 1998.

60. Barnitt R, Roberts L. Facilitating ethical reasoning in student physical therapists. *J Phys Ther Educ.* 2000;14:35–41.

61. Swisher LL. Environment, Professional Identity, and the Roles of the Ethics Educator: An Agenda for Development of the Professional Ethics Curriculum. In: Purtilo RB, Jensen GM, Brasic Royeet C, eds. *Educating for Moral Action: A Sourcebook in Health and Rehabilitation Ethics.* Philadelphia: FA Davis; 2005:225–238.

62. Triezenberg HL. Teachings ethics in physical therapy education. *J Phys Ther Educ.* 1997;11:16–22.

63. Triezenberg HL, Davis C. Beyond the code of ethics: educating physical therapists for their role as moral agents. *J Phys Ther Educ.* 2000;14:48–58.

64. Edwards I, Delany C. Ethical reasoning. In: Higgs J, Jones M, Loftus S, Christensen N, eds. *Clinical Reasoning in the Health Professions.* 3rd ed. Amsterdam: Elsevier; 2008.

65. Triezenberg HL, McGrath JH. The use of narrative in an applied ethics course for physical therapist students. *J Phys Ther Educ.* 2001;15:49–56.

66. Griffin D. *Emergence of Leadership: Linking Self-Organization and Ethics.* London: Routledge; 2002.

67. Stacey R. *Complex Responsive Processes in Organizations.* London: Routledge; 2001.

68. Mostrom E. Teaching and learning about the ethical and human dimensions of care in clinical education: exploring student and clinical instructor experiences in physical therapy. In: Jensen G, Purtilo R, Brassic Royeen C, eds. *Educating for Moral Action: A Sourcebook in Health and Rehabilitation Ethics.* Philadelphia: FA Davis; 2005:265–283.

69. Purtilo RB. New respect for respect in ethics education. In: Purtilo R, Jensen G, Brassic Royeen C, eds. *Educating for Moral Action: A Sourcebook in Health and Rehabilitation Ethics.* Philadelphia: FA Davis; 2005:1–10.

70. Cranton P. *Understanding and Promoting Transformative Learning: A Guide for Education of Adults.* San Francisco: Jossey-Bass; 1994.

71. American Physical Therapy Association. *Professionalism in Physical Therapy: Core Values.* Available at: http://www.apta.org/AM/Template.cfm?Section=Policies_and_Bylaws&TEMPLATE=/CM/ContentDisplay.cfm&CONTENTID=36073; 2008 Accessed 19.03.08.

72. Beauchamp T, Childress J. *Principles of Biomedical Ethics.* 5th ed. New York: Oxford University Press; 2001.

73. Marcus R. Moral dilemmas and consistency. *J Philos.* 1980;77: 121–136.

PATIENT EDUCATION AND HEALTH LITERACY

Elizabeth Mostrom

CHAPTER OUTLINE

The following excerpts are drawn from reflective journals of students as they learn important lessons about patient education during clinical internships:

- *I had this one patient with neck and arm pain and she seemed really stressed out about the problem and worried that she might get worse with therapy. So I decided to keep her initial home exercise program really simple at first and I gave her only three very mild stretching exercises to do. Well, the next session she came back and I asked her to show me her exercises like she was doing them at home. I couldn't believe what I saw!! I could hardly recognize what she was doing! From now on, I am going to go very slowly when teaching exercises—I am going to have the patient show me the exercises several times in therapy and make sure that they have written home programs with pictures and simple explanations on them. I think I rushed my teaching with this patient and was too timid in my instructions because she was so worried about getting worse.[1(p 308)]*

- *If I have a hard time finding time to do trunk strengthening exercises [that I need to do], then don't my patients have a hard time finding time to do a home exercise program? I think that therapists, including me, forget that parents who have a child who needs to do a HEP have busy lives and may not have time to do the program with their child. If I can keep this in mind, I think I will have better success when it comes to designing a HEP and having the patient actually do it. Also, when I ask a parent or child if they have been doing the HEP, I have to be prepared for the "no's" and armed with the "why's" to do the program and the "how's" to fit it in.[1(p 309)]*

- *Another time I felt good was when I was describing to the patient what was happening with her. I got out the model of the spine and showed her the area from which the problem stemmed. I educated her on the discs and nerve roots.*

She really seemed to benefit from the discussion and learned a lot. She said it made her understand the purpose of her exercise program and of the treatments we were doing with her. It made me feel good because I felt effective.[1(p 309)]

LEARNING GOALS

After completing this chapter, the reader will be able to:

1. Describe the scope and breadth of the "literacy problem" in the United States and accurately identify specific patient populations seen in physical therapy who are at risk for low literacy.

2. Define and distinguish between the following terms: general literacy, literacy domains, literacy levels, health literacy, readability, suitability, and comprehension.

3. Discuss risk factors and behavioral cues that might indicate low health literacy in patients and identify appropriate methods for assessing and addressing their literacy needs to achieve desired educational and health-related outcomes.

4. Describe characteristics of effective verbal and nonverbal communication with patients that can create a shame-free clinical environment, facilitate the development of positive relationships, enhance learning, and foster comprehension.

5. Assess the literacy demands, readability, and suitability of written educational materials developed for patients using selected informal methods or formal tools and instruments.

6. Identify or develop home programs, instructional materials, or media resources that are appropriately designed to meet the learning needs and goals of patients and their care providers.

7. Describe and implement several teaching/learning activities that can link classroom instruction about patient education and health literacy with experiential learning in clinical settings.

8. Describe, design, and implement teaching/learning activities that provide opportunities for reflection and dialogue about patient education and health literacy during clinical experiences.

Through these excerpts we hear students reflecting on both failures and successes in patient education. How could an understanding of health literacy further inform the practice and teaching effectiveness of these students and of physical therapy clinicians? This is a question we will explore and address in this chapter.

CENTRALITY OF PATIENT EDUCATION TO EFFECTIVE CLINICAL PRACTICE AND ACHIEVEMENT OF DESIRED HEALTH OUTCOMES

Numerous documents directly related to physical therapy practice and education emphasize the centrality and importance of patient education in the everyday work of physical therapists.[2–6] The American Physical Therapy Association (APTA) *Guide to Physical Therapy Practice*[2] identifies patient/client instruction as a key component of intervention in the patient/client management model and defines patient/client related instruction as follows: "The process of informing, educating, or training patients/clients, families, significant others and caregivers is intended to promote and optimize physical therapy services. Instruction may be related to the current condition; specific impairments, functional limitations, or disabilities; plan of care; need for enhanced performance; transition to a different role or setting; risk factors for developing a problem or dysfunction; or need for health, wellness, or fitness programs. Physical therapists are responsible for patient/client related instruction across all settings for all patients/clients."[2(p 47)] This definition highlights the depth and breadth of a therapist's responsibility for effective teaching and promoting learning in clinical encounters in a wide variety of practice settings.

In addition, The Joint Commission standards for accreditation of hospitals and other health care organizations require that individual providers and organizations provide effective, "patient-centered" communications to optimize the quality of care delivered and ensure patient understandings and safety.[7] Those standards require, among other

things, that education provided to patients is based on assessment of patient and family/caregiver needs (both clinical and communication needs), addresses their needs, is appropriate and adapted to the patient's level of understanding and abilities, and is delivered using a variety of instructional tools or methods, and that patient comprehension of educational information provided is evaluated. During the past decade, as the standards for patient-provider communication have been further developed and elaborated, The Joint Commission has also spearheaded several initiatives in this area that have culminated in reports that highlight the importance of addressing literacy issues and concerns as health care professionals and organizations serve an increasingly diverse and aging citizenry in the United States.[8–10]

Finally, the new *Healthy People 2020*[11] (HP 2020) framework and objectives encourage increased emphasis on health communication and the effective use of information technology to achieve the overarching goals of HP 2020. The broad goals of HP 2020 and selected health communication and information technology objectives are shown in Box 12–1.

Clearly, the time for focused attention on the health literacy of the patients, family members, and care providers we encounter in our daily work as physical therapists is here. Furthermore, as our scope of practice continues to expand in the realms of community-based education, health promotion, and wellness, attention to the health literacy of the larger population of individuals in our society is essential for us to be effective health educators. (See also Chapters 13 and 15.)

SCOPE AND MAGNITUDE OF THE "LITERACY PROBLEM" IN THE UNITED STATES

Surprisingly, focused attention on general literacy concerns, and more recently health literacy concerns, in the United States is a relatively recent trend in our history. In response to these concerns, however, the first nationwide assessment of adult literacy, the National Adult

---

BOX 12–1   Healthy People 2020 Overarching Goals and Selected Related Health Communication and Health Information Technology Objectives

HEALTHY PEOPLE 2020 OVERARCHING GOALS

- Attain high-quality, longer lives free of preventable disease, disability, injury, and premature death.
- Achieve health equity, eliminate disparities, and improve the health of all groups.
- Create social and physical environments that promote good health for all.
- Promote quality of life, healthy development, and healthy behaviors across all stages of life.

SELECTED HEALTH COMMUNICATION AND HEALTH INFORMATION TECHNOLOGY OBJECTIVES

- Improve the health literacy of the population.
- Increase the proportion of persons who report that their health care provider always gave them easy-to-understand instructions about what to do to take care of their illness or health condition.
- Increase the proportion of persons who report that their health care provider always asked them to describe how they will follow the instructions.

- Increase the proportion of persons who report that their health care provider's office always offered help in filling out a form.
- Increase the proportion of persons who report that their health care providers have satisfactory communication skills.
- Increase the proportion of persons who report that their health care provider always listened carefully to them.
- Increase the proportion of persons who report that their health care provider always explained things so that they could understand them.
- Increase the proportion of persons who report that their health care provider always showed respect for what they had to say.
- Increase the proportion of persons who report that their health care provider always spent enough time with them.
- Increase the proportion of persons who report that their health care provider always involved them in decisions about their health care as much as they wanted.
- Increase the proportion of persons whose doctor recommends personalized health information resources to help them manage their health.

BOX 12–2   Functional Tasks Needed to Access, Understand, and Use Information

- Prose tasks: The knowledge and skills needed to understand and use information from text materials such as newspapers, magazines, books, brochures, etc.
- Document tasks: The knowledge and skills needed to find, interpret, and use information from documents such as applications, forms, maps, transportation schedules, charts, etc.
- Quantitative tasks: The knowledge and skills required to read, interpret, and work with numerical information and apply mathematics to calculate or reason numerically such as reading nutrition labels and calculating calories, computing restaurant bills and tips, balancing a checkbook, etc.

Literacy Survey (NALS), was conducted by the U.S. Department of Education in 1992. That survey and a 10-year follow-up study, the 2003 National Assessment of Adult Literacy (NAAL), revealed a high prevalence of illiteracy and low literacy in the United States.[12–14] The NALS and the NAAL defined general literacy as, "Using printed and written information to function in society, to achieve one's goals, and to develop one's knowledge and potential."[14]

In the 2003 NAAL, the literacy skills of a representative sample of about 20,000 adults (defined as 16 years or older) were measured in three domains. These domains represent three functional tasks that individuals would need to access, understand, and use information (Box 12–2).

In the NAAL, the degrees of difficulty for literacy tasks in these the domains were identified as below basic, basic, intermediate, or proficient. Brief descriptions of these levels and the findings from the 2003 NAAL are shown in Table 12–1. Note that 55% of the sample population was determined to be at the basic or below basic level for quantitative tasks; 43% of the sample population was determined to be at the basic or below basic level for prose tasks; and 34% of the sample population was determined to be at the basic or below basic level for document tasks. If you think about the kinds of tasks patients are required to do in the course of clinical care, those individuals at the basic or below basic level (55% in the quantitative category, 43% in the prose category) might experience significant difficulty completing intake forms, comparing drug plans, identifying what they may or may not drink or eat before a medical test, or following written instructions on prescriptions to determine correct dosages. Even those individuals at the intermediate level (53% in the document category, 44% in the prose category) may have difficulty fully understanding insurance forms and plans, consent forms, and medication and other health care instructions.

In the 2003 NAAL, a health literacy scale was included, and tasks specific to health literacy were assessed nationwide for the first time. The development of this scale and the tasks included in the assessment were guided by a definition of health literacy that had been adopted by the Institute of Medicine[15] and used by Healthy People 2010.[16] Health Literacy was defined as, "[t]he degree to which individuals have the capacity to obtain, process, and understand basic health information and services needed to make appropriate health decisions."[15(p 32)] The health literacy tasks in the NAAL were distributed across three domains of health care services or information:

1. Clinical care (e.g., understanding health or medication dosing instructions or filling out a form)
2. Prevention services and information (e.g., following guidelines for prevention services such as immunizations)
3. Navigation of the health care system (e.g., understanding an insurance plan or determining eligibility for assistance)

In each of those domains, literacy tasks were identified as primarily prose, document, or quantitative tasks.

The health literacy results of the NAAL were published in 2006[17] and underscored the need for health care professionals, health care organizations, and the health care system as a whole to "take health literacy seriously."[18,19] The overall findings are shown in Figure 12–1 and indicated that 36% of adults in the sample (representing more than 75 million adults) had basic or below basic levels of health literacy: this means their overall literacy skills were at about an 8th-grade level or below. Of these individuals, 14% were measured at the below basic level and would be considered functionally illiterate when dealing with health information. Fifty-three percent of the individuals in the sample (representing about 114 million adults) were rated in the intermediate level of health literacy (about 10th- to 12th-grade level), and only 12% of the population was considered proficient (see Figure 12–1). Two percent of the individuals in the NAAL sample (representing about 4 million adults) had language barriers that prevented participation and were unable to be measured. Those individuals were categorized as nonliterate in English, although it is important to note that they may be literate in their

---

TABLE 12–1   Descriptions of Literacy Levels and Findings from the 2003 National Assessment of Adult Literacy

Literacy Level	Prose (%)	Document (%)	Quantitative (%)	Approximate Grade Level (Prose)
Below basic: non-literate in English or only able to complete easy, concrete literacy tasks	14	12	22	About 5th grade or below
Basic: able to complete simple everyday literacy tasks	29	22	33	About 8th grade
Intermediate: able to complete moderately challenging literacy tasks	44	53	33	About 10th grade to high school
Proficient: able to perform complex and challenging literacy tasks	13	13	13	About high school graduate–to college

From National Center for Education Statistics. 2003 National Assessment of Adult Literacy (NAAL). Available at: http://nces.ed.gov//naal/resources/execsumm.asp.

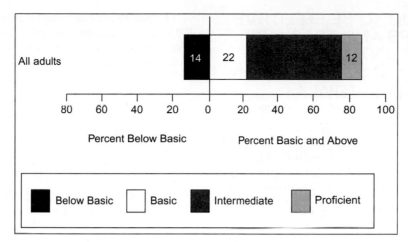

FIGURE 12–1 Percentage of adults in each health literacy level. (From National Center for Education Statistics. The Health Literacy of America's Adults: Results from the 2003 National Assessment of Adult Literacy. Washington, DC: U.S Department of Education, Institute for Education Sciences, 2006.)

primary language. The findings also identified several risk factors and populations at risk for low health literacy, and these will be discussed further in the next sections of this chapter.

The good news that emerges from these rather disturbing findings is that there has been increasing attention given to addressing the health literacy problem in the United States, and many initiatives have been undertaken to make health information more accessible, clear, and understandable in all forms (oral, visual, and textual) so that a much larger percentage of the population can evaluate, use, and benefit from the information provided by health care professionals. There is a clear realization that we must not only address health literacy concerns but also move as rapidly as possible toward solutions at the level of individual providers, health care organizations and systems, and health policy makers. This vision and commitment are captured in a summary in the National Action Plan to Improve Health Literacy: "By focusing on health literacy issues and working together, we can improve the accessibility, quality, and safety of health care; reduce costs; and improve the health and quality of life of millions of people in the United States."[20]

IMPLICATIONS OF LOW LITERACY FOR INDIVIDUAL AND PUBLIC HEALTH

It is likely that the readers of this chapter are individuals who have at least college-level education and beyond. Think about some of your own encounters in the health care system over the past few years. Have there been times when you were uncertain about or confused by health information provided to you? When, exactly, to take a medication? What food or drink you should avoid before a medical test? How and when, exactly, to do a prescribed activity? Have you ever been befuddled by the language used in various forms you were asked to sign when consenting to care? Or explaining your HIPAA rights? Now, think about individuals trying to understand the complex instructions often given by health care providers or

navigating the health care system with substantially lower literacy skills than you have. What might be their understandings—or misunderstandings? Could misunderstandings have serious consequences? What happens if the "signals" they receive from health care providers are confusing or not accurately interpreted as they were intended?

The reader is encouraged to view several videos available on health literacy at the American Medical Association (AMA) website entitled, "Low Health Literacy: You Can't Tell by Looking" and "Health Literacy and Patient Safety: Help Patients Understand." An additional video by the Institute of Medicine entitled, "Health Literacy: A Prescription to End Confusion" is available on YouTube. These videos will help students and clinicians gain a clearer sense of the personal experiences of individuals with low literacy skills in our health care system.

There is a large and growing body of literature that suggests links between low literacy and poor health outcomes, but it is beyond the scope or intent of this chapter to review all of that literature. A report from the Agency for Health Care Research and Quality (AHCRQ), however, provides a review of evidence and a summary of the many links between low literacy and poor health outcomes, health status, and health disparities.[21,22] What we do know from the literature is that low health literacy can lead to low health knowledge and understanding and thus less healthy behaviors, safety concerns for patients and others involved in their care, disparities in access to and quality of care delivered, and greater health costs for individuals and society. We also know that "literacy skills are a stronger predictor of an individual's health status than age, income, employment status, educational level, and racial or ethnic group."[23,24] Given the high prevalence of low health literacy skills in our population and the health and societal consequences associated with low literacy, it is incumbent on all health professionals to respond. We must do this in order to address the patient's right to and need for clear communication about their health, to reduce the potential for error and increase patient safety, to enhance the quality of health care services, and to contain health care costs.

WHAT CAN WE DO TO BE EFFECTIVE COMMUNICATORS AND TEACHERS AND FOSTER PATIENT LEARNING?

RECOGNIZING POPULATIONS AT RISK, RISK FACTORS, AND HEALTH LITERACY CHALLENGES

Based on the findings from the health literacy component of the 2003 NAAL,[14,17] we know several groups of individuals are at higher risk for health literacy concerns (Table 12–2).

A quick review of the list in Table 12–2 suggests that many of the individuals we see in our clinics on a daily basis may fall into several of these groups or present with several risk factors for low health literacy concurrently. Being aware of the potential for health literacy concerns is a first step toward responding appropriately but much more is needed. In the following section, we will discuss several strategies and tools clinicians can use for assessing health literacy.

ASSESSING HEALTH LITERACY: INFORMAL ASSESSMENTS

Physical therapists and rehabilitation and health professionals in general are excellent observers. Combined with our recognition of the prevalence of low health literacy in the U.S. population, we can use our keen observational and interviewing skills to identify clues for low literacy or alert us to "red flags." Picking up on these clues and identifying red flags will allow us to adapt our educational interventions to better meet the needs of our patients. Table 12–3 provides a list of some red flags that you may have encountered in your interactions with patients. Can you identify others?

Some of the behaviors and responses described in Table 12–3 may be due to many patients with low literacy feeling ashamed about their difficulty reading and trying to hide it—even from family members in some cases.[25,26] Because of the potential for shame or stigma, patients may also be hesitant to admit to health professionals that they have difficulty reading or understanding health information. Therefore, we need to develop strategies for assessing and addressing literacy concerns by creating clinical environments and encounters that are "shame free" and reduce the potential for embarrassment or humiliation of the patient.

Therapists can use the social history and the subjective portion of their examination to screen for possible literacy concerns for their patients. For example, as you review information available to you in the medical chart, intake forms, or referrals, be alert for the risk factors identified in Table 12–2. If any of those factors are or may be present, then be on heightened alert for the behaviors listed in Table 12–3. It is also important to remember that stress associated with illness, injury, and disability, in and of itself, can create barriers to communication and understanding of complex health information.

As you conduct the subjective portion of the examination, try to ask questions that would get at the potential for literacy problems while being as nonthreatening as possible to the patient. Some suggestions for questions that may be useful and help to open the door for the patient to discuss their abilities in this realm are shown in Box 12–3.

The last three questions in Box 12–3 were identified by Chew and colleagues[27] as effective screening questions for identifying patients with insufficient health literacy (below basic level), although they were less effective in identifying individuals with marginal health literacy (5th- to 8th-grade level, basic level). In a follow-up study, Wallace and colleagues[28] found that the single most useful question for screening for limited and marginal literacy was the last question in Box 12–3 regarding confidence in filling out medical forms.

Finally, it is worth noting that merely asking the patient's highest school grade completed or educational level is not always the best indicator of their actual literacy skills. There can be a 2- to 5-year discrepancy between grade level attained and a patient's true reading abilities.[29] That is, someone could have completed 10th grade but still read at 5th- or 6th-grade level (basic or below basic). It is also important to note that oral communication skills may be far better than reading skills for an individual with low literacy.

Another informal method for assessing literacy skills is to complete a medication review with the patient. Although some may view this activity as more the purview of nurses, physicians or physician's assistants, or pharmacists, in today's health care environment where therapists have direct access to patients/clients and responsibility for medical screening and keep-refer decision making, a medication review can be an invaluable clinical and literacy screening tool. Completing a medication review simply requires that you ask patients to bring their medications to therapy and then spend time talking with your patients about their medications. During the discussion, you can assess the patients' understanding of what medications they are taking, why they are taking them, when they are taking them, and how they are taking them (e.g., with or without food). Once completed, you will have valuable information that will guide the development of appropriate interventions and monitoring strategies from both a clinical *and* literacy perspective. As noted earlier, patients with low health literacy may rely on the visual appearance of the pill or a few letters in the name of the medication to identify what they are taking. They may not know what the medication is for or how or when to take it and may become confused when asked about their medications. An excellent example of a medication review conducted with a patient with low health literacy can be viewed in the AMA video referred to earlier in this chapter, "Health Literacy and Patient Safety: Help Patients Understand" and available on YouTube.

ASSESSING HEALTH LITERACY: FORMAL ASSESSMENTS

There are also formal testing tools that have been developed to screen for low health literacy skills in patients. Many of the tools are used primarily for research purposes and are too lengthy or unwieldy to realistically use in clinical practice. Furthermore, the administration of some tests for literacy may be threatening to individuals with low literacy skills and increase the potential for feelings of shame or stigmatization. For the purposes of this chapter, I introduce two tools that are brief and easy to use in clinical settings: The Newest Vital Sign (NVS) and several versions of the Rapid Estimate of Adult Literacy in Medicine (REALM)

TABLE 12–2   Individuals at Higher Risk for Health Literacy Concerns

Population	Characteristics
Older adults	Adults who are 65 years old or greater had lower average health literacy than those who were younger. The physical changes associated with aging are likely to contribute to or compound this problem—visual changes, hearing loss, cognitive changes, etc. More than 60% of individuals 65 years or older were at the basic or below basic level.
People with low incomes or living at or below the poverty line	Adults living at or below the poverty line had lower average health literacy than those above the poverty line.
People with less than a high school degree	Average health literacy increases with each higher level of education attained starting with high school graduates or individuals with a GED. Below basic health literacy comprised 49% of adults who had never attended or completed high school.
Racial and ethnic minorities	Hispanic adults had lower average health literacy than black, American Indian/Alaska Native, and multiracial adults. Whites and Asian/Pacific Islander adults had higher average health literacy than all of those groups.
Non-native speakers of English	Individuals who spoke only English before starting school had higher average health literacy than those who spoke English and another language or only another language before starting school.
Male Gender	Men had lower average health literacy than women. Sixteen percent of men were in the below basic category compared with 12% of women.
Persons on Medicare, Medicaid, or uninsured	Adults who received Medicare or Medicaid and adults who had no insurance had lower average health literacy than adults who were covered by other types of insurance (employer provided, privately purchased, or military).
Individuals with chronic disease or disability	Adults who had chronic disease or disability had lower average health literacy than those who did not.

TABLE 12–3   Some Clues and Red Flags that Might Suggest Low Health Literacy

	Behaviors You Might Observe	Things a Patient Might Say
Reading behaviors	Lifts texts closer to face when reading Points to and follows text with finger while reading Eyes wander over page without finding central focus Slow reading; asks someone else to read text/form for them Signs forms without reading Struggles with more than one piece of information or paper at a time May get frustrated with multiple forms, leave the clinic or waiting room	"I forgot (lost, broke) my glasses, can you read this to me?" "My eyes are tired, I'll read this when I get home." "I'm having trouble seeing." "The lighting is not good." "I don't feel well, will you read this for me?"
Self-care behaviors	Unable to name medications, explain why they take them or when/how to take them. Identifies medications by color and size of pill, not by name or reading labels Makes errors or lacks follow-though on self-care instructions such as exercise prescriptions, therapy recommendations, or medication regimens; may appear or be labeled nonadherent/noncompliant Misses appointments or arrives at the wrong times for appointments Resists filling out forms or activity logs; forms are incomplete or incorrectly filled out Waits until illness or problem is advanced before seeking help	"I just put them in my daily/weekly container—I don't need to know the names of my pills." "I lost/can't find my instruction sheet." (exercise or activity log) "Could you just draw pictures of the exercises for me?" "I lost my appointment card." "Could I have my appointments on the same days and at the same time?" "I was too busy to get help." "I don't have time."
Communication behaviors	Shows signs of nervousness or frustration May not answer questions or incorrectly answer questions; demonstrates differences between what is heard and read Is very quiet, passive Nods head in response to information but doesn't ask any questions in follow-up Asks a lot of questions, possibly out of context, about information provided previously or in written materials	In response to questions from the health care provider like "Do you understand?" or "Does that make sense?" always answers "Yes" without further questions In response to questions like "Do you have any other questions?" frequently answers "No"

Data from Area Health Education Clear Health Communication Program, The Ohio State University. You Can't Tell By Looking: Assessing a Patient's Ability to Read and Understand Health Information. Columbus, OH: The Ohio State University, Office of Outreach and Engagement, 2007.

(revised and short forms). Information on other literacy assessment instruments can be found in Appendix 12-A.

The Newest Vital Sign

The NVS is a tool developed by Weiss and colleagues[30] to be used as a quick screen for literacy in primary care settings. As indicated by the name of the instrument, the authors suggest that this screen could be something included in routine intake assessments with many patients in the same way we assess other vital signs like blood pressure, heart rate, and respiratory rate. The NVS has been found to be a "reliable and accurate measure of literacy with high sensitivity for detecting persons with limited literacy."[30,31]

The NVS consists of an ice cream nutrition label that the patient is asked to review and then answer a series of six questions regarding information in the label (Figure 12–2). The NVS instrument is also available in Spanish. A glance at the label and questions will reveal that the NVS assesses all three dimensions of literacy: prose, document, and quantitative (or numeracy). The NVS takes only about 3 minutes to administer, and a laminated copy of the labels, score sheets, and administration and interpretation instructions are available from the Pfizer Clear Health Communication Initiative.

Rapid Estimate of Adult Literacy in Medicine

The original version of the REALM was a 66-item (medical and health related terms) instrument that a patient was asked to read.[32,33] Terms were listed in three columns, and the tester then scored the individual based on his or her ability to read and correctly pronounce words on the lists. A revised and abbreviated form of the REALM, the REALM-R, was introduced in 2003.[33] This shortened version correlated with other literacy assessments and the longer REALM but had only 8 items (medical terms)

and took only 2 minutes or less to administer. The terms included osteoporosis, allergic, jaundice, anemia, fatigue, directed, colitis, and constipation. Testers could also add words pertinent to specific realms of care, such as terms related to the management of hypertension, and still keep the time for administration under 2 minutes.

Based on research conducted for an Agency for Health Care Research and Quality (AHRQ) grant, an additional shortened version of the REALM was posted to the agency website in 2008—the REALM Short Form or REALM-SF. This form of the REALM includes only 7 items and is shown in Figure 12–3. The REALM-SF and another assessment of health literacy for adults who are Spanish speaking, the Short Assessment of Health Literacy for Spanish Adults (SAHLSA-50) can be found online at the AHRQ website. Both of these instruments have been field-tested and have been shown to have excellent agreement with the longer 66-item REALM instrument in terms of grade-level assignments.

DEVELOPING APPROPRIATE EDUCATIONAL INTERVENTIONS AND MATERIALS

How many times have you experienced the same kind of feelings and thoughts expressed by the student in the first vignette at the beginning of this chapter? You thought you had explained an exercise program very clearly to a patient, but when they return to the clinic and you ask them to demonstrate their exercises, there was clearly some confusion! Something was definitely "lost in translation." Could limited health literacy have been one possible reason?

Now that you have some strategies and tools for recognizing literacy concerns in your patients, we'll turn to other techniques and strategies you can use to enhance communication, learning, and understanding for your patients in face-to-face encounters and through the development or identification of appropriate, accessible, easy-to-read patient educational materials.

FACE-TO-FACE COMMUNICATION AND TEACHING STRATEGIES

As noted earlier, many individuals with low literacy skills are embarrassed and ashamed about their inability to read and understand health-related information.[26] This may lead to attempts to hide their lack of understanding resulting in poorer health outcomes from both the provider and patient perspectives. To be most effective in our communication with patients with low literacy skills, we need to create shame-free and patient-centered environments and adopt approaches to interaction and teaching that diminish the potential for patient embarrassment or humiliation. For that matter, if we adopt such approaches in our interaction with *all patients*, we, and they, would likely realize more positive clinical outcomes.

To create a shame-free environment, it is important to be attentive to the continuum of the experience of the patient in the health care system—from the initial referral and scheduling of an appointment with a provider, to check-in procedures, through the clinician-patient

Nutrition Facts

Serving Size	½ cup
Servings per container	4

Amount per serving		
Calories 250	Fat Cal	120

	%DV
Total Fat 13g	20%
Sat Fat 9g	40%
Cholesterol 28mg	12%
Sodium 55mg	2%
Total Carbohydrate 30g	12%
Dietary Fiber 2g	
Sugars 23g	
Protein 4g	8%

*Percentage Daily Values (DV) are based on a 2,000 calorie diet. Your daily values may be higher or lower depending on your calorie needs.

Ingredients: Cream, Skim Milk, Liquid Sugar, Water, Egg Yolks, Brown Sugar, Milkfat, Peanut Oil, Sugar, Butter, Salt, Carrageenan, Vanilla Extract.

Score Sheet for the Newest Vital Sign
Questions and Answers

READ TO SUBJECT:
This information is on the back of a container of a point of ice cream.

	ANSWER CORRECT?	
	yes	no

1. If you eat the entire container, how many calories will you eat?
   Answer: 1,000 is the only correct answer

2. If you are allowed to eat 60 grams of carbohydrates as a snack, how much ice cream could you have?
   Answer: Any of the following is correct: 1 cup (or any amount up to 1 cup), half the container. Note: If patient answers "two servings," ask "How much ice cream would that be if you were to measure it into a bowl?"

3. Your doctor advises you to reduce the amount of saturated fat in your diet. You usually have 42 g of saturated fat each day, which includes one serving of ice cream. If you stop eating ice cream, how many grams of saturated fat would you be consuming each day?
   Answer: 33 is the only correct answer

4. If you usually eat 2,500 calories in a day, what percentage of your daily value of calories will you be eating if you eat one serving?
   Answer: 10% is the only correct answer

READ TO SUBJECT.
Pretend that you are allergic to the following substances: penicillin, peanuts, latex gloves, and bee stings.

5. Is it safe for you to eat this ice cream?
   Answer: No

6. (Ask only if the patient responds "no" to question 5): Why not?
   Answer: Because it has peanut oil.

Number of correct answers:

Interpretation
Score of 0-1 suggests high likelihood (50% or more) of limited literacy.
Score of 2-3 indicates the possibility of limited literacy.
Score of 4-6 almost always indicates adequate literacy.

Pfizer Working together for a healthier world**

February 2011

FIGURE 12–2 Newest Vital Sign label **(A)** and Score Sheet **(B)**. (From Pfizer Clear Health Communication Initiative, 2007. Available at: http://www.clearhealthcommunication.com/public-policy-researchers/NewestVitalSign.aspx.)

REALM-SF Form

Patient name _____ Date of birth _____ Reading level _____

Date _____ Examiner _____ Grade completed _____

Menopause ☐

Antibiotics ☐

Exercise ☐

Jaundice ☐

Rectal ☐

Anemia ☐

Behavior ☐

Instructions for Administering the REALM-SF

1. Give the patient a laminated copy of the REALM-SF form and score answers on an unlaminated copy that is attached to a clipboard. Hold the clipboard at an angle so that the patient is not distracted by your scoring Say:

   "I want to hear you read as many words as you can from this list. Begin with the first word and read aloud. When you come to a word you cannot read, do the best you can or say, 'blank' and go on to the next word".

2. If the patient takes more than 5 seconds on a word, say "blank" and point to the next word, if necessary, to move the patient along. If the patient begins to miss every word, have him or her pronounce only known words.

FIGURE 12–3 REALM Short Form (From Agency for Healthcare Research and Quality. Available at: http://www.ahrq.gov/populations/sahlsatool.htm.)

encounter itself, and to follow-up procedures. During the initial scheduling of the appointment, ensure that patients have simple directions or maps to locate the clinic if needed and be clear about what you would like them to bring to their first appointment (e.g., medications or medication lists, copies of any test reports or health records that they have). Look around the agency and your clinic space. Are building markers, signage, directions, and maps simple, clear, and easily visible? Are information desks or reception areas clearly marked, easily accessible, and staffed by people willing and able to direct patients to where they need to go? Is your clinic area clearly marked and identifiable? Making changes to decrease the stress associated with just getting to a clinic appointment will help all patients. One strategy that is widely used in very large clinical settings is colored stripes on walls or floors or other visual images that direct patients to various areas of the hospital or clinic.

Once patients arrive at your clinic, reception staff and others who interact with the patient need to be aware of - patient populations that might be at risk for literacy concerns (see Table 12–2) and watch for signs that would indicate literacy problems (see Table 12–3) during check-inprocedures. With all patients, but especially patients with low literacy, it is important to convey an attitude of respect, caring, and sensitivity, and a willingness to assist patients as needed. Because reading and filling out forms (registration, insurance, HIPAA, intake, and consent forms) can be very challenging for individuals with low literacy, offer to assist patients in the completion of forms. If providing assistance, move to a private area away from the immediate waiting room area. It would also be helpful to re-evaluate the forms used during check-in and simplify them as much as possible by using plain language and formatting them to make them easy to read. Writing in plain language requires that information presented is clear, simple, to the point, and directed toward the target audience. There are numerous resources available with principles, guidelines, and tips for the use of plain language in both written and oral communication.[24,33-38] One example of these, specifically related to health forms, is a resource available through the Health Resources and Service Administration (HRSA) on making HIPAA privacy notices more readable.[39]

Once you meet your patient and begin the therapy session, there are several communication and teaching strategies you can employ to help your patient feel comfortable and to facilitate learning and understanding (Box 12–4). Two of these suggestions will be discussed in more detail: (1) the key elements of plain language, and (2) the *teach-back technique*, also referred to as the *interactive communication loop*.

Plain Language

Although the term *plain language* might seem self-explanatory, there are several important elements of plain language that you can use when interacting with patients in the clinic. As noted in Box 12–4, it is important to limit the amount of new information provided to the patient in one teaching session; try to determine what is essential—what the patient truly needs to know or do right now. Once priorities are determined, slow down when

---

> **BOX 12–4   "Shame-Free" Communication and Teaching Strategies**
>
> - When gathering and providing information, move to a private area to decrease the potential for embarrassment.
> - Reassure the patient that many people have difficulty understanding complex health information and medical terms; convey patience through verbal and nonverbal messages when talking with the patient and be willing to repeat or rephrase information if indicated.
> - Sit down with the patient at their level and face them when speaking to them.
> - Observe and listen carefully to the patient and invite questions in follow-up to information you provide; be attentive and respond to quizzical looks or other nonverbal messages that suggest confusion or a lack of understanding.
> - Don't overwhelm the patient with too much information. Identify the priority information and try not to present more than three key points at a time.
> - Use "plain language" that is clear, simple, and direct.
> - Use the "teach-back" method to check for patient understanding. Ask the patients to tell you or show you what they have learned.
> - Provide easy-to-read materials to support and reinforce information you have given.
>
> From Area Health Education Clear Health Communication Program, The Ohio State University. Creating a Shame-Free and Patient-Centered Environment for Those with Limited Literacy Skills. Columbus, OH: The Ohio State University, Office of Outreach and Engagement; 2007; and Pfizer Clear Health Communication Initiative. Help Your Patients Succeed. 2007.

---

delivering information and instructions and frame the information. Think of framing as the front and back cover of an informational pamphlet. On the front page, you want to let the readers (learners) know what you are going to tell them and why it is important to them. On the back page, you want to reiterate the message and re-emphasize the importance to the patient. This is exactly what you can do in your teaching sessions with patients.

When delivering new information or instructions, use short and simple terms that would be familiar to the patient and used in their everyday language as opposed to using medical terms, physical therapy lingo, or jargon. One strategy that is useful in physical therapy is to use analogies to name and describe exercises you are teaching the patient. For example, when assessing or teaching patients tandem walking, you might demonstrate and call this activity "heel-to-toe walking" or "walking the tight rope." What simple name can you give a shoulder flexion exercise that uses terms most people would be familiar with? Another strategy for increasing understanding and fostering remembering is to let patients name the exercise using their own words once they understand the movement you are asking them to perform. Just ask them: "If you were naming this exercise, what would you like to call it?" For example, a cervical rotation movement to the left for a patient with vestibular dysfunction might become "checking your blind spot" if the patient drives a car.

Sometimes even simple terms that we might use in therapy can be confusing because they have more than one meaning. For example, when we talk about "gait" with our patients, they may be thinking "gate." Most people will understand "walking" pattern before they will understand gait pattern or the term *ambulation*. An excellent resource on the types of words that can create misunderstandings for patients (medical words, concept words, category words, and value judgment words) and examples of "problem words" to avoid ("Words to Watch") and words to use instead can be found at the National Patient Safety Foundation's website.

Although using plain language will help your patients at the outset, it is still helpful to repeat and rephrase information to assure that the message was received as intended. Other supports to the verbal delivery of information are the use of demonstration, visual images or models, audio-visual resources, and written materials.

At the conclusion of a session, make sure to allow time for the patient to ask questions but try not to ask, "Do you have any questions?" This question invites a "no" response if the patient is confused by information and potentially embarrassed by the fact that they don't fully understand what has just been said or taught. Instead you might say: "I have given you a lot of information today! What questions do you have for me now?"

One clear health communication initiative that focuses on encouraging patient questions about their health care is the "Ask Me 3" intervention.[40] This patient education program promotes three questions that patients should ask their physicians or other health care providers:

1. What is my main problem? (focus on diagnosis or major problem)
2. What do I need to do? (focus on instructions or interventions)
3. Why is it important for me to do this? (focus on creating a context for instructions and adherence)

The other important component of this initiative, of course, is to encourage health care providers to formulate clear and direct answers to these questions from patients.

In addition to providing patients with opportunities to ask questions for clarification, it is helpful to verify understanding of information using a teach-back technique.

Teach-Back Technique

The teach-back technique, also referred to as the interactive communication loop, is a strategy you can use to assess or verify a patient's understanding of instructions or information you have provided to them.[41,42] A similar technique has also been referred to as a *tell-back collaborative inquiry* method.[43]

An example of a physician using a teach-back technique with a patient following instructions regarding medication can be seen in the AMA video referred to earlier in this chapter, "Health Literacy and Patient Safety: Help Patients Understand" and available on YouTube. The following is an example of how the teach-back technique might be used in a physical therapy session for a patient with low back pain due to poor posture in prolonged sitting (Box 12–5).

An excellent Clear Health Communication Checklist for health care providers that incorporates the principles of plain language and the teach-back method described earlier can be found at the Health Literacy section of the Pfizer website. This simple resource would be an excellent tool for all therapists who wish to ensure they are communicating with their patients in a way to optimize patient learning and understanding.

BOX 12–5   Example of the Teach-Back Technique in a Therapy Session

- Step 1—Clinician explains new concept:
  - The therapist introduces the concept of the importance of maintaining lumbar lordosis (a "forward curve in your low back") in sitting, provides a lumbar support cushion, and demonstrates its use when sitting at work, at home, and in the car. She also explains to the patient why this position should help decrease his postural back pain and when the cushion should be used throughout the day.
- Step 2—Clinician assesses patient recall and comprehension:
  - Near the conclusion of the session, the therapist says, "I want to be sure I explained things well in therapy today and that you don't have any further questions at this time. Can you tell me, in your own words, why changing your sitting position and using the cushion might help decrease your back pain?" The therapist also asks the patient to demonstrate the placement of the cushion in a chair and asks the patient to tell her when and where they will use the cushion when they return home. The patient is able to correctly explain why the use of the cushion might help and demonstrates correct placement of the cushion, but is confused about when, where, and how long he should use the cushion.
- Step 3—Clinician clarifies and tailors the explanation to the patient:
  - Because the patient had most discomfort after long periods of time sitting at work and when driving more than 1 to 2 hours, the therapist now reviews her recommendations for using the cushion at all times when at work and when driving and clarifies her suggestions for standing or taking a brief break from driving at least every hour.
- Step 4—Clinician reassesses patient recall and comprehension:
  - After additional instruction and review, the therapist asks the patient to tell her, in his own words, when he will be using the cushion when he goes to work or gets in the car. This time the patient responds correctly, and the therapist reinforces the response using positive feedback.
- Step 5—Patient correctly recalls and comprehends the instruction:
  - This recall and reinforcement should increase the possibility for adherence to the therapist's recommendations and hopefully lead to a reduction in the patient's back pain.

DESIGNING AND EVALUATING PATIENT EDUCATION MATERIALS: HELPING YOUR PATIENTS TO LEARN FROM WRITTEN MATERIALS

As noted previously, an important support to and extension of teaching and learning in the clinic is the provision of written materials or resources for your patients to take with them when they leave the clinic. These materials can take many forms, such as patient information sheets or brochures, home exercise programs, activity or exercise logs, or audiovisual materials. In some cases, you will develop your own patient education materials, and in other cases, you will be selecting other prepared patient education materials to use with and for your clients. In either situation, it is important to create or choose materials that will be easy to read, accessible, and understandable for your patients. In this section, we review three types of assessments you can use to evaluate the clarity, difficulty, and suitability of patient education materials: (1) the use of checklists of attributes of written materials, (2) some commonly used readability formulas to determine literacy demands and grade level estimates of textual materials, and (3) suitability assessments of materials (SAM).[37]

CHECKLISTS OF ATTRIBUTES OF WRITTEN MATERIALS

Simple checklists provide one method for determining whether written materials you are developing or considering for adoption, purchase, and dissemination have attributes that will make them easy to read and effective educational tools.[37]

These checklists help you to assess attributes of written materials in four general categories: (1) organization of the materials (including amount of information provided), (2) writing style (including the use of active voice and plain language), (3) appearance (including print type and size and use of illustrations), and (4) appeal and suitability. Although this checklist was originally developed for print materials, it can be adapted for use with audiovisual materials as well. Doak and colleagues' book[37] and the checklist can be accessed online at the Harvard School of Public Health website.

Another useful checklist is a "Plain Language Checklist" developed through the Ohio State University AHEC Clear Health Communication Program. This checklist is also available online. It identifies criteria to assess in written materials that also fall into four main categories: content, organization, language and writing style, and design and appeal.

READABILITY ASSESSMENTS: THE SMOG AND FRY FORMULAS

Given the demographic data on literacy of the U.S. population discussed earlier in this chapter, it should be evident that patient education materials that are written at the 4th- to 5th-grade level would be more likely to improve readability and subsequent understanding for many of our patients and thus increase health literacy. Most patient education materials, however, are often written at the 8th-grade level or higher, with the average falling between the 10th- and 12th-grade levels.

Readability formulas can help you to specifically assess the reading difficulty of written materials, and most formulas are easy to use. Readability formulas usually look at two key features of text (vocabulary difficulty as assessed by the number of polysyllabic words and sentence length) to determine the level of difficulty and result in a numerical score that represents a grade level approximation for the material (plus or minus one grade level). It is important to note, however, that readability formulas test only readability. They do not tell you whether the material is accurate, organized, formatted to make it appealing and attractive, or appropriate for various populations (i.e., address gender, ethnic, cultural, language, age, or developmental issues). Thus, readability is just part of the overall assessment of educational materials, albeit an important part.

There are numerous readability formulas available, but for the purpose of this chapter, we review two common and easy-to-use tools: the Simple Measure of Gobbledygook (SMOG) formula and the FRY readability test/graph.

SMOG Grading Formula

The SMOG is one of the easiest, fastest, and most accurate predictors of readability. It was developed in 1969 by G. Harry McLaughlin[44] and can be applied to long texts (30 sentences or greater) and shorter texts (less than 30 but greater than 10 sentences). It can be easily calculated by hand in a short amount of time or can be completed by using a SMOG calculator available online at Dr. McLaughlin's website. (See Box 12–6 for instructions for hand calculation of SMOG values).

An alternative to the last two steps described in Box 12–6 is to use SMOG Conversion Tables to find the grade level of materials. SMOG Conversion Tables for long texts (conversion table I) and short texts (conversion table II) and additional guidelines for completing SMOG assessments can be found online or in a resource from the Ohio State University AHEC Clear Health Communication Program entitled, "Who's Reading Your Writing: How Difficult is Your Text?"[45]

FRY Graph Readability Formula

The FRY readability assessment method was first introduced in 1968[46] and was further refined and extended in 1977[47] so that it could assess reading levels ranging from grades 1 through 17. Like the SMOG formula, this method is easy to use and can be completed manually in less than 15 minutes. The FRY looks at similar features of text materials (word syllables and sentence length), but grade levels are assessed by plotting values on a FRY Readability Graph rather than by using mathematic calculations or conversion tables.

The extended FRY graph for estimating readability is provided in Figure 12–4. Additional guidelines for use of the FRY assessment are shown in Box 12–7 and a Fry Graph Readability Calculator is available online.

SUITABILITY ASSESSMENT OF MATERIALS

The SAM was developed and validated in the early 1990's.[37] It is a comprehensive, systematic process and scoring instrument that can be used to evaluate several factors (and related criteria) that can affect whether print materials are appropriate, attractive, and readable for

---

BOX 12–6   SMOG Value Calculation for Written Materials of 30 Sentences or Longer

- Select and count off 10 consecutive sentences at the beginning, middle, and end of your material (30 sentences total).
- In each of these three sections, circle all of the words that contain three or more syllables (polysyllabic words). Add up the number of words circled in each section. Repetitions of polysyllabic words should be counted as separate words.
- Estimate the square root of the total number of polysyllabic words counted in the entire sample. (Find the nearest perfect square and take its square root.)
- Add 3 to the square root. This number will be the SMOG reading level or the expected grade level the reader would need to have completed to understand the material.

GRAPH FOR ESTIMATING READABILITY—EXTENDED
by Edward Fry, Rutgers University Reading Center, New Brunswick, N.J. 08904

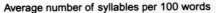

Average number of syllables per 100 words

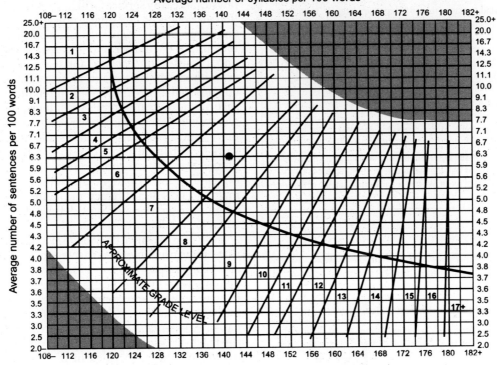

Expanded Directions for Working Readability Graph

1. Randomly select three (3) sample passages and count out exactly 100 words each, beginning with the beginning of a sentence. Do count proper nouns, initializations, and numerals.
2. Count the number of sentences in the hundred words, estimating length of the fraction of the last sentence to the nearest one-tenth.
3. Count the total number of syllables in the 100-word passage. If you don't have a hand counter available, an easy way is to simply put a mark above every syllable over one in each word, then when you get to the end of the passage, count the number of marks and add 100. Small calculators can also be used as counters by pushing numeral 1, then push the + sign for each word or syllable when counting.
4. Enter graph with *average* sentence length and *average* number of syllables; plot dot where the two lines intersect. Area where dot is plotted will give you the approximate grade level.
5. If a great deal of variability is found in syllable count or sentence count, putting more samples into the average is desirable.
6. A word is defined as a group of symbols with a space on either side; thus, *Joe, IRA, 1945,* and & are each one word.
7. A syllable is defined as a phonetic syllable. Generally, there are as many syllables as vowel sounds. For example, *stopped* is one syllable and *wanted* is two syllables. When counting syllables for numerals and initializations, count one syllable for each symbol. For example, *1945* is four syllables, *IRA* is three syllables, and & is one syllable.

Note: This "extended graph" does not outmode or render the earlier (1968) version inoperative or inaccurate; it is an extension. (REPRODUCTION PERMITTED—NO COPYRIGHT)

FIGURE 12–4 The extended FRY graph for estimating readability. (From Fry E. Fry's readability graph: clarifications, validity, and extension to level 17. J Read. 1977;21:242–252.

BOX 12–7   Instructions for Completing a FRY Assessment on Written Materials Greater than 300 Words

- Select three 100-word passages randomly from the material. Do not count proper nouns or numbers in the word count. If there are different content areas in the material, try to select a passage from those different areas.
- Count the number of sentences in each passage. If the last sentence is not complete, estimate the fraction of the last sentence to the nearest 10th.
- Calculate the average number of sentences in the passages: (s1 + s2 + s3) divided by 3.
- Count the total number of syllables in each 100-word passage. Add these values to get a total syllable count.
- Calculate the average number of syllables in the passages: (w1 + w2 + w3) divided by 3.

Use the FRY readability graph (see Figure 12–4) by locating the average number of syllables on the horizontal axis and the average number of sentences on the vertical axis. The intersection of these two points will fall in a section of the graph indicating a grade level.

TABLE 12–4 Factors Evaluated in the Suitability Assessment of Materials (SAM)

Factor	Selected Related Criteria
Content	Purpose is clear; scope is focused and limited; focus is on behaviors; summary is included.
Literacy demand	Readability; use of common words; use of active voice; context for material is provided
Graphics	Cover shows purpose; graphics are simple, appropriate, and relevant to content; captions provided
Layout and typography	Layout uses "white space"— not cluttered; typography is simple; subheadings used to "chunk" content
Learning stimulation and motivation	Material is interactive; behaviors are specific and are modeled; behaviors seem achievable to promote self-efficacy and motivation
Cultural appropriateness	Concepts and ideas presented are appropriate for the target cultural audience; language, images, and examples convey the cultural group in a positive way.

From Doak CC, Doak LG, Root JH. Teaching Patients with Low Literacy Skills, 2nd ed. Philadelphia: JB Lippincott, 1996.

target audiences (Table 12–4). Detailed instructions for completion of a SAM and a SAM scoring sheet can be found in Doak and colleagues' book[37] or online at the Harvard School of Public Health website.

Briefly, the SAM evaluates six primary factors that influence the suitability and potential effectiveness of written materials for various patient populations. Once the SAM instrument is completed according to the instructions and criteria, the evaluator will calculate a numerical percentage score for the material that will fall into one of the following categories: superior (70% to 100%), adequate (40% to 69%), or not suitable (0% to 39%). If the evaluator is also the developer of the educational material, a close analysis of subsection scores on the SAM can provide suggestions for revision of materials to increase suitability for target audiences and purposes.

SUMMARY

Given the enormity of the literacy problem in the United States and the likelihood that many patients receiving physical therapy services will have general literacy or health literacy concerns, the time is now to ensure that all students and clinicians are aware of and responsive to literacy issues they might encounter in clinical settings. There are many opportunities for teaching and learning about health literacy in both classroom and clinic settings. Once informed about populations at risk for limited literacy and behaviors that might indicate literacy problems, students and therapists can use their keen observational and listening skills to more quickly identify concerns and address them as they work with patients on a day-to-day basis. Integrate some of the literacy screening questions into your subjective evaluations for all patients. In addition to informal assessments of potential literacy problems, you might consider administering the NVS or REALM-SF in your clinics when deemed appropriate.

This chapter also provides several strategies and tools that can be used to create shame-free clinical environments and promote positive and supportive interactions with our patients with limited health literacy. Evaluate the signage in your clinical environments and your check-in procedures and forms. When you are working with your patients, use plain language to facilitate learning and use the teach-back technique to verify understanding of information you have provided in therapy sessions. Complete reviews of the educational materials you are currently providing to patients. Do they meet checklist suggestions or suitability criteria? Are they written at a 4th- to 8th-grade level so that they can be accessible and useful to a wide range of individuals? Findings from these assessments will help you to individualize your instructions and care to meet the needs of patients with limited health literacy, and they are also likely to improve the quality and effectiveness of the care you provide to all patients.

THRESHOLD CONCEPTS

Threshold Concept #1: Patient education and assessment of patient learning are essential components of all clinical interventions provided by physical therapists and serve as an important building block for attaining desired goals.

Threshold Concept #2: Without individualized communication and effective teaching in clinical settings, patient learning and desired therapy goals and health outcomes for clients may not be fully realized.

Threshold Concept #3: Limited general literacy and health literacy can be a significant barrier to patient learning and health behavior change and should be assessed to some degree, informally or formally, in all patient encounters.

ANNOTATED BIBLIOGRAPHY

Doak CC, Doak LG, Root JH. *Teaching Patients with Low Literacy Skills.* 2nd ed. Philadelphia: JB Lippincott; 1996.

  A classic and ground-breaking, frequently cited text that provides clear, concise, and practical suggestions for health professionals on ways to assess and address health literacy concerns in their everyday work with clients. The book includes several tools and guidelines for assessing the suitability and readability of health education materials and for developing materials that are accessible and useful to individuals with low general and health literacy.

Falvo DR. *Effective Patient Education: A Guide to Increased Adherence.* 4th ed. Sudbury, MA: Jones and Bartlett; 2011.

A comprehensive overview of numerous aspects of patient education authored by a highly regarded health professional who is a registered nurse, licensed psychologist, rehabilitation counselor, and former Chair of the Society of Teachers of Family Medicine. The text offers an explicit patient-centered approach to patient education that urges the creation of practitioner-patient partnerships. In addition to all of the excellent chapters in this volume, there is a chapter specifically devoted to "Health Literacy in Patient Education and Patient Adherence" (Chapter 10).

Osborne H. *Health Literacy from A to Z: Practical Ways to Communicate Your Health Message.* 2nd ed. Burlington, MA: Jones and Bartlett; 2012.

As stated in the preface to the book, this edition of *Health Literacy from A to Z* is "written for someone who cares a lot about communicating health messages clearly and simply. It is also written for someone to whom health literacy is just one of many projects competing for your time and attention. In other words, this book is written for you." Indeed it is. A simple and straightforward, practical guide to health literacy and strategies you can use to assess and address health literacy in your clinical practice. Chapters are brief, stand-alone, and organized by topic from A to Z as the book title suggests.

Zarcadoolas C, Pleasant AF, Greer DS. *Advancing Health Literacy: A Framework for Understanding and Action.* San Francisco: Jossey-Bass; 2006.

Another frequently cited and accessible text that provides an overview of health literacy and then moves to specific descriptions and evaluation of health education programs designed to address health concerns that incorporated attention to health literacy as part of their design and implementation. The text concludes with 11 "Guidelines for Advancing Health Literacy" (Chapter 14) that span the areas from use of vocabulary to graphics to web design. The guidelines would be useful to any health professional interested in providing effective health education whether it is delivered primarily in face-to-face oral, written, visual, or media formats.

REFERENCES

1. Mostrom E, Shepard K. Teaching and learning about patient education. In: Shepard KF, Hensen GM, eds. *Handbook of Teaching for Physical Therapists.* Boston: Butterworth-Heinemann; 2002.
2. American Physical Therapy Association. *Guide to Physical Therapist Practice.* 2nd ed. Alexandria, VA: American Physical Therapy Association; 2003.
3. American Physical Therapy Association. *A Normative Model of Physical Therapist Professional Education: Version 2004.* Alexandria, VA: American Physical Therapy Association; 2004.
4. American Physical Therapy Association. *Evaluative Criteria for Accreditation of Education Programs for the Preparation of Physical Therapists.* Alexandria, VA: Commission on Accreditation in Physical Therapy Education; Updated May, 2011. Available at: http://www.capteonline.org/AccreditationHandbook/; Accessed 20.10.2011.
5. American Physical Therapy Association. *Minimum Required Skills of Physical Therapist Graduates at Entry-Level.* Alexandria, VA: American Physical Therapy Association; Updated December 14, 2009. Available at: http://www.apta.org/Educators/Curriculum/APTA/; Accessed 20.10.2011.
6. American Physical Therapy Association. *Physical Therapist Clinical Performance Instrument for Students.* Alexandria, VA: American Physical Therapy Association; 2006.
7. Joint Commission. *Comprehensive Accreditation Manual for Hospitals (CAMH): The Official Handbook.* Oakbrook Terrace, IL: The Joint Commission; 2011.
8. Joint Commission. *What Did the Doctor Say? Improving Health Literacy to Protect Patient Safety.* Oakbrook Terrace, IL: The Joint Commission; 2007.
9. Wilson-Stronks A, Lee KK, Cordero CL, et al. *One Size Does Not Fit All: Meeting the Health Needs of Diverse Populations.* Oakbrook Terrace, IL: The Joint Commission; 2008.
10. Joint Commission. *Advancing Effective Communication, Cultural Competence, and Patient- and Family-Centered Care: A Roadmap for Hospitals.* Oakbrook Terrace, IL: The Joint Commission; 2010.
11. Healthy People 2020. U.S. Department of Health and Human Services. *Office of Disease Prevention and Health Promotion.* Available at: http://www.healthypeople.gov/2020/; Accessed 19.10.2011.
12. National Center for Education Statistics. *Adult Literacy in America: National Adult Literacy Survey.* Washington, DC: U.S. Department of Education; 1993.
13. National Center for Education Statistics. *Adult Literacy in America: A First Look at the National Adult Literacy Survey.* 3rd ed. Washington, DC: U.S. Department of Education. Available at: https://nces.ed.gov/pubs93/93275.pdf.
14. National Center for Education Statistics. *2003 National Assessment of Adult Literacy (NAAL).* Available at: http://nces.ed.gov//naal/resources/execsumm.asp.
15. Institute of Medicine. *Health Literacy: A Prescription to End Confusion.* Washington, DC: National Academies Press; 2004.
16. U.S. Department of Health and Human Services. *Health People 2010: Understanding and Improving Health.* Washington, DC: U.S. Department of Health and Human Services; 2000.
17. National Center for Education Statistics. *The Health Literacy of America's Adults: Results from the 2003 National Assessment of Adult Literacy.* Washington, DC: U.S Department of Education, Institute for Education Sciences; 2006. Available at: http://nces.ed.gov/naal/health_results.asp.
18. Area Health Education Clear Health Communication Program, The Ohio State University. *Health Literacy: It's Time to Take it Seriously.* Columbus, OH: The Ohio State University, Office of Outreach and Engagement; 2006.
19. American Medical Association Foundation. *Assessing the Nation's Health Literacy: Key Concepts and Findings of the National Assessment of Adult Literacy (NAAL).* Available at: http://www.amafoundation.org/go/healthliteracy; 2008. Accessed 20.06.2009.
20. U.S. Department of Health and Human Services. *National Action Plan to Improve Health Literacy.* Available at: http://www.health.gov/communication/HLActionPlan; 2010. Accessed 18.01.2011.
21. Berckman ND, DeWalt DA, Pignone MP, et al. *Literacy and Health Outcomes.* Evidence Report/Technology Assessment Number 87: Available at: http://archive.ahrq.gov/clinic/eparch.htm; 2004; Accessed 19.10.2011.
22. DeWalt ND, Berkman ND, Sheridan S, et al. Literacy and health outcomes: a systematic review of the literature. *J Gen Intern Med.* 2004;19:1228–1239.
23. Area Health Education Clear Health Communication Program, The Ohio State University. *You Can't Tell By Looking: Assessing a Patient's Ability to Read and Understand Health Information.* Columbus, OH: The Ohio State University, Office of Outreach and Engagement; 2007.
24. Weiss BD. *Health Literacy: A Manual for Clinicians.* 2nd ed. Chicago: American Medical Association Foundation; 2007.
25. Marcus EN. The silent epidemic: the health effects of illiteracy. *N Engl J Med.* 2006;3555:339–341.
26. Parikh NS, Parker RM, Nurss JR, et al. Shame and health literacy: the unspoken connection. *Patient Educ Couns.* 1996;27:33–39.
27. Chew LD, Bradley KA, Boyko EJ. Brief questions to identify patients with inadequate health literacy. *Family Med.* 2004;36:588–594.
28. Wallace LS, Rogers ES, Roskos SE, et al. Brief report: screening items to identify patients with limited health literacy skills. *J Gen Intern Med.* 2006;21:874–877.
29. Area Health Education Clear Health Communication Program, The Ohio State University. *Creating a Shame-Free and Patient-Centered Environment for Those with Limited Literacy Skills.* Columbus, OH: The Ohio State University, Office of Outreach and Engagement; 2007.
30. Weiss BD, Mays MZ, Martz W, et al. Quick assessment of literacy in primary care: the Newest Vital Sign. *Ann Family Med.* 2005;3:514–522.
31. Davis TC, Long SW, Jackson RH, et al. Rapid estimate of adult literacy in medicine: a shortened screening instrument. *Family Med.* 1993;25:391–395.
32. Bass PF, Wilson JF, Griffith CH. A shortened instrument for literacy screening. *J Gen Intern Med.* 2003;18:1036–1038.
33. U.S. National Archives and Records Administration. *Plain Language Tools.* Available at: http://www.archives.gov/federal-register/write/plain-language/.
34. Plain Language Association International (PLAIN). Available at: http://www.plainlanguagenetwork.org; 2011.
35. *Pfizer Principles for Clear Health Communication.* 2nd ed. Available at: www.aspiruslibrary.org/literacy/PfizerPrinciples.pdf.
36. Health Literacy Innovations. *The Health Literacy and Plain Language Resource Guide.* 2008. Available at: www.HealthLiteracyInnovations.com
37. Doak CC, Doak LG, Root JH. *Teaching Patients with Low Literacy Skills.* 2nd ed. Philadelphia: JB Lippincott; 1996.

38. Wickland K, Ramos K. Plain language: effective communication in health care settings. *J Hospital Librarianship.* 2009;9:177–185.

39. Health Resources and Services Administration. *Plain Language Principles and Thesaurus for Making HIPAA Privacy Notices More Readable.* Available at: ftp://ftp.hrsa.gov/hrsa/hipaaplainlang.pdf.

40. National Patient Safety Foundation. *Ask Me 3.* Available at: http://www.npsf.org/askme3/.

41. Schillinger D, Piette J, Grumbach K, et al. Closing the loop: physician communication with diabetic patients who have low health literacy. *Arch Intern Med.* 2003;163:83–90.

42. Osborn H. *Health Literacy from A to Z: Practical Ways to Communicate Your Health Message.* 2nd ed. Burlington, MA: Jones and Bartlett Learning; 2011.

43. Kemp EC, Floyd MR, McCord-Duncan E, Lang F. Patients prefer the method of "Tell Back-Collaborative Inquiry" to assess understanding of medical information. *J Am Board of Fam Med.* 2008;21:24–30.

44. McLaughlin GH. SMOG grading: new readability formula. *J Read.* 1969;12:639–646.

45. Area Health Education Clear Health Communication Program, The Ohio State University. *Who's Reading Your Writing: How Difficult is Your Text?* Columbus, OH: The Ohio State University, Office of Outreach and Engagement; 2007.

46. Fry E. A readability formula that saves time. *J Read* 1968;11:513–516, 575–578.

47. Fry E. Fry's readability graph: clarifications, validity, and extension to level 17. *J Read.* 1977;21:242–252.

Appendix 12-A Selected Health Literacy Tools, Reports, and Additional Resources

Selected Tools and Instruments for Assessing Health Literacy

Newest Vital Sign (NVS)
http://www.clearhealthcommunication.com/public-policy-researchers/NewestVitalSign.aspx

Rapid Estimate of Adult Literacy in Medicine (REALM) (long version)
Contact: Terry Davis, PhD
LSU Medical Center
1501 Kings Hwy
Box 598
Shreveport, LA 71130-3932

Rapid Estimate of Adult Literacy in Medicine—Revised (REALM-R)
http://www.ahrq.gov/pharmhealthlit/documents/realm-r.htm

Rapid Estimate of Adult Literacy in Medicine—Short Form (REALM-SF)
http://www.ahrq.gov/populations/sahlsatool.htm

Short Assessment of Health Literacy for Spanish Adults (SAHLSA-50)
http://www.ahrq.gov/populations/sahlsatool.htm

Test of Functional Health Literacy in Adults (TOFHLA) (long version)
Contact: Peppercorn Books and Press
PO Box 693
Snow Camp, NC 27349
http://www.peppercornbooks.com

Short Test of Functional Health Literacy in Adults (S-TOFHLA)
http://nmmra.org/resources/Physician/152_1485.pdf

Selected Health Literacy Guides, Reports and Resources:

Quick Guide to Health Literacy: Fact Sheets, Strategies, Resources
U.S. Department of Health and Human Services
Office of Disease Prevention and Health Promotion
http://www.health.gov/communication/literacy/quickguide/

Literacy and Health in America
Policy Information Report—Educational Testing Service

Policy Information Center
Mail Stop 19-R
ETS
Rosedale Road
Princeton, NJ 08541-0001
pic@ets.org
http://www.ets.org/research/policy_research_reports/pic-health

Health Literacy: A Prescription to End Confusion
Institute of Medicine of the National Academies Report
The National Academies Press
500 Fifth St. NW
Washington, DC 20001
http://www.nap.edu

Pfizer Principles for Clear Health Communication: A Handbook for Creating Patient Education Materials that Enhance Understanding and Promote Health Outcomes (2nd edition)
http://www.aspiruslibrary.org/literacy/PfizerPrinciples.pdf

Assessing the Nation's Health Literacy: Key Concepts and Findings of the National Assessment of Adult Literacy (NAAL)
American Medical Association Foundation
http://www.ama-assn.org/ama/pub/about-ama/ama-foundation/our-programs/public-health/health-literacy-program/assessing-nations-health.page

The Health Literacy of America's Adults: Results From the National Assessment of Adult Literacy (2006)
U.S. Department of Education
National Center for Education Statistics
http://nces.ed.gov/pubsearch/pubsinfo.asp?pubid=2006483

Proceedings of the Surgeon General's Workshop on Improving Health Literacy National Institutes of Health (2006)
http://www.surgeongeneral.gov/topics/healthliteracy/toc.htm

"What Did the Doctor Say?": Improving Health Literacy to Protect Patient Safety
The Joint Commission (2007)
http://www.jointcommission.org/assets/1/18/improving_health_literacy.pdf

Just What Did the Doctor Order? Addressing Low Health Literacy in North Carolina
North Carolina Institute of Medicine (2007)

The Health Literacy and Plain Language Resource Guide
Health Literacy Innovations (2008)
http://www.HealthLiteracyInnovations.com

One Size Does Not Fit All: Meeting the Health Care Needs of Diverse Populations
The Joint Commission (2008)
www.jointcommission.org/assets/1/6/HLCOneSizeFinal.pdf

National Standards for Culturally and Linguistically Appropriate Services in Health Care
U. S. Department of Health and Human Services
Office of Minority Health
http://www.minorityhealth.hhs.gov/assets/pdf/checked/executive.pdf

Health Literacy Information Resources
U.S. National Library of Medicine
National Institutes of Health
http://www.nlm.nih.gov/services/queries/health_literacy.html

Improving Health Literacy Guide
University of Michigan Library
http://guides.lib.umich.edu/healthliteracy

Harvard School of Public Health—Health Literacy Website
http://www.hsph.harvard.edu/healthliteracy/

Ohio State University—AHEC Clear Health Communication Program
http://medicine.osu.edu/orgs/ahec/CHCP

Improving Readability in Health Care
U-Write.com
http://www.u-write.com/

chapter 13

APPLIED BEHAVIORAL THEORY AND ADHERENCE
MODELS FOR PRACTICE

Judith R. Gale ☯ Teresa M. Cochran ☯ Gail M. Jensen

CHAPTER OUTLINE

Ruby is an 82-year-old woman with some 'senior' dementia (forgetfulness, slight confusion) and cardiac arrhythmia. She was residing in assisted living and recently lost her husband of 65 years. She fell at home, fracturing her left hip, and required a hemiarthroplasty. She was hospitalized for 5 days but received no physical therapy or occupational therapy during that time. She did not stand or walk while hospitalized. She was transferred to a rehabilitation center to receive daily physical and occupational therapy and after 3 weeks had made very little progress. She was labeled nonadherent.

Why was she "nonadherent"? How can we, as physical therapists, help this patient to be successful with her rehabilitation program? Are there tools to assist us? The goal of this chapter is to provide therapists with practical ideas and strategies to enhance patient learning and motivation to follow treatment recommendations. These will be based on sound theoretical concepts and evidence in the literature. We will present concepts related to the patient-practitioner collaborative model and behavioral theories to promote adherence and health behavior change.

Therapists identify the role of educator, teacher, or facilitator as a large part of their overall responsibilities. During the examination process, they are likely to focus on identifying the problems and the patient's goals, generating a working hypothesis regarding the cause of the patient's

symptoms, establishing the diagnosis, and developing an intervention plan to be implemented within a limited number of visits. Although they consider the patient's goals, physical therapists are less likely to assess the patient's beliefs and health behaviors as they relate to adherence to the intervention plan. Experienced therapists, however, will talk about "reading the patient" or "connecting with the patient." What does that mean? Are such things simply aspects of evaluation and intervention that are part of communicating well and being nice to the patient, or is there more to it?

If a physical therapist wants to be an effective practitioner, he or she must become an influential person in each patient's life. Technical competence in assessment and intervention planning, although very important, means little if patients do not follow the home program or continue unhealthy habits that contribute to their current problems. Experienced therapists know that many patients present with neuromusculoskeletal problems that are the result of lifestyle choices that can put them at risk for serious illness and even premature death. Although the therapist cannot control what the patient does at home, he or she can influence the patient so that there is a greater likelihood that what is prescribed is followed at home. The challenge is to negotiate the most efficacious intervention or prevention plan that the patient will be motivated to follow.

CHANGES IN THE HEALTH CARE ENVIRONMENT: HEALTH CARE DELIVERY AND REIMBURSEMENT

Some physical therapists may object to the view that part of their responsibility is to work with the patient's nonadherence or lifestyle risks, believing that the patient is responsible for intervention implementation and that the therapist's responsibility ends with providing the best advice possible regarding intervention or healthy lifestyle habits. However, structural changes in the delivery and reimbursement of health care services have affected, and will continue to affect, how physical therapists work with patients.

One stimulus focusing more attention to lifestyle modification during the clinical encounter is the increasing use of the Health Plan Employer Data and Information Set (HEDIS).[1] This is a set of common data indicators for the examination of managed care organization performance that was initially developed in the 1990s by the National Committee on Quality Assurance (NCQA). The latest version of HEDIS requires managed care organizations to report on more than 75 prevention-oriented indicators across eight domains of care (e.g., obesity, diabetes, hypertension).[1]

In 2006, the Tax Relief and Health Care Act (TRHCA, PL 109-432) established the physician quality reporting system under the jurisdiction of the Centers for Medicare and Medicaid Services (CMS). This plan identified Physician Quality Reporting Indicators (PQRI) to incentivize payment for practitioners (including physical therapists) to monitor and report on health-related symptoms in patients (e.g., blood pressure, balance risk) in order to identify costly conditions earlier and implement prevention strategies.[2] This focus on prevention offers physical therapists increasing opportunity to apply adherence and health behavior change strategies with patients.

The Balanced Budget Act of 1997 (established by PL 105-33) was enacted to reduce health care spending by $160 billion between the years 1998 and 2002.[3] Since that time, physical therapists, especially those providing care for Medicare beneficiaries, have been required to focus on facilitating adherence and producing successful and effective patient outcomes under increasing conditions of cost-containment and payment scrutiny. More recent federal legislation promises to further influence the delivery of health care service models in the United States. The Patient Protection and Affordable Care Act (PL 111-148)[4] of 2010 offers three major programs that directly affect physical therapists:

- Accountable care organizations
- Medicare innovation models
- Centers for Medicare and Medicaid services' medical home or patient-centered medical home models

ACCOUNTABLE CARE ORGANIZATIONS

Accountable care organizations (ACOs) are a direct response to Congress' continued efforts to reduce spending in health care, by authorizing the development of ACOs under both Medicaid and Medicare programs. ACOs would authorize specific groupings of health professions to provide care while saving on unnecessary expenditures. At this time, physical therapists are not expressly included as eligible participants in ACOs, but advocacy groups such as the American Physical Therapy Association are supporting inclusion among eligible practitioners because interventions have been shown to decrease overall patient care costs.[4]

MEDICARE INNOVATION MODELS

The Patient Protection and Affordable Care Act (PL 111-148) also establishes the Medicare and Medicaid Innovation Center "to research, develop, test, and expand innovative payment and delivery arrangements to improve the quality and reduce the cost of care provided to patients,"[5] especially in situations such as outpatient settings, that do not require referral by or plan of care established by a physician.[5] Physical therapists with the ability to facilitate patient adherence will be well positioned to demonstrate improved efficiency in the delivery of quality care.

MEDICAL HOME OR PATIENT-CENTERED MEDICAL HOME MODELS

The final promising model proposed in the Patient Protection and Affordable Care Act of 2010 is the CMS Medical Home or Patient-Centered Medical Home model designed to provide comprehensive primary care partnerships between individual patients or families and their health providers.[6] Like the Direct Access model, the purpose is to develop and test service delivery models to decrease health care costs. Although unknown at this time, the impact on physical therapy could be significant if physical therapists become participants in the medical home model.[6] Although the effects of current and future health care legislation are uncertain, it is clear that practitioners will be required to produce effective and economical patient outcomes. This will require physical therapists to facilitate adherence and the patient's ability to self-manage conditions.

ROLE OF LIFESTYLE IN MORBIDITY AND MORTALITY

Physical therapists often see patients with neuromusculoskeletal problems related to chronic inactivity, poor diet, obesity, and tobacco use. Those who present with one or more of these lifestyle risk factors are likely to benefit from attempts to modify their health risks. Physical therapists are in a unique position to support their patients' efforts to change.

There is significant evidence that lifestyle risks can contribute to premature morbidity and mortality. Healthy People 2020 targets several determinants of health, including diet, physical activity, and tobacco use.[7] More than 60% of the deaths in the United States in 2007 are attributable to chronic illnesses such as heart disease, stroke, diabetes, cancer, and chronic lower respiratory diseases.[8] Lifestyle-related behaviors can contribute to all of these diseases.

Research has demonstrated that intervening with inactive patients is likely to be helpful because virtually all individuals can benefit from some form of regular activity. According to the Surgeon General's *Vision for a Fit Nation 2010*, about two thirds of adults and one third of children are overweight or obese.[9,10] Non-Hispanic blacks and Hispanics are more likely to be obese than non-Hispanic whites. The prevalence of obesity in adults was almost 34% in 2007-2008 and was slightly higher in women than in men.[9] The annual medical-related costs are estimated at $147 billion. Each year, obese workers cost their employers an estimated $644 more than their counterparts of normal weight.[11]

The U.S. Department of Health and Human Services reports that more than 80% of adults do not meet the 2008 Physical Activity Guidelines for aerobic and strengthening exercise.[12] Factors associated with participation in physical activity include postsecondary education, higher income, social support, safe place to exercise, and self-efficacy (belief in ability to perform the exercises). Conversely, those who are overweight or obese or who have lower income or perception of poor health are less likely to engage in physical activity. People who reside in rural communities or have a lack of motivation are also less inclined to perform regular exercise.[7]

FUNDAMENTAL RELATIONSHIP BETWEEN PATIENT AND PRACTITIONER IN THE THERAPEUTIC PROCESS

Physical therapists should integrate adherence and lifestyle counseling into their practices for a variety of reasons. Reports of adherence rates to supervised exercise, as is seen in cardiac rehabilitation or other outpatient programs, range from 70% to 94%,[13,14] whereas adherence to home exercise programs is significantly less. Taal and associates,[15] in a study of patients with rheumatoid arthritis, found that 6% had difficulty adhering to a physical therapy regimen in the clinic, whereas 28% had difficulty adhering to a home exercise program. Nonadherence can take the form of the patient doing less or more of the prescribed intervention, never starting, or quitting prematurely. Each of these variations might represent a potential threat to the patient's recovery and level of function. Degree of adherence should be assessed at each visit to help determine risk versus benefits to overall recovery. Factors related to adherence include the patient's personal characteristics, variables associated directly with the disease or injury, intervention variables, and those having to do with the relationship between the patient and the practitioner (Table 13-1).

Physical therapists know that they are more likely to achieve patient cooperation or adherence when they try to understand the patient's perspective about the condition and its effects. This perspective is the patient's unique

TABLE 13-1 Thirty-Six Factors Related to Treatment Nonadherence

Variables	Factors
Personal variables (patient)	Characteristics of the individual Sensory disturbance Forgetfulness Lack of understanding Conflicting health benefits Competing sociocultural concepts of disease and treatment Apathy and pessimism Previous history of nonadherence Failure to recognize need for treatment Health beliefs Dissatisfaction with practitioner Lack of social support Family instability Environment that supports nonadherence Conflicting demands (e.g., poverty, unemployment) Lack of resources
Disease variables	Chronicity of condition Stability of symptoms Characteristics of the disorder
Treatment variables	Characteristics of treatment setting Absence of continuity of care Long waiting time Long time between referral and appointment Timing of referral Absence of individual appointment Inconvenience Inadequate supervision by professionals Characteristics of treatment Complexity of treatment Duration of treatment Expense
Relationship variables (patient-practitioner)	Inadequate communication Poor rapport Attitudinal and behavioral conflicts Failure of practitioner to elicit feedback from patient Patient dissatisfaction

From Meichenbaum D, Turk DC. Facilitating Treatment Adherence. New York: Plenum, 1987.

interpretation that incorporates sociocultural, emotional, and cognitive factors as well as sense of uniqueness, or the perceived probability that he or she is like or different than others with the same condition, all of which determine the patient's response to illness.[16-20] The patient's perspective and the process of trying to understand it can be contrasted to the student-teacher model, in which the student is the "empty vessel" into which the teacher pours his or her wisdom and knowledge. Using the same model with patients and practitioners, then, the practitioner gives the patient information (through teaching, written materials, or classes) about the condition, and if the patient does not improve, the practitioner may conclude that the "vessel" is not yet full and more information needs to be provided. However, more information does not necessarily lead to a change in behavior.[21,22] Following a treatment plan requires that the patient

- Chooses to do so
- Knows when to enact the plan
- Has the psychomotor skills to perform the plan, and
- Remains motivated to follow through until the problem resolves.

Thus, although knowledge of the condition is important, the patient's initial and long-term motivation are critical elements. To understand them, the therapist must understand the patient's perspective. Therapists are more likely to facilitate change in the patient's health behaviors by understanding the patient's belief system, which is usually rational and based on culture, past experiences, and support systems.[21–23]

The ability to effectively understand the patient's perspective will be increasingly important as changes in health care affect practice. Because of decreases in health care resources, therapists will be under increased pressure to maximize those scarce resources and yet continue to provide quality care for their patients. This will undoubtedly transfer much of the responsibility to the patients themselves and to their families. Designing therapeutic interventions with the highest likelihood of patient follow-through and adherence will be an essential factor in assessing patient outcomes.[21,23] In response to societal needs and demands, increased emphasis on patient education, prevention, and health promotion is found in federal guidelines (Table 13–2) and in the policies and guidelines of the American Physical Therapy Association.[7,10,24]

EXPLANATORY MODELS IN CLINICAL PRACTICE

Kleinman initiated the concept of explanatory models to analyze problems that may arise between the patient and therapist during the clinical encounter.[25] Kleinman defined explanatory models as the "notions patients, families, and practitioners have about a specific illness episode."[25] These explanatory models represent the patient's attempt to make sense of the change from "ease" to "disease." These beliefs often incorporate an attempt by the patient to self-disprove and ascribe a course to the condition. The patient's diagnosis and causal beliefs bring into play beliefs about the likely consequences of the condition, the time before the condition resolves, and the interventions (both prescribed and home remedies).[25] Kleinman and others[22,25,26] speculate that the effectiveness of clinical communication and the patient's health outcome may be a function of the extent of discrepancy between the patient's and the practitioner's explanatory model. For example, if a patient comes to physical therapy with the expectation that the therapist will fix the problem using massage for muscle pain, but the therapist expects to engage the patient in a home exercise program in a single visit, there will likely be a conflict in their interactions, or disappointment when either realizes the other is not meeting expectations.

Every therapist has one or more explanatory models in mind when working with patients. These models usually develop by thinking about the patient's goals and needs, strategies to understand more about a patient's receptivity to change, and strategies to engage the patient in his or her self-care at home. Just as a patient comes to the clinic with ideas about his or her condition, its immediate and long-term consequences, and the types of treatment that have and have not helped, therapists have their own beliefs for explaining the cause of the patient's condition and

TABLE 13–2 Examples of Guidelines for Patient Education, Health Promotion, and Prevention

Source	Examples
U.S. Department of Health and Human Services. Healthy People 2020. Available at: www.healthypeople.gov/2020	*Overarching goals:* • Attain high-quality, longer lives free of preventable disease, disability, injury, and premature death. • Achieve health equity, eliminate disparities, and improve the health of all groups. • Create social and physical environments that promote good health for all. • Promote quality of life, healthy development, and healthy behaviors across all life stages.
American Physical Therapy Association. Interactive Guide to Physical Therapist Practice, 2003. Available at: www.apta.org/Guide.	Progression from a healthy state to pathology—or from pathology or impairment to disability—does not have to be inevitable. The physical therapist may prevent impairments, functional limitations, or disabilities by identifying disablement risk factors during the diagnostic process and by buffering the disablement process. The patient/client management described in the Guide includes three types of prevention: • *Primary prevention.* Prevention of disease in a susceptible or potentially susceptible population through specific measures such as general health promotion efforts. • *Secondary prevention.* Efforts to decrease duration of illness, severity of disease, and sequelae through early diagnosis and prompt intervention. • *Tertiary prevention.* Efforts to decrease the degree of disability and promote rehabilitation and restoration of function in patients with chronic and irreversible diseases. In the diagnostic process, physical therapists identify risk factors for disability that may be independent of the disease or pathology.
Commission of Accreditation in Physical Therapy Education, American Physical Therapy Association, 2011	*Evaluative criteria for accreditation of physical therapist education programs:* • Physical therapists provide prevention [services] and promote health, wellness, and fitness. • Physical therapists provide prevention services that forestall or prevent functional decline and the need for more intense care. • Through timely and appropriate screening, examination, evaluation, diagnosis, prognosis, and intervention, physical therapists frequently reduce or eliminate the need for costlier forms of care and also may shorten or even eliminate institutional stays. • Physical therapists also are involved in promoting health, wellness, and fitness initiatives, including education and service provision that stimulate the public to engage in healthy behaviors.
A Normative Model of Physical Therapist Professional Education, Version 2004. Alexandria, VA: American Physical Therapy Association, 2004.	*Practice management expectations:* • Provide culturally competent physical therapy services for prevention, health promotion, fitness, and wellness to individuals, groups, and communities. • Promote health and quality of life by providing information on health promotion, fitness, and wellness within the scope of physical therapy practice.

BOX 13-1   Kleinman's Questions

1. What do you think caused the problem?
2. Why do you think it happened when it did?
3. What do you think your sickness does to you? How does it work?
4. How severe is your sickness? Will it have a short course?
5. What kind of treatment do you think you should receive?
6. What are the most important results you hope to receive from this treatment?
7. What are the chief problems your sickness has caused for you?
8. What do you fear most about your sickness?

Data from Kleinman A, Eisenberg L, Good B. Culture, illness, and care: clinical lessons from anthropologic and cross-cultural research. Ann Intern Med 1978;88:251-258.

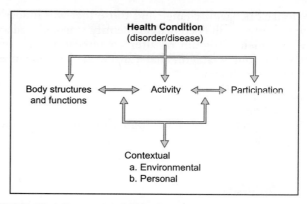

FIGURE 13-1 International Classification of Functioning, Disability, and Health (ICF) Model. (From Towards a Common language for Functioning, Disability and Health: ICF. Geneva: World Health Organization, 2002, p 9.)

anticipating the patient's response to intervention. The therapist uses this explanatory framework, or model, to guide patient evaluation and decision making about patient management. These models may reflect beliefs about teaching and learning or motivation and behavioral change. The patient also comes with certain beliefs and expectations about what he or she wants from the provider about the sources and consequences of the illness. Using a set of simple questions proposed by Kleinman[25] (Box 13-1) can help clarify the patient's beliefs and goals.

The biomedical model has dominated the explanatory frameworks shared by many health care practitioners in Western societies. It focused on pathology and the disease process, the physical symptoms that resulted from the disease, and the medication interventions intended to resolve the problem.[27] Although this model was initially useful, its deficiencies as a comprehensive framework for patient management have become increasingly apparent. The model became more focused on the critical importance of patient outcomes and addressing the patient's functional needs and health status rather than just documenting changes in physical impairment measures (e.g., range of motion or strength) and assuming those changes will result in a positive functional outcomes in patients' lives.[28,29] Such emphasis draws the therapist's attention to the patient's perspective because it requires that the therapist know the patient's functional goals. However, this emphasis ignores other elements of the patient's explanatory model that may affect treatment adherence (see Box 13-1).

Another example of an explanatory model is an enablement schema, such as the International Classification of Functioning, Disability, and Health (ICF). This model was endorsed by all 191 member states of the World Health Organization (WHO) at its 54th World Health Assembly in 2001.[30] A model like the ICF provides therapists with common terms used to clearly illustrate the importance of facilitating physical function (i.e. altering body structure) to allow personal or social engagement (i.e., participation) (Figure 13-1). For example, a patient who has a disease like diabetes, which results in peripheral vascular disease and a subsequent lower extremity amputation, has several bodily structures and functions involved as a result of the pathology and the medical intervention. In turn, these may lead to limitations in the person's ability to participate in certain activities. As seen in Figure 13-1, enablement not only involves the physical levels of changes in body systems but also reflects ability for engagement and participation in society and the fulfillment of social roles. The physical therapist's

primary role in facilitating patient movement and enhancing function has to do with change at both the individual and societal levels.[30] Achieving these goals requires that the therapist explore the patient's treatment goals and explanatory model to determine potential intervention barriers.

As health care providers strive to become patient centered, an increased emphasis on the quality of the therapeutic encounter between the patient and provider is necessary; therefore, therapeutic intervention must be skillfully implemented from the initial contact.

BEHAVIORAL THEORIES TO INFORM PRACTICE, PROMOTE ADHERENCE, AND FACILITATE HEALTH BEHAVIOR CHANGE

In today's managed care environment, in which time to work directly with patients is limited, it is important that efforts to promote adherence and lifestyle modification be efficient and effective. Three models of behavior theory will be presented in this chapter: the Health Belief Model, the Five A's Behavioral Intervention Protocol, and the Transtheoretical Model of Change. All three of these models presume that the beliefs of patients are major determinants of their behavior. These approaches all draw on Social Learning Theory as described by Bandura.[31]

SOCIAL LEARNING THEORY

Social Learning Theory proposes that people learn through direct observation of the beliefs and actions of others and outcomes of those actions. Through these observations, people form their own ideas of how to behave and what to believe. A major component of Social Learning Theory is the concept of self-efficacy, which refers to a person's belief that he or she can accomplish a behavior.[31]

Self-Efficacy

Many of the areas for exploration, renegotiation, and problem solving with the patient have to do with the concept of *self-efficacy*. It is the responsibility of the physical therapist to help the patient recognize those beliefs that will assist in the desired behavior change and those that will hinder it. Often a patient will need help to identify reasons to adhere to a treatment program or alter an unhealthy behavior. There are four strategies that can be used to enhance a patient's self-efficacy:

- Skills mastery
- Modeling
- Reinterpretation of physiologic signs and symptoms
- Persuasion

Skills Mastery

This concept involves ensuring that the patient is able perform the task. It can entail breaking a more complex task into smaller pieces that can be more easily learned and accomplished successfully. The patient will need feedback about his or her performance to increase the likelihood of mastery of the skill. Goal setting and contracting are other methods of providing feedback.[21,31]

Modeling

Modeling is a second strategy for increasing self-efficacy. The physical therapist is often the model in patient care settings. In group education courses, however, the model will often be someone much like the patient. This can include ethnicity, gender, age, diagnosis, and socioeconomic status. Group educational intervention can be successful because patients are modeling to each other, thereby enhancing their own self-efficacy.[21] In order for modeling to be effective, the therapist must make sure that the patient is attentive to the model, motivated to and able to perform the requested activity, and able to retain the new information.[32]

Reinterpretation

The reinterpretation of physical signs and symptoms can be a powerful strategy for patients. First, the therapist must find out what patients believe about their conditions or how they interpret their present symptoms. For example, if the patient believes that pain with exercise is a sign of more damage to a joint, he or she is not likely to exercise. This patient must be taught to reinterpret the beliefs about exercise and symptoms. The therapist may need to teach the patient to distinguish between different types of pain.

Persuasion

Persuasion is a common method used by physical therapists. Verbal persuasion involves urging the patient to do more by giving verbal support and encouragement. As a last resort, the therapist might emphasize the negative consequences of not participating in the program. This strategy of stressing what a patient might lose should be used with care and only after trying other methods. An initial focus on the positive consequences of the intervention program is an important aspect of patient-practitioner collaboration.

BOX 13–2   Key Concepts of the Health Belief Model

- Perceived threat (susceptibility): belief that it is possible to get the disease or condition
- Perceived severity: belief in the gravity of the consequences of having the condition
- Perceived benefits: belief that the recommendations or behavior change will be helpful
- Perceived barriers: beliefs about the costs (monetary, time, psychological, etc.) of initiating the recommended action or behavior change
- Perceived self-efficacy: belief in one's ability to change a behavior

Adapted from Champion VL, Skinner CS. The health belief model. In Glanz K, Rimer BK, Viswanath K (eds). Health Behavior and Health Education: Theory, Research and Practice, 4th ed. San Francisco: Jossey-Bass, 2008, p 48.

HEALTH BELIEF MODEL

In the Health Belief Model (Box 13–2), the individual must believe that he or she is susceptible to a disease or condition, that the disease has consequences, that changing a behavior can reduce the threat, that the benefits of changing the behavior outweigh the costs or barriers, and that he or she is capable of making the change (perceived self-efficacy).[22,32] One way of applying these concepts is to ask the patient about the possible adverse consequences of poor adherence to a treatment program or continuing an undesired behavior. Ascertaining whether the patient believes the intervention will help is also important. Discussion of costs and barriers versus benefits will provide additional information to assist the therapist in designing a program that is reasonable in terms of costs and time, yet effective in managing the patient's condition. The final construct in the Health Belief Model is the belief in the ability to make the desired change. This is a most important piece of the model. The therapist can assist with increasing the patient's confidence in successfully making the change by setting small, attainable goals.

FIVE A'S BEHAVIORAL INTERVENTION PROTOCOL

The Five A's process is a sequenced, systematic process that is applied during the initial visit and at subsequent visits to promote adherence (Figure 13–2). Each step has a purpose and, if performed well, is likely to achieve its intended effect (Box 13–3). Skipping a step because of time constraints may be necessary but may diminish the overall effectiveness of the process.[22,33]

Step One: Address the Issue

Patients come to physical therapy with an agenda or concern, typically seeking symptom relief. This means that they are willing to discuss the problems that brought them but may not have come thinking about behavior change. Following the history and examination, the therapist will develop a plan of care. It is imperative at this point to address adherence as part of negotiating the most efficacious

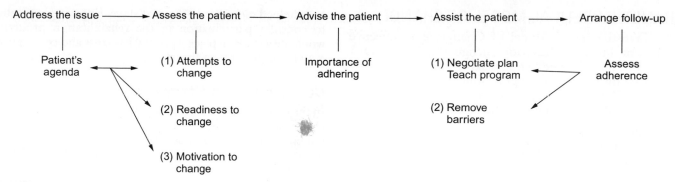

FIGURE 13–2 The steps in the Five A's Behavioral Intervention Protocol. Each step is sequenced to achieve maximal effectiveness as the patient moves through the stages.

BOX 13–3   Steps of the Five A's Process

- Step one: address the issue
- Step two: assess the patient
- Step three: advise the patient
- Step four: assist the patient
- Step five: arrange for follow-up

From Fiore MC, Bailey WC, Cohen SJ, et al. Treating tobacco use and dependence. Clinical Practice Guideline. Rockville, MD: U.S. Department of Health and Human Services; 2000.

---

intervention that the patient is willing to follow. For example, the therapist might ask, "What do you think is the problem?" or "What kinds of things do you feel will help you get better?" These questions open the door to discussions of healthy behavior changes.

Step Two: Assess the Patient

At least three main areas should be assessed: recent attempts to follow a home program or change an unhealthy behavior, the patient's readiness to change, and the patient's motivation to perform the program or make the desired behavior modification. The patient should be encouraged to reveal what has worked and what has not worked in the past and barriers to success. Asking simple questions like, "Can you think of any problems with carrying out this program?" or "What kinds of things are you unable to do now that you would like to be able to do?" can help focus the intervention, identify motivational factors, and direct the intervention in a way that will encourage success.

Step Three: Advise the Patient

In this step, the physical therapist is exerting his or her influence as a knowledgeable health care provider to advise the patient of the importance of adhering to the therapeutic program or initiating a lifestyle change. The physical therapist conveys this advice not only by what is said but also by how it is said. Social pressure, especially if exerted by persons viewed as important in the patient's life, can

be an important influence. Addressing adherence and advising the patient can begin with stating the value of the interventions prescribed: "Completing your home program regularly and correctly is important to getting you back to the activities you enjoy. We need to agree on what you feel you can do on a daily basis to accomplish that."

Step Four: Assist the Patient

Assisting the patient consists of three major activities: negotiating a plan, educating the patient about the program or correcting any mistaken beliefs or assumptions, and identifying and problem-solving any barriers to following the plan. Once a program has been agreed on, educate the patient on how to do it, when to do it, what side effects to expect and what to do if they occur, the time frame in which an improvement should be noticed, and what changes will be evidence of improvement. Give the patient enough resources, practice, and direction in the clinic so that he or she can perform the program correctly at home. Because commitment to change can be tenuous, negotiating what is reasonable for the patient to accomplish is necessary, as is recognizing and problem-solving barriers to success.

Developing an initial program based on what the patient tells you, rather than simply informing him or her of the program, increases the likelihood that the patient will be adherent and successful. Such success is based, in part, on the fact that the patient helped decide on what to do him or herself.

Step Five: Arrange for Follow-Up

In addition to reassessing the patient's medical condition, this step allows the therapist to address the patient's adherence to the negotiated plan. Arranging for follow-up discussions on adherence helps convey that the patient is accountable. This can be conveyed easily by stating, "When you come back in 2 weeks, we will talk about how you are doing and what problems you have had in following your home program."

TRANSTHEORETICAL MODEL OF CHANGE

The Transtheoretical Model of Change is an effective model for initiating behavior change. As Figure 13–3 shows, this model suggests that making a behavior change such as following a home program follows a nonlinear progression of five stages, also known as the Stages of Change Model.[22,32] The stages include the following:

1. Precontemplation
2. Contemplation
3. Preparation
4. Action
5. Maintenance[34]

Application of this stage process implies that the therapist first assesses a patient's stage and then uses education and persuasion to move the patient closer to the action stage.

Precontemplation Stage

In this beginning stage, the patient has no intention to make a behavior change within the near future, usually within the next 6 months. There may be a lack of knowledge about the consequences of continuing with an unhealthy behavior. It is also possible that the patient may have been unsuccessful in changing the behavior in the past or perceives the change as being too difficult. At this stage, it is appropriate for the physical therapist to provide information about the potential risks of continuing the behavior and the benefits of change. There may be times that this information and education are all it takes to move patients to another stage. Often, however, they can be resistant to or fearful of change, and they may need time to assimilate the information and the emotions associated with it. Therapists should be empathetic and encouraging at this stage. Helping the patients to believe in their ability to make the desired change is a good strategy; that is, efforts to increase perceived self-efficacy are beneficial in this stage.

Refer back to the case of Ruby, our 82-year-old patient with a fracture of the left hip. It seems likely that she remained in the precontemplative stage while in the hospital and during most of her stay in the rehabilitation center. This could be a woman who has never exercised regularly, and now the rehabilitation team is asking her to exercise several times each day. This would probably seem daunting to her because it is very unfamiliar. Perhaps spending some extra time with her discussing the possible consequences of nonadherence, the benefits of adherence, and how this could positively influence her goals and providing some of the details of the rehabilitation program itself would have helped move her to the next stage. Encouraging Ruby to consider participation in the rehabilitation program would be a starting place. Gaining her trust and confidence are very important in this stage.

Contemplation Stage

In the contemplation stage, the patient is beginning to think about making a positive change in behavior within the next 6 months or so but is not wholly committed to carrying it out. The patient may vacillate between feeling confident that the change is good and necessary and feeling that it might be too difficult to achieve and might not be necessary after all. The therapist can assist in this stage by clarifying the possible risks involved in resisting change and highlighting the benefits of making it. Coercion should be avoided even if the patient remains in this stage for a period of time. However, expressing concern about continuation of a risky behavior is often a good strategy to move the patient along.

If Ruby were to say that she has been thinking about trying to assist more with transfers or participating in the group exercise class, it is the perfect time for the physical therapist to elaborate further on the benefits of these activities and reinforce her consideration of participating more. Encouragement is the key to "hooking" her in this stage.

Preparation Stage

Making plans to change occurs in the preparation stage. The patient is moving toward making a change and plans to do so within the next 30 days. This stage is also called the determination stage as the patient has now made a commitment to the change. The role of the physical therapist is to assist in developing and supporting a plan of action. This should include realistic implementation strategies and attainable goals. The patient must be intimately involved in setting these goals and strategies in order to "own" the proposed program. Asking him or her to the articulate reasons for changing can get the ball rolling. Weighing the perceived benefits against the perceived barriers at this stage might be helpful.

For Ruby, it would have been beneficial to assist her in remembering the important things in her life that she was missing by her lack of progress while in the rehabilitation setting. There were undoubtedly things she missed doing because she was unable to get out and about, and desire to be able to do these things again might serve as a motivation to begin the rehabilitation program. Supporting a more positive thought process might have served as an impetus to initiate a plan of action.

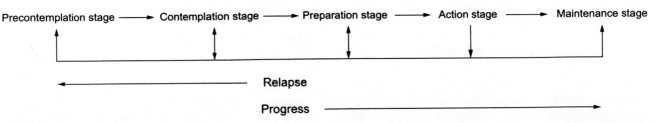

FIGURE 13–3 The Transtheoretical Model of Change. Relapse can occur at any stage. Strategies for facilitating change are stage dependent. (Adapted from Rollnick S, Mason P, Butler C. Health Behavior Change: A Guide for Practitioners. Philadelphia: Churchill Livingstone, 1999.)

Action Stage

The implementation of the plan occurs during the action stage. Patients begin actively participating in their treatment programs. It is here that the therapist can support the patient, first by promoting the patient's self-confidence in his or her ability to achieve desired goals, and second by outlining the steps to reach their goals. These goals should be small enough to be accomplished yet large enough to enable the patient to see positive change. The implementation plan, as well as the goals, is revisited as the patient progresses through the anticipated steps. There can be many iterations of the program as the patient begins to demonstrate changes in behavior. Part of the support the therapist can offer is to aid the patient in developing the skills needed to overcome unanticipated barriers to progress. Without these problem-solving skills, the patient is vulnerable to relapse into old, more comfortable behavior patterns.

After her hip fracture, if the rehabilitation team members spent time with Ruby dedicated to increasing her motivation, she might have been able to reach the action stage. Planning the steps needed to leave the rehabilitation center and visit her daughters and grandchildren might have started with encouraging her desire to do this. The next step might have entailed building her confidence that this was possible. Finally, breaking down the steps to reach that larger goal into small, measurable steps would have served as reinforcement that she could do this. She might have begun by strengthening her upper and lower extremity musculature to enable her to transfer more easily, then standing in the parallel bars, and finally beginning to ambulate. Along the way, she would have needed lots of encouragement and ongoing support.

Maintenance Stage

If the behavior change has persisted for more than about 6 months, the patient is moved from the action stage to the maintenance stage. The main goal in this stage is prevention of relapse. Relapse is common and can occur at any time and to any prior stage. It is an integral part of the change process. There is always the temptation to return to prior behaviors, especially when support is decreased.

Discussion between the physical therapist and the patient to help maintain the new behavior can include such things as problem-solving potential new barriers, identifying new rewards for adherence or behavior change, or reminding the patient of the risks of nonadherence. Patients will typically not need quite as much support during this stage, but it needs to be available if needed. As time goes on, however, they require less and less support, reinforcement, and encouragement as the new behaviors "take hold" and become part of a changed lifestyle.[22,32]

COMPARING THE THREE MODELS

Figure 13–4 provides a schematic comparison of the three models discussed earlier: the Transtheoretical Model of Behavior Change, the Health Belief Model, and the Five A's model. There are many similarities and considerable overlap between the models.

THE PATIENT-PRACTITIONER COLLABORATIVE MODEL

A patient-practitioner collaborative model (Figure 13–5) can be use to help physical therapists and physical therapist assistants focus their interventions on the patient's needs and improve adherence to treatment. This model integrates concepts from several other models in medicine and physical therapy.[22,23,27,32,35,36]

At the center of this model is the patient in the context of his or her life. This includes the patient's beliefs, attitudes, skills, and feelings, shaped by a lifetime of experiences, his or her diseases, others diseases and illnesses, and his or her support system. It is helpful here to distinguish two conceptualizations of ill health: disease and illness. Disease represents what went wrong with the body as a machine, whereas illness represents a person's experience of the disease and its effect on his or her life. Diseases are diagnosed by the physician or physical therapist using a biomedical model of health care. On the other hand, patients come to physical therapy with many beliefs about their illness experiences, which may or may not be scientifically sound. Although the focus of

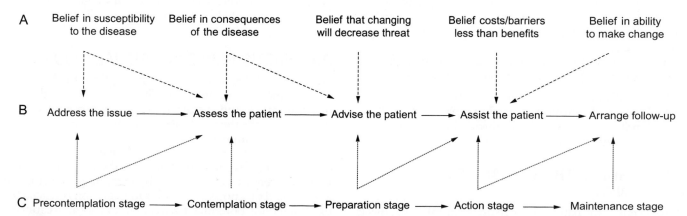

FIGURE 13–4 Similarities among the Transtheoretical Model of Change **(A)**, the Five A's Behavioral Intervention Protocol **(B)**, and the Health Belief Model **(C)**.

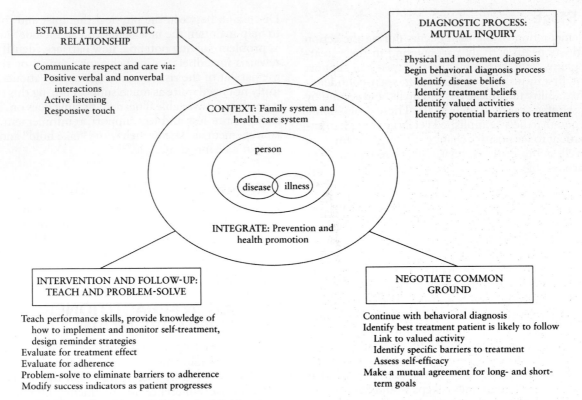

FIGURE 13–5 The Patient-Practitioner Collaborative Model.

the practitioner's examination and evaluative process is finding out the diagnosis, the patient's illness experience may not be explicitly explored or fully understood by the practitioner. As a consequence, the therapist's goals and explanations may not align with the patient's goals and understanding of the problem. Connecting with the patient involves developing a relationship that allows probing the patient's beliefs as a first step in negotiating a treatment. We propose here that understanding disease *and* illness is a critical aspect of successful therapeutic intervention. Essential to the therapist's role as a professional is understanding the context of the patient's life and the health care system, as well as how these contexts influence manifestations of the patient's disease and illness. Finally, through the process of education, support, and persuasion, therapists need to teach patients how to prevent disease or relapse and to promote health.

The model has four phases and can be easily integrated into the physical therapy evaluation process:

1. Establishing the therapeutic relationship
2. Diagnosing through mutual inquiry
3. Finding common ground through negotiation
4. Intervening and following up

ESTABLISHING THE THERAPEUTIC RELATIONSHIP

The concept of the patient as a person is central to all aspects of therapeutic intervention. The evaluative process begins with establishing a therapeutic relationship or connecting with the patient during the interview. Doing so is crucial for fostering the trust and mutual respect necessary to allow

the patient to reveal his or her beliefs and feelings about the disease, illness, evaluation, and treatment. Verbal and nonverbal behaviors contribute to establishing this therapeutic relationship. Although some may think that these behaviors are common sense, when practitioners are focused on gathering evaluative data regarding signs and symptoms, they are often unaware of their behavior. For example, when the therapist is pressed for time, he or she may not make eye contact or may cut off a person's story and gather only disease data. Not allowing the patient to fully express concerns sends the message that the disease is important, not the patient. Table 13–3 provides an overview of key behaviors that facilitate or impede the therapist's connection with the patient.[23,36–38] Consistent and timely use of behaviors that facilitate connection has a great influence on whether the patient reveals his or her beliefs and becomes a willing partner.

DIAGNOSTIC PROCESS: MUTUAL INQUIRY

Some form of diagnostic process is usually at the heart of a physical therapy examination. This process begins the second the patient and therapist meet. The process typically intensifies as the therapist interviews the patient and begins the physical examination. We recommend that, along with inquiring about the movement dysfunction, the therapist begin to do an explicit assessment of the potential for patient adherence or cooperation by beginning to formulate a behavioral diagnosis.[22,23,32] This information is crucial for understanding potential barriers to the ideal treatment. Typical barriers include lack of education as to how and when to perform the treatment, lack of confidence in ability to perform it, beliefs or values incompatible with the treatment and lack of time, resources or support.

TABLE 13-3 Interactional Behaviors that Facilitate or Impede the Therapist's Ability to Connect with Patients

Behavior Type	Behaviors
Connecting behaviors	Verbal
	Greeting the patient in a friendly manner
	Making positive comments
	Inquiring about the patient
	Reflecting on the patient's feelings
	Clarifying the patient's needs
	Nonverbal
	Facing the patient
	Making eye contact
	Leaning toward patient
	Displaying an open posture
	Using nonverbal cues to acknowledge active listening
Impeding behaviors	Acting busy
	Reading notes
	Doing tasks
	Using medical jargon
	Cutting off patient's story
	Responding only to disease information
	Failing to give feedback
	Showing little empathy
	Not asking about the patient's concerns

Data from Meichenbaum D, Turk DC. Facilitating Treatment Adherence. New York: Plenum, 1987; Jensen GM, Lorish C. Promoting patient cooperation with exercise programs: linking research, theory, and practice. Arthritis Care Research, 1994;7:181; Carkuff R. The Art of Helping (7th ed.) Amherst, MA: Human Resources Press, 1993.

Assessing what the patient knows and believes about his or her condition and treatment is a good place to start. This assessment includes identification of the patient's beliefs about the condition and what treatments he or she is likely to follow.[21,23,27] The therapist needs to identify the patient's beliefs about positive and negative consequences of the disease or condition and how it is affecting his or her life (Box 13–4).

It is important to gather information about the patient's treatment beliefs, including past treatment, home remedies, and future treatments. The therapist should also identify any potential barriers to the treatment.

- What seems to help? Are there things you are not willing to try?
- What are the worst things you anticipate about treatment?
- Have you ever tried exercise?
- If you were given a home program, what difficulties do you think would you have doing it?

BOX 13–4   Sample Questions that Could Be Used during this Diagnostic Process

- How would you describe the problem that brought you to physical therapy?
  - What do you think caused the problem?
  - Why do you think this happened to you?
- Inquiring about the patient's symptoms and activity limitations includes these types of questions:
  - What things can you no longer do as a result of this condition?
  - What daily activities would you like to return to as quickly as possible?
  - How does your family react to your condition?
- How do you know whether you are better or worse? What causes these changes?

The answers to questions like these reveal much about what the patient knows and does not know about the condition, what activities the patient wants to regain that might serve to increase motivation and promote adherence, and what alternative treatments the patient may be doing in addition to those prescribed. Physical therapists are ultimately interested in facilitating patients' self-care in terms of their movement problems. Exercise is likely to be one of the health behaviors that is part of the treatment regimen carried out at home. As the therapist asks the patient to reveal more about his or her understanding and beliefs, the patient is also gaining information about the therapist by observing the questions and responses, then developing or modifying beliefs about the therapist's competence and trustworthiness.[15,27] By inquiring about beliefs, the therapist demonstrates interest in the patient as a person as well as the patient's illness and disease process.

FINDING COMMON GROUND THROUGH NEGOTIATION

During the course of the evaluation and behavioral diagnosis process, the physical therapist is also negotiating treatment goals with the patient. The essential question is not what is the best intervention for this condition but what is the best intervention that the patient is likely to follow. To answer this question, the therapist must continue with the behavioral diagnosis and find out more specifically about other potential barriers (e.g., physical, sociocultural, and psychological) that were not revealed by the other questions.[23,32] To discover barriers, the therapist should begin by acknowledging that it can be difficult to follow a home program and that many people have trouble doing it. Possible questions to ask the patient include the following:

- What problems do you anticipate?
- What are your beliefs or feelings about exercise?
- What are the best and worst things about exercise?
- What can I do to help you succeed?

A central aspect of the behavioral diagnosis process is the assessment of the patient's motivation to improve. It is hoped that the patient has some important activity or symptom that will serve as a factor to motivate treatment behavior. The therapist should determine what activity the patient wants most to return to, or what symptom he or she wants most to control or eliminate.[22] In addition to the goal, the concept of self-efficacy, as discussed earlier, is a good predictor of motivation and behavior.[31] A patient is also more likely to follow the intervention if he or she believes there is high likelihood that the intervention will result in achieving the goal. The patient's belief that the treatment will result in the desired outcome can be developed by reference to other successful patients, graded success, and mastery experiences with treatment. If the patient is not confident in his or her ability to perform the intervention, then practice opportunities must be provided. Good questions for assessing the patient's motivation include the following:

- What is the most important activity that you wish to return to?

- What symptoms do you want to minimize first?
- How confident are you in your ability to perform the program?
- Do you think these exercises will help you recover?

The physical therapist should link the intervention to improving the patient's condition. The patient and the therapist can then decide on reasonable short- and long-term goals and make a mutual agreement on the intervention regimen.

TEACHING AND PROBLEM SOLVING DURING INTERVENTION AND FOLLOW-UP

One of the most common mistakes when teaching a treatment program is making it too complex.[21,39] Although the therapist may believe that doing the entire program would be most beneficial, the likelihood that the patient will be able to complete a very complex home program is quite low. Patients should receive specific instruction in the psychomotor aspects of the activities, clearly written directions accompanied by illustrations or some other visual representations, and specific tailoring of the program to the patient's literacy level, lifestyle, and valued activities. Inclusion of reminder strategies can also increase adherence. These could include use of daily exercise logs, setting a specific time of day to exercise, or engaging a family member or friend to be an "exercise buddy." The therapist should find out about social support and teach the family the exercises if necessary. The following questions might be helpful in assessing the patient's understanding of the program.

- Are there exercises you already do at home? How often do you do them?
- Can you demonstrate them?
- Are there problems fitting the program into your daily activities?
- Do you have the necessary equipment? Can we find things around the house to use for the exercises?
- Do you have a place to do the program?

When the patient returns for follow-up, the therapist should evaluate the patient for change in body function and structure and activities and participation as well as for adherence.

- Can you show me the exercise?
- What changes have you noticed since starting the program?
- Have there been any negative consequences of doing the exercises?
- Have you had problems remembering to do them?

With follow-up the patient and the physical therapist have the opportunity to renegotiate and problem-solve. These steps are necessary because the patient's beliefs can change during the intervention. As the patient's experiences with illness and with treatment change, previous motivations or barriers may no longer play the same role. The therapist must be able to identify these changes in the patient, explore the new motivational factors, and problem-solve ways to eliminate the barriers. The treatment plan may need to be modified to meet new goals.

REMOVING BARRIERS TO INTERVENTION

The patient-practitioner interaction is an essential element in adherence to an intervention program.[22,32] If the patient has trouble adhering to the program, the therapist is responsible for identifying any barriers that stand in the way of success. He or she might need to modify or completely change the intervention plan to accommodate barriers that cannot be removed. Lorig and colleagues[21] outlined a decision chart that can be used by the physical therapist to explore with the patient how to improve adherence (Table 13–4).

MOTIVATIONAL INTERVIEWING

A tool that therapists can use to elicit behavior change is motivational interviewing. Its purpose is to allow the patient to arrive at the conclusion that a behavior change is necessary or desirable. When using this technique, the therapist is no longer using persuasion or suggesting methods of change.[40] Motivational interviewing is defined as a "directive, client-centered counseling style for eliciting behaviour change by helping clients explore and resolve ambivalence."[41] Motivational interviewing requires careful

TABLE 13–4   Suggestions for Improving Patient Adherence

Problem	Patient's Response	Suggestion
Can the patient tell you why he or she is not doing the exercise?	Yes	Listen and problem solve.
Does the patient believe that adherence to the regimen will help the problem?	No	Explore the patient's belief system. Expand on the patient's current belief system.
Does the patient understand the exercise program?	No	Teach the patient why exercises are important.
Does the patient have the skills to do the exercises?	No	Teach the patient the skills. Break the regimen into smaller parts. Give the patient feedback on his or her performance.
Does adherence to the exercise program have negative consequences for the patient?	Yes	Adapt the regimen to the patient's complications. Reinterpret the patient's symptoms (if necessary).
Does nonadherence have positive consequences for the patient?	Yes	Problem-solve with the patient. Provide a support structure for the patient.
Does the patient forget to do the exercises?	Yes	Design memory strategies.
Does the patient believe that he or she cannot do the exercises?	Yes	Increase the patient's self-efficacy.
What if the patient does not want to adhere to the regimen?	—	That is okay. You have tried your best.

Adapted from Lorig K (ed). Patient Education: A Practical Approach, 2nd ed. Thousand Oaks, CA: Sage, 1996.

listening, encouraging the desire to change *from the patient* by eliciting cognitive dissonance, and instilling confidence in the patient's ability to make the change, thus reducing or resolving the cognitive dissonance.[42,43] Showing empathy and encouragement throughout the process helps to support the patient's self-efficacy. Channon and coworkers[44] described the sequence of steps in motivational interviewing as awareness building (helping the patient to recognize the pros and cons of continuing the behavior), creating alternatives to the current behavior, problem solving, making choices between alternative behaviors, goal setting, and avoidance of confrontation. This last concept is very important in motivational interviewing. The therapist should ask open-ended questions to encourage the patient to identify the problem behaviors, alternatives, and choices. In this way, the process is patient centered, not therapist driven.[44]

SUMMARY

Little research has been done in physical therapy regarding patient-centered communication, but there have been several studies in medicine investigating whether patient-centered communication has any effect on patient satisfaction and health outcome. There is strong evidence that more patient-centered communication does lead to a higher degree of patient satisfaction and more positive outcomes.[15-17] The following are suggestions for effective patient-practitioner communication:

- Ask questions about the patient's complaints, concerns, understanding of the problem, expectations, and feelings.
- Show support and empathy.
- Let the patient tell his or her story.
- Encourage the patient to ask questions.
- Provide educational materials.
- Share decision making with the patient.

In this chapter, we have discussed ways to promote adherence and presented a model of patient-practitioner collaboration, both of which can be useful in clinical practice. Understanding what patients believe, how they act relative to lifestyle changes, and how they respond to the health care provider are necessary components of successful physical therapy interventions. Attention to and integration of effective patient-practitioner communication and employing strategies to promote adherence should be part of every physical therapist's interaction with all patients.

THRESHOLD CONCEPTS

Threshold Concept #1: Physical therapists work to facilitate and support patients' ability to engage in behavior change. In order to do this, physical therapists must recognize that they are not just purveyors of information and treatments. Uncovering and assessing elements of health beliefs and values that underlie patients' behaviors must be a standard part of the physical therapy examination and evaluation.

Learn to "read" your patients. This involves asking enough questions and listening carefully to the answers to get a feel for what motivates them, what is important

to them, what they are afraid of, what misconceptions they might have, and what interventions they feel are likely to be beneficial. Careful listening is the beginning step in facilitating patients' ability to make healthy behavior changes.

Threshold Concept #2: In this current health care environment, now more than ever, successful outcomes are contingent on the patients' ability to self-manage. Central to this is robust patient-practitioner communication. Be honest at all times with your patients. They should be able to trust you completely.

Trust is earned by being forthright, thoughtful, considerate, and open. Ask open-ended questions designed to help the patient to discover what behaviors need to change. Be encouraging and supportive. Do not overload your patients with exercises. Try to link successful exercise to gains in function that will enable them to do activities that they value. Discuss what they are willing to do and what activities they value, and tailor your exercise interventions to their answers.

ANNOTATED BIBLIOGRAPHY

Dreeben O. *Patient Education in Rehabilitation.* Sudbury, MA: Jones and Bartlett; 2010.
> Written primarily by physical therapists, this text is very useful text for those who want more in-depth information regarding patient education. Divided into five sections, each has a summary and complementary case study. Sections include Basic Concepts of Patient Education, Patient Education Variables, Teaching and Learning Theories, and Ethical, Legal and Cultural Variables.

Glanz K, Rimer B, Viswanath K. *Health Behavior and Health Education: Theory, Research and Practice.* 4th ed. San Francisco: Jossey-Bass; 2008.
> Written for students as well as practitioners in multiple disciplines, this book explains the theories and application of health education and health promotion practices. It describes how health education changes when dealing with different populations, from the individual patient through the community groups. The tables and figures support the text well.

Mason P, Butler C. *Health Behavior Change: A Guide for Practitioners.* 2nd ed. New York: Churchill Livingstone Elsevier; 2010.
> This text provides strategies for the health care professional to assist patients in making healthy behavior changes. Various examples of desired behavior changes, techniques to encourage active patient participation, and pitfalls to avoid are scattered throughout the book. These apply to many health care disciplines. The approach presented in this easy-to-read book strongly supports the patient-practitioner collaborative model.

Redman B. *The Practice of Patient Education: A Case Study Approach.* 10th ed. St. Louis: Mosby Elsevier; 2007.
> This is a great book for those in clinical practice. The early chapters touch on the many theoretical models of behavior change and the principles, objectives, instructional methods, and program evaluation that guide patient education. These chapters are full of examples, tables, and figures that help the reader easily grasp the content. The latter chapters are dedicated to education about specific health conditions. Study questions at the end of each chapter highlight major points.

REFERENCES

1. Health Plan Employer Data and Information Set (HEDIS). *National Committee on Quality Assurance (NCQA).* Available at: http://www.ncqa.org. Accessed 22.07.11.
2. Physician Quality Reporting System (PQRS). *Centers for Medicare and Medicaid Services (CMS).* Available at:https://www.cms.gov/PQRS. Accessed 22.07.11.
3. Balanced Budget Act of 1997. *Centers for Medicare and Medicaid Services (CMS).* Available at: https://www.cms.gov; 1997. Accessed 10.07.11.
4. Issue in Focus. *Physical Therapy in a Reformed Health Care System: Accountable Care Organizations.* American Physical Therapy Association; June 2010.

5. Issue in Focus. *Physical Therapy in a Reformed Health Care System: Center for Innovation (Direct Access)*. American Physical Therapy Association; June 2010; 1.

6. Issue in Focus. *Issue in Focus. Physical Therapy in a Reformed Health Care System: Medical Home*. American Physical Therapy Association; December 2010.

7. Healthy People 2020. *Determinants of Health*. U.S. Department of Health and Human Services. Available at http://www.healthypeople.gov/2020. Accessed 03.05.11.

8. Xu J, Kochanek MA, Murphy SL, Tejada-Vera B. Deaths: final data for 2007. U.S. Department of Health and Human Services. *Vital Statistics Reports*. 2010;58:1–2.

9. Flegal KM, Carroll MD, Ogden CL, Curtin LR. Prevalence and trends in obesity among US adults, 1999-2008. *JAMA*. 2010;303:235.

10. *Surgeon General's Vision for a Healthy and Fit Nation*. Rockville, MD: U.S. Department of Health and Human Services; 2010.

11. Goetzel RZ, Gibson TB, Short ME, et al. A multi-worksite analysis of the relationships among body mass index, medical utilization, and worker productivity. *J Occup Environ Med*. 2010;52:S52–S58.

12. 2008 Physical Activity Guidelines for Americans. *U.S. Department of Health and Human Services*. Available at: http://www.health.gov/PAGuidelines. Accessed 03.05.11.

13. Pollock M, Carroll J, Graves J, et al. Injuries and adherence to walk/jog and resistance training programs in the elderly. *Med Sci Sports Exerc*. 1991;23:1194–1200.

14. Malounin E, Potvin M, Prevost J, et al. Use of an intensive task-oriented gait training program in a series of patients with acute cerebrovascular accidents. *Phys Ther*. 1992;72:781–789.

15. Taal E, Rasker JJ, Seydel ER, Wiegman O. Health status, adherence with health recommendations, self-efficacy and social support in patients with rheumatoid arthritis. *Patient Educ Couns*. 1993;20:63–76.

16. Atreja A, Bellam N, Levy SR. Strategies to enhance patient adherence: making it simple. *Med Gen Med*. 2005;7:4.

17. LaPointe NMA, Fang-Shu O, Calvert SB, et al. Association between patient beliefs and medication adherence following hospitalization for acute coronary syndrome. *Am Heart J*. 2011;161:855–863.

18. Rau JL. Determinants of patient adherence to an aerosol regimen. *Respir Care*. 2005;50:1346–1359.

19. George J, Kong CM, Stewart K. Adherence to disease management programs in patients with COPD. *Int J Chron Obstruct Pulmon Dis*. 2007;2:253–262.

20. Veazie PJ, Cai S. A connection between medication adherence, patient sense of uniqueness, and the personalization of information. *Med Hypotheses*. 2007;68:335–342.

21. Lorig K, ed. *Patient Education: A Practical Approach*. 3rd ed. Thousand Oaks, CA: Sage; 2000.

22. Glanz K, Rimer BK, Viswanath K. *Health Behavior and Health Education: Theory, Research and Practice*. 4th ed. San Francisco: Jossey-Bass; 2008.

23. Jensen GM, Lorish C. Promoting patient cooperation with exercise programs: linking research, theory and practice. *Arthritis Care Res*. 1994;7:181.

24. American Physical Therapy Association. *Interactive Guide to Physical Therapist Practice 2003*. Available at: http://www.apta.org. Accessed 03.05.11.

25. Kleinman A. *The Illness Narratives: Suffering, Healing, and the Human Condition*. New York: Basic Books; 1987.

26. Levanthal H. The role of theory in the study of adherence to treatment and doctor-patient interactions. *Med Care*. 1985;23:556.

27. Stewart M, Brown J, Weston W, et al. *Patient-Centered Medicine: Transforming the Clinical Method*. Thousand Oaks, CA: Sage; 1995.

28. Jette A. Physical disablement concepts for physical therapy research and practice. *Phys Ther*. 1994;74:380.

29. Jette A. Outcomes research: shifting the dominant research paradigm in physical therapy. *Phys Ther*. 1995;75:965.

30. International Classification of Functioning. *Disability and Health*. Geneva: World Health Organization; 2001.

31. Bandura A. *Social Foundations of Thought and Action: A Social Cognitive Theory*. Englewood Cliffs, NJ: Prentice-Hall; 1986.

32. Dreeben O. *Patient Education in Rehabilitation*. Boston: Jones and Bartlett; 2010.

33. Fiore MC, Bailey WC, Cohen SJ, et al. *Treating tobacco use and dependence. Clinical Practice Guideline*. Rockville, MD: U.S. Department of Health and Human Services; 2000.

34. Prochaska JO, Norcross JC, DiClemente CC. *Changing for Good*. New York: W Morrow; 1994.

35. Miller WL, Crabtree BF. Clinical research: conversing the wall. In: Denzin NK, Lincoln YS, eds. *Handbook of Qualitative Research*. 2nd ed Thousand Oaks, CA: Sage; 2000:618.

36. Meichenbaum D, Turk DC. *Facilitating Treatment Adherence*. New York: Plenum; 1987.

37. Turk D. Correlates of exercise compliance in physical therapy [commentary]. *Phys Ther*. 1993;73:783.

38. Carcuff R. *The Art of Helping*. 7th ed. Amherst, MA: Human Resources Press; 1993.

39. Mason P, Butler CC. *Health Behavior Change: A Guide for Practitioners*. 2nd ed. Edinburgh: Churchill Livingstone/Elsevier; 2010.

40. Rollnick S, Butler CC, Stott N. Helping smokers make decisions: the enhancement of brief intervention for general medical practice. *Patient Educ Couns*. 1997;31:191–203.

41. Rollnick S, Miller WR. What is motivational interviewing? *Behav Cog Psychother*. 1995;23:326.

42. Rollnick S, Butler CC, Kinnersley P, et al. Competent novice motivational interviewing. *Br Med J*. 2010;340:c1900.

43. Redman BK. *The Practice of Patient Education: A Case Study Approach*. 10th ed. St. Louis: Mosby Elsevier; 2007.

44. Channon SJ, Huws-Thomas MV, Rollnick S, et al. A multicenter randomized controlled trial of motivational interviewing in teenagers with diabetes. *Diabetes Care*. 2007;30:1390–1395.

45. Grotle M, Garratt AM, Klokkerud M, et al. What's in team rehabilitation care after arthroplasty for osteoarthritis? Results from a multicenter, longitudinal study assessing structure, process and outcomes. *Phys Ther*. 2010;90:121–131.

46. Trummer UF, Mueller UO, Nowak P, et al. Does physician-patient communication that aims at empowering patients improve clinical outcome? A case study. *Patient Educ Couns*. 2006;61: 299–306.

47. Matthias MS, Blair MJ, Nyland KA, et al. Self-management support and communication from nurse care managers with primary care physicians: a focus group study of patients with chronic musculoskeletal pain. *Pain Manag Nurs*. 2010;11:26–34.

TEACHING AND LEARNING PSYCHOMOTOR SKILLS

Lisa Kenyon ✺ **Diane Nicholson**

CHAPTER OUTLINE

Last summer I worked with a 5-year-old boy who had left hemiparesis secondary to cerebral palsy. He was able to perform many skills independently, including walking, running, and jumping; however, he had difficulty using his left hand and arm in functional tasks. This was especially problematic when he was attempting activities on the playground at school. The child's ability to climb the ladder to the playground slide was specifically concerning to his mother and teacher because they worried that he could fall and get hurt when attempting this task. When I observed the child attempting to climb the ladder to the slide, I too had concerns for the child's safety. I noted that he led the activity with his right extremities, such that his body was rotated, with the right side of his body close to the ladder and the left side turned away from it. He did not use his left upper extremity at all during the activity, but instead held his left arm in shoulder adduction and internal rotation, elbow flexion, forearm pronation, and wrist flexion. He had difficulties propelling his body up the ladder and was unable to coordinate the reciprocal nature of the task. Instead he used a step-to pattern in which he grasped the ladder with his right hand, stepped up a rung with his right foot, then stepped up with his left foot, placing only his forefoot in contact with the rung. He then leaned the right side of his body into the ladder for support while releasing the ladder with his right hand to grasp the next rung. He almost fell multiple times when ascending the ladder and required physical assistance to regain his balance on two of those occasions. The child expressed his desire to be able to climb the ladder to the slide and play with his classmates. This goal was added to his care plan and became the focus of his intervention over the following weeks.

As his physical therapist, one of my primary roles with this child was to be an educator. In fulfilling this role, I established a physical therapy program that focused on the task and environmental demands of being able to climb the ladder to the slide with lots of other children on the playground during a busy recess period. I provided abundant practice opportunities that were challenging to the child but not too challenging. I considered ways to motivate the child and provide feedback while at the same time identifying methods that promoted active, discovery learning. The child worked diligently in therapy and in his home exercise program. His hard work paid off, and at the end of several months, he was able to ascend the ladder to the playground slide using a functional and safe movement pattern.

Motor learning focuses on the processes to develop new strategies, to retain strategies, and to generalize strategies. An understanding of these motor learning principles is as important to the practitioner in physical therapy as are the elements of didactic and clinical teaching presented in Chapters 2, 3, and 8 to 11. The primary purpose of this chapter is to present variables related to motor learning that therapists can manipulate to facilitate acquisition of psychomotor skills.

LEARNING GOALS

After completing this chapter, the reader should be able to:
1. Differentiate between motor performance and motor learning.
2. Differentiate amongst Adams', Schmidt's, and Newell's motor learning theories.
3. Describe processes that influence motor performance and motor learning.
4. Identify stages of motor learning as described by Fitts and Posner.
5. Discuss the application of Gentile's taxonomy of tasks to physical therapy practice.
6. Describe individual, task, and environment influences on motor performance and motor learning.
7. Manipulate prepractice, practice, and feedback variables to optimize motor learning based on learner characteristics and task demands.
8. Adapt motor learning principles to meet the unique needs of various patient populations.

DISTINCTION BETWEEN MOTOR LEARNING AND MOTOR PERFORMANCE

Physical therapist practice centers on helping patients to learn or relearn motor skills. *Motor learning* is an internal process associated with practice or experiences that results in a relatively permanent change in a person's ability to perform a motor skill. Because it is an internal process, motor learning cannot be directly measured and must be indirectly assessed through observation of motor behavior. In physical therapy, motor learning can be indirectly evaluated by measuring change in a patient's performance of a motor task.

Motor performance may be influenced by a number of variables, including motivation and the use of pharmacologic agents. Maturation and practice are factors that may influence both motor performance and motor learning. A common method of separating the permanent effects of maturation and practice is to measure changes across days or weeks instead of years. However, this method is often ineffective when attempting to measure learning in pediatric and elderly populations because maturation can result in significant changes over days or weeks in children and older adults. To separate maturation and practice influences on performance in these populations, comparisons of practice and nonpractice groups are often necessary. For example, several studies have used two group experimental designs to separate performance changes due to maturation and participation in early intervention programs.[1,2]

Temporary factors, such as motivation, physical or verbal guidance, fatigue, stress, and boredom during long therapy sessions, may also influence motor performance. To measure motor learning, the effects of temporary factors on performance should be minimized. The most common method used to reduce the temporary effects of variables on performance is to allow a rest interval between the practice and the evaluation session. In physical therapy settings, the effects of temporary factors can be minimized by evaluating a patient's performance after he or she rests, or by evaluating performance at the beginning of a subsequent therapy session.

Separating the effects of temporary and permanent factors on performance is critical for documentation. As therapists, we often document changes in patient function based on our observations of a patient's best performance during a therapy session. The patient's performance during the session, however, may have been influenced by the temporary effects of our therapy (e.g., hands-on guiding or facilitation techniques). Evaluating and documenting the patient's performance of a practiced skill at the onset of a subsequent therapy session will more accurately reflect the long-term impact of our interventions.

Physical therapy goals often focus on a patient's ability to function in various settings under a variety of conditions. For example, goals for gait training might include the ability to walk at slow, medium, and fast velocities; on tile, carpet, grass, or snow; or in a crowded or dimly lit hallway. The field of motor learning distinguishes between assessments in practiced and new or differing environments. Evaluation in the same environment used during a practice or therapy session is termed a *retention test*, whereas evaluation in a different environment than that used during a practice session is termed a *transfer test*. For example, if a patient practices walking on a tiled surface during therapy, he or she would undergo a retention test when evaluated on tile, and a transfer test when evaluated on carpet. Retention and transfer tests are used for measures of learning. Retention tests measure how well performers learn practiced tasks. Transfer tests measure how well performers generalize learning to perform the task unpracticed in a different environment.

OVERVIEW OF PROCESSES OF MOTOR LEARNING

The processes of motor learning extend beyond conquering the mere motor demands of a task. Motor learning involves developing strategies to cope with the complexities of performing a specific task under specific environmental conditions. Learners must be able to solve motor problems (i.e., process information and engage in sensory encoding and memory retrieval processes) and respond to changes in the task and the environment. To optimize learning, therapists must provide patients with practice conditions that encourage (or possibly force) them to engage in problem-solving processes.[3] This suggests that patients should be active participants not only in the production of their movements but also in planning their movements. Instead of providing patients with solutions to motor problems, therapists should act as educators and guide patients through learning processes that allow the patients to actively explore and discover solutions to motor problems.[3] A summary of the processes of motor learning is given in Box 14–1.

MOTOR LEARNING THEORIES

Various theories attempt to explain motor learning.[4-6] Table 14–1 provides a brief summary of several popular theories: Adams' Closed-Looped Theory,[4] Schmidt's Schema

---

BOX 14–1   Summary of Processes of Motor Learning

- Learners remember processes, not specific movement patterns.
- Relative to guidance, problem solving enhances learning.
- The three sequential stages of learning are cognitive, associative, and autonomous.
- Automaticity develops by learning to focus on a critical subset of perceptual cues and motor strategies and by reorganizing information in units (termed chunking).
- The capability to detect and correct errors enhances learning. Error detection and correction occur online or during, slow, positioning movements. They occur after the movement in fast, timing tasks.

- Sensory and motor memories are thought to be stored in memory.
- Retrieval practice enhances learning more than repetitive drills.
- Instead of focusing on individual elements of a functional task, performers should focus on the goals of a task.
- With practice, actions become more efficient when performers learn to exploit the biomechanics of a task.
- Categorizing tasks based on task goals and environmental context and learner characteristics can enhance understanding of task requirements.

TABLE 14–1 Summary of Theories of Motor Learning

Theory	Defining Characteristics
Adams' Closed-Looped Theory	Sensory feedback is required for movement (now known to be false).
	Exemplar (or individual) sensory and motor memories are stored each time an action is performed.
	Enhancing sensory feedback will enhance learning.
	Errors will always interfere with learning (now known to be false).
	Emphasizes practicing tasks to be performed at a later time (termed *specificity of learning*).
Schmidt's Schema Theory	Defines a class of tasks as actions having identical relative timing and amplitude.
	Generalized sensory and motor memories are stored for a class of tasks.
	Novice actions should be performed as well as practiced actions within the same class of tasks.
	Errors can enhance learning.
	Emphasizes benefits of practicing several variations of a class of tasks (termed *variability in practice*).
Newell's Ecological Theory	Emphasizes performer, task, and environment constraints and relationships.
	Emphasizes relationships between sensory (perceptual) cues and motor (action) strategies.
	Emphasizes relationships between sensory and motor processes.
	Emphasizes the importance of variable practice related to task demands and environmental conditions.

Theory,[5] and Newell's Ecological Theory.[6] Each of these theories has limitations and varying levels of research support as well as clinical implications. For example, clinical application of Schmidt's Schema Theory[5] may consist of practicing a task under a variety of conditions to assist learners in developing a set of rules or schema related to the specific task. Application of Newell's Ecological Theory[6] would suggest that practicing a task under variable conditions will assist learners in understanding the relationship between perceptual cues and motor action (i.e., the glass looks heavy and therefore will require more force to lift).

STAGES OF LEARNING

According to Fitts and Posner,[7] the process of motor learning can be divided into three sequential stages: (1) the cognitive stage, (2) the associative stage, and (3) the autonomous stage. During the cognitive stage, the learner focuses on understanding the task, developing strategies to execute the task, and determining ways to evaluate task success. Performance during this stage is often characterized by inaccuracies, slowness, and movements that appear stiff and uncoordinated. Because this stage is characterized by rapidly improving and variable performance, it is thought to require a high degree of attention and other cognitive processes.

My teenager's first attempts at driving a car provide a classic example of the cognitive stage of learning. While sitting stiffly and tightly gripping the steering wheel, my daughter would intently focus on the road ahead. As the car moved forward and it came time to shift into a higher gear, her eyes would dart back and forth between the road and the gear shift as she slowly attempted to shift. Engaging in a conversation with me or trying to listen to a traffic update on the radio were too taxing at this stage. All of her attention was directed at trying to keep the car on the road and on understanding the relationships amongst the gas pedal, the clutch, and the brake. Basically, driving demanded all of her attention.

Each time we attempt a new motor task (e.g., juggling, knitting, or snowboarding), and often when we perform a well-learned task in an infrequently practiced environment (e.g., driving a car on icy, snowy roads, or skiing down a steeper hill than we are used to), we find ourselves in this cognitive stage of learning. Our patients often display similar processes during therapy sessions. After a shoulder injury, for example, patients may need to relearn motor tasks such as dressing or brushing their hair.

Therapists can actively promote learning during the cognitive stage by facilitating the patient's understanding of the task and organizing practice in ways that will specially encourage early learning.[8] Emphasizing the purpose of the activity within a context that is functionally relevant to the individual patient may help the patient to better understand the task.[8,9] Structuring the environment to reduce distractions may help the learner to better attend to learning. Clear, concise instructions should be provided in a manner that does not overwhelm the learner. Demonstrations of how the task should ideally be performed and providing hands-on guidance as needed will assist the patient in developing a cognitive map of the correct performance of the task. The use of feedback and practice schedules to promote learning at the various stages will be discussed later in this chapter.

After the initial cognitive stage, learners enter the associative stage of learning. Here, the goal is to fine-tune a skill. During this stage, the focus is on how to produce the most efficient action. Relative to the cognitive stage, this stage is characterized by slower gains in performance and reduced variability. To continue with the previous example of learning to drive a car, the first year or so of driving represents the associative stage of learning. After time, my daughter learned to smoothly accelerate and decelerate the car at intersections and to smoothly change gears using the gearshift, clutch, and gas pedals. The associative stage is represented in physical therapy when patients practice a skill to increase the safety or efficiency of a task. For example, when a person with a transfemoral amputation is learning to use a lower extremity prosthesis, the slow transition from taking a few uncoordinated steps to walking smoothly across the floor represents the associative stage. In essence, the patient needs practice time to enhance performance of the skill. Therapists can enhance learning in the associative stage by reducing the amount of hands-on guiding or assistance provided to the patient.[8] The environment should be structured to gradually promote variations in practice conditions and demands.[8]

The autonomous stage of learning is also described as the *automatic stage*. Relative to the first two stages, performance in this stage requires very little attention and information processing. After several years of driving practice, my teenager's driving style characterizes the autonomous stage. She is now able to follow the verbal directions provided by a GPS unit, hold a conversation with a friend in the car, drink from a water bottle, and change lanes on the highway all at the same time. In therapy sessions, this autonomous stage is often achieved over the course of an episode of care when a patient progresses from ambulating with an assistive device, to ambulating independently in select closed environments, to ambulating independently in a community setting under dual task demands (e.g., walking while holding a conversation).

ERROR DETECTION

The capability to detect errors is another process that is thought to develop with learning. Error detection capabilities are thought to require memory of sensory feedback from previously performed actions and are used differently for slow-positioning and fast-timing tasks. In slow-positioning tasks, sensory feedback is used to guide the action to its endpoint. Thus, learners move until feedback from the present action matches the memory of sensory feedback for the desired action. In fast-timing tasks, learners are unable to use sensory feedback to alter an action online, or during an action. In such tasks, sensory feedback is used to detect errors after the action has ended.[10]

Reaching for a cup while reading the newspaper is an example of a slow-positioning task. People will often reach toward the general direction of a cup, then use shoulder abduction and adduction until the hand hits the cup. They will then grasp the cup and bring it to their lips. In contrast, trying to catch a glass of juice that is falling off a table is an example of a fast-timing task. A movement such as this is too fast for sensory feedback to be used during the movement. Sensory feedback can be used only after the movement to determine the accuracy of the action—that is, the person is holding the glass or looking at a puddle on the floor.

MOTOR MEMORIES

Memory is an essential aspect of effective motor learning.[11] Three distinct memory systems are thought to exist: short-term sensory store (STSS), short-term memory (STM), and long-term memory (LTM).[11] In STSS, numerous segments or streams of sensory information entering the system are briefly stored by sensory modality (e.g., visual, tactile, kinesthetic). Information in STSS is not thought to reach a conscious level and is only retained for a matter of milliseconds. Selected information from STSS is selected for further processing in STM. Selection is thought to be based on the relevance and pertinence of the information. Some authors conceptualize STM as a temporary workspace and may term STM as a form of working memory.[11] People hold onto information in STM for only as long as they direct their attention to the information.

LTM is memory system that stores information and experiences accumulated over a life time.[11] LTM is thought to consist of two basic forms: declarative (explicit) learning and nondeclarative (implicit) learning. Explicit learning is associated with knowledge that can be consciously recalled and stated, such as facts and events. It requires attention, awareness, and reflection.[12] Implicit learning refers to memories that are less accessible to conscious recollection and verbal recall. Several forms of implicit learning are exemplified by fairly passive learning processes in which learners acquire knowledge through exposure to information. The attentional and cognitive demands of such learning processes are limited. Implicit learning includes the following forms of learning: nonassociative, associative, and procedural.[11,12]

Nonassociative learning occurs when individuals are repeatedly exposed to a single stimulus.[11] Simple forms of nonassociative learning include habituation and sensitization and are often utilized in clinical practice. For example, patients with certain vestibular disorders have been shown to benefit from exercises that center on repeated performance of activities that provoke their dizziness.[13,14] Although the neuromechanisms behind habituation are not fully understood, over time, these patients habituate to the stimulus and experience a reduction in their symptoms.[13,14]

Through associative learning, a person learns to predict relationships such as the relationship of one stimulus to another (classical conditioning) or the relationship of a behavior to a consequence (operant conditioning).[11] In therapy sessions, if we repeatedly provide a patient with a verbal cue and a physical prompt when performing a transfer, we may see that over time, the patient will begin to associate the verbal and physical cueing and begin to perform the transfer with verbal cues only. In operant conditioning, a patient may learn that behaviors leading to rewards should be repeated and that behaviors that have negative results should be avoided. This may be a factor for our elderly patients who have recently experienced a fall (a *negative consequence*) in that such patients may choose to decrease their activity in order to decrease their chances of falling again. Fear of falling may thus become an obstacle that must be conquered in our therapy sessions.

Procedural learning relates to learning tasks though intense practice to the point at which the task can be performed without conscious thought or active attention.[11] Such learning occurs with repetition across varying environmental conditions and happens gradually over a period of time. Once the learner learns the "rules" to performing the task, the task is executed with very little conscious attention.[11] In therapy, achieving such comfort with motor skills is often a desired outcome. For example, when teaching a patient with a spinal cord injury to perform transfers, our long-term goal may relate to achieving a level of automaticity and generalizability that will allow the patient to transfer safely under a variety of plausible conditions.

Many intervention approaches rely on explicit learning techniques. When teaching crutch use on stairs, for example, therapists often use strategies that involve explicit directions: "Up with the right foot; down with the left foot." When gait-training with a patient, we often give the patient verbal instructions: "Take a longer step on the right" or "Lift your knee higher." For patients who are able to process verbal information, maintain attention, and concurrently perform motor and cognitive tasks (listening to the therapist while walking), such strategies may be successful and appropriate. Yet for patients who have cognitive, attentional, or language deficits, such explicit learning strategies may pose difficulties. For example, Orrell and coworkers[15] compared explicit and implicit learning strategies for teaching a dynamic balance task and found that the provision of explicit information may actually be detrimental for some patients after a stroke. A study by Boyd and Winstein[16] further found that regardless of whether subjects had sustained a stoke involving the basal ganglia or the sensorimotor cortex, the provision of explicit information had a negative impact on learning and skill retention.

FOCUSING ON ACTIONS, NOT MOVEMENTS

Many motor behaviorists argue that memories for movements focus on task goals.[17] There is little evidence that learners store and retrieve memories for individual segments of an action (e.g., extend the elbow, open the fingers, close the fingers, then grasp an object), without regard for the task goal or the environment. This principle suggests that patients should practice tasks or actions, not individual movements. For example, a child with cerebral palsy may be learning to ride a tricycle during therapy sessions. The therapeutic goal may be to enhance interlimb coordination between her legs. During practice, however, the therapist and child focus on an outcome goal (moving the tricycle forward as fast as possible), and not on the movements required for interlimb coordination.

LEARNING TO EXPLOIT BIOMECHANICS

Increased consistency in kinematics and coordination also occurs with practice. Learners are taught to discover ways to take advantage of the passive inertia properties of muscles, joints, and limbs.[3] With practice, performers demonstrate increased speed and decreased energy costs because they have learned to optimize the peripheral sensory and

motor requirements of the task. Therapists must be able to help patients exploit biomechanics to achieve a goal. This is especially important during the associative stage of learning when patients are trying to fine-tune a skill and should be exposed to different variations of the same skill. For example, therapists most often teach a force-control strategy for sit-to-stand transfers. Although this strategy is relatively safe, a momentum strategy is more efficient.[9] Shumway-Cook and Woollacott[9] advocate that patients be allowed to explore several strategies for transfers so that they have choices available. When patients seek safety over efficiency, they may choose a force-control strategy, whereas when efficiency is the primary goal, a momentum strategy may be chosen.

VARIABLES THAT INFLUENCE SKILL LEARNING

The purpose of this section is to provide information on applying motor learning principles to clinical situations. As reflected in Figure 14–1, structuring our therapy sessions to best promote motor learning requires consideration of characteristics related to the task, the environment, and the individual. Determining the specific practice variables that will facilitate an individual's motor learning requires careful consideration of research findings from both the general and clinical populations.

GENTILE'S TASK TAXONOMY

Given that therapeutic goals and outcomes strive to optimize patient function and independence across a variety of settings, therapists must consider the characteristics of both the task and the environment when planning instructional strategies. Task attributes can be classified based on whether an activity is a discrete task with a discernible beginning and endpoint, such as moving from sit to stand, or a continuous task with a variable endpoint, such as walking or biking. An additional task attribute relates to whether the base of support is stationary or changing.

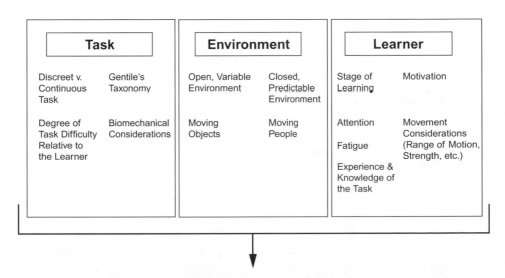

Determination of Teaching Strategies to Promote Motor Learning

FIGURE 14–1 Factors that influence the selection of teaching strategies in motor learning.

For example, in quiet standing, the base of support is still, but in ascending stairs, the base of support changes with each step. Other considerations include upper extremity manipulation requirements, the amount of attention demanded by a task, and the variability of the movement.[9,12] When analyzing movement tasks, physical therapists must also consider biomechanical factors of the specific muscle groups and muscle actions involved in an activity; the range of motion requirements for the movement; and the coordination, power, and speed demands of the task.[9,18]

What processes are critical for a particular task? Gentile[12] attempted to answer this question by classifying tasks. Her hypothesis was that the sensory, motor, and cognitive demands of a task are dependent on task goals and on environmental and performer contexts. Table 14–2 lists Gentile's taxonomy of tasks. The rows are classified into one of four environmental contexts. In the first two categories, termed *stationary*, the environment is stable while the task is being performed. In the last two categories, termed *motion*, the environment is moving while the task is being performed. In the first and third categories, termed *no intertrial variability*, the environment remains constant from trial to trial. In the second and fourth categories, termed *intertrial variability*, the environment changes from trial to trial. Examples of tasks are provided in Tables 14–3 and 14–4.

As shown in the top of Table 14–2, tasks with little or no variation that are performed in a stable environment are termed *closed tasks*. These tasks require consistent patterns of movement and can be done automatically (or with little attention). Tasks that vary with each repetition, or that are performed in a changing environment, are termed *open tasks* (see Table 14–3). These tasks require attention and a relatively high amount of information processing. Examples of functional closed-skill tasks are climbing a familiar flight of stairs and transferring from a wheelchair to a therapy mat. Examples of functional open-skill tasks are walking down a crowded corridor and maintaining balance while standing on a moving bus.

With the columns, Gentile[12] separates tasks into one of four performer contexts. In the two categories on the left, termed *body stability*, the person focuses on maintaining a posture. In the two categories on the right, termed *body transport*, the person focuses on transporting himself or herself to another location. In the first and third categories, termed *no manipulation*, the person focuses on one task (e.g., holding a posture, or transporting herself or himself to another location). In the second and fourth categories, termed *manipulation*, the person is required to perform two tasks simultaneously (e.g., holding a posture and manipulating an object, or transporting himself or herself to another location while manipulating an object).

How does Gentile's taxonomy relate to physical therapy? Therapists can use the taxonomy to identify the degree of difficulty associated with a movement task and to progress the complexity of a task by altering its taxonomy. Categorizing tasks within Gentile's taxonomy allows therapists to (1) understand the processes required for different activities and goals, (2) evaluate the types of tasks likely to be less challenging and those more likely to be difficult for an individual patient, (3) design an effective exercise program based on an individual's needs and the tasks he or she would like to perform, and (4) educate patients and families on the types of tasks that are safe and unsafe for patients to perform.

PREPRACTICE VARIABLES

Supporting a patient's motor learning starts before actual motor practice begins. Prepractice variables that therapists must consider include motivation and goal setting. Patients and families should direct the goal setting process so that therapy goals are meaningful to the individual patient. Goals should be motivating and challenging, yet focused and achievable. Goals should be objective and measurable (e.g., walk independently without losing balance for 80 meters in 1 minute). The goal "do the best you can" should be avoided because it may be less effective for learning than

TABLE 14–2 Gentile's Taxonomy of Tasks

Environmental Context		Performer Context			
		Body Stability		**Body Transport**	
Condition	**Variability**	**No Manipulation**	**Manipulation**	**No Manipulation**	**Manipulation**
Stationary	No intertrial variability	Closed Consistent Motionless Body stability No manipulation	Closed Consistent Motionless Body stability Manipulation	Closed Consistent Motionless Body transport No manipulation	Closed Consistent Motionless Body transport Manipulation
	Intertrial variability	Variable Motionless Body stability No manipulation	Variable Motionless Body stability Manipulation	Variable Motionless Body transport No manipulation	Variable Motionless Body transport Manipulation
Motion	No intertrial variability	Consistent Motion Body stability No manipulation	Consistent Motion Body stability Manipulation	Consistent Motion Body transport No manipulation	Consistent Motion Body transport Manipulation
	Intertrial variability	Open Variable Body stability No manipulation	Open Variable Body stability Manipulation	Open Variable Body transport No manipulation	Open Variable Body transport Manipulation

Adapted from Gentile AM. Skill acquisition: action, movement and neuromotor processes. In Carr J, Shepherd R, Gordon J, et al (eds). Movement Science: Foundations for Physical Therapy in Rehabilitation, 2nd ed. Rockville, MD: Aspen Press, 2000.

TABLE 14–3 Examples of Intertrial Variability Tasks in Gentile's Taxonomy of Tasks

Environmental Condition	No Intertrial Variability	Intertrial Variability
Stationary	**Closed Tasks** *Definition: Spatial features of the environment do not change from one attempt to the next.* Examples: • Climbing stairs at home • Brushing teeth • Unlocking the front door • Stepping onto a bathroom scale	**Variable Motionless Tasks** *Definition: Spatial features of the environment vary from one attempt to the next.* Examples: • Walking on different surfaces • Climbing stairs of various heights • Drinking from cups, mugs, or glasses
Motion	**Consistent Motion Tasks** *Definition: Objects or supporting surface is in motion, but conditions do not change across trials.* Examples: • Stepping onto an escalator • Lifting a suitcase from an airport conveyor belt • Moving through a revolving door	**Open Tasks** *Definition: Other persons, objects, or supporting surface is in motion and conditions change across trials.* Examples: • Sitting in a moving car • Catching a ball • Walking through a crowded hallway • Carrying a wiggling child

Adapted from Gentile AM. Skill acquisition: action, movement and neuromotor processes. In Carr J, Shepherd R, Gordon J, et al (eds). Movement Science: Foundations for Physical Therapy in Rehabilitation, 2nd ed. Rockville, MD: Aspen Press, 2000.

TABLE 14–4 Examples of Manipulation Tasks in Gentile's Taxonomy of Tasks

Body Orientation	No Manipulation	Manipulation
Stability	**Body Stability** *Definition: The body is not moving.* Examples: • Sitting • Standing • Leaning on table	**Body Stability Plus Manipulation** *Definition: The body is not moving but is accomplishing simultaneous tasks.* Examples: • Holding an object while standing • Reaching for a glass while sitting • Writing at a desk
Transport	**Body Transport** *Definition: The body is moving from one place to another.* Examples: • Walking • Running • Crawling	**Body Transport Plus Manipulation** *Definition: The body is moving from one place to another while accomplishing simultaneous tasks.* Examples: • Carrying child while walking • Running to catch a ball • Driving a car

Adapted from Gentile AM. Skill acquisition: action, movement and neuromotor processes. In Carr J, Shepherd R, Gordon J, et al (eds). Movement Science: Foundations for Physical Therapy in Rehabilitation, 2nd ed. Rockville, MD: Aspen Press, 2000.

objective, measurable goals. Goals should also be focused on the action or task level (e.g., walk up the steps) rather than related to performing specific motions or movement patterns (e.g., bend your hip and knee).

Therapists may find individualized patient-centered measures such as the Canadian Occupational Performance Measure (COPM)[19] or the Perceived Efficacy and Goal Setting System (PEGS)[20] to be helpful when establishing collaborative goals and patient outcomes. The COPM[19] is administered as a semistructured interview through which activity limitations and participation restrictions are identified. The patient and family also rate their perception of current performance or satisfaction with a variety of tasks at the onset of therapy, and when readministered at the end of an episode of care, the COPM[19] provides an outcome measure for intervention activities. The COPM[19] was designed for use with people with a variety of diagnoses and conditions across all developmental levels

and has been used with adults and children as young as 8 years of age. For children 6 to 9 years of age, the PEGS[20] may be used to set goals for intervention. In addition to caregiver and teacher questionnaires, the PEGS[20] utilizes a picture-based system that helps the therapist guide the child through a process to pinpoint tasks that the child finds challenging and to identify tasks that the child would like to work on in therapy. It is important that therapists work with both children and caregivers to establish goals because children may have goals that differ from those of their parents and teachers.[20,21]

PRACTICE VARIABLES

Intensity of Practice

A critical factor in learning or relearning motor skills is the amount of practice. Within a practice session, the number of repetitions performed is more critical than the actual amount of time spent practicing. How many repetitions are needed for learning to occur? More research is needed to determine the ideal number of repetitions. Many studies focused on motor learning require subjects to complete a high number of repetitions. For example, in a study designed to investigate the interaction between feedback and motor adaption, healthy adults performed 300 repetitions of a simple reaching task.[22] When examining the impact of explicit feedback on motor learning following a stroke, Boyd and Winstein[16] required subjects to perform 150 trials of two separate motor tasks. Learning complex skills such as those required for high-level athletic or musical performance may require thousands of repetitions. In a study by Lang and colleagues,[23] however, the average number of repetitions performed during outpatient therapy sessions for patients following a stroke was found to be much lower. These authors observed that in sessions addressing the lower extremity, an average of 33 active exercise movements, 6 passive exercise movements, and 8 purposeful movements were practiced. In sessions addressing gait, an average of 292 steps were taken. Based on the need to provide practice opportunities, therapists should consider alternative means to increase the number of repetitions patients perform, such as task-specific home programming and use of virtual reality or robotic training.[24,25]

Schmidt and Lee[26] describe a logarithmic relationship between practice and the rate of improvement. This relationship suggests that the rate of improvement at any point during practice is related to the amount of improvement left to achieve. Based on this concept, learners in the early stages of practice would be expected to experience more rapid improvement than learners who have already undergone a large amount of practice. This relationship has been suggested as a possible explanation for the success of constraint-induced therapy programs for patients with hemiplegia following a stroke. The sheer number of practice trials performed during these intensive therapy programs is thought to accelerate the learning process and result in rapid improvements in performance.[26]

Massed versus Distributed Practice

Given the importance of practice and repetition, therapists must consider the potential impact of different practice schedules. During *massed practice*, the amount of actual practice time is much greater than amount of rest time between practice trials. In a *distributed practice* schedule, the amount of time allotted for rest is equal to or even greater than the amount of time spent practicing. Which is better: massed or distributed practice? The answer depends on factors related to the learner and the task to be learned because there are both limitations and advantages to each of these types of practice schedules.

Mental and physical fatigue are often concerns when using massed practice schedules. Patients who have endurance issues or limitations in their ability to perform without rest breaks may find massed practice interferes with learning as the demands are too taxing. When practicing continuous tasks, massed practice may decrease performance but the real issue may relate to the impact of fatigue on patient safety. Massed practice may thus be better suited for patients who have sufficient stamina, attention, and concentration.

Massed practice has been used in several studies involving patient populations.[27-29] Constraint-induced movement therapy (CIMT) programs targeting upper extremity function in adults and children with hemiplegia have used massed practice to create intensive practice scenarios.[27] Shumway-Cook and colleagues[28] used massed practice as a component of an intervention program addressing balance recovery in children with cerebral palsy and found that subjects' improvements were sustained even after the completion of the intervention program. Beekhuizen and Field-Fote[29] examined the effect of massed practice versus massed practice plus somatosensory stimulation in subjects with chronic incomplete tetraplegia. These investigators found that subjects in the massed practice plus somatosensory stimulation group demonstrated greater improvements in pinch strength and timed functional test scores than subjects in the massed practice only group.

Distributed practice schedules may be beneficial for patients with short attention spans or poor concentration abilities. Tasks that conform well to a distributed practice schedule include highly complex tasks, tasks that are very energy consuming, and tasks that require a large amount of time to complete.

Constant Practice and Variable Practice

The ability to generalize learning allows us to perform tasks under unique or varied conditions. *Variable practice* may assist learners in adapting to novel situations and demands. Within variable practice conditions, learners practice different versions of the same task within the same practice session and thus develop competence in creating parameters for various dimensions of the motor actions required to perform a task.[11] For example, practice sessions involving throwing a ball at various distances to a target of varying size allow a learner to discover how throwing force influences the distance the ball is thrown and how accuracy changes at different throwing speeds. In therapy sessions, this may involve situations such as practicing sit-to-stand transfers from surfaces of varying heights and firmness (a mat table versus a soft couch) or practicing spoon feeding with different types of foods (yogurt versus soup).

Another example of variable practice relates to the speed at which tasks are practiced. Movement tasks practiced in therapy sessions are often performed functionally at varying speeds. For example, my typical gait speed when walking in a dimly lit theater is different from my typical gait speed when walking to my mailbox. To assist in developing such generalizable skills, therapists should encourage patients to practice functional tasks at varying speeds so as to promote responses to the changing demands of performing a task at a slow versus a faster pace.

Variability in practice may be most valuable when learning is focused on a task that will be performed under a variety of conditions. For tasks requiring minimal variation that will be performed under stable, predictable conditions, *constant practice* may be beneficial. Constant practice refers to practice sessions focused on one version of a single task.[11] Skills that aim at exactly replicating a task each and every time, such as executing a complex dive from the high board, would benefit most from constant practice.

Contextual Interference

Patients may practice several skills during a typical therapy session. Often, several trials of one task are practiced before initiating practice of a second task. This type of scheduling is termed *blocked practice*. An alternative way to schedule practice is to practice different tasks on consecutive trials. This scheduling is termed *random practice*. Both blocked and random practice involve the same number of repetitions and tasks, but in random practice, the order of tasks is nonrepetitive and unpredictable. The term *contextual interference* is used to refer to the intertrial inconsistency that is generated by practice order.[11,26] Blocked practice thus produces low contextual interference whereas random practice yields high contextual interference.[11,26] Not surprisingly, repeatedly rehearsing the same task in blocked practice typically results in improved motor performance. However, actual motor learning of a skill (e.g., long-term skill retention and transfer) has been shown to be facilitated by random practice. Random practice appears to be most effective when the sequence of skills being practiced involve different patterns of coordination and movement.[11]

Many studies involving the benefits of contextual interference have focused on healthy adult populations.[11,30,31] Ste-Marie and associates,[37] however, conducted a series of experiments to examine the impact of blocked versus random practice on handwriting skills in elementary school children. A random practice schedule was found to enhance transfer and retention of handwriting skills. Hanlon[33] explored the impact of random versus blocked practice in subjects who had chronic stroke and found that subjects who practiced under random conditions performed better on retention tests than subjects who had practiced under blocked conditions.

Despite these findings, random practice schedules may not always be beneficial. Findings by Dick and coworkers[34] suggest that subjects with Alzheimer disease learned best under constant practice conditions. In a study by Lin and colleagues,[35] subjects with early Parkinson disease (Hoehn and Yahr stages I and II) were found to benefit from a blocked practice schedule over random practice. Shumway-Cook and Woollacott[9] further suggest that random practice may not be beneficial in the early stages of learning and should not be undertaken until the learner exhibits an understanding of the characteristics of the task to be learned. Therapists should thus consider individual learner characteristics when deciding to implement a blocked versus a random practice sequence.

Part- and Whole-Task Practice

Depending on the skill and experience of the learner, the complexity of certain skills may be initially overwhelming to learners. For certain tasks, learners may benefit from breaking down the task and practicing individual components.[11] Such part-task practice is felt to be most beneficial to learning tasks that involve a serial skill. In such tasks, the actions are akin to a series of discrete skills in that one part of the task is not affected by the actions of the next part of the task. A wheelchair transfer can be viewed as a serial skill in which locking the brakes is one discrete component of the overall task.

When the task to be learned involves information, part-task practice may also prove to be beneficial.[11] For example, the task of going from home to a downtown therapy location requires strategies for understanding spatial directions. The focus is on learning how to solve a maze of streets, and then making appropriate left and right turns to arrive at the location. Because information processing is the item to be learned, the focus of practice should be on learning segments of the task (e.g., directions from my house to the freeway, directions for freeway intersections, and directions from the freeway exit to the therapy setting).

When the task to be learned is a continuous task or requires timing between segments, then whole-task practice has been found to enhance learning. For example, when my teenager was learning to drive, she found it easy to learn to depress the clutch and to move the gear stick from one gear to another; the difficult part of the task was coordinating depressing the clutch while changing gears. Because coordination (or timing) is an essential component of the task, her practice sessions focused on the whole task. Examples of tasks in which whole-task practice is recommended include wheelchair wheelies and momentum transfers.

Mental Practice

Mental practice is an active process in which a learner mentally rehearses a task with the intent of enhancing motor learning. During mental practice, learners do not physically practice a skill. Instead they focus on cognitive processes such as seeing and feeling themselves performing the skill.[36] Several authors suggest that mental practice can be an effective adjunct to physical practice and that such practice activates the same neural structures as physical practice of the same skills.[36–38]

Several studies have examined the effects of mental practice on patient populations.[39–41] Page and colleagues[39] used a randomized, placebo-controlled trial to examine the effects of mental practice on specific upper extremity movements in subjects with chronic stroke. Subjects in the therapy plus mental practice group exhibited significant improvements in upper extremity impairments and in daily arm function compared with the therapy-only group. A study by Liu and colleagues[40] found that subjects after stroke who were trained to perform mental practice of specific daily living tasks demonstrated significant improvement in household and community tasks compared with subjects who did not perform mental practice. A pilot study by Tunney and associates[41] examined the influence of mental practice on retention of a newly learned functional motor task in community-dwelling older adults (ages 66 to 89 years) and found that subjects in the mental practice group were found to perform better on retention tests than those who did not use mental practice techniques.

When considering the use of mental practice methods, therapists must consider patient-related factors such as familiarity with the task, cognition, and the ability to engage in motor imagery.[36] Dickstein and Deutsch[36] suggest that patients who are familiar with the motor task to be learned generally will experience greater benefit from mental practice than patients who are not familiar with the task. Although not an absolute contraindication for the use of mental practice, several authors caution that patients with cognitive deficits may have difficulties with mental practice techniques.[36,41,42] Dickstein and Deutsch[36] further advocate that a patient's ability to engage in motor imagery should be evaluated before such techniques are employed. Tools such as the Kinesthetic and Visual Imagery Questionnaire (KVIQ)[43] may be used to assess a patient's abilities in the visual and kinesthetic dimensions of motor imagery. The KVIQ has been found to be valid and reliable for use with patients after stroke as well as patients with Parkinson disease.[42,43]

Use of Guidance Techniques

Intervention techniques frequently involve the use of physical cueing to assist patients in learning or relearning motor skills. Therapists may use physical prompts or even hand-over-hand assist to help patients perform tasks and movements during therapy sessions. Although such guidance in the very early stages of learning may help introduce the learner to the characteristics of the task to be learned, long-term use of physical guidance and assistance techniques may promote dependency and affect task retention and transferability.[9,11] Such concepts do not imply that therapists should never use guidance techniques during therapy sessions. Instead, these ideas suggest that guidance should be withdrawn as soon as possible to help promote long-term learning and retention.

Use of Feedback

Feedback has also been shown to be an essential aspect of the learning process. Feedback is typically divided into two subclasses: intrinsic and extrinsic feedback. Intrinsic feedback comes from various sensory systems as the result of the production of the movement. Extrinsic feedback acts as a supplement to intrinsic feedback and is provided to the learner by an outside source (e.g., a therapist, a stop watch). Extrinsic feedback may be provided concurrently during the execution of a task or at the end of the task and is often classified as either knowledge of results (KR) or knowledge of performance (KP). KR is defined as terminal feedback about the outcome of a movement as related to the goal of the movement.[26] In some learning situations, KR may be redundant because it provides the learner with the same information as intrinsic feedback.

KP is feedback related to the kinematics or quality of the movement pattern used to achieve the goal. KP should provide the learner with information related to the essential components of the movement pattern. Thorpe and Valvano[44] use the task of broad jumping to illustrate this concept. The essential components of broad jumping include bending the knees to at least 45 degrees and propelling forward using the legs, using the arms to assist in propelling the trunk forward, and using a two-footed takeoff and landing. Meaningful KP would thus provide learners with feedback directed at these components of the jumping pattern.

Video Feedback

Although much of the feedback provided to learners during physical therapy sessions is verbal in nature, visual feedback in the form of video replay may also assist learning.

Schmidt and Wrisberg[11] even suggest that a split-screen display may be beneficial in providing video feedback to learners. This technology allows the learner's movements to be displayed on the screen alongside a model of correct or optimal performance. Whether the video uses a split screen or a display of the learner only, effective videotape feedback has been found to relate to both the learner's skill level and the use of verbal cues.[11] Advanced learners have been found to benefit from videotape feedback, regardless of the provision of verbal cues. In contrast, to be effective for learning, novice learners needed verbal cues to focus their attention to pertinent information on the videotape. Given that therapy sessions typically focus on the early stages of skill learning, videotape replay may be an effective method for learning. To optimize learning, therapists should focus a client's attention on critical aspects of the videotape. Similar to augmented feedback, videotape feedback should be provided frequently early in practice and less often as practice continues.

Gilmore and Spaulding[45] explored the impact of videotaped feedback plus occupational therapy on the ability to don socks and shoes in patients who had sustained a stroke. Although no group differences were found between subjects receiving occupational therapy only and subjects receiving video feedback plus occupational therapy, the authors noted that the group receiving video feedback reported a perception of performing the task better and were more satisfied with their ability to perform the task. The authors thus concluded that the use of video feedback may improve satisfaction with task performance, which may influence motivation and effort during therapy activities.

Motivation and Reinforcement

In addition to information about performance and results, feedback can serve to motivate and reinforce learning. Learners may find that feedback makes the learning experience more enjoyable and encourages continued practice and effort.[11] Without feedback, learners may lack the incentive to continue practicing: practice efforts may wane, and learners may even discontinue training all together.

Feedback may also provide reinforcement to the learner.[11] Positive reinforcement increases the likelihood that a learner will repeat the performance on subsequent trials. Negative reinforcement occurs when an aversive condition or stimulus is removed following performance, thus increasing the chances that the action will be repeated. The buzzer that sounds when a car is started and continues until all seat belts are buckled is an example of negative reinforcement. Punishment differs from negative reinforcement in that punishment decreases the likelihood that a response will be repeated. Negative reinforcement and punishment are often difficult for learners to interpret and do not provide the learner with information to improve performance. Positive reinforcement is thus thought to generate greater improvements in learning than negative reinforcement or punishment.

Frequency and Timing of Feedback

In addition to the type of feedback provided, the frequency and timing of feedback have been shown to influence learning. As stated by Ezekiel and colleagues,[46] therapists should consider ways of providing feedback that discourage patients from becoming dependent on the feedback. Such methods may include allowing learners time to think about an action before feedback is provided, asking learners to estimate their own errors before feedback is provided, and withholding feedback on some practice trials (especially near the end of practice).[11,46]

Concurrent or immediate feedback may create dependence on the feedback and thus may become an impediment to learning.[46,47] Delaying extrinsic feedback allows the learner time to process the intrinsic feedback created by the execution of a task. In this way, intrinsic information is not lost or left unused, and the learner is able to benefit from both the intrinsic and extrinsic feedback. This concept can be extended to include nontherapist forms of extrinsic feedback such as use of a mirror. The visual feedback and information provided by the mirror may cause learners to shift their focus away from the proprioceptive feedback and information provided by the movement.[46] In discussing the use of augmented sensory cues to enhance learning in patients with Parkinson disease, Nieuwboer and coworkers[48] suggested that therapists incorporate a weaning-off stage to assist such patients in dissociating the task learned from the cues provided.

Providing feedback on a reduced or faded schedule is another means to reduce the likelihood of a learner becoming dependent on feedback to enhance performance.[49] Such feedback is again thought to enhance the information-processing demands of a practice session and is associated with skill retention. Therapists should recognize, however, that reduced feedback schedules may not always be beneficial to motor learning. Sullivan and associates[50] found that motor learning in typically developing children between 8 and 14 years of age required longer periods of practice with a more gradual reduction in feedback compared with healthy young adults. The authors surmised that the increased cognitive demands created by a reduced feedback schedule created an optimal challenge for young adults and helped to focus their learning. The children in the study, however, were though to be too challenged by the demands of a reduced feedback schedule, therefore surpassing the children's optimal level of challenge.

A study by Chiviacowsky and Wulf[51] creates an interesting idea related to the provision of feedback. In this study, healthy undergraduate students were divided into two groups: one group received KR only on "good" trials, whereas the other group received KR only on "poor" trials. The group receiving KR only on good trials showed better performance on delayed retention tasks. The authors believed that receiving KR only after good trials created a more successful experience for learners, which perhaps motivated the learners and enhanced their learning.

Focus of Attention

Numerous studies suggest that a learner's focus of attention may be an important influence on both motor performance and motor learning.[52-54] In a study involving healthy high school and university students, Wulf and coworkers[53] found that the effectiveness of feedback for learning complex motor skills is influenced by the focus of attention

induced by the feedback. Providing an external focus of attention using feedback directed at the effects of movement ("Hit the ball as if using a whip") was more effective than feedback that provided an internal focus of attention directed at the movement itself ("Snap your wrist when hitting the ball"). Adopting an external focus of attention has been found to be an effective strategy for healthy individuals when learning a variety of skills, such as balance tasks, sports skills, and movement skills.[53,54]

Several studies in patient populations support the concept of providing feedback to promote an external focus of attention.[55,56] Fasoli and associates[55] looked at the impact of attentional focus on reaching tasks in patients following a stroke and in age-matched controls. Both groups were found to perform tasks more effectively when provided with instructions that promoted an external focus of attention ("Think about the size and shape of the mug"). Wulf and colleagues[56] found that subjects with idiopathic Parkinson disease who were in Hoehn and Yahr stages II and III showed less postural sway (e.g., reduced postural instability) when instructions and feedback promoted an external versus an internal focus of attention.

Clinically, we can use an external focus of attention to assist patients in learning a variety of tasks. When working on weight shifting, for example, we may ask the patient to reach for strategically placed objects rather than to focus on the weight shift itself. Using gait-training strategies such as instructing the patient to imagine kicking a ball during terminal swing may be more effective in improving heel strike than simply asking the patient to "Hit the ground with your heel."[52] Placing lines on the floor and instructing a patient to "Step over the line" may help to improve stride length.[57] Techniques such as these may help patients to focus on the effects of movement and perhaps may function in ways that permit more unconscious control processes to emerge.[52]

A FRAMEWORK FOR MOTOR LEARNING

What can be done to best facilitate motor learning in a clinical setting? The answer to this question is dependent on numerous factors, including learner-specific characteristics, the demands of the specific task to be learned, environmental conditions, and factors related to the interplay among the task, the environment, and the learner. The Challenge Point Framework developed by Guadagnooli and Lee[58] is a theoretical framework that helps to conceptualize the optimal challenge point for motor learning by considering characteristics of the learner, the task to be learned, and the condition of practice. Under the Challenge Point Framework, learning is related to the amount of information available to the learner compared with the amount of information viewed as a challenge to the learner. Optimal levels of information leads to optimal learning, whereas too little or too much information can inhibit learning.

Within the Challenge Point Framework, the difficulty of the task to be learned is said to relate to both nominal and functional factors. Nominal task difficulty reflects the perceptual and motor requirements of the task and is constant regardless of who is performing the task. Functional task difficulty refers to how challenging the task is relative to the skill level of the person attempting the task and the conditions under which the task is being performed. For a task such as walking on a level surface in a quiet, unchanging environment, the functional task difficulty might be low for a typical, healthy young person but high for a patient recovering from a brainstem stroke.[9] In accordance with the Challenge Point Framework, as the patient's skill level progresses, the functional difficulty associated with this walking task decreases. The patient may then be ready for the therapist to increase the difficulty of the task by changing the environment of practice (adding obstacles or people).

Onla-or and Winstein[59] tested the predictions of the Challenge Point Framework in individuals with moderately severe Parkinson disease compared with a control group. In this study, nominal task difficulty and the conditions of practice were manipulated. Under conditions of low demand, subjects with Parkinson disease displayed learning comparable to controls. Under high-demand situations, however, subjects with Parkinson disease demonstrated learning deficits in generalizing and transferring skills and were only able to perform comparably to controls when the recall test was exactly the same as during practice. Although further research is needed to validate the Challenge Point Framework in patient populations, it serves as an excellent reminder that therapists must consider characteristics of the task to be learned, the environment, and the patient when planning and organizing therapy sessions to enhance motor learning.

THRESHOLD CONCEPTS

Threshold Concept #1: Therapists should consider factors related to the environment, the task, and the learner when teaching psychomotor skills.

As identified throughout this chapter, successful application of motor learning principles involves consideration of multiple factors related to the learner, the task, and the environment. Although physical therapist practice may often focus on patient-specific body impairments and the activity restrictions that influence a patient's ability to execute motor tasks, contemplating the potential impact of factors related to the task and environment will assist therapists in planning and organizing intervention sessions that enhance and support motor learning.

Threshold Concept #2: Gentile's taxonomy of tasks provides a framework to assist in increasing or decreasing the level of challenge provided to a patient.

As a clinical instructor, I noticed that students often had difficulties modifying interventions to meet patients' changing needs. I found that Gentile's taxonomy of tasks provided students with a framework from which to identify ways to modify both the task and the environment to increase or decrease the demands of intervention activities.

ANNOTATED BIBLIOGRAPHY

Schmidt RA, Wrisberg CA. *Motor Learning and Performance: A Situation-Based Learning Approach.* 4th ed. Champaign, IL: Human Kinetics; 2008.
  This text expands on the fundamentals of motor learning and provides multiple examples related to the application of motor learning

concepts within a variety of settings. Included are chapters that focus on integration and application of motor learning principles and provide checklists to evaluate characteristics related to the learner, the task, and environment that should be considered when designing learning experiences. Case studies further illustrate the application of theory in various motor learning situations.

Magill RA. *Motor Learning and Control: Concepts and Applications.* 9th ed. Dubuque, IA: McGraw-Hill; 2011.
  This book provides an introductory study of motor learning and control. It includes chapters on motor learning principles for several types of tasks, learners, and environments. It focuses on performance and learning effects of several variables while providing theoretical explanations of motor learning phenomena.

REFERENCES

1. Dirks T, Blauw-Hospers CH, Hulshof LJ, et al. Differences between the family-centered "COPCA" program and traditional infant physical therapy based on neurodevelopmental treatment principles. *Phys Ther.* 2011;91:1303–1322.
2. Blauw-Hospers CH, Dirks T, Hulshof LJ, et al. Pediatric physical therapy in infancy: from nightmare to dream? A two-arm randomized trial. *Phys Ther.* 2011;91:1323–1338.
3. Higgins S. Motor skill acquisition. *Phys Ther.* 1991;71:123–139.
4. Adams JA. A closed-loop theory of motor learning. *J Mot Behav.* 1971;3:111.
5. Schmidt RA. A schema theory of discrete motor skill learning. *Psychol Rev.* 1975;82:225.
6. Newell KM. Motor skill acquisition. *Annu Rev Psychol.* 1991;42:213–237.
7. Fitts PM, Posner MI. *Human Performance.* Belmont, CA: Brooks/Cole; 1967.
8. O'Sullivan SB. Examination of motor function: motor control and motor learning. In: O'Sullivan SB, Schmitz TJ, eds. *Physical Rehabilitation.* 5th ed. Philadelphia: FA Davis; 2007:227–271.
9. Shumway-Cook A, Woollacott MH. *Motor Control: Translating Research into Clinical Practice.* 4th ed. Philadelphia: Lippincott Williams & Wilkins; 2012.
10. Schmidt RA, White JL. Evidence for an error detection mechanism in motor skills: a test of Adams' closed-loop theory. *J Mot Behav.* 1972;4:143–153.
11. Schmidt RA, Wrisberg CA. *Motor Learning and Performance: A Situation-Based Learning Approach.* 4th ed. Champaign, IL: Human Kinetics; 2008.
12. Gentile AM. Skill acquisition: action, movement and neuromotor processes. In: Carr J, Shepherd R, Gordon J, et al. *Movement Science: Foundations for Physical Therapy in Rehabilitation.* 2nd ed. Rockville, MD: Aspen Press; 2000.
13. Clendaniel RA. The effects of habituation and gaze stability exercises in the treatment of unilateral vestibular hypofunction: a preliminary results. *J Neurol Phys Ther.* 2010;34:111–116.
14. Cohen HS, Kimball KT. Increased independence and decreased vertigo after vestibular rehabilitation. *Otolaryngol Head Neck Surg.* 2003;128:60–70.
15. Orrell AJ, Eves FF, Masters RS. Motor learning of a dynamic balancing task after stroke: implicit implications for stroke rehabilitation. *Phys Ther.* 2006; 86:369–380.
16. Boyd LA, Winstein CJ. Explicit information interferes with implicit motor learning of both continuous and discrete movement tasks after stroke. *J Neurol Phys Ther.* 2006;30:46–57.
17. Bernstein N. *The Coordination and Regulation of Movements.* Oxford, UK: Pergamon Press; 1967.
18. Fell DW. Progressing therapeutic intervention in patients with neuromuscular disorders: a framework to assist clinical decision making. *J Neurol Phys Ther.* 2004;28:35–46.
19. Law M, Baptiste S, Carswell A, et al. *Canadian Occupational Performance Measure.* 3rd ed. Ottawa: CAOT Publications ACE; 1998.
20. Missiuna C, Pollock N, Law M. *Perceived Efficacy and Goal Setting System.* San Antonio, TX: Pearson Corporation; 2004.
21. Dunford C, Missiuna C, Street E, et al. Children's perceptions of the impact of developmental: coordination disorder on activities of daily living. *Br J Occup Ther.* 2005;68:207–214.
22. Fine MS, Thoroughman KA. Motor adaptation to single force pulses: sensitive to direction but insensitive to within-movement pulse placement and magnitude. *J Neurophysiol.* 2006;96:710–720.

23. Lang CE, MacDonald JR, Gnip C. Counting repetitions: an observational study of outpatient therapy for people with hemiparesis post-stroke. *J Neurol Phys Ther.* 2007;31:3–10.

24. Sandlund M, Hoshi K, Waterworth EL, et al. A conceptual framework for design of interactive computer play in rehabilitation of children with sensorimotor disorders. *Phys Ther Rev.* 2009;14: 348–354.

25. Brokaw EB, Murray T, Nef T, et al. Retraining of interjoint arm coordination after stroke using robot-assisted time-independent functional training. *J Rehabil Res Dev.* 2011;48:299–316.

26. Schmidt RA, Lee TD. *Motor Control and Learning: A Behavioral Emphasis.* 5th ed. Champaign, IL: Human Kinetics; 2011.

27. Wolf SL, Winstein CJ, Miller JP, et al. Effect of constraint-induced movement therapy on upper extremity function 3 to 9 months after stroke. *JAMA.* 2006;296:2095–2104.

28. Shumway-Cook A, Hutchinson S, Kartin D, et al. Effect of balance training on recovery of stability in children with cerebral palsy. *Dev Med Child Neurol.* 2003;45:591–602.

29. Beekhuizen KS, Field-Fote EC. Massed practice versus massed practice with stimulation: effects on upper extremity function and cortical plasticity in individuals with incomplete cervical spinal cord injury. *Neurorehabil Neural Repair.* 2005;19:33–45.

30. Boutin A, Blandin Y. On the cognitive processes underlying contextual interference: contributions of practice schedule, task similarity and amount of practice. *Hum Mov Sci.* 2010;29:910–920.

31. Ollis S, Button C, Fairweather M. The influence of professional expertise and task complexity upon the potency of the contextual interference effect. *Acta Psychol (Amst).* 2005;118:229–244.

32. Ste-Marie DM, Clark SE, Findlay LC, et al. High levels of contextual interference enhance handwriting skill acquisition. *J Mot Behav.* 2004;36:115–126.

33. Hanlon RE. Motor learning following unilateral stroke. *Arch Phys Med Rehabil.* 1996;77:811–815.

34. Dick MB, Hsieh S, Dick-Muehlke C, et al. The variability of practice hypothesis in motor learning: does it apply to Alzheimer's disease? *Brain Cogn.* 2000;44:470–489.

35. Lin C, Sullivan KJ, Wu AD, et al. Effect of task practice order on motor skill learning in adults with Parkinson disease: a pilot study. *Phys Ther.* 2007;87:1120–1131.

36. Dickstein R, Deutsch JE. Motor imagery in physical therapist practice. *Phys Ther.* 2007;87:942–953.

37. Decety J. The neurophysiological basis of motor imagery. *Behav Brain Res.* 1996;77:45–52.

38. Lacourse MG, Turner JA, Randolph-Orr E, et al. Cerebral and cerebellar sensorimotor plasticity following motor imagery based mental practice of a sequential movement. *J Rehabil Res Dev.* 2004;41: 505–524.

39. Page SJ, Levine P, Leonard A. Mental practice in chronic stroke: results of a randomized, placebo-controlled trial. *Stroke.* 2007; 38:1293–1297.

40. Liu KP, Chan CC, Lee TM, et al. Mental imagery for promoting relearning for people after stroke: a randomized controlled trial. *Arch Phys Med Rehabil.* 2004;85:1403–1408.

41. Tunnery N, Billings K, Blakely BG, et al. Mental practice and motor learning of a functional motor task in older adults: a pilot study. *Phys Occup Ther Geriatr.* 2006;24:63–80.

42. Randhawa B, Harris S, Boyd LA. The kinesthetic and visual imagery questionnaire is a reliable tool for individuals with Parkinson disease. *J Neurol Phys Ther.* 2010;34:161–167.

43. Malouin F, Richards CL, Jackson PL, et al. The kinesthetic and visual imagery questionnaire (KVIQ) for assessing motor imagery in persons with physical disabilities: a reliability and construct validity study. *J Neurol Phys Ther.* 2007;31:20–29.

44. Thorpe DE, Valvano J. The effects of knowledge of performance and cognitive strategics on motor skill learning in children with cerebral palsy. *Pediatr Phys Ther.* 2002;14:2–15.

45. Gilmore PE, Spaulding SJ. Motor learning and the use of videotape feedback after stroke. *Top Stroke Rehabil.* 2007;14:28–36.

46. Ezekiel HJ, Lehto NK, Marley TL, et al. Application of motor learning principles: the physiotherapy client as a problem-solver, III. Augmented feedback. *Physiother Can.* 2001;53:33–39.

47. Winstein CJ, Pohl PS, Cardinale C, et al. Learning a partial-weight-bearing skill: effectiveness of two forms of feedback. *Phys Ther.* 1996; 79:985–993.

48. Nieuwboer A, Rochester L, Müncks L, et al. Motor learning in Parkinson's disease: limitations and potential for rehabilitation. *Parkinsonism Relat Disord.* 2009;15:S53–S58.

49. Winstein CJ, Schmidt RA. Reduced frequency of knowledge of results enhances motor skill learning. *J Exp Psychol Learn Mem Cogn.* 1990; 16:677–691.

50. Sullivan KJ, Kantak SS, Burtner PA. Motor learning in children: feedback effects on skill acquisition. *Phys Ther.* 2008;88:720–732.

51. Chiviacowsky S, Wulf G. Feedback after good trials enhances learning. *Res Q Exerc Sport.* 2007;78:40–47.

52. McNevin NH, Wulf G, Carlson C. Effects of attentional focus, self-control, and dyad training on motor learning: implications for physical rehabilitation. *Phys Ther.* 2000;80:373–385.

53. Wulf G, McConnel N, Gärtner M, et al. Enhancing the learning of sport skills through external-focus feedback. *J Mot Behav.* 2002;34:171–182.

54. Totsika V, Wulf G. An external focus of attention enhances transfer to novel situations and skills. *Res Q Exerc Sport.* 2003;74:220–225.

55. Fasoli SE, Trombly CA, Tickle-Degnen L, et al. Effect of instructions on functional reach in persons with and without cerebrovascular accident. *Am J Occup Ther.* 2002;56:380–390.

56. Wulf G, Landers M, Lewthwaite R, et al. External focus instructions reduce postural instability in individuals with Parkinson disease. *Phys Ther.* 2009;89:162–168.

57. Morris ME, Iansek R, Matyas TA, et al. Stride length regulation in Parkinson's disease: normalization strategies and underlying mechanisms. *Brain.* 1996;119:551–568.

58. Guadangnoli MA, Lee TD. Challenge point: a framework for conceptualizing the effects of various practice conditions in motor learning. *J Mot Behav.* 2004;36:212–224.

59. Onla-or S, Winstein CJ. Determining the optimal challenge point for motor skill learning in adults with moderately severe Parkinson's disease. *Neurorehabil Neural Repair.* 2008;22:385–395.

COMMUNITY HEALTH PROMOTION
EVOLVING OPPORTUNITIES FOR PHYSICAL THERAPISTS

15

Julie Gahimer ☉ David Morris

CHAPTER OUTLINE

In 2005, the University of Indianapolis, Krannert School of Physical Therapy initiated a campus-community partnership between the Baxter YMCA and the University of Indianapolis to integrate health promotion practices into clinical education experiences for second year Doctor of Physical Therapy (DPT) students. The purpose of the program is to provide adults with long-term neurologic disability a weekly social and leisure experience that also enhances their physical activity and wellness.

The format of the class is 12 weeks with four students per week working with adults with neuromuscular disabilities. The class meets 1.5 hours per week. The neurologic diagnostic groups represented include spinal cord injury (paraplegia and tetraplegia), Guillain-Barré syndrome, multiple sclerosis, Parkinson disease, stroke, and traumatic brain injury. The program consists of 20 to 30 minutes of warm-up, in a circle and to music, in which each student and each participant choose an exercise or activity. In addition, medicine balls, free weights, Thera-Band, and gymnastic balls are used. This is followed by 30 to 45 minutes of individualized exercise programs to meet each person's needs. The purpose of the exercise portion of the program is to improve balance, coordination, endurance, flexibility, strength, and mobility. The program is advertised on the INSHAPE Indiana website as a success story.[1]

Feedback from the participants of the program include "an improved sense of well-being," "socialization," "increased community involvement," "feeling better," and "feeling stronger." Feedback from the students participating in the program is very positive. The students experience opportunities to apply such exercise prescription and program planning principles as mode, intensity, duration, frequency, rate of progression, warm-up, and cool-down related to exercise, communication skills with persons with different neuromuscular diagnoses, professional behaviors, intervention planning, cultural sensitivity, and safety awareness.

Our star participant is a 91-year-old woman with past history of stroke who lives alone. She drives to the class and states that she loves the social aspect of coming to see her friends once a week. She says that the class reminds her how important exercise is during the rest of her week.

The experience brings to life aspects related to the International Classification of Function, Disability, and Health (ICF) because it classifies health-related domains and describes body structures, functions, activities and participation, and interaction with environmental and personal factors.[2] The experience also helps students understand the importance of the Surgeon General's Call to Action (SGCA), which was developed in July 2005 to improve the quality of life for individuals with disabilities through acceptance and better health care.[3] In addition, the students are exposed to Healthy People 2020,[4] a government initiative that targets those with disabilities as a subgroup of the population. The goals of Healthy People 2020 include elimination of health disparities and reduction of the number of barriers to participation. Finally, the *students are exposed to the National Center on Physical Activity and Disability (NCPAD), a web-based research and information center devoted to physical activity and disability.[5] The NCPAD is a clearinghouse of resources for exercise, recreation, and other forms of physical activity for persons with disabilities. As such, it is an important tool for rehabilitation professionals and the patients and clients they serve.*

LEARNING GOALS

After completing this chapter, the reader will be able to:

1. Discuss the role of community health promotion in meeting contemporary health care needs.
2. Describe and apply the language and focus of community health promotion.
3. Discuss how health care practitioners have integrated community health promotion into their professional duties.
4. Identify the roles of the physical therapist in promoting community health.
5. Discuss opportunities for incorporating community health promotion into one's professional activities.
6. Identify strategies and skills physical therapists can use to design and implement community health promotion programs for people with and without disabilities.
7. Describe evidence-based examples of community health promotion programs relevant to physical therapy practice.

When considering the health issues facing American society, modifiable lifestyle and behavior factors underlie many of the problems challenging our health care system.[6] Despite the many efforts to educate U.S. citizens about the importance of healthier lifestyles, the nation's health still needs significant attention. For example, in 2010 about one third (33.8%) of U.S. adults were obese, and 17% of children between 2 and 9 years of age were obese.[7] In any 2-week period of 2005, about 7.3% of Americans reported experiencing clinical depression. Eighty percent of these individuals reported some level of functional impairment, and 27% reported serious difficulties in work and life.[8] Only 3 of 10 U.S. adults regularly perform the recommended amount of physical activity, and 37% are

not active at all.[9] Despite irrefutable evidence of the dangers of cigarettes, almost 18% of adults still smoked in 2009.[10] Damaging lifestyle choices are not exclusive to adults. An increasing number of U.S. children have one or more risk factors for one or more unhealthy lifestyle conditions. Some believe that the life expectancy of children in the United States will be less than that of their parents if drastic measures are not taken to change their health choices.[11] Table 15–1 summarizes eight modifiable risk factors and their link to some of the leading causes of death and disability.[12] The table illustrates how poor lifestyle choices directly and substantially increase the risks for multiple devastating medical conditions. Particularly vulnerable to the negative effects of unhealthy lifestyles are the 40 million Americans currently living with disabilities.[13] If one considers those currently living with disabilities, those who will be developing disabilities in the future, and the families of these individuals, a great majority of U.S. citizens will be directly affected by the negative effects of disability if dramatic efforts are not undertaken soon.

Clearly, health care practitioners must look beyond their patients'/clients' medical diagnoses and related impairments or changes in body structure and function and encourage healthier lifestyle choices using effective health promotion strategies. The purposes of this chapter are to define community health promotion, discuss the importance of community health promotion in today's health care system, discuss the physical therapist's roles in providing community health promotion services, propose the skills and competencies needed to fulfill these roles, and provide effective examples of evidence-based community health promotion programs with which the physical therapist can engage. Although the physical therapist is the focus of this chapter, many of the concepts addressed are also applicable to activities carried out by physical therapist assistants.

In many ways, the U.S. health care system can be described as reactive; most efforts are directed at addressing health problems after they are manifested as illness and disease. Also, health care is traditionally delivered primarily in the clinic or institutional setting on a one-to-one

---

TABLE 15–1   Modifiable Risk Factor of the Lifestyle Conditions

Risk Factor	Cardiovascular Disease	Cancer	Obstructive Lung Disease	Stroke	Diabetes	Osteoporosis
Smoking	X	X (↑Risk for all-cause cancer*)	X	X	X	X
Physical inactivity	X	X		X	X	X
Obesity	X	X	X	X	X	
Nutrition	X	X		X	X	X
High blood pressure	X			X	X	
Dietary fat†/blood lipids	X	X		X	X	
Elevated glucose levels	X	X		X	X	
Alcohol‡	X	X		?	X	X

Modified from Bradberry JC, Peripheral artery disease: Pathophysiology, risk factors, and role of antithrombotic therapy. Journal of the American Pharmaceutical Association 2004; 44:S37-S44, Charkoudian N, Joyner MJ. Physiologic considerations for exercise performance in women. Clinics in Chest Medicine 2004; 25:247-255, Heart and Stroke Found of Canada. Canada 2003, http://www.heartandstroke.ca (Accessed on August 28, 2011)
*Smoking not only is related to cancer of the nose, mouth, airways, and lungs but also increases the risk for all-cause cancer.
†Partially saturated, saturated, and trans-fats are the most injurious to health.
‡Alcohol can be protective in moderate quantities, red wine in particular.

basis between health care practitioner and patient. Further, the primary care physician has been held largely responsible for addressing general health and lifestyle issues with those under their care. Many have come to believe that all members of the health care team should adopt a community-based approach to change unhealthy lifestyle choices (e.g., smoking, obesity, inactivity).[14] Also, leaders in many health care professions, including physical therapy, have called on their colleagues to accept responsibility to promote healthier lifestyles among their patients/clients.[15,16] This approach to health care, commonly referred to as *health promotion*, is believed by many to be most likely to significantly improve the health of the U.S. population.

HEALTHY PEOPLE INITIATIVE

A major driving force behind this different perspective about the nation's health is the Healthy People initiative—the disease prevention agenda for the United States.[4] Healthy People has as its origin the 1979 Surgeon General's Report, also called Healthy People, which stated that the nation's health strategy must emphasize the prevention of disease.[17] Healthy People 2020 is addressed in detail here because it represents a major touchstone and resource for health care professionals, including physical therapy practitioners, interested in applying their unique professional skills to positively influence the health of U.S. citizens. The Healthy People initiatives provide science-based 10-year national objectives for improving the health of all Americans. The program does this by establishing benchmarks and monitoring progress over time in order to accomplish the following:

- Encourage collaborations across a wide variety of organizations and stakeholders
- Guide individuals toward making informed health decisions
- Measure the impact of prevention activities

Preceded by Healthy People 2000 and Healthy People 2010, Healthy People 2020 (HP 2020) was launched in December of 2010 and strives to accomplish four overarching goals within the context of the program's mission (Box 15–1).

Like the previous healthy people programs, the HP 2020 Framework was developed through an exhaustive collaborative process among the U.S. Department of Health and Human Services and federal agencies, public stakeholders, and professional organizations, including the American Physical Therapy Association (APTA).[18–20]

The HP 2020 framework focuses on population disparities, including those categorized by race/ethnicity, socioeconomic status, gender, age, disability status, sexual orientation, and geographic location. Four foundation health measures will serve as an indicator of progress towards achieving these goals:

- General health status
- Health-related quality of life and well-being
- Determinants of health
- Health disparities

BOX 15–1   Goals and Mission of the Healthy People 2020 Initiative

PROGRAM GOALS

1. Attain high-quality, longer lives free of preventable disease, disability, injury, and premature death.
2. Achieve health equity, eliminate disparities, and improve the health of all groups.
3. Create social and physical environments that promote good health for all.
4. Promote quality of life, healthy development, and healthy behaviors across all life stages.

PROGRAM MISSION

"Identify nationwide health improvement priorities; Increase public awareness and understanding of the determinants of health, disease, and disability and the opportunities for progress; Provide measurable objectives and goals that are applicable at the national, state, and local levels; Engage multiple sectors to take actions to strengthen policies and improve practices that are driven by the best available evidence and knowledge; and Identify critical research, evaluation, and data collection needs."

From U.S. Department of Health and Human Services. Healthy People.gov. Available at healthypeople.gov/2020. Accessed August 28, 2011.

The National Prevention, Health Promotion, and Public Health Council was established in June 2010 with the intent to move the nation's focus from sickness and disease to prevention, wellness, and health promotion. The Council uses the following guiding principles[19]:

- Prioritize prevention and wellness
- Establish a cohesive federal response
- Focus on prevention of the leading causes of death and the factors that underlie them
- Prioritize high-impact intervention
- Promote high-value preventive care practices
- Promote health equity
- Promote alignment between the public and private sectors
- Ensure accountability

THE LANGUAGE OF HEALTH PROMOTION

To understand how the health of a community can be positively influenced, one must first understand the language of health promotion. The term *health promotion* is really an umbrella term that encompasses a wide range of concepts. Green and Kreuter[21] describe health promotion as any combination of health education and related organizational, economic, and environmental supports for behavior of individuals, groups, or communities conducive to health. Fair describes it as the science and art of helping people change their lifestyle to move toward a state of optimal health.[22] As the ultimate goal of health promotion, health is defined by the APTA as not only being free of disease and illness but also including a positive component (wellness) that is associated with quality of life and a positive well-being.[23] Fair elaborates on the term *wellness*, describing it as a lifestyle that promotes physical, mental, and social health in the cognitive, psychomotor, and affective domains, both internally and externally.[24] Others include additional aspects of health in their definition of wellness. For example, Hettler describes the dimensions of wellness as including emotional, intellectual, spiritual, occupational, social, physical, environmental, and cultural.[25] Jonas added the environment and culture as important dimensions for wellness that should be considered.[26] Wellness is not a fixed state of being; instead, it is a dynamic process in which most individuals experience hills and valleys in their state of wellness. Additionally, no dimension of wellness functions in isolation. For example, one's social wellness likely influences one's physical wellness. Physical therapists can, and should, address all dimensions of their patients' wellness. Of these dimensions, physical wellness is most closely related to the physical therapist's scope of practice. The term *fitness* is closely related to the dimension of physical wellness. The *Guide to Physical Therapist Practice* describes fitness as "a dynamic physical state—comprising of cardiovascular/pulmonary endurance, muscle strength, power, endurance, and flexibility; relaxation and body composition—that allows optimal and efficient performance of daily and leisure activities."[27] Many health promotion efforts incorporate aspects of prevention. The *Guide* defines prevention as activities that are directed toward the following[27]:

- Achieving and restoring optimal functional capacity
- Minimizing impairments, functional limitations, and disabilities
- Maintaining health (thereby preventing further deterioration or future illness
- Creating appropriate environmental adaptations to enhance function.

The *Guide* goes on to describe three types (levels) of prevention incorporated into the physical therapists practice; primary, secondary, and tertiary (Box 15–2).

A variety of strategies are used to foster health promotion. Health education is any combination of learning experiences designed to facilitate voluntary adaptations of behavior conducive to health.[28] A related activity is consultation; rendering professional or expert opinion or advice.[27] Finally, health promotion can be provided through advocacy or organized activism related to a particular issue—in this case, improved health for target populations. Taking a comprehensive approach to health promotion would involve integrating all these activities into one's professional duties.

As explained by Green and Kreuter, health promotion can be delivered at the individual, group, or community level.[21] *Community* can be defined as a group of people with diverse characteristics who are linked by social ties, share common perspectives, and engage in joint action in geographic locations or settings.[29] As such, a community can

BOX 15–3 Principles of Effective Health Education

1. Tailor to a specific population within a particular setting
2. Involve the participants in planning, implementation, and evaluation
3. Integrate efforts aimed at changing individuals, social and physical environment, communities, and policies
4. Link participants' concerns about health to broader life concerns and to a vision of a better society
5. Use existing resources within the environment
6. Build on the strengths found among participants and their communities
7. Advocate for the resources and policy changes needed to achieve the desired health objectives
8. Prepare participants to become leaders
9. Support the diffusion of innovation to a wider population
10. Seek to institutionalize successful components and to replicate them in other settings

be described in terms of such diverse characteristics as geography, race, age, gender, sexual orientation, and socioeconomic status.

Freudenberg and colleagues listed 10 principles of effective health education programs (Box 15–3).[30] These principles can also be applied to all health promotion initiatives. The principles are designed to build the capacity and guide actions of individuals and communities to promote health and prevent disease. Note that the key element in these principles is active participation from the target audience in planning, implementing, and maintaining health promotion programs. Reviewing these principles gives the therapist a sense of the skills needed to engage in community health promotion.

In summary, physical therapists engage in health promotion by using such strategies as health education, consultation, and advocacy to promote health, wellness, and fitness in their patients/clients. Physical therapists can deliver these services at the individual, group, or community level.

COMMUNITY HEALTH PROMOTION AND HEALTH CARE PROFESSIONALS

Although addressing the chief medical complaint is most frequently the primary focus for the health care provider, activities that promote a healthier lifestyle are increasingly apparent in the day-to-day practice of most health care professionals. Although most health care providers provide the bulk of their services in the clinical setting, many are also providing health promotion in the community. A 1998 Pew Health Professions Commission Report advocated the inclusion of such activities.[14] The Commission proposed the characteristics and needs of the health care system of the 21st century that clearly speak to promoting health at the community level. They include the following:

- Incorporating the multiple determinants of health into clinical care
- Improving access to health care for those with the unmet health needs
- Partnering with communities in health care decisions
- Rigorously practicing preventive care

BOX 15–2 Three Levels of Prevention

- Primary prevention involves using health promotion strategies to avoid disease, before it occurs, in a susceptible or potentially susceptible population.
- Secondary prevention includes efforts to decrease the impact of existing disease states through early diagnosis and intervention.
- Tertiary prevention works to slow down or limit the degree of disability for persons with chronic and irreversible diseases.

- Integrating population-based care and services into practice
- Working in interdisciplinary teams
- Balancing individual, professional, system, and societal needs
- Advocating for public policy that promotes and protects the health of the public

These concepts are further supported in the more recent Core Competencies for Interprofessional Collaborative Practice.[16]

Helvie compared and contrasted the differences between clinic-based and community health practices in nursing.[31] This comparison has been adapted for physical therapy services as shown in Table 15–2. In nursing professional education, alternative settings are commonly used for community health clinical experiences. These sites include

TABLE 15–2 Differences in Clinic-Based Physical Therapy and Community-Based Physical Therapy

	Clinic Based	Community Based
Unit of service	Individual focused; hospitalized patient	Community groups and subgroups specific to age, health problem, condition, or setting
Activity focus	Treatment of disease, short-term intervention for restoration of health	Multiple focuses: health promotion, screenings, rehabilitation, and consideration given to socioeconomic and cultural factors that affect health conditions
Range and variability of work	Works with disease classifications, acutely ill patients	Works with entire spectrum of health and illness, all settings, all ages
Boundaries of service	One institution, treatment, and recovery	All institutions (e.g., schools, industries)
Coordination	Within the institution	Between a variety of medical and nonmedical personnel
Legal and medical authority	Institutional policy and state practice acts; always under medical care; diagnosis and treatment orders from referring physician provide framework for care	Health officer, health regulations and laws, and political jurisdiction; frequently no medical diagnosis from referring physician; services obtained through multiple public agencies
Autonomy	Physician is medical authority, workload regulated by admissions	Medical management and authority shared by multiple professionals
Family and patient autonomy	Individual autonomy of patient is restricted and must fit into institutional routine	Complete autonomy and control
Predictability of events	Treatment of patient in one time and place	Interplay of home environment; social, physical, and emotional climate; cultural background

public health agencies, schools, adult day care senior centers, neighborhood clinics, occupational health centers, social service clubs for boys and girls, hospices, homeless shelters, child day care centers, and day care centers for special needs children. Similar examples of alternative clinical education settings for physical therapy students are also becoming more common.

Several articles have been published related to the role of the primary care physician in community health. Study results suggest that physicians are inconsistent in promoting physical activity with their patients.[32-34] These studies suggest that although most physicians ask their patients about their exercise habits, significantly fewer actually counsel their patients about exercise and rarely assist them with exercise prescription. Also concerning, surveys have found only a small percentage of physician participants were familiar with the American College of Sports Medicine (ACSM) recommendations for exercise. More recently, however, theory-based health promotion intervention strategies are being promoted among physicians in hope of positively influencing the adoption of healthier lifestyles with their patients.[35]

Referring to occupational therapists, Baum and Law[36] point out that, because of changes in the U.S. health care system, practitioners must focus on the long-term health needs of clients so that clients can develop healthy behaviors and thus minimize the health care costs associated with disabling conditions.[36,37] They state, however, that doing so requires a shift in thinking from a biomedical to a sociomedical framework and taking an active role in building health communities.

In response to the need for more professionals to address these issues, several certifications have been designed. Certified Health Educator Specialists (CHES) are health educators who have met the standards and passed the CHES examination established by the National Commission for Health Education Credentialing (NCHEC).[38] They have skills and knowledge in the following areas: performing needs assessments of individual and community health education and planning, implementing, and evaluating research on effective health education strategies, interventions, and programs. In addition, they serve as resources and advocates for health and health education. They work in various settings, including schools, governmental agencies, and health care facilities. Their titles range from patient educators, to health coaches, to community organizers, to public health educators and managers.

The ACSM and the National Center of Physical Activity and Disability (NCPAD) have recently developed a specialty certification entitled the Certified Inclusive Fitness Trainer (CIFT).[39] The CIFT is a fitness professional who conducts assessments and develops and implements exercise programs for persons with physical or cognitive disabilities who are medically stable to perform independent physical activities. A CIFT has knowledge of exercise physiology, exercise testing, programming, and inclusive facility design and awareness of social inclusion for people with disabilities and the Americans with Disabilities Act (ADA). The CIFT is trained to lead safe, effective, and individually adapted methods of exercise and understands precautions for persons with particular disabilities.

PHYSICAL THERAPIST'S ROLE IN COMMUNITY HEALTH PROMOTION

Physical therapists have much to offer to address community health, health promotion, and disease prevention efforts in the United States and globally. As early as 1970, Helen Blood wrote about the importance of developing community health content in physical therapy educational curricula.[40] Over the ensuing years, however, physical therapist education and practice continued to be concentrated primarily on curative approaches for their patients'/clients' chief movement complaint, with less attention paid to health promotion and community health. In 1999, Rimmer called for a greater emphasis to be placed on community-based health promotion initiatives for people with disabilities.[41] He charged all rehabilitation professionals to participate in these initiatives but highlighted the physical therapist's role as an important collaborator, educator, researcher, and program provider for individuals with disabilities. His conceptual model of health promotion for people with disabilities illustrates how physical therapists must extend their services beyond the clinical setting into community-based fitness centers (Figure 15–1).

As experts on movement dysfunction, physical therapists have a key role in collaborating with fitness professionals to ensure that these services are available for persons with disabilities. In a recent special issue of *Physiotherapy Theory and Practice on Physical Therapy in the 21st Century*, Elizabeth Dean claimed that physical therapists are uniquely positioned to promote health to both individuals and the community at large.[15] The physical therapist is uniquely positioned to participate in health promotion because of the following qualifications:

- Educational background in pathology and pathophysiology in relation to anatomy and exercise
- Ability to apply this knowledge functionally
- Lengthy and frequent contact with patients
- Often close and trusting relationship with patients/clients.[15]

Her recommendations for assisting physical therapists to fulfill this need are addressed later in this chapter.

In recent years, documents that directly influence physical therapy professional education and curricula, such as the *Guide to Physical Therapist Practice*,[27] the Evaluative Criteria for Accreditation of Education Programs for the Preparation of Physical Therapists,[42] and the *Normative Model of Physical Therapist Professional Education*[43] all advocate the preparation of physical therapists for their roles in health promotion, disease prevention, and community health. The *Guide* states that part of the physical therapist's practice is to "provide prevention and promote health, wellness, and fitness."[27] The *Guide* also describes specific activities commonly carried out by physical therapists that can apply to the concept of community health promotion (Table 15–3). Specific standards within the Evaluative Criteria for Accreditation of Education Programs for the Preparation of Physical Therapists speak to educational content required of entry-level physical therapist educational programs (Box 15–4).

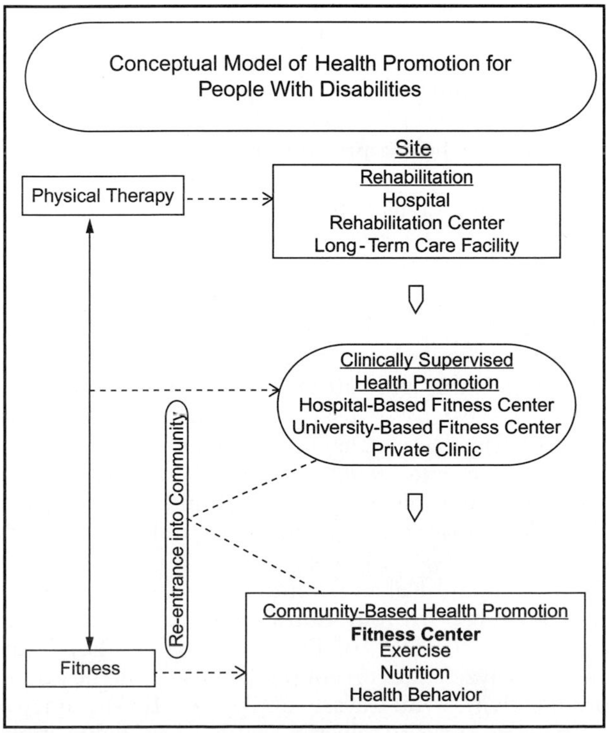

FIGURE 15–1 Rimmer's Conceptual Model of Health Promotion for People with Disabilities. (From Rimmer JH. Health promotion for people with disabilities: the emerging paradigm shift from disability prevention to prevention of secondary conditions. Phys Ther 1999;79:495-502.)

TABLE 15–3 Health Promotion and Disease Prevention Content from the *Guide to Physical Therapist Practice*

Type of Activity	Examples
Screening activities	Identification of lifestyle factors that may lead to increased risk for serious health problems
	Identification of elderly individuals in a community center or nursing home who are at high risk for falls
	Identification of workplace risk factors
Prevention and wellness activities	Identification of workplace risk factors
	Back schools
	Workplace redesign
	Strengthening, stretching, and endurance exercise programs
	Postural training to prevent and treat low back pain
	Exercise programs, including weight bearing and weight training, for those at risk for osteoporosis
	Exercise training, gait training, and balance and coordination activities for those older adults at risk for falls
	Exercise programs, cardiovascular conditioning, and instruction in ADL and IADL to prevent dysfunction for women who are pregnant
	Broad-based consumer education and advocacy programs to prevent problems
Community settings	Schools
	Hospices
	Corporate or industrial health centers
	Industrial, workplace, or other occupational environments
	Athletic facilities, fitness centers, and sports training facilities

Data from Guide to Physical Therapist Practice, 2nd ed. Phys Ther 2001;81:31-102.
ADL, activities of daily living; IADL, instrumental activities of daily living.

BOX 15-4   Health Promotion Educational Criteria for Physical Therapist Educational Programs

- Standard CC-5.50. Graduates should be prepared to "provide culturally competent physical therapy services for prevention, health promotion, fitness and wellness to individuals, groups, and communities."
- Standard CC-5.51. Graduates should also be prepared to "promote health and quality of life by providing information on health promotion, fitness, wellness, disease, impairment, functional limitation, disability, and health risks related to age, gender, culture, and lifestyle within the scope of physical therapist practice."
- Standard CC-5.52. Graduates should be prepared to apply principles of prevention to defined population groups.

From capteonline.org/uploadedFiles/CAPTEorg/About_CAPTE/Resources/
Accreditation_Handbook/EvaluativeCriteria_PT.pdf. Accessed on December 6, 2011.

The physical therapist's role in community health promotion also appears in many professional positions and standards. In 2000, the APTA developed a vision sentence and vision statement to guide their practice into the future.[44] The vision sentence reads: "By 2020, physical therapy will be provided by physical therapists who are doctors of physical therapy, recognized by consumers and other health care professionals as the practitioners of choice to whom consumers have direct access for the diagnosis of, interventions for, and prevention of impairments, functional limitations, and disabilities related to movement, function, and health." The statement goes on to add that patients will have direct access to therapists in all environments for services in patient/client management, prevention, and wellness.[44]

This view has been supported by several APTA House of Delegates standard positions including HOD P06-93-25-50: Health Promotion and Wellness by Physical Therapists and Physical Therapist Assistants[45] and HOD P06-04-22-18: Physical Education, Physical Conditioning, and Wellness Advocacy.[46] The recent APTA Branding Initiative not only encourages physical therapists to embrace their role in health promotion but also includes careful messaging to consumers and other health care providers that physical therapists are available for and competent to provide such services.[47] Finally, as the result of a 2006 APTA House of Delegates motion, the Physical Therapy and Society Summit (PASS) was convened in February of 2009 to focus on how physical therapists can meet current, evolving, and future societal health care needs.[48] Discussion took place related to the way that physical therapists can be leaders in the integration of innovative technologies and practice models. The emphasis was also to promote the establishment of collaborative and interdisciplinary partnerships. Participants in the summit included leaders in physical therapy, public and health policy, academia, engineering and bioscience, theology, and information technology. Issues related to the leveraging of the determinants of health, improved management of chronic disease, improve population health, community-based practice models of care, and preventative health were among the themes discussed at the conference. The conference encouraged imagination, inspiration, and innovation in approaches to meet the future health care needs of society. One of the most emphatic recommendations coming from PASS was that physical therapists not only needed to demonstrate proficiency in health promotion, fitness, and wellness but also needed to develop leadership among the health care professions in this area.

Are physical therapists currently meeting the health promotion needs of their patients/clients and the communities in which they live? Several studies suggest that many U.S. physical therapists are not adequately addressing health promotion with their patients/clients.[49-54] These studies are summarized in Table 15-4.

Although leaders in the physical therapy profession believe that physical therapists should be incorporating health promotion into their professional duties, studies suggest that these practices are currently incompletely developed and integrated into physical therapy practice for many clinicians. To fulfill this need, physical therapy educators and practitioners must enhance their understanding of effective community health promotion practices. A variety of resources exist, many outside of the physical therapy literature, to guide this growth.

STRATEGIES FOR EFFECTIVE COMMUNITY HEALTH PROMOTION

Contemporary health care has evolved from a model that was almost exclusively directed at the treatment of patients' and clients' impairments and delivering services exclusively in clinical and institutional settings to a more holistic approach directed at the community level that emphasizes education and prevention strategies. To participate in these kinds of services, contemporary physical therapists need an understanding of effective community health promotion practices as well as the skills and confidence to execute them successfully. Recent literature and resources from health promotion experts serve as guides for preparing physical therapists to meet this role. Dean proposed components of health-focused practice for physical therapists. She recommends that in addition to a more traditional focus on physical activity and exercise, physical therapists should also routinely and systematically address smoking cessation, nutrition optimization, weight control, stress reduction and management, sleep hygiene and optimization, and substance abuse cessation.[12,15] She provides an extensive list of knowledge competencies needed to effectively manage these issues. Included in this list are theories and models of health behavior, effectively using screening tools for a variety of unhealthy behaviors, and evidence-based management of unhealthy lifestyle choices.

Goodstadt and Kahan from the University of Toronto, Centre for Health Promotion developed The Interactive Domain Model (IDM) of Best Practices.[55] They created a way to analyze your current public health and health promotion activities and ways to apply their IDM framework to current response to selected health issues, delineation of criteria, and guiding principles, including values, goals, beliefs, assumptions, strategies, and processes. They include health promotion strategies/activities, health promotion processes, and health promotion research and evaluation

TABLE 15-4 Summary of Studies about Health Promotion Practices by Physical Therapists

Study	Purpose/Method	Findings
Gahimer & Domholdt, 1996[49]	Audiotaped 37 physical therapy practitioners during 137 patient treatments and counted the frequency and types of patient education statements made during the encounters	They found a low frequency of health promotion–related statements per session; on average there were 2.54 statements on general advice, 0.38 statements on health education, and 0.021 statements on stress counseling.
Fruth et al., 1998[50]	Examined 96 physical therapy treatment sessions to assess the frequency of health promotion and disease prevention statements made	Found that the mean frequency of health promotion statements used by the physical therapists was only 2.44. When such statements were made, 79% of the time they addressed physical aspects of wellness. Other aspects of health (e.g., emotional, mental, or spiritual health) were rarely addressed at all.
Rea et al., 2004[51]	Surveyed physical therapists about their perception about the frequency with which they address four focus areas of Healthy People 2010: physical activity, psychological well-being, nutrition and weight management, and smoking cessation	The investigators discovered that the respondents believed that they were addressing these issues in varying degrees and in lower than desirable percentages based on Healthy People 2010 goals. In this study, the health promotion behavior most commonly thought to be practiced was assisting patients to increase physical activity (54% of the time). Less frequent behaviors were addressing psychological well-being (41% of the time), nutrition and overweight issues (19% of the time), and smoking cessation (17% of the time). The researchers also asked the respondents to rank their self-efficacy (i.e., confidence in performing each behavior) and their outcome expectation (i.e., personal judgment that a behavior will result in a desired goal) related to addressing health promotion topics. They found that greater self-efficacy was predictive of more frequent health promotion practices by the respondents and recommended that future efforts attempt to build physical therapists' confidence in their capabilities in this area of practice.
Goodgold, 2005[52]	Surveyed pediatric physical therapists to examine their professional and personal wellness beliefs and practices	She found that most of the respondents valued the promotion of wellness to patients, had considered incorporating wellness into their physical therapy practice, and were incorporating wellness into their personal life. However, only 54.5% of the respondents were actually incorporating wellness promotion in their daily physical therapy practice. The author concluded that professional development opportunities were needed to assist pediatric physical therapists to fulfill their role in wellness promotion among their patients/clients.
Shirley et al., 2010[53]	Studied Australian physical therapists and physical therapist students in relation to their promotion of nontreatment physical activity for better health. She examined factors related to therapist and student knowledge, confidence, barriers, perception of role, counseling practices, and feasibility of these practices	She found that both groups consider giving patients nontreatment activity advice as part of their role. She concluded that a very important public health role can be played by physical therapists by promoting a physically active lifestyle during patient clinic visits.
Perrault, 2008[54]	Conducted a review of literature concerning health promotion, physical therapy, and interventions for people with low back pain	She found that health education was overwhelmingly the most frequently cited strategy used for health promotion by physical therapists. She also found examples of secondary and tertiary prevention activities by physical therapists but few examples of physical therapists engaging in primary prevention.

activities. The Goodstadt and Kahan model is presented in Figure 15-2.

Prevention of secondary conditions in persons with disabilities by developing innovative strategies to promote healthy living has emerged as an important public health issue. These secondary health issues often include weight gain, fatigue, depression, pressure sores, and pain and often are not related to the primary disability but rather are acquired issues related to lifestyle. Persons with disabilities require much more attention to architecturally, attitudinal, and programmatic barriers that face them. Rimmer and Rowland discuss health domains that can be inaccessible to persons with disabilities.[56] These include exercise, nutrition, employment, self-efficacy, stress, access to medical care, and spirituality, to name a few. They suggest many ways in which health care professionals can empower the person as well as enable the environment as solutions for overcoming barriers to health promotion.

Another valuable resource for health professionals interested in developing community-based health promotion programs comes from guidelines and criteria developed by the Expert Panel on Health Promotion Programs for People with Disabilities convened at the Rehabilitation Research and Training Center on Health and Wellness (RRTC) at Oregon Health and Science University. In a 2009 publication, the RRTC Expert Panel provided an optimal set of "best practices" for health professionals and educators to consider before implementing a health promotion program for persons with disabilities[57]:

- Criterion 1: Health promotion programs for people with disabilities should have an underlying conceptual or theoretical framework.
- Criterion 2: Health promotion programs should implement process evaluation.
- Criterion 3: Health promotion programs should collect outcomes data using disability-appropriate outcomes measures.
- Criterion 4: People with disabilities and their families or caregivers should be involved in the development

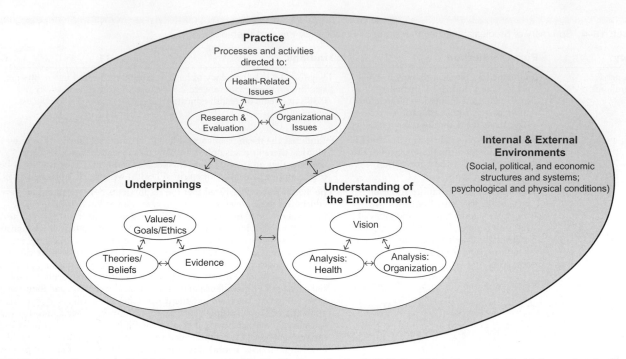

FIGURE 15–2 Best Practices in Health Promotion and Public Health. From Goodstadt M, Kahan B. Best Practices in Health Promotion, Application of the Interactive Domain Model of Best Practice in Health Promotion Practice. Workbook, 2006. Available at www.bestpractices-healthpromotion.com. Accessed on August 28, 2011.

and implementation of health promotion programs for people with disabilities.

- Criterion 5: Health promotion programs for people with disabilities should consider the beliefs, practices, and values of their target groups, including support for personal choice.
- Criterion 6: Health promotion programs should be socially, behaviorally, programmatically, and environmentally accessible.
- Criterion 7: Health promotion programs should be affordable to people with disabilities and their families or caregivers.

The seven criteria for best practices are discussed briefly below.

Criterion 1: Health Promotion Programs for People with Disabilities Should Have an Underlying Conceptual or Theoretical Framework

Health behavior is complex, and a variety of theoretical models are available to assist program administrators to develop and evaluate health promotion programs that will be more likely to produce the desired behavior change. Selection of the most appropriate theoretical model will depend on the specific health behavior change desired, and program planners often successfully mix and match constructs from more than one theoretical model to plan and evaluate their program. Health behavior theories commonly employed for health promotion program design and implementation are described in Table 15–5.[12] In addition

to health behavior theory, evidence-based program planning models like the PRECEDE-PROCEED model or the Social Marketing model can also be used by program administrators to design, implement, and evaluate health promotion programs.

Criterion 2: Health Promotion Programs Should Implement Process Evaluation

Process evaluation employs a variety of techniques to monitor how program elements are delivered and received by program participants. Using this type of evaluation can determine which program elements work and which ones do not. In the case of ineffective programs, process evaluation shows whether a program is truly ineffective or simply was not delivered as intended. In this situation, remediation of those poorly delivered elements can prevent premature rejection of a potentially effective program. The Centers for Disease Control and Prevention provide a framework for effective process evaluation strategies that should prove helpful to program administrators wishing to employ this type of evaluation.[58]

Criterion 3: Health Promotion Programs Should Collect Outcomes Data Using Disability-Appropriate Outcomes Measures

The RRTC expert panel emphasized that the larger program evaluation should not be a separate but rather a tandem process to program implementation. Evaluation

TABLE 15-5 Predominant Behavior Change Theories and Models with Reference to Health Behavior Change

Theory or Model	Premise or Construct	Examples of Health Application
Social Cognitive Theory Bandura, 1977[15]*; Bandura, 1986[15]; Bandura, 1997[15] Baranowski, 2001[15]; Stretcher et al., 1986[15]; Whitehead, 2001[15]	Addresses social cognitive component of health behavior change, including knowledge, belief, motivation, drive, attitude, and self-efficacy Triadic: behavior, personal, and environmental determinants Dependent on "cognitive processes in the acquisition of and retention of new behavioral patterns" Predominant construct: self-efficacy Cognitive behavioral therapy integrates behavioral modification principles	Schwarzer & Fuchs, 1995[15]; Allen, 2004[15] Smoking cessation Exercise promotion Nutrition and weight control
Theory of Reasoned Action or Planned Behavior (perceived behavioral control construct), Ajzen, 1991[15]; Armitage & Conner, 2001[15]; Glanz, 2001[15]	An individual's decision to engage in a health behavior such as exercise is based on his or her intention Intention is a function of the person's attitudes, perceived control and self-efficacy, and social factors	Armitage & Conner, 2001[15]; Corneya, 2001[15]; Norman, 1999[15] Exercise promotion Smoking cessation
Self-Determination Theory Deci & Ryan, 1985[15]; Ryan and Deci, 2000[15]; Sheldon, 2003[15]	Motivation to change, participate in, and maintain a specific behavior Role of intrinsic motivation and social influence	AHRQ, 2000[15]; Williams et al., 2002[15] Smoking cessation Weight loss
Transtheoretical Model of Change Prochaska, 1982[15]; Prochaska, 1997[15]	Directly associated with health behavior change vs. predictors of behavior	Prochaska et al., 2005[15]; Snow et al., 1994[15]; Henry et al., 2006[15]; Kim, 2006[15]; Jones et al., 2003[15] Nutrition and dietary change Exercise promotion Smoking cessation Alcohol consumption control
Behavior Modification Skinner, 1988[15]; Wierenga & Oldham, 2002	Extrinsically conditioned motivation Feedback Stimulus control and antecedent events to the behavior Reinforcement of the behavior—positive and negative and reinforcement schedules, i.e., continuous or intermittent Consequent events Shaping with the reinforcement of small progressive steps toward a larger goal Principles can be incorporated into a model of lifestyle modification that incorporates other factors such as culture (e.g., Guise, 2000[58ZB]; Wierenga & Oldham, 2002[58ZC])	Srinath et al., 1995; Granath et al., 2006; van der Ven et al., 2005; Herning et al., 2005.[15] Smoking cessation Nutritional counseling and glycemic control Weight control Exercise Stress management
Health Belief Model Stetcher & Rosenstock, 1997[15]; Beeker, 1974[15] Rosentstock et al., 1994[15]	Readiness to take health action depend on: Perceived susceptibility to the disease Perceived severity or seriousness of the disease Perceived benefits of the health action Perceived barriers to performing the action General health motivation Demographic variables Psychosocial variables Structural variables (e.g., knowledge of the disease and contact with the disease) "Cues to action," i.e., related to stimuli in the one's environment to participate	Applications incorporated into the literature on the application of the transtheoretical model and decisional analysis
Extension to the Health Belief Model Dishman, 1986[15]	Main perceived barriers: Effort Time Health limitations Obstacles	Proposed that these reported barriers are more justification for lack of participation rather than explanations for it; do not emerge as important factors predictive of exercise participation.

*From Dean E. Physical therapy in the 21st century. Part II: evidenced based practice within the context of evidence-informed practice. Physiother Theory Pract 2009;25:354-368.

strategies should be directed specifically to each program objective using psychometrically sound outcome measures. The panel also cautioned against using outcome measures that are inappropriate for the target population for which the program was designed. Although well-designed, some generic health-related quality-of-life measures are not useful for evaluating improvements in persons with disabilities. For example, the 36-item Short

Form Health Survey (SF-36) uses the ability to walk long distances and climb stairs as measures of health.[59] These activities are not feasible for persons with certain disabilities regardless of their health status. Therefore, care should be taken to select disability-specific outcome measures whenever possible. The panel also cited a great need for the development of more disability-specific outcome measures.

Criterion 4: People with Disabilities and Their Families or Caregivers Should Be Involved in the Development and Implementation of Health Promotion Programs for People with Disabilities

A commonly accepted principle in health promotion is that the "client knows best" when it comes to anticipating needs and potentially effective strategies for improving health. As such, participants and their families should be involved in all levels of program planning and implementation. The Jakarta Declaration on Leading Health Promotion into the 21st Century states that, "health promotion is carried out by and with people, not on or to people."[60] This philosophy is consistent with patient-centered care (i.e., when patients and their families are integrated into the health care team) and patient activation principles (i.e., the process of providing the skills, knowledge, and motivation to patients to be part of the health care team). Both principles are believed to be important for effective health promotion programs.

Criterion 5: Health Promotion Programs for People with Disabilities Should Consider the Beliefs, Practices, and Values of Their Target Groups, Including Support for Personal Choice

For optimal effectiveness, programs should be specifically tailored to the target population with consideration to trends in motives, preferences, perceived barriers, and other shared experiences of the target population. In addition to these shared experiences, the panel encouraged program administrators to enhance their awareness of the culture of disability in general. Insights learned from examining these factors should be used in all program elements, including methods of delivery and marketing materials.

Criterion 6: Health Promotion Programs Should Be Socially, Behaviorally, Programmatically, and Environmentally Accessible

The lack of accessibility to health promotion programs has been cited as a significant negative factor on the health of persons with disabilities. Program administrators should constantly look for accessibility barriers of all kinds and rectify them whenever possible. Helpful resources for identifying and reducing such barriers include Closing the Gap: A National Blueprint to Improve the Health of Persons with Mental Retardation and the Surgeon General's Call to Action to Improve Health and Wellness of Persons with Disabilities.[3,61]

Criterion 7: Health Promotion Programs Should Be Affordable to People with Disabilities and Their Families or Caregivers

Because many people with disabilities face financial constraints, health promotion programs should strive to keep costs for participating as reasonable as possible. Program administrators should constantly be on the lookout for unneeded and costly program elements and eliminate them whenever possible.

Two recently published textbooks serve as excellent references for promoting health and wellness from an evidence-based approach. Durstine and associates have published a third edition of a text entitled, *ACSM's Exercise Management for Persons with Chronic Disease and Disabilities*.[62] In this text, the intention is to assist exercise professionals in managing exercise programs for persons with chronic disease and disabilities. Fair, in her recently published text, *Wellness and Physical Therapy*,[22] addresses various aspects of wellness, including physical wellness, nutrition, fitness, body composition, mental wellness, and social wellness. She specifically describes the physical therapists' role in community wellness.

EVIDENCE-BASED PROGRAMS

During the past decade, many evidence-based programs have been developed and may be replicated and administered in the community setting. In this section, we discuss several of these programs:

- Chronic Disease Self-Management Program (CDSMP)
- Osteofit
- Tai Chi: Moving for Better Balance
- Stepping On
- Silver Sneakers

CHRONIC DISEASE SELF-MANAGEMENT PROGRAM

The U.S. Department of Health and Human Services has allotted $27 million dollars in grants to help older Americans with chronic diseases learn how to manage their chronic diseases and conditions.[63] The grants are funded by the American Recovery and Reinvestment Act of 2009 and allow states to provide self-management programs for older adults with chronic diseases. These programs are intended to develop into statewide programs and train a workforce to deliver these programs. The current secretary of Health and Human Services, Kathleen Sebelius, has stated that "prevention activities can strengthen the nation's healthcare infrastructure and reduce healthcare costs. These new grants will provide an important opportunity for states, tribes, territories and communities to advance public health across the lifespan and to help reduce or eliminate health disparities."[64(p 1)] The Administration on Aging will administer the grants.

The Stanford University CDSMP serves as a model for this initiative. The program emphasizes the patients' role in managing their illness and building their self-confidence in order to be successful in adopting healthy behaviors. CDSMP is a program that is led by lay people. It is offered in communities, and participants are adults experiencing chronic health conditions, including hypertension, arthritis, heart disease, stroke, lung disease, and diabetes. Family members, friends, and caregivers can also able to participate. Information and practical skills related to managing chronic health problems are the focus. Building confidence and fostering motivation are the hallmarks of the CDSMP program. Participants are taught to manage their challenges of living with a chronic health condition. Lorig and colleagues[63] found that, comparing baseline measures, the CDSMP participants exercised more often, had better symptom management and coping strategies, had better communications with their primary health care providers, showed improvement in areas related to health distress, experienced less fatigue, had more energy, and had overall decreased disability.

OSTEOFIT

Osteofit is another evidence-based program that offers safe exercise and education for persons with osteoporosis and osteopenia and those at risk for falling.[65] The program was developed in British Columbia and is designed to improve strength, balance, coordination, functional ability, independence, and quality of life. Osteofit provides a link between individual physical therapy and community group programming for those at risk for falls. Participants in the Osteofit program do not need a physician's referral, and most programs are located in community centers.

TAI CHI: MOVING FOR BETTER BALANCE

Li and coworkers developed a program entitled, Tai Chi: Moving for Better Balance.[66] They developed a package of training materials, including an instructors manual, videotape, and user's guidebook. The content of the program was shown to support the outcome measures of program feasibility and patient satisfaction. The package of materials now provides a solid foundation for implementing the program on a larger scale in community settings.

STEPPING ON

Stepping On is a program developed in Wisconsin to address the prevalence of falls in that state.[67] The program is designed to empower older adults to engage in healthy behaviors that reduce the risk for falls, improve self-management skills, and increase their quality of life. It is a community-based workshop that promotes the development of skills related to risks for falls and addresses fears of falling. Specific skills include activities for improving balance and strength, safety for the home and their personal environment, vision, and review of medications. The effectiveness of the program is based on the fact that the classes are highly participative, and mutual support is built as the participants learn to manage their health behaviors that contribute to risk for falls.

SILVER SNEAKERS

Silver Sneakers is a program designed to improve the health of seniors and to promote physical activity and thus decrease health care costs.[68] The program studied seniors enrolled in a Medicare Advantage plan that provides a health club membership. Specifically, there were three goals of the study: to determine the association between health care costs of older adults who used a health plan–sponsored health club benefit, determine the association between persons with diabetes and depression, and the determine the impact of the use of a health plan–sponsored health club benefit. It was found that as a result of providing a health club benefit through the health plan, the members participated in organized physical fitness activities. After 2 years, participants began seeing a significant decrease in health care costs

FUTURE DIRECTIONS OF COMMUNITY HEALTH EDUCATION

O'Donnell reported that despite the increase in amateur athletes and the increase in fitness centers in the United States, the proportion of the population who are sedentary has not improved.[69] Success has been found by assisting persons who are already living a healthy lifestyle to continue in that fashion.

Chapman and colleagues reported that incentives have been a part of the health promotion and wellness landscape for a number of decades.[70] They commented that the needs for engagement and risk mitigation are changing the role that incentives play in programming strategies and describe the importance of incentives, factors related to effectiveness, what consumers desire from incentives, the changing role of incentives, ideal incentives, and the future of incentives. They concluded that incentives are the key to successful health promotion and wellness programs. Chapman has published a guide entitled "Using Wellness Incentives" and claims that material goods and merchandise as well as coupons that have merchandise as their endpoint are excellent motivators for participation in health promotion programming.[70] Chapman reports that trends for wellness incentives in the future will include things such as following a pay-or-play philosophy, including spouses and families, having a strong set of outline interventions, and record keeping, to name a few.

e-Health is bound to become popular in the coming years. Evers described the growth trends of the Internet, general applicability, and evaluation strategies for online interventions for health promotion.[71] He described evaluation tools and their use in online programming and proposed that e-Health is playing an increasingly important role in health promotion because it is a source of low-cost and effective solutions to health issues. A recent issue of the *Art of Health Promotion* focused on the use of e-health technologies, including the growth of the Internet, e-health and health promotion, the use of the Internet for health promotion, online health promotion information, evaluation of e-health promotion interventions and tools, application of evaluation tools to online websites, and population use of e-health promotion. Annang and associates[72] discussed the use of technology in health promotion. In addition to the newer technologies, including e-mail, text messaging, websites, and online support groups, the online virtual worlds such as Second Life and Whyville can be innovative possibilities for reaching a broader population with health promotion.

SUMMARY

There are many local, national, and international initiatives related to community health promotion that may assist physical therapists in their evolving role as health and wellness educators. In 2008, The federal government issued the first-ever Physical Activity Guidelines for Americans.[73] These guidelines describe types and amounts of physical activity that offer substantial health benefits to Americans. Scientifically based guidelines provide information related to active children and adolescents, active adults, and older adults. They assist persons from all walks of life in learning about the benefits, procedures, and risks of physical activity. The Guidelines have been consolidated into a one-page desk reference that physical therapists can use.

Dean states that, "Without question, physical therapy will play a major role in setting and tackling the objectives of Healthy People 2020—in many instances leading the way."[12] She suggests that all physical therapists should be involved in lifestyle and public health issues. Many of the causes of premature death and substantial morbidity are lifestyle related and can be addressed by physical therapists, who are uniquely positioned to educate the public. Healthy People 2020 goals can be addressed through a number of initiatives, including screenings, taskforces, forums, community involvement, research, and programs and activities within clinics, to name a few. *Mobility disability* is defined in the literature as the inability to walk one fourth of a mile. Scherer described *public health* as a term that encompasses multiple factors that influence people's health, not just individual behaviors, but social supports and structures and the physical environment.[18] She also stated that of the 38 topic areas of HP 2020, physical therapists can make a difference in at least 15. A statement from the APTA claims that "all qualified health care professionals licensed within their scope of practice" be included in an objective that currently reads, "Increase the proportion of physician office health care provider visits for chronic health diseases or conditions, including visits for counseling or education related to exercise." Physical therapists are movement specialists and should use their skills in proactive ways.[18]

THRESHOLD CONCEPTS

Threshold Concept #1: Physical therapists are experts on promoting physical activity, especially for individuals with movement dysfunction and those who are prone to movement dysfunction.

Threshold Concept #2: Physical therapists are also important for educating individuals about other health and wellness issues that influence movement dysfunction.

Threshold Concept #3: Community health education is important for:

- Preventing movement dysfunction
- Promoting the physical therapy profession

Threshold Concept #4: Community health education is:

- The physical therapist's responsibility
- Challenging yet feasible because of the many tools and resources available to the physical therapist
- Beneficial for both consumers and physical therapists

> ## BOX 15–5   Sample Of Assignments for Teaching and Learning About Health Promotion
>
> ### THEORETICAL MODELS
>
> Study and learn about theoretical models commonly used in health behavior change of individuals and communities. Describe their commonalities and differences (e.g., Health Belief Model, Prochaska Stages of Change, Social Cognitive Model, Health Locus of Control, Social Support, and Self-efficacy).
>
> ### PERSONAL VISION OF HEALTH PROMOTION AND WELLNESS
>
> Develop your own personal description of wellness. Write a one- to two-page summary of your personal vision of health promotion and wellness. This paper should discuss your current wellness philosophy and what has contributed to the development of this philosophy. Support your opinions with at least two references from the current literature.
>
> ### PERSONAL HEALTH BEHAVIOR CHANGE ASSIGNMENT
>
> Assess your personal health behaviors through completion of a health risk appraisal, a readiness questionnaire, a food log, and a fitness assessment to develop and initiate a personal health behavior change project. Use self-selected models of behavior change, providing a detailed, efficacious plan and objectives for this process. First, complete a personal health risk assessment from the National Wellness Institute: Health Risk Assessment. Second, complete a three-day food log and access mypyramid.gov and review the new pyramid and its components. Then go to mypyramid.gov/professionals and read the information for professionals about the pyramid. Third, from the results of your health risk assessment and food plan, choose one lifestyle behavior you would like to change that would improve your health or decrease or eliminate a risk factor for poor health. For example, identify a behavior you want to eliminate, add, or enhance. Complete the Stages of Change Questionnaire to determine your readiness to change the behavior that you have selected.
>
>   Specifically:
>
> 1. Collect baseline data on the behavior you want to change (self-assessment).
> 2. Identify the behavior change model(s) you will use in developing your project.
> 3. Develop one or two specific behavioral objectives. These are the specific outcomes you expect from participating in this health behavior change project.
> 4. Develop several specific plans that will help you succeed in making this health behavior change, and that follow your selected health behavior change theory or theories. Use your literature and readings as resources to get "good ideas" about identifying the most efficacious plans to put in place that will help you to be successful in changing this health behavior. In our example, the plans could include reminder notes to yourself in the car, reactivating the alarm in the car that reminds you to wear your seat belt, reminders from your kids that you are supposed to wear a seat belt, and so forth.
> 5. Include a system of supports and rewards as part of your plan.
> 6. Follow the plan for 6 weeks by journaling, recording data of daily progress, and then reflect on your outcomes.

Threshold Concept #5: A variety of strategies can be employed to engage student learners in health promotion activities (Box 15–5).

ANNOTATED BIBLIOGRAPHY

Bensley RJ, Brookings-Fisher J. *Community Health Education Methods: A Practical Guide.* 3rd ed. Sudbury, MA: Jones and Bartlett; 2009.

   The purpose of this text is to provide concepts and theories that can be used when implementing community health interventions. Techniques for communicating and implementing health education messages positively at the individual as well as the community level are presented. Real-world perspectives from health educator practitioners in the field are included. Practical applications assist in improving understanding of the topics presented. Didactic techniques, essential tools for various audiences, are provided to assist health educators deliver positive messages related to influencing norms, behaviors, and healthy lifestyles. Issues related to facilitating groups and selecting and delivering effective presentations, print materials, and electronic media are included. Vignettes and practical steps for implementing change, addressing barriers, and measuring outcomes are included. Persons involved in health education or health promotion would find this book full of useful practical information.

Durstine JL, Moore GE, Painter PL, Roberts SO. *ACSM's Exercise Management for Persons with Chronic Diseases and Disabilities*. 3rd ed. Champagne, IL: Human Kinetics; 2009.

Now in its third edition, *ACSM's Exercise Management for Persons with Chronic Diseases and Disabilities* offers both exercise and health professionals the latest research and applications for integrating exercise into the treatment of 49 chronic diseases and disabilities. Developed by the American College of Sports Medicine (ACSM), the text was written by contributors with significant clinical and research experience in exercise programming for people with chronic conditions. This book contains tools to assist in the coordination of exercise within an integrated model of patient care. The updated edition presents a framework for determining functional capacity in persons with chronic diseases and disabilities and offers guidance in developing appropriate exercise programming to optimize functional capacity and reduce the compounding effects of exercise intolerance.

Fair SE. *Wellness and Physical Therapy*. Sudbury, MA: Jones and Bartlett; 2011.

The focus of this text is the application of wellness principles to the practice and profession of physical therapy. This one-of-a-kind textbook addresses wellness within the realm of the Normative Model of Physical Therapist Professional Education: Version 2004 and the criteria for the Commission on Accreditation of Physical Therapy Education. The text consists of foundational knowledge, theoretical models, empirical research, and application of material to physical therapy practice. Evidence-based practice is emphasized through a mixed approach of formalist and reader response. Complete with chapter objectives and useful appendices and resources, this is an important text for all physical therapy practitioners and students.

McKenzie JF, Pinger RR, Kotecki JE. *An Introduction to Community Health*. 7th ed. Sudbury, MA: Jones and Bartlett; 2012.

An Introduction to Community Health is a comprehensive, user-friendly textbook that contains current trends and statistics related to specific communities. The purpose of the text is to provide the introductory knowledge and skills for persons interested in pursuing a career in health education or community health; however, many health professionals could benefit from the immense amount of material presented in this book. Specific topics of the book range from global topics, including epidemiology, community organizing, and program planning to specific age group health topics related to maternal health, infants and children, adolescents, young adults, adults, and elders. Contemporary issues related to minority health, health care, mental health, environmental health, drugs, safety, and occupational health are also included. Each chapter contains short scenarios for application to real-life, key ideas, terminology and definitions, and Internet activities.

REFERENCES

1. State of Indiana Governors Council for Physical Fitness and Sports. *INShape Indiana website*. Available at: http://www.inshapeindiana.org/; Accessed 28.08.2011.
2. World Health Organization. *International Classification of Functioning, Disability and Health: ICF*. Geneva: World Health Organization; 2001.
3. U.S. Department of Health and Human Services. *The Surgeon General's call to action to improve the health and wellness of persons with disabilities*. Washington, DC: Office of the Surgeon General, U.S. Department of Health and Human Services; 2005.
4. U.S. Department of Health and Human Services. *Healthy People.gov*. Available at: http://www.healthypeople.gov/2020; Accessed 28.08.2011.
5. University of Chicago Department of Disability and Human Development. *The National Center for Physical Activity and Disability*. Available at: http://www.ncpad.org/; Accessed 28.08.2011.
6. Mokdad AH, Marks JS, Stroup DF, Gerberding JL. Actual causes of death in the United States, 2000. *JAMA*. 2004;291:1238–1245.
7. Centers for Disease Control and Prevention. *Overweight and Obesity: Data and Statistics*. Available at: http://www.cdc.gov/obesity/data/index.html; Accessed on 28.08.2011.
8. Centers for Disease Control and Prevention. *Faststats: Depression*. Available at: http://www.cdc.gov/nchs/fastats/depression.htm; Accessed on 28.08.2011.
9. U.S. Department of Health and Human Services, Presidents Council on Physical Fitness and Sports. *Resources: Physical Activity Facts*. Available at: http://www.fitness.gov/resources_factsheet.htm; Accessed on 28.08.2011.
10. Centers for Disease Control and Prevention. *Faststats: Smoking*. Available at: http://www.cdc.gov/nchs/fastats/smoking.htm; Accessed on 28.08.2011.
11. Olshansky SJ, Pessaro DJ, Hershow RC, et al. A potential decline in life expectancy in the United States in the 21st Century. *N Engl J Med*. 2005;352:1138–1145.
12. Dean E. Physical therapy in the 21st century. Part I: toward practice informed by epidemiology and the crisis of lifestyle conditions. *Physiother Theory Pract*. 2009;25:330–353.
13. Institute of Medicine. *Future of Disability in America*. Available at: http://www.iom.edu/Reports/2007/The-Future-of-Disability-in-America.aspx; Accessed on 28.08.2011. 2007.
14. O'Neil EH. for the Pew Commission for the Health Professions. *Recreating Professional Practice for a New Century*. San Francisco: Pew Health Professions Commission; 1998.
15. Dean E. Physical therapy in the 21st century. Part II: evidenced based practice within the context of evidence-informed practice. *Physiother Theory Pract*. 2009;25:354–368.
16. Interprofessional Education Collaborative. *Core Competencies for Interprofessional Collaborative Practice*. Available at: http://www.aacn.nche.edu/education/pdf/IPECReport.pdf; Accessed on 28.08.2011.
17. U.S. Department of Health, Education, and Welfare. *Healthy People: The Surgeon General's Report of Health Promotion and Disease Prevention*. Washington, DC: U.S. Department of Health, Education, and Welfare; 1979.
18. Ries E. A healthy role for physical therapy. *PT in Motion*. 2010;7:20–26.
19. U.S. Department of Health and Human Services. *Understanding the Affordable Care Act*. Available at: http://www.healthcare.gov/law/introduction/index.html; Accessed 28.08.2011.
20. American Physical Therapy Association. *Health Care Reform 2009: A Physical Therapist's Perspective*. Available at: http://www.apta.org/uploadedFiles/APTAorg/Advocacy/Federal/Health_Care_Reform/APTA_Position/PTPerspectiveonHealthCareReform.pdf; Accessed 28.08.2011.
21. Green LW, Kreuter MW. *Health Promotion Planning: An Educational and Ecological Approach*. 3 rd ed. Mountain View, CA: Mayfield; 1999.
22. Fair SE. *Wellness and Physical Therapy*. Boston: Jones and Bartlett; 2010.
23. American Physical Therapy Association. *Physical Fitness, Wellness, and Health Definitions*. Available at: http://www.apta.org/uploadedFiles/APTAorg/About_Us/Policies/BOD/Practice/PhysicalFitnessWellnessHealth.pdf#search=%22definition of health%22; Accessed on 28.08.2011.
24. Fair SE. *The humanistic model of wellness*. A paper for the Southern California University for Professional Studies, Palo Alto, CA.
25. National Institute of Wellness. *The Six Dimensions of Wellness Model*. Available at: http://www.nationalwellness.org/index.php?id_tier=2&id_c=25; Accessed on 28.08.2011.
26. Jonas S. *Talking about Health and Wellness with Your Patients*. New York: Springer; 2000.
27. American Physical Therapy Association. *The Guide to Physical Therapist Practice*. 2nd ed. Available at: http://guidetoptpractice.apta.org/; Accessed on 28.08.2011.
28. Glanz K, Rimer BK, Lewis FM. *Health Behavior and Health Education: Theory, Research and Practice*. 4th ed. San Francisco: John Wiley and Sons; 2007.
29. MacQueen KM, McLellan E, Metzger DS, et al. What is community? An evidence-based definition for participatory public health. *Am J Public Health*. 2001;91:1929–1938.
30. Freudenberg N, Eng E, Ray B, et al. Strengthening individual and community capacity to prevent disease and promote health: in search of relevant theories and principles. *Health Educ Q*. 1995;22:290–306.
31. Helvie C. *Community Health Nursing: Theory and Process*. Philadelphia: Harper and Row; 1981.
32. Walsh JM, Swangard DM, Davis T, McPhee SJ. Exercise counseling by primary care physicians in the era of managed care. *Am J Prev Med*. 1999;16:307–313.
33. Bauman A, Mant A, Middleton L, et al. Do general practitioners promote health? A needs assessment. *Med J Aust*. 1989;151 (262):265–269.
34. Pinto BM, Goldstein MG, Marcus BH. Activity counseling by primary care physicians. *Prev Med*. 1998;27:506–513.

35. Harvard Medical School. *Lifestyle Medicine Education*. Available at: http://www.harvardlifestylemedicine.org/index.php; Accessed on 28.08.2011.

36. Baum C, Law M. Community health: a responsibility, an opportunity and a fit for occupational therapy. *Am J Occup Ther*. 1998; 52:8–10.

37. Baum C, Law M. Occupational therapy practice: focusing on occupational performance. *Am J Occup Ther*. 1997;51:277–288.

38. National Commission for Health Education Credentialing, Inc. Available at: http://www.nchec.org/; Accessed on 28.08.2011.

39. National Center on Physical Activity and Disability. *Certified Inclusive Fitness Trainer*. Available at: http://www.ncpad.org/exercise/fact_sheet. php?sheet=679&view=all&print=yes; Accessed on 28.08.2011.

40. Blood H. Developing community health content in a physical therapy curriculum. *Phys Ther*. 1970;50:1226–1238.

41. Rimmer J. Health promotion for people with disabilities; the emerging paradigm shift from disability prevention to prevention of secondary conditions. *Phys Ther*. 1999;79:495–502.

42. Commission on Accreditation in Physical Therapy Education. *Evaluative Criteria for Accreditation of Education Programs for the Preparation of Physical Therapists*. Alexandria, VA: American Physical Therapy Association; 2006.

43. *Normative Model of Physical Therapist Professional Education, Version 2000*. Alexandria, VA: American Physical Therapy Association; 2000.

44. American Physical Therapy Association. *Vision 2020*. Available at: http://www.apta.org/Vision2020/; Accessed on 28.08.2011.

45. American Physical Therapy Association. *Health Promotion and Wellness by Physical Therapists and Physical Therapist Assistants, HOD P06-04-22-18*. Available at: http://www.apta.org/uploadedFiles/ APTAorg/About_Us/Policies/HOD/Health/HealthPromotion.pdf .pdf; Accessed on 28.08.2011.

46. American Physical Therapy Association. *Physical Education, Physical Conditioning, and Wellness Advocacy HOD P06-22-18*. Available at: http://www.apta.org/uploadedFiles/APTAorg/About_Us/Policies/ HOD/Practice/PhysicalEducation.pdf; Accessed on 28.08.2011.

47. American Physical Therapy Association. *BrandBeat: "Move Forward" Branding Campaign*. Available at: http://www.apta.org/BrandBeat/; Accessed on 28.08.2011.

48. Kigin CM, Rodgers MM, Wolf SL. The physical therapy and society summit (PASS) meeting: observations and opportunities. *Phys Ther*. 2010;90:1555–1567.

49. Gahimer JE, Domholdt E. Amount of patient education in physical therapy practice and perceived effects. *Phys Ther*. 1996;76:1089–1096.

50. Fruth SJ, Ryan JJ, Gahimer JE. The prevalence of health promotion and disease prevention education within physical therapy treatment sessions. *J Phys Ther Educ*. 1998;12:10–16.

51. Rea BL, Hopp II, Neish C, Davis N. The role of health promotion in physical therapy in California, New York, and Tennessee. *Phys Ther*. 2004;84:510–523.

52. Goodgold S. Wellness promotion beliefs and practices of pediatric physical therapists. *Pediatr Phys Ther*. 2005;17:148–157.

53. Shirley D, Van Der Ploeg H, Bauman A. Physical Activity Promotion in the Physical Therapy Setting: Perspectives from Practitioners and Students. *Phys Ther*. 2010;90:1311–1322.

54. Perreault K. Linking health promotion with physiotherapy for low back pain: a review. *J Rehabil Med*. 2008;40:401–409.

55. Goodstadt M, Kahan B. *Best Practices in Health Promotion, Application of the Interactive Domain Model of Best Practice in Health Promotion Practice. Workbook, 2006*. Available at: www.bestpractices-healthpromotion. com; Accessed on 28.08.2011.

56. Rimmer JH, Rowland J. Health promotion for people with disabilities: implications for empowering the person and promoting disability-friendly environments. *Am J Lifestyle Med*. 2008;10:1–12.

57. Drum CE, Peterson JJ, Culley C, et al. Guidelines and criteria for implementation of community-based health promotion programs for individuals with disabilities. *Am J Health Prom*. 2009;24:93–101.

58. Framework for program evaluation in public health. *MMWR Recomm Rep*. 1999;48:1–40.

59. Ware JE, Kosinski M, Grandek B. *SF-36 Health Survey: Manual and Interpretation Guide*. Lincoln, RI: Quality Metric Inc; 2000.

60. World Health Organization. *Jakarta Declaration on Leading Health Promotion into the 21st Century*. Geneva: World Health Organization; 1997.

61. U.S. Department of Health and Human Services. *Closing the Gap: A National Blueprint to Improve the Health of Persons with Mental Retardation*. Washington, DC: Office of the Surgeon General, U.S. Department of Health and Human Services; 2002.

62. Durstine JL, Moore GE, Painter PL, Roberts SO. *ACSM's Exercise Management for Persons with Chronic Diseases and Disabilities*. 3rd ed. Human Kinetics. 20CDSMP. Available at: http://patienteducation.stanford. edu/programs/cdsmp.html; Accessed on 28.08.2011.

63. Lorig KR, Sobel DS, Stewart AL, et al. Evidence suggesting that a chronic disease self-management program can improve health status while reducing hospitalization: a randomized trial. *Med Care*. 1999;37:5–14.

64. U.S. Department of Health and Human Services. *Obama administration releases national prevention strategy*. Available at: http://www.hhs .gov/news/press/2011pres/06/20110616a.html; June 16, 2011 Accessed on 30.08.2011.

65. *Osteofit*. Available at: http://www.osteofit.org/osteofit.htm; Accessed on 28.08.2011.

66. *Tai Chi*. Available at: http://holistichealinginstitute.org/tai_chi_ instructor_training; Accessed on 28.08.2011.

67. *Stepping On*. Available at: http://www.gwaar.org/index.php/; Accessed on 28.08.2011.

68. *Silver Sneakers*. Available at: http://www.silversneakers.com/; Accessed on 28.08.2011.

69. O'Donnell M. Health Promoting Community Design [editor's notes]. *Am J Health Prom*. 2003;18:iv–v.

70. Chapman LS, Whitehead D, Connors MC. The changing role of incentives in health promotion and wellness. *Am J Health Prom*. 2008;23:1–11, iii.

71. Evers KE. eHealth promotion: the use of the Internet for health promotion. *Am J Health Prom*. 2006;20:1–7, iii.

72. Annang L, Muilenburg JL, Strasser SM. Virtual worlds: taking health promotion to new levels. *Am J Health Prom*. 2010;24:344–346.

73. U.S. Department of Health and Human Services. *Physical Activity Guidelines for Americans*. Available at: http://www.health.gov/ paguidelines/; Accessed on 28.08.2011.

POST-PROFESSIONAL CLINICAL RESIDENCY AND FELLOWSHIP EDUCATION

J.B. Barr ✷ Carol Jo Tichenor

When I came to the residency program, I wanted to learn many different examination and treatment techniques so that I would have a large "bag of tricks" to use with my patients. Day after day over a year, I had the opportunity to work with my clinical supervisors. They challenged me to "think on my feet" and to respond to the emerging data from the patient. I learned how to conduct a focused examination; systematically prioritize problems for the difficult, multifactorial patient; justify a treatment plan; and reassess the effects of treatment. Although I came to the residency program to advance my skills and knowledge within a clinical specialty area, I also became a "generalist." I strengthened my patient management skills in a manner that would impact all types of patients. I learned how to listen to my patients and understand their perception of the disease or dysfunction, so that I could better judge their readiness to learn and their ability to change in response to my recommendations. Doing so has changed the manner in which I listen and communicate in my professional, as well as personal, life. The changes from the manner in which I originally practiced physical therapy are far beyond my initial expectations. After this year of intensive clinical supervision and didactic education, I believe that I have gained the tools that will enable me to continue to grow throughout the rest of my career. I am confident that I am prepared to meet the rapid changes in service delivery models that are happening in physical therapy and throughout health care.

LEARNING GOALS

After completing this chapter, the reader will be able to:
1. Discuss the history and philosophy of residency and fellowship education for physical therapists in the United States.
2. Identify key components of residency and fellowship curricula.
3. Compare and contrast residencies and fellowships.
4. Describe various models for design of residency and fellowship educational programs.
5. Discuss learning needs of residents and fellows compared with physical therapy students.
6. Design mentoring strategies to facilitate the development of clinical reasoning skills in residents and fellows.
7. Describe residency and fellowship teaching strategies to facilitate the development of efficient, systematic, patient-centered clinical reasoning skills and provide a rationale for their use.
8. Identify resources that can be used in the design of residency and fellowship curricula.

CLINICAL RESIDENCY AND FELLOWSHIP EDUCATION TODAY

Our country is undergoing health care changes unlike any in the history of medicine. Health care reform legislation will likely bring changes in reimbursement and new regulations governing practice delivery. Projections regarding the future of medicine suggest that health care professionals will face the challenge of needing to see more patients with fewer resources and to develop service delivery models that preserve quality while providing cost-effective, clinically effective, accessible, consumer-oriented care. Physical therapists are being asked to seriously re-examine their paradigm of practice without ethical compromise. How can the patient's needs be addressed in fewer visits, with group interventions and/or with telemedicine to decrease costs and improve accessibility to care? Are there any other practitioners who can serve patients in conjunction with, or in place of, the physical therapist? Are there new venues to which physical therapists can expand practice? Some physical therapists respond to these challenges by becoming paralyzed, unable and unwilling to change their paradigm of practice. Others respond by seeking clinical and academic education that will enable them to be more effective and efficient in their examination and treatment skills and to stay competitive in the current health care environment.

In their desire to attain advanced clinical skills, some therapists seek postprofessional clinical doctorates in physical therapy (DPT degrees), but emphasis on *advanced clinical training* is highly variable in many existing programs. Others turn to certifications or weekend continuing education courses. Physical therapists, frustrated by a piecemeal approach to weekend continuing education courses, are rethinking their professional goals to establish sound, cohesive, professional plans for themselves—plans that will have a major impact on their level of clinical competence over time.[1] Postprofessional clinical residency and fellowship education can assist physical therapists to significantly advance their knowledge and skills in a defined area of clinical practice. The educational principles and teaching strategies presented in this chapter and the resources outlined in Appendix 16-A can assist educational institutions and health care organizations in the design of residency and fellowship curricula and in the development of effective mentoring strategies. The concepts presented are also applicable to aspects of physical therapy professional curricula. Potential applicants to residency and fellowship programs may also use the concepts in this chapter to determine whether the scope and intensity of residency and fellowship education meet their career objectives and may also be used to assess the quality of the programs to which they may wish to apply.

WHAT ARE RESIDENCY AND FELLOWSHIP PROGRAMS?
MISSION AND PHILOSOPHY OF RESIDENCY AND FELLOWSHIP EDUCATION

Although it is difficult to articulate a single mission statement or philosophy that can cross many clinical specialty areas and include a broad range of models, individual residency and fellowship programs should compose a mission statement that fits with their umbrella organization's mission and the specific program's core philosophical approach.[2,3] In addition, key program outcome objectives should be carefully constructed to help guide the curriculum and to choose effective teaching strategies. Residency and fellowship education is directed toward the development of a therapist's ability to link theory and practice

through a combination of didactic and clinical coursework and through supervised and unsupervised clinical practice. In this chapter, *didactic coursework* will refer to instruction in the basic and applied sciences (e.g., anatomy, neurophysiology, biomechanics, research methods), whereas *clinical coursework* will refer to instruction in patient-centered topics and the development of psychomotor skill (e.g., lab practice, case discussion, clinical seminars). Beyond instruction in these areas and refinement of advanced intervention strategies, the core of residency and fellowship curricula is the development of a systematic clinical reasoning process.

Residency and fellowship education is founded on the premise that the development of advanced clinical practice requires a significant commitment of time and practice over an extended period of time. It is also based on the tenet that clinical mentoring involving ongoing, constructive critique and feedback is necessary for the development and refinement of advanced examination and management skills.[4-6] Residency and fellowship programs also seek to educate clinicians who will be able to critically review current literature and to creatively integrate relevant evidence into clinical practice. Some programs seek to have their graduates contribute to literature through research. At the foundation of residency and fellowship curricula is the goal to develop clinicians who will substantially advance the practice of physical therapy, provide expertise to the patients they serve, and make lasting contributions to their professional communities through clinical practice, teaching, consultation, and community service.

RESIDENCIES VERSUS FELLOWSHIPS

Physical therapists interested in formal postprofessional clinical training with overarching goals of specialization and the development of expertise have two primary options supported by a credentialing process: clinical residencies and clinical fellowships. Neither of these experiences is considered to be synonymous with the term *clinical internship*, which may refer to any supervised clinical experience. The American Board of Physical Therapy Residency and Fellowship Education (ABPTRFE), which determines requirements, policies, and procedures for the credentialing process, proposes the following definition of clinical residencies: "A clinical residency is a planned program of post-professional clinical and didactic education for physical therapists that is designed to significantly advance the physical therapist resident's preparation as a provider of patient care services in a defined area of clinical practice. It combines opportunity for ongoing clinical supervision and mentoring with a theoretical basis for advanced practice and scientific inquiry."[6]

Whereas residency programs are designed to foster initial development of expertise in one of the primary areas of physical therapy practice, fellowships train professionals to advance their skills in a subspecialty area. The primary specialty areas for residency training tend to coincide with the eight board certification areas offered through the American Board of Physical Therapy Specialties (ABPTS) (Box 16–1). Because residency training is not required for entry into a fellowship, some individuals may elect to go directly into a fellowship after achieving the experience

BOX 16-1 Primary Physical Therapy Practice Specialty Areas*

- Neurology
- Pediatrics
- Orthopedics
- Sports
- Clinical electrophysiology
- Geriatrics
- Women's health
- Cardiovascular and pulmonary physical therapy

Data from American Board of Physical Therapy Specialties: www.abpts.org.
*Recognized by the American Board of Physical Therapy Specialities.

TABLE 16-1 Residency and Fellowship Comparison

	Residencies	Fellowships
Content area	Physical therapy specialty area (e.g., pediatrics, sports)	Physical therapy subspecialty area (e.g., neonatal care, Division I athletics)
Participant characteristics	Typically entry-level or recent graduates; pre-ABPTS board certification	Two to six years of practice experiences[7]; may be ABPTS board certified and/or residency trained
Curricular focus	Based on DSP in specialty area	Based on practice analysis in specialty area (e.g., DASP for OMPT)
Credentialing requirements	1500 total hours Didactic training (minimum, 75 hr) One-on-one clinical mentoring (minimum, 150 hr)	1000 total hours Didactic training (minimum, 50 hr) One-on-one clinical mentoring (minimum, 100 hr)
Length	Minimum, 9 mo (typical range, 9-18 mo)	Minimum, 6 mo (typical range, 6-36 mo)
Outcomes	Advanced clinical practice in specialty area; ABPTS certification	Advanced clinical practice in subspecialty area

From American Board of Physical Therapy Residency and Fellowship Education. Application for Credentialing of Residency and Fellowship Programs. Alexandria, VA: American Physical Therapy Association Residency and Fellowship Credentialing, 2010.
ABPTS, American Board of Physical Therapy Specialties; DSP, Description of Specialty Practice; DASP for OMPT, Description of Advanced Specialty Practice for Orthopedic Manual Physical Therapy.

and coursework required by a particular program. ABPTRFE's definition of a clinical fellowship is: "... a planned program of post-professional clinical and didactic education for physical therapists who demonstrate clinical expertise, prior to commencing the program, in a learning experience in an area of clinical practice related to the practice focus of the fellowship. (Fellows are frequently post-residency prepared or board-certified specialists)."[6]

Clinical residencies and fellowships are similar in many respects, including training models that include a didactic curriculum, clinical curriculum, and one-on-one clinical mentoring, but they differ in focus and in the background of their participants. ABPTRFE credentialing requirements and program outcomes also differ somewhat. The important similarities and differences between clinical residencies and fellowships are summarized in Table 16-1.[6] For the remainder of this chapter, unless specifically stated, for simplicity the term *residency* will be used to refer to both types of post-professional training. Similarly, the term *resident* will refer to the learning needs of a resident or fellow unless otherwise stated.

THE CREDENTIALING PROCESS

In addition to medicine,[8] which has had ambulatory care residencies since the early 1870 s, psychology,[9] podiatry,[10] optometry,[11] and pharmacy[12] are among the many professions that have recognized the knowledge, clinical competence, and confidence that can be attained through residency education for entry into the profession and for specialization. Each of these professions has established an accreditation or credentialing process for clinical residencies. For physical therapy, the concept of residency training dates back to the 1960s, with the development of the University Affiliated Programs that incorporated formalized, interdisciplinary, long-term training in pediatrics.[13] In the late 1970s, the lack of opportunities for advanced training in manual therapy in the United States led some American physical therapists to travel to such countries as Norway and Australia to receive long-term mentoring and advanced coursework.[1]

In 1993, the American Academy of Orthopedic Manual Physical Therapists (AAOMPT) created the Standards for Orthopaedic Manual Physical Therapy Residency Education[14] and a formal recognition process to assess manual

therapy programs. APTA developed a credentialing process for post-professional clinical residencies in 1998 and for fellowship programs in 2000.[2,15] The APTA credentialing process merged with the AAOMPT recognition process in 2002 and with the Sports Medicine Section's process for credentialing sports physical therapy residencies in 2004.[2]

Since 2000, the number of credentialed residency and fellowship programs in the United States has expanded rapidly. There are now credentialed residency programs in the specialty areas of orthopedics, neurology, pediatrics, sports, geriatrics, women's health, and cardiovascular and pulmonary physical therapy. Credentialed fellowship programs now exist in orthopedic manual therapy, hand therapy, movement science, and Division I athletics. In response to demand from the growing number of programs requesting credentialing, support, and continued assessment, in 2009, APTA established the ABPTRFE and the related Credentialing Services Council and Program Services Council.[2] The Credentialing Services Council conducts the review of programs, oversees site team visits, and implements training for reviewers and onsite visitors. The Program Services Council promotes the development of additional residency and fellowship programs by developing resources and marketing plans to increase awareness of residency and fellowship education.[2]

The credentialing process for new residency and fellowship programs ensures a level of consistency among programs and guarantees a high-quality experience for participants. The process requires programs to submit a formal application and receive an onsite visit by residency education experts. Among other elements, the application requires programs to develop a program mission statement, outcome objectives, formal didactic and clinical curricula, a clinical mentoring plan, and formal assessment plan for participants. During the site visit, the program's director, faculty, clinical facilities, and other resources are examined. APTA offers extensive supporting material and short courses to support individuals and facilities who are either in the credentialing process or considering development of a residency or fellowship. Refer to Appendix 16-A for a compilation of resources.

OVERVIEW OF RESIDENCY AND FELLOWSHIP MODELS

A variety of residency models exist in the United States today, which can all meet the requirements of credentialing. Some of the options, which are highlighted in Table 16–2, include the following:

- Full-time or part-time
- Employment offered through the sponsoring organization or tuition based
- Affiliated with a university or residing in a hospital system or private practice

TABLE 16–2   Overview of Common Residency and Fellowship Models

Characteristic	Options (Any Combination of Characteristics Is Possible)	
Full vs. part time	*Full-time:* Curriculum is continuous, linear Typically 9-18 months Patient care 20-30 hr/wk within normal work week Participants reside at program's home location	*Part-time:* Curriculum may be blocked in short segments May take longer to complete Participants probably not employed by sponsoring institution Participants may travel for instruction and mentoring
Employment	*Employment through sponsoring institution:* Compensation based on hourly rate for patient care or percentage of regular starting salary	*Tuition based:* Participants pay program for instruction provided and continue to work outside of program
Affiliation	*University affiliated:* Program housed in university setting where entry-level physical therapy education program exists Graduate credit may be offered toward post-professional clinical doctorate or other graduate degree	*Hospital system or private practice affiliated* Program housed in hospital system or private practice Programs may contract with universities to provide some didactic content to residents

RESIDENCY FACULTY AND CLINICAL MENTORS

Residency faculty members are generally physical therapy senior clinicians, coordinators, or clinical specialists on staff at the sponsoring institution. Other residency faculty may be private practitioners in the community who come to the residency on a regular basis to provide lectures or laboratory instruction. Some residency faculty may serve the program primarily or exclusively as clinical mentors; these individuals are expert clinicians providing one-on-one mentoring to residents in a clinical practice setting. These mentors may live at a distance from the program's home location, particularly in part-time models. Residency faculty usually teach the clinical lectures and laboratory sessions, provide clinical mentoring, and conduct the examinations. Having one or more faculty members with prior residency experience on staff or as consultants can be valuable in designing all components of the curriculum, particularly the clinical mentoring and examination components. Physical therapy academic faculty members from a clinical doctorate (DPT or tDPT) or PhD program may also serve as residency faculty or clinical mentors, bringing a strong education background to a program. Physicians and other non–physical therapy practitioners may provide medical lectures or other clinical seminars.

FULL-TIME VERSUS PART-TIME MODELS

In a full-time model, residents complete the residency in a continuous, linear fashion, working and learning around a normal work week. In contrast, part-time models often allow residents to live at a distance from the program's home location. The resident must then travel regularly to a designated residency clinic during weekdays, evenings, or weekends to receive instruction, provide patient care, and receive one-on-one clinical mentoring. As a result of the less linear structure, part-time residencies are highly variable in duration. In either format, ABPTRFE requires that both residency and fellowship programs be completed in a maximum of 36 months.[2]

EMPLOYMENT- VERSUS TUITION-BASED PROGRAMS

A variety of possibilities exist relative to a resident's employment while completing a residency program. A resident may be employed by the health system, private practice, or university that houses the program. Under this arrangement, compensation will typically depend on the number of weekly clinical hours a resident works. This model is commonly used for full-time programs in which the resident works in the same facility that houses the residency program. Or, the facility housing the program may contract with outside clinics to provide clinical practice opportunities. The contracted clinic may hire the resident directly, or may compensate the residency's home facility for the resident's billable practice hours.

Other residency programs are tuition based. Under this arrangement, a resident pays tuition for the learning experiences provided by the program. The resident is not employed by the facility housing the program, but rather continues to work at a facility of his or her choosing. This model is typical of part-time residency programs in which the resident lives somewhere other than the program's home facility. Hybrid models also exist whereby some tuition is required, but the resident is also compensated for billable hours worked.

UNIVERSITY-AFFILIATED PROGRAMS VERSUS HEALTH SYSTEM– OR PRIVATE PRACTICE–BASED PROGRAMS

An increasing number of residency programs are housed within formal university settings. For instance, a physical therapy department whose primary function is entry-level physical therapy education may also house a credentialed residency program. Residents participating in this type of residency have access to university resources like formal coursework, teaching opportunities, and university-affiliated clinics. Also, programs housed within hospital systems or private practices may contract with universities to provide some of the residency's didactic content. The collaboration of physical therapy academic faculty and residency faculty can result in tremendous short- and long-term benefits to the curricula of both organizations. Academic faculty bring expertise in teaching and examination methodology, in the basic and applied sciences, and in research to assist the residency program in developing a sound educational framework for the entire curriculum.

USE OF TECHNOLOGY

Some residency programs are now using information technology tools for the delivery of portions of their curricular content and to enhance communication among residents, mentors, and other residency faculty. Whether they are at a distance or located at the program's home location, residents may take online coursework for some didactic components of the curriculum. These online education modules may be contracted out to a third party or developed by the residency faculty. Other residency programs are linking to university programs that may have a distance education component. Within this type of arrangement, some distance-based coursework might be completed for university credit and count toward a graduate degree.

Communication at a distance can be a challenge for programs with residents spread around the country geographically. Technology tools like video conferencing, discussion boards, blogs, wikis, and cloud-based sharing websites can facilitate communication. These tools make discussion about cases and didactic content more convenient and more immediate. The resident may, for example, travel to the program's home location periodically for coursework or clinical mentoring in an intensive format. In between these intensive experiences, residents and mentors can maintain contact through web-based applications that provide avenues for informal or formal interaction as well as synchronous or asynchronous discussions.

KEY COMPONENTS IN THE DESIGN OF RESIDENCY CURRICULA
DESCRIPTIONS OF SPECIALTY PRACTICE

The APTA credentialing process requires residency programs to demonstrate that curricula reflect practice dimensions identified through a valid and reliable practice analysis.[2] All of the clinical practice areas for which residencies or fellowships have been developed are based on a document called the Description of Specialty Practice (DSP), Description of Advanced Clinical Practice (DACP), or Description of Advanced Specialty Practice (DASP). The document is used to both guide the curriculum and ground the credentialing process. Resources for obtaining existing DSPs are included in Appendix 16-A. The DSP of the specialty area should provide the framework for determining the major curricular components of the program (e.g., examination, evaluation, diagnosis). Practice dimensions of the DSP, which are stated in behavioral terms, can be used to define the performance outcomes of the program and instructional objectives in individual courses.

CURRICULAR STRUCTURE

The didactic portion of a residency curriculum must follow the areas outlined in the DSP and ultimately meet the program's outcome objectives. The actual structure and sequence of the didactic curriculum, however, may be constructed in a variety of ways. For example, choices like the ordering of content and the mix of classroom instruction, laboratory teaching, online learning modules, readings, and discussions are made by individual programs based on their resources and the program's mission and philosophy.

The grid presented in Figure 16–1 provides a temporal illustration of the curriculum of a year-long, full-time fellowship program in Orthopedic Manual Physical Therapy (OMPT) based in a hospital system. Although the actual content would differ, the curriculum components and design in this example can apply to other clinical specialty areas.

The program is divided into four teaching modules, which are reflected in Figure 16–1. OMPT clinical lectures and laboratory instruction are presented during a 1-week introductory intensive to establish a foundation for examination and treatment in the clinic. Selected anatomy and biomechanical lectures are also presented during the initial week and during periodic lectures over the first 4 months of the program, from January through April. Clinical coursework and laboratory instruction occur about 2 to 3 weekends each month and cover the major curricular topics shown in Figure 16–1 (e.g., planning the objective examination, re-examination, implementation of plan of care, and medical lectures). Clinical practice in an outpatient clinic and clinical supervision begin the second week of the program and continue throughout the program. Small group tutorials focused on refinement of clinical reasoning concepts, review and critique of the literature, case study review, and handling skills are held about every 3 weeks during nonclinic days. Clinical examinations occur at the end of every module.

When a joint complex (e.g., the hip) is covered, all aspects of hip examination and implementation of a plan

	Jan	Feb	Mar	Apr	May	June	July	Aug	Sept	Oct	Nov	Dec
	Module One			Module Two			Module Three			Module Four		
Orientation and introductory clinical lectures												
Introduction to anatomy/biomechanical concepts												
Patient exam, evaluation, and diagnosis												
Planning the objective exam, re-examination, establishing a prognosis												
Implementation of plan of care, treatment selection/progression, re-examination												
Anatomical, neurophysiological, and biomechanical basis of OMPT												
Medical lectures												
Review and critique of the literature/research design												
Research												
Clinical rotation I: Spine and shoulder complex												
Clinical rotation II: Pelvis, hip, knee, foot, and ankle												
Clinical rotation III: Elbow, wrist, hand, and TMJ												
Clinical rotation IV: Review and refine spine and all peripheral joints												
Clinical mentoring												
Small group tutorials												
Clinical exams												
Final clinical exams												
Clinical projects/case studies												

OMPT, Orthopedic manual physical therapy; TMJ, Temporomandibular joint.

FIGURE 16–1 Temporal illustration of curriculum schedule for full-time, hospital-based orthopedic manual physical therapy (OMPT) clinical fellowship.

of care are covered during lecture and laboratory sessions. During each module, although the overall aim is to prepare the fellow to examine and manage the patient globally, lectures, laboratory, and clinical mentoring emphasize the concepts of that module. For example, lectures on the hip complex emphasize concepts related to planning the physical examination and establishing a prognosis. During clinical mentoring, the fellow is supervised on all aspects of his or her patient care delivery; however, the clinical mentor will emphasize the identified patient management concepts. When examinations occur at the end of each module, the clinical mentor scores the fellow on all aspects of patient care, but points are weighted toward planning the examination and establishing a prognosis. In later modules, the mentoring and examination would focus on selecting, justifying, and progressing management (e.g., manual therapy, exercise, self-mobilization, and ergonomics) for more complex patients.

Throughout the program, assigned readings and ongoing clinical projects relate to the lectures and laboratory sessions being taught. Coursework in anatomy, neurophysiology, and biomechanics is taken online through a university distance learning program or through special lectures provided by academic faculty from affiliating universities. Program faculty also reinforce the basic and applied science concepts during ongoing lectures.

Laying out the program in a bar graph format allows the program director and faculty to assess the vertical and horizontal relationships between curriculum components. In assessing the horizontal relationships between elements of coursework, the faculty need to determine how course material and learning activities are building on one another. For example, initially the fellow receives instruction in patient examination, evaluation, and diagnosis, and then progresses to concepts related to establishing a prognosis and implementing a plan of care. When looking at the vertical relationships of the program, the bar graph enables the faculty to determine how different components reinforce each other. For example, lecture concepts are reinforced with tutorial and clinical mentoring experiences.

An example of the curricular layout for a year-long, full-time pediatric residency program housed in a university setting is provided in Figure 16–2. The concepts described previously for the OMPT curriculum still apply, but note the differences in content and in structure with a program using a university calendar as its basis. The clinical teaching component is also different, giving the resident opportunities to learn through preparation and execution of teaching experiences. The resident's responsibilities for teaching gradually build throughout the year from primarily assisting faculty early on to eventually planning and leading class sessions and laboratories at the end of the year.

CLINICAL PRACTICE

A significant number of hours per week must be devoted to clinical practice. As licensed practitioners, residents typically spend most of this practice time unsupervised

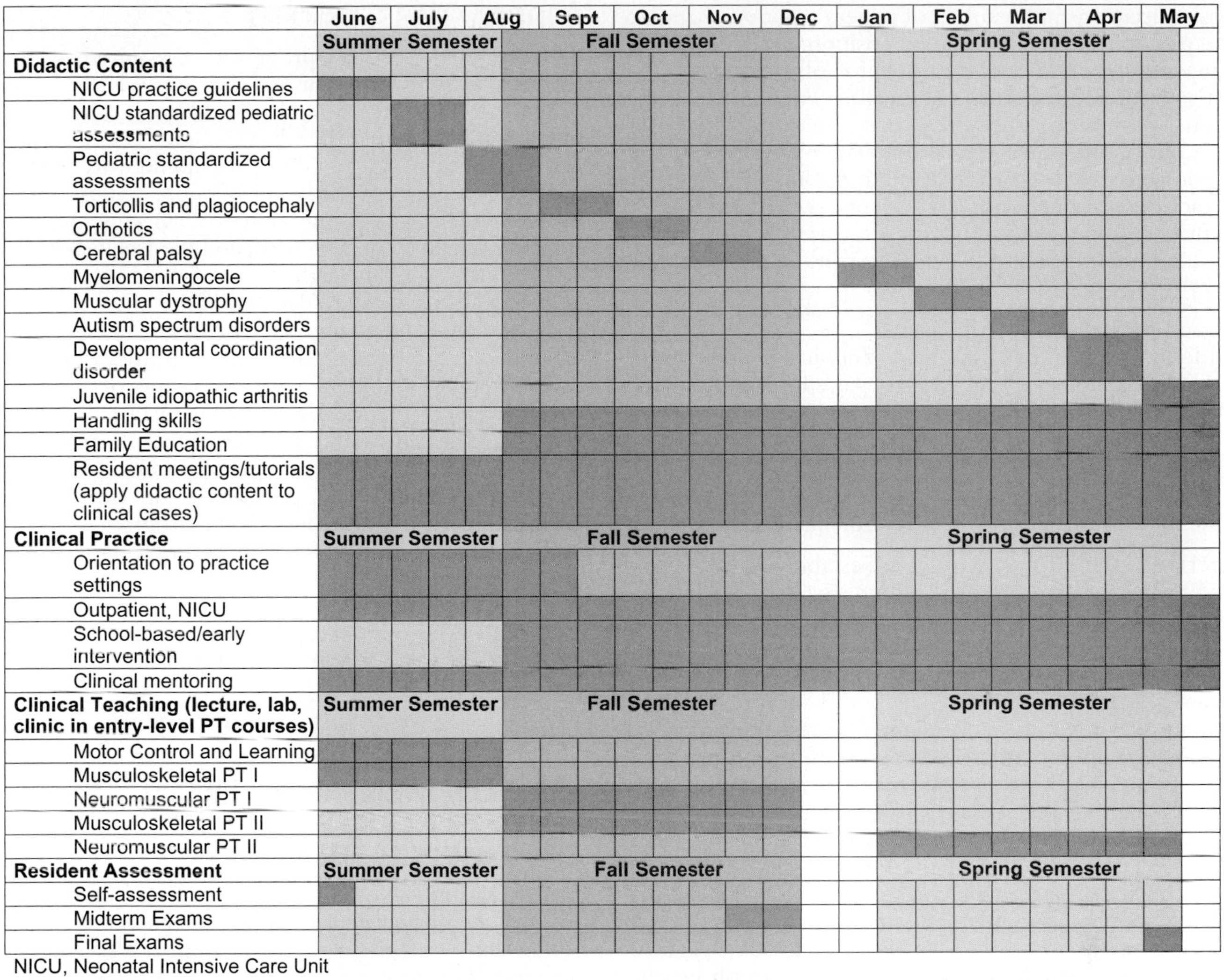

	June	July	Aug	Sept	Oct	Nov	Dec	Jan	Feb	Mar	Apr	May
	Summer Semester			Fall Semester					Spring Semester			
Didactic Content												
NICU practice guidelines												
NICU standardized pediatric assessments												
Pediatric standardized assessments												
Torticollis and plagiocephaly												
Orthotics												
Cerebral palsy												
Myelomeningocele												
Muscular dystrophy												
Autism spectrum disorders												
Developmental coordination disorder												
Juvenile idiopathic arthritis												
Handling skills												
Family Education												
Resident meetings/tutorials (apply didactic content to clinical cases)												
Clinical Practice	Summer Semester			Fall Semester					Spring Semester			
Orientation to practice settings												
Outpatient, NICU												
School-based/early intervention												
Clinical mentoring												
Clinical Teaching (lecture, lab, clinic in entry-level PT courses)	Summer Semester			Fall Semester					Spring Semester			
Motor Control and Learning												
Musculoskeletal PT I												
Neuromuscular PT I												
Musculoskeletal PT II												
Neuromuscular PT II												
Resident Assessment	Summer Semester			Fall Semester					Spring Semester			
Self-assessment												
Midterm Exams												
Final Exams												

NICU, Neonatal Intensive Care Unit

FIGURE 16–2 Temporal illustration of curriculum schedule for full-time, university-based pediatric physical therapy residency program. *NICU*, neonatal intensive care unit.

(without a mentor present), engaged in regular physical therapy practice. This unmentored practice time provides experiences to draw on for self-reflection and discussion with other clinicians and colleagues. It also serves the practical purpose of generating clinical revenue for the facilities participating in the program so that the resident's position may be funded.

In the example provided in Figure 16–1, the fellows training in this program are employed by a medical center and receive a salary and reduced benefit package for 12 months. In a typical week, the resident provides 26 hours of patient care in a large outpatient orthopedic setting and receives 5 hours per week of one-on-one mentoring. When the fellows begin clinical practice, patient types are scheduled according to the clinical lecture and laboratory instruction within the curriculum. Hence, in Clinical Rotation I, fellows primarily see patients with spinal and shoulder complex dysfunctions while they concurrently receive lectures on examination and treatment of spinal and shoulder complex dysfunctions. Clinical Rotation II focuses on patients with hip, knee, foot, and ankle dysfunctions. These patient types are then added to the fellow's schedule.

MENTORING

A portion of a resident's clinical practice time must include one-on-one mentoring from a member of the residency faculty. This mentoring is done in the context of actual patient care, with both the mentor and resident participating in the patient's care. Most mentoring sessions are done such that the patients are part of the resident's caseload, but some mentoring sessions may be done with the mentor as the primary therapist. Clinical mentoring is a crucial component of all residency programs and is dealt with in detail in the following section of this chapter.

RESIDENT EVALUATION

Residents should be evaluated at periodic intervals using a variety of methods. Common ways to assess resident performance include written examinations, technique examinations, and practical patient examinations. Written exams are typically case based with questions designed to assess clinical reasoning. Technique exams involve evaluation of specific patient handling skills as they are performed on a residency faculty member. Feedback is provided on such areas as accuracy and comfort of patient position, therapist hand position, and therapist body position. Practical patient exams are done with a clinical mentor observing the resident's performance during an actual patient clinical examination. Whatever the methods, these exams need to directly relate to the program's overall outcome objectives and any specific objectives for a given learning module or unit.

Practical examinations with patients involve performing an entire examination and intervention as the clinical mentor scores the resident on such factors as the following:

- Thoroughness and accuracy of the patient interview and physical examination
- Identification and justification of clinical hypotheses on which the management decisions are based
- Selection, justification, and progression of the management plan
- Patient education
- Time management
- Identification and justification of the patient's prognosis

Criteria for practical evaluations are established by the residency faculty, based on the program's graduation competencies and specific course objectives. Efforts should be made to establish intra-tester and inter-tester reliability among evaluators for practical examination criteria within a given program.

As another measure of resident progress, performance summaries can be completed by clinical mentors at defined intervals and shared with other mentors who are working with the same resident so that problems with clinical performance are identified early and strategies and timelines for remediation are identified. Performance summaries should be benchmarked against the defined objectives for each component, module, or rotation of the program. These expectations should have been discussed and agreed on by the mentors. It can be helpful to establish benchmarks for performance based on expectations at defined points in the program. An example of a form that can be used to provide feedback to a resident and shared with other mentors who are working with the same resident is included in Appendix 16-B.

Finally, development of a portfolio is another valuable process for use in summative and formative assessment of resident learning, mentor, and program performance.[15] A resident may engage in a collaborative, reflective process of setting goals, assessing his or her own performance and planning for further learning, and in so doing, builds habits of critical self-assessment. Resident portfolios may consist of documents, or exemplars, that demonstrate a resident's performance or progress at a given point in time. The portfolio may include such components as the resident's professional goals, projects and assignments, practical and written examinations, and ongoing self-reflection on his or her performance throughout the program. A portfolio can also include the development of written case studies, which provide valuable insight into a resident's ability to plan, progress, and justify an intervention plan and to interpret relevant outcomes measures. Faculty and program directors are encouraged to also explore how to use the portfolio for mentor and program assessment,[15] how portfolios may be scored,[16] and existing evidence and its implications for residency curriculum design.[17]

PROGRAM ASSESSMENT

Residency and fellowship programs are required to demonstrate a process for regular and ongoing evaluation of the program's goals, faculty, and curriculum, including examples of how the curriculum has changed as a result of the review process.[2] Program directors should work with their faculty to review the program mission, philosophy, and goals and identify potential sources of assessment information, how the data may be used, and the frequency of data collection. This plan might include program evaluations from residents, academic faculty, and clinical mentors at mid term and at the end of the program, interviews with training site coordinators and administrators who oversee the program goals and funding, and surveys of patients and employers of graduates. All such data must be obtained following the confidentiality policies of the practice settings involved. Graduates of the program should also be surveyed periodically for a perspective on the program's effectiveness over the long term. Program assessment information is provided formally through the credentialing, recredentialing, and annual report processes. The ABPTRFE *Application Resource Manual* includes numerous examples of how residencies and fellowships across several specialty areas conduct this ongoing program evaluation process.[3]

DEVELOPMENT OF CLINICAL REASONING IN RESIDENCY AND FELLOWSHIP EDUCATION

Residency and fellowship curricula focus on curricular components and strategies that will enable the practitioner to develop strategies to move toward advanced clinical practice. The progression to advanced clinical practice does not occur only during the 1 to 3 years of residency training. Instead, achievement of this high level of practice is based on the development, refinement, and consolidation of a systematic clinical reasoning process that occurs over subsequent years of experience. The following attributes, which are cultivated during the residency years, are linked with advanced clinical reasoning: evolution of the clinician's knowledge base[18]; personal attributes, values, and attitudes[19]; involvement of the patient in collaborative decision making[20]; organization, efficient retrieval, and refinement of knowledge[18,21,22]; refinement of technical skills; development and articulation of a philosophy of practice; and cognitive and meta-cognitive skills.[23]

Beginning in the 1980s, various models of clinical reasoning have been proposed and investigated in the health professions. The reader is referred to Chapter 11 of this book and the work of Edwards and Jones[24] for an overview of definitions, clinical reasoning models, or strategies that underlie expert practice. Regardless of which clinical reasoning model an individual uses, Gale and Marsden[25] point out that active interpretation and evaluative thinking processes are essential elements that occur throughout the clinical reasoning process. Development of these skills is the focus of the clinical mentoring process and is facilitated when the clinical mentor works collaboratively with the resident with multiple patients over an extended period of time.

Residency programs need to consider how they will integrate evidence appraisal into their facilitation of clinical reasoning. The frequently cited evidence pyramid of Sackett and colleagues[26] places the meta-analysis of randomized controlled trials at the top, descriptive studies lower, and expert opinion at the bottom. The research that physical therapists are now contributing to the medical literature is affecting the credibility of our profession in ways that has not existed in prior decades. Sackett and colleagues[26] reinforce the need for external evidence to be combined with clinical expertise and patient values and expectations to achieve optimal clinical outcomes and to best serve the patient. This therapeutic alliance derives from gathering and critically appraising the patient's stories, symptoms, and signs and incorporating this information with their values and expectations. The works of several authors reinforce the importance of the clinician's ability to effectively use knowledge throughout the clinical reasoning process.[18,21,22,24] Knowledge from the literature, however, does not always apply to real patients. Of critical importance is facilitating development of the critical thinking that will enable a clinician to make decisions about when current evidence related to tests, measures, and interventions cannot be easily applied to an individual patient's presentation or goals. Schön[27,28] calls book knowledge "technical rationality" and argues that this knowledge usually does not address the uncertain and frequently complex problems in professional practice. Professionals need to solve the problems of practice by thinking about why something does not work, solving the problem, and consequently adapting their knowledge and skills.

The role of experience and its relationship to the development of clinical expertise is well described.[29-32] Benner and associates[29-32] use the Dreyfus and Dreyfus model[33] of skill acquisition, a framework that has been applied by many educators in the health professions.[34-36] Benner and associates[29-32] propose that, in acquiring and developing skill, the clinician passes through five levels of proficiency: novice, advanced beginner, competent, proficient, and expert. Movement through these five levels of expertise reflects the following changes in several general aspects of skill performance:

- Movement from reliance on abstract principles and rules to use of past concrete experiences as guides
- Change in the perception and understanding of a situation (i.e., seeing the situation less as a compilation of equally relevant bits of information and more as a complete and complex whole)
- Shift from reliance on analytic, rule-based thinking to intuitive judgment
- Passage from a detached observer to an involved and fully engaged participant

The research of Jensen and coworkers[37] takes the Dreyfus and Dreyfus model[33] and Benner's work[29-32] to another level of application to physical therapy. The dimensions of expert practice derived from their study of clinical expertise in pediatric, orthopedic, neurologic, and orthopedic physical therapy are presented along with practical strategies that can be used in training mentors and in developing activities to enhance residents' clinical reasoning processes.

KEY STEPS IN DESIGNING MENTORING SESSIONS

Physical therapists come to residencies for the opportunity to receive clinical mentoring over an extended period of time. These sessions are truly the core of residency education. For mentoring to be dynamic, effective, and efficient, there must be ongoing planning and communication among the mentors and the program director. The timing and design of mentoring sessions directly affects the value of the sessions for the resident. Careful consideration should be given to creating a mentoring schedule that balances the productivity needs of the organization with sufficient time for the resident to receive feedback and ask questions of the mentor. The amount of mentoring that occurs each week will depend on the duration of the program, the availability of the clinical mentors, and total hours allocated by the program.

In full-time programs, clinical mentoring is frequently provided once per week over an extended period of time. If a program, for example, plans to provide 130 hours of one-on-one mentoring over a year, a typical mentoring schedule might be 3 to 4 hours per week. Part-time programs may complete mentoring in blocks of time over a few weeks. Other part-time programs may require a resident to bring in a patient to demonstrate and receive feedback from faculty and classmates. Alternatively, a resident may be asked to evaluate and treat patients who are on the caseload of the faculty member at the residency clinic. With these latter mentoring strategies, the resident may not have the opportunity to receive ongoing feedback throughout the course of the patient's episode of care. The resident can maintain contact with the faculty member regarding the progress of his or her caseload through ongoing phone contacts, webinars, e-mail, or other electronic discussions. e-Mentoring options[34] are emerging in the health professions and will likely become a significant training avenue in the near future.

An example for a 4-hour block of mentoring time is provided in Box 16-2. This resident is seeing two new patients for evaluations and two patients for follow-up visits. Initially, the number of patient evaluations and follow-up visits may be lower until the resident is clearly able to manage that number while being mentored. If productivity requirements limit weekly discussion time, it is important to schedule electronic or brief phone communication after the session so that the resident will have an avenue for the mentor to address questions that have arisen during the session.

BOX 16-2	Example of Clinical Mentoring Schedule
8:00 AM	New physical therapy evaluation
9:00 AM	Follow-up visit
9:30 AM	Discussion of two prior patients
10:00 AM	New physical therapy evaluation
11:00 AM	Follow-up visit
11:30 AM	Discussion and prioritization of expectations until next session
12:00 PM	Completion of mentoring

INTERACTION BETWEEN CLINICAL MENTORS AND RESIDENTS

Before beginning a mentoring process, the clinical mentor and resident should have an open discussion about the following issues in order to create a time-efficient, interactive, and supportive process:

- How will the mentor be introduced to the patient so that the resident is viewed as a colleague and not an instructor?
- How can the clinical mentor communicate to the resident in a manner that will support excellent service to the patient? For example, the mentor and resident need to communicate *with* the patient, not *over* the patient.
- What types of issues might require the clinical mentor and resident to step out of the room for discussion?
- How can the treatment room be organized to efficiently accommodate resident, mentor, and patient (e.g., Are the treatment tables, computer, and other physical therapy equipment arranged to promote efficiency and communication?)
- What cues can the mentor use when additional questioning or testing is necessary? What cues can the resident use when seeking assistance related to complex or confusing patient care issues?

The clinical mentor faces a complex decision-making process regarding when and how he or she will skillfully intervene during the mentoring session. Bowen[38] describes how clinical teachers must diagnose the patient's disorder while concurrently diagnosing the resident's teaching and learning needs and promoting the resident's abilities. What issues will require immediate intervention? This might include safety issues such as failure to rule out "red flag" conditions, questioning that might lead to inaccurate management decisions, and behaviors by the resident that could contribute to the patient's perception of poor service. The clinical mentor will need to decide which areas can be addressed through written instructions to the resident that can be reviewed after the patient leaves. If the mentor elects to intervene during the patient care session, he or she should do so without disrupting the thinking process of the resident and causing the patient to lose respect for the resident's care.

Although many residents are relatively inexperienced practitioners, some residents and fellows come to a program after many years of practice. Clinical mentoring of an experienced physical therapist poses complex and sometimes difficult challenges. Although physical therapists come to a program because of the clinical mentoring they will experience, working side by side with a mentor may be threatening, depending on the resident's expectations of the mentor, the resident's performance anxiety, the ability of the clinical mentor to articulate his or her clinical reasoning process, and the educational atmosphere that the program and the clinical mentor create. The resident who is an experienced practitioner brings a much broader base of clinical experience than a physical therapy student brings to a clinical internship. The experienced resident has also developed some level of self-esteem and self-perception as a professional, which may include a significant level of expertise in selected areas of physical therapy.

He or she may now be asked to rethink prior learning or clinical reasoning approaches, change prior patient interview and examination habits, and refine and expand on aspects of patient management. Residents' ability to make these clinical practice changes depends in large part on their flexibility and adaptability in thinking patterns and willingness to reassess previously held beliefs, thinking, clinical reasoning, and clinical practice patterns.

Although residents are adult learners, some are not able to articulate their learning needs because they have never received this intense level of mentoring before. The clinic coordinator or program director can play a valuable role in ensuring an effective and supportive clinical mentoring process by encouraging ongoing feedback from the program director, clinical mentor, and resident and by recognizing the teaching strengths and weaknesses of the clinical mentor in relation to the resident's learning style and needs. Regardless of the experience level of the mentor or resident, the success of this mentoring partnership requires that each individual contribute equally to its success.[39]

DEVELOPING PATIENT-CENTERED INTERVIEW SKILLS

Excellent observation and communication skills are well accepted as attributes of effective health care practitioners. Jensen[40] describes the expert clinician's ability to focus on verbal and nonverbal communication with the patient and caregivers as one of the attributes that differentiates expert from novice clinicians. Benner[29,31] reports that the effective clinician integrates "the implications of [a patient's] illness and recovery into their lifestyle" and "most important, captures the patient's readiness to learn." Furthermore, experts strive for collaborative solutions to the patient's problems rather than labeling or blaming the patient. In seeking the best possible care for the patient, experts take seriously the responsibility of advocacy for the patient. Viewing the patient as a trusted source of knowledge begins with the expert's communication with the patient.[29] The expert's data-gathering process begins the moment the patient and therapist meet and includes careful observation of the patient's overall appearance, facial expression, spontaneous postures, and manner of movement. The information gained from these early interactions is used by the expert to recognize and formulate an initial hypothesis as to the nature of the patient's problems and their relevance to the patient's goals.

During the interview process, a resident may frequently have difficulty obtaining accurate, meaningful data. A common fault lies in the manner in which questions are asked. The resident may be too intent on obtaining the data to fill in the evaluation instead of listening carefully and guiding the patient in telling his or her story (Box 16–3).

Maitland[41] considered the patient as the "expert" from whom the therapist must seek information from a totally nonjudgmental manner, actively listening to and believing in whatever the patient conveys in his or her story and symptoms describing the movement disorder. An adept clinical mentor can role-model an efficient, patient-centered questioning style by rephrasing questions or interjecting a question that facilitates more useful dialogue

<table>
<tr><td>

BOX 16–3 Typical Errors in Patient Questioning

- Asking biased questions
- Asking more than one question at a time
- Making assumptions as to the nature of the patient's problems
- Failing to allow or make use of the patient's spontaneous comments
- Repetitively asking questions or pursuing responses that do not yield useful information
- Failing to pursue a response in sufficient detail

</td></tr>
</table>

with the patient, family, or caregiver. In some cases, when persistent questioning yields no useful data, the clinical mentor may urge the resident to "move on" and later explain why the questioning was unnecessary.

PHYSICAL EXAMINATION AND PRIORITIZING THE MANAGEMENT PLAN

Residents need to continually use data to predict or plan the next step in the process—the physical examination. Throughout the interview process, residents need to ask themselves: What interview data have I gained that will enable me to focus my physical examination? What are the key tests and measures that I *must* complete on day 1? What data might I expect from each test? What tests and measures must I complete on day 1, and what can be deferred to day 2? This thinking process trains residents to consider all possible contributing factors and to approach the physical examination in a systematic manner because, early in the training process, they may tend to overexamine or underexamine the patient or examine in an almost rote manner. This characteristic is common even with experienced fellows as they are learning the examination schema taught by the program.

A key skill in the clinical reasoning process is the ability to identify salient interview information when there are multiple impairments or multiple functional problems. By *salient*, we mean clinically relevant data (i.e., information pertaining to the provocation of the patient's symptoms or relief of symptoms, to the patient's main participation restrictions or activity limitations, or to prognosis or management of the problem). The clinical mentor plays a vital role in assisting the resident in this identification of interview data that can be used to plan the physical examination and initial interventions on day 1. Residents early in the educational process often have difficulty knowing what information to gather from the patient's history and may view all data as being of equal value. They also have difficulty prioritizing what data are important to use in making decisions for further examination and in developing their management plan. The clinical mentor may need to selectively intervene, assisting the resident while establishing the relationship among impairments, activity limitations, functional limitations and family or social issues. Box 16–4 provides examples of strategies and questions a mentor may use to guide the resident's examination process.

In addition, Bowen[38] provides examples of problems in clinical reasoning that may occur in medical education and recommendations as to how the clinical teacher can help organize the resident's clinical reasoning process.

<table>
<tr><td>

BOX 16–4 Examination-Guiding Strategies

- Point out meaningful diagnostic information in the interview and physical examination that will help the resident determine the nature of the patient's problem and encourage the resident to revise his or her hypotheses according to this data.
- Selectively intervene to assist the resident in identifying relationships among impairments, relevant social and family issues, and activity and functional limitations that may affect the patient's prognosis and ongoing management plan.
- Help the resident eliminate irrelevant information.
- Highlight discriminating features and how to weigh these features in the diagnostic or management process. Questions might include:
  - What questions and tests did you include that would support your primary hypothesis?
  - In your physical examination, what tests constitute a significant positive test to support your hypothesis?
  - What negative responses might be significant in ruling out a particular hypothesis?
  - Are there red or yellow flags that make referral to another provider important at this time?
  - Are there family or social issues that will impact the patient's prognosis for recovery?

</td></tr>
</table>

Further recommendations are outlined by Carraccio and associates,[35] who take the reader through the developmental steps to expertise of the Dreyfus and Dreyfus model, provides brief case study examples of a clinician in each step of development and recommends clinical teaching strategies.

CLINICAL MENTORING GUIDES AND FEEDBACK FORMS

A key element of successful mentoring is to develop guides or feedback forms on which the mentor can document questions, concerns, and recommendations *during* the mentoring process and residents can be challenged to make their thought process explicit. The program should identify the major components of the examination and management for which they would like to provide consistent feedback. A sports residency will have different priorities for its form than a geriatric or pediatric residency. Because the mentor must continually decide which issues need to be addressed immediately during the mentoring process (e.g., safety issues, poor technique performance, or questioning that might lead to inaccurate decisions) as opposed to issues that can wait for later feedback, a good mentoring feedback form is crucial for ensuring that a resident eventually receives a complete critique. The form may include the following elements:

- *Interview feedback.* Identify components of the interview that your program has prioritized for residents to be thorough and systematic.
- *Physical examination critique.* Include choice of tests/measures, exam organization, and performance of skills.
- *Outcomes measures*
- Areas that require *clarification or referral*
- *Prognosis with justification*
- *Intervention plan and rationale*
- *Areas to work on* until the next mentoring session
- *Strategies for change* until the next mentoring session

The program may elect to define several categories as demonstrated previously to elicit more specific feedback from the mentor or have more open-ended feedback. An example of a mentoring guide for a pediatric physical therapy residency is located in Appendix 16-C. Many other examples from several specialty areas can also be obtained from the ABPTRFE's *Application Resource Manual*.[3]

The most important section of the mentoring feedback form is the identification of problem areas that are to be the focus of the resident's learning until the next mentoring session. The feedback form becomes a vehicle by which the resident can reflect on his or her strengths and areas for improvement. The mentoring feedback form can also be used to provide feedback to the resident when it is inappropriate for the mentor to interrupt the resident with the patient present. There may be relatively minor issues, such as repetitive questioning or unclear wording of interview questions that can be addressed later through the mentoring form. The mentor can use the form to write alternative questions like, "You could have asked the question in the following manner" or additional questions like, "Next time, also ask the following." The mentor can also provide specific strategies to help the resident change his or her questioning style. Similarly, the mentor can document additional or more vigorous testing that could have been done during the physical examination if he or she elects not to interrupt and demonstrate these with the patient present. This type of feedback can be very effective without compromising the patient care session.

SELF-REFLECTION AFTER MENTORING SESSIONS

The program may wish to develop a separate clinical reasoning form that identifies components of the examination and management plan for the resident to engage in critical self-reflection on his or her clinical reasoning and performance between mentoring sessions. Examples of a retrospective case analysis form might include some of the questions listed in Appendix 16-D. The resident would answer these questions for the patients who were seen during the mentoring process for a given day and keep these forms in a binder for ongoing self-reflection.

REFLECTION BY THE MENTOR

Because the clinical mentoring process takes place in the context of practice, the mentor and resident are both involved in thinking more deeply about the patient. As clinical mentors mature in their skill development, it is important for them to receive ongoing feedback on how they interact with their resident and to make a commitment to self-assess their own teaching skills and behaviors throughout the mentoring process. Common questions a mentor may ask: Am I intervening too often or too little? Are my written instructions readable and clear? What else can I do to help the resident be more comfortable with the mentoring process? A common pitfall of new clinical mentors is to interrupt the resident too often during a given session and provide too many recommendations for change, leaving the resident overwhelmed and lacking confidence.

Mentors must be able to clearly identify and prioritize areas for change along with strategies for change during *each* mentoring session. For example, a resident who is having difficulty with time management may be asked to time each segment of his interview and physical examination in order to determine where he is losing time. A resident who is having difficulty making decisions about which tests and measures to choose may be asked to meet with classmates to role-play various patient scenarios. Clinical mentors who are "agile" and flexible in their ability to respond to residents' varying learning styles create a dynamic and collaborative mentoring environment. Extensive research on the qualities of effective clinical educators is available in the literature[42-44] and is discussed in Chapters 9, 10, and 11.

MENTORING RESIDENTS VERSUS PHYSICAL THERAPIST STUDENTS

Educators frequently ask how mentoring in a residency or fellowship differs from the clinical supervision of a physical therapist student in a physical therapist professional program. This can be viewed along a continuum of professional development in which students fall at the beginner stage, whereas residents fall at the competent or proficient stage.

In general, mentoring a physical therapy student is of shorter duration and focuses on safety, basic physical therapy management, and skill acquisition in how to examine and manage a broad range of patient presentations. The physical therapy student has limited practical clinical knowledge and tends to be more rule-governed, whereas residents are beginning to be more intuitive. Physical therapy students may not fully appreciate the context of clinical data, so the recommendations of the clinical supervisor will tend to focus on basic management decisions. Black and associates[45] describe in detail the learning and development of physical therapists in their first year of physical therapy practice. Their findings support the need for facilitating structured learning experiences and mentoring in the early years of practice.

In contrast, residents will generally receive extended periods of mentoring over several weeks or months with the opportunity to focus on expanded problem solving, analysis, and multifaceted selection and progression of interventions. Residents may be initially more rote in their communication but are able to move toward a more focused interview and physical examination process, using a broader range of tests and measures. Whereas the mentor for a physical therapy student may serve primarily as an instructor or guide, the mentor for a resident tends to assume a greater role as facilitator and colleague.

STRATEGIES FOR LINKING ACADEMIC AND CLINICAL CURRICULUM COMPONENTS

A key characteristic of experts is their superior ability to recognize common clinical presentations, which in turn influences their subsequent clinical reasoning and development of intervention strategies.[46,47] In addition to exposing the resident to a broad range of current evidence related to tests, measures, and current interventions in a specialty area, using published patient cases from the literature and informal cases written by the clinical mentor can be an excellent way to link didactic knowledge with clinical practice. Cases can be presented during role-playing, as live patient demonstrations, or as online webinars with video. They may be one-on-one sessions or small group tutorials.

A common theme that underlies all of these strategies is teaching residents to reflect on performance or to continually self-monitor practice, during and after seeing patients. According to Cross,[48] for any experience to have lasting meaning, it must be followed at some appropriate distance by a period of reflection—mere involvement is not enough. Schön[27,28] refers to these actions as "reflection-in-action" and "reflection-about action" and views self-correction and adaptation processes as essential to the development of expertise. The process of articulating clinical reasoning draws the often subconscious or tacit skill of clinical reasoning to the participant's awareness, exposing it to self-critique and critical feedback from others and helping the learner to critique and defend his or her clinical reasoning,[49,50] and allows the learner to make a "decision based on the resulting insight."[51]

Case presentation and discussion can follow a number of effective formats. As an example, residents could be given selected data from one of the clinical mentor's cases and then would be asked facilitating questions in class or during a synchronous webinar or asynchronous online discussion forum to stimulate discussion. Other uses of case studies might involve sequential presentation of written case study data in which the mentor role-plays as the patient and one resident role-plays as a therapist with a small group or another classmate observing. As data are revealed about the patient through the interview (of the mentor), the small group critiques how to reword, clarify, and focus interview questions or tests and measures and identifies missing data and its importance.

Role-playing scenarios enable the mentor to present cases of varying degrees of difficulty and enables residents to respond to emerging data and "think on their feet," which is frequently a challenge in the clinical setting. Benner and Wrubel[52] note that use of case studies can assist residents in achieving a shift in their clinical reasoning processes. They state that the "interaction of the learner's prior knowledge creates experience, a turning point in understanding." Role-playing case studies, combined with questions requiring the resident to articulate and justify their clinical reasoning processes with classmates, enhances the clinician's awareness and deliberate attention to relevant clinical information. This collaborative learning within a supportive practice environment can be an important step in the development of clinical reasoning.[53]

Another strategy includes live demonstrations with patients who have given signed consent or simulated patients.[54] These sessions enable the mentor or simulated patient to role-model excellent examination and patient management skills. Mentors can also display the subtle nuances of skilled communication, listening, instructing, and confident patient handling that are crucial in providing excellent patient service. Observations of subtle changes in movement patterns, impairments, and functional limitations missed by the resident can be reinforced by the mentor, followed by discussions of how this information will contribute to management decisions.

SUMMARY

In post-professional residency and fellowship education, physical therapists can link theory with clinical practice and receive ongoing clinical mentoring over an extended period of time. Residency and fellowship curricula are directed toward teaching practitioners examination and intervention strategies that will enable them to continually monitor and critique their performance and develop clinical expertise over time. As stated by Rivett and Higgs,[55] "[T]o achieve expertise ... is to 'rise above mediocrity.' The structured learning environments of residencies and fellowships help clinicians develop and practice relevant strategies to turn their experience into learning."

The curriculum and teaching strategies presented in this chapter are derived from our knowledge of post-professional residency and fellowship programs and are grounded in the literature concerning the development of sound judgment and clinical reasoning and expert practice. We hope that the ideas in this chapter will stimulate academic faculty and clinicians alike to plan for the expansion of residency and fellowship programs to meet a growing demand for such experiences. The range of recommendations presented in this chapter for developing mentoring schedules, creating learning activities, and developing questions to facilitate self-reflection by the resident reinforces the amount of time residents and fellows may need to advance their clinical reasoning. Also, the timing and specificity of the reflections are crucial in optimizing the impact of the mentoring process.[56] Health care changes are placing high demands on novice therapists, who must "hit the ground running" after graduating from entry-level physical therapist education programs, and on experienced physical therapists, who must assume new roles with greater responsibility and autonomy. In this new environment, a commitment to clinical residency and fellowship education is a commitment to clinical excellence.

THRESHOLD CONCEPTS

Threshold Concept #1: Residency and fellowship education is more about improving *thinking and clinical reasoning* than it is about adding more hands-on *skills*.

Many physical therapists have a misconception that residency education is about learning new techniques. Even those who explore residencies and decide to apply to programs may continue to hold this misconception until they finally begin a program. The resident story at the beginning of this chapter reflects this common thinking. Eventually, participants in a residency program come to understand that it is more important to improve clinical reasoning skills (i.e., thinking) than to add more intervention tools to the toolbox. There are a number of effective strategies for helping residents develop better reasoning skills outlined in this chapter in the sections on clinical mentoring. Most mentoring strategies challenge residents to reflect on their thought process before, during, or after a patient interaction or role-playing exercise.

The following mentoring technique can help foster a resident's ability to examine his or her thinking during a patient encounter. The technique is commonly referred to as *thinking aloud*. Initially, it is best incorporated during role-plays, during simulated patient encounters, or with patients the resident already knows. It can also be done in a separate room immediately after a portion of a patient encounter is completed, such as just after a patient interview or immediately after a physical examination. The mentor asks the resident a specific question about the encounter. The question may pertain to a hypothesis the resident generated, a prioritization of patient limitations, or an intervention choice that was made. The mentor then challenges the resident to verbally describe or justify the thinking that lead to his or her decision. The technique, although simple, is critical for developing residents' meta-cognitive skills, or ability to examine their own thought processes. Only by doing critical self-reflection can a practitioner recognize and correct thinking errors.

Threshold Concept #2: Role-modeling is a key aspect of mentorship.

Mentorship from an expert clinician is critical to the process of facilitating growth in residents. This chapter addresses incorporation of mentoring into all aspects of a residency program. Various clinical mentoring strategies are discussed in the chapter, including role-playing, forum discussions, patient demonstrations, and preparation of written retrospective analysis forms. Besides providing critical analysis of, and feedback concerning, residents' performance, mentors can also role-model good technique or efficient performance of a particular task.

One example of a role-modeling activity occurs within the context of a live patient examination. The experienced therapist allows the resident to complete an entire patient interview, gathering all the data the resident deems important and appropriate. The mentor makes notes about areas the resident did not address, areas that were unnecessary to cover in detail, and items the resident should have explored in more depth. Then, before giving any specific feedback, the mentor immediately repeats the interview with the patient. The experienced therapist role-models an efficient, thorough interview. In so doing, the mentor might use different language to make a question clearer, ask follow-up questions the resident missed, or ignore some pieces of information deemed irrelevant. This technique can be more effective than giving simple feedback because the resident immediately experiences a counter-example to what just transpired. The resident can "see" alternative approaches that enable the mentor to succeed where he or she struggled. This type of role-modeling can be used for any aspect of patient care.

ANNOTATED BIBLIOGRAPHY

Bowen JL. Educational strategies to promote clinical diagnostic reasoning. *N Engl J Med.* 2006;355:2217–2235
    Bowen provides excellent examples of problems in clinical reasoning (e.g., how a novice resident versus an expert resident might solve a clinical problem in medicine) and presents strategies for diagnosing a learner's skill and for addressing problems in clinical reasoning. Although examples relate to medical residency education, the article has great applicability to residents, fellows, or students in physical therapy.

Carraccio CL, Bradley JB, Nixon J, Derstine PL. From the educational bench to the clinical bedside: translating the Dreyfus Developmental Model to the learning of clinical skills. *Acad Med.* 2008;83:761–767
    This article provides a discussion of the different steps of the Dreyfus Model of Skill Development using cases to show the progression of skill level and implications for developing teaching and learning strategies for the clinical teacher. The characteristics demonstrated in the physician cases can easily be applied to physical therapy. The article makes the Dreyfus Model come alive and become useful for clinical mentors in a broad range of practice settings.

Kilminster S, Cottrell D, Grant J, Jolly B. AMEE Guide 27. Effective educational and clinical supervision. *Med Teach.* 2007;29:2–19
    This article provides a literature review of characteristics of educational and clinical supervision practice. Definitions; how effective supervision can be determined in a clinical setting; skills, qualities, and activities of effective supervisors; how supervisors can be trained; and common challenges of supervision are discussed in a clear, practical manner. This article would provide a very good background for developing expectations for novice as well as experienced mentors.

REFERENCES

1. Tichenor CJ. Clinical residency: another turning point for our profession? *PT Mag.* 1995;3:49.
2. American Board of Physical Therapy Residency and Fellowship Education. *Application for Credentialing of Residency and Fellowship Programs.* Alexandria, VA: American Physical Therapy Association Residency and Fellowship Credentialing; 2010.
3. American Board of Physical Therapy Residency and Fellowship Education. *Application Resource Manual.* Alexandria, VA: American Physical Therapy Association Clinical Residency and Fellowship Program Credentialing; 2011.
4. American Academy of Orthopaedic Manual Physical Therapists. *Standards for Orthopaedic Manual Physical Therapy Residency Training.* Biloxi, MS: American Academy of Orthopaedic Manual Physical Therapists; 1999.
5. American Physical Therapy Association Task Force on Accreditation of Clinical Residencies. Alexandria, VA: American Physical Therapy Association; 1994.
6. *APTA Residency vs. Fellowship page.* American Physical Therapy Association website. Available at http://www.apta.org/ResidencyFellowship/ResidencyvsFellowship/; Accessed 28.07.11.
7. Smith KL, Tichenor CJ, Schroeder M. Orthopaedic residency training: a survey of the graduates' perspective. *J Orthop Sports Phys Ther.* 1999;29:635–655.
8. Stoeckle JD, Leaf A, Grossman JH, et al. A case history of training outside the hospital and its future. *Am J Med.* 1979;66:1008.
9. American Psychological Association. *Accreditation Handbook.* Washington, DC: American Psychological Association; 1986.
10. Council on Podiatric Medical Education. *Standards, Requirements and Guidelines for Approval of Residencies in Podiatric Medicine.* Bethesda, MD: American Podiatric Medical Association; 1993.
11. Council on Optometric Education Residency Standards. *Accreditation Handbook.* St. Louis: American Optometric Association; 1994.
12. Horton ER, Upchurch H, Michelucci A. Development of a postgraduate year 1 pharmacy residency program at a large teaching hospital. *Am J Health Syst Pharm.* 2011;68:1245–1250.
13. Long TM, Sippel K. A pediatric clinical residency. *PT Mag.* 1995;3:57.
14. American Academy of Orthopaedic Manual Physical Therapists. *Standards for Orthopaedic Manual Physical Therapy Residency Training.* Gulfport, MS: American Academy of Orthopaedic Manual Physical Therapists; 1993.
15. Paschal KA, Jensen GM, Mostrom E. Building portfolios: a means for developing habits of reflective practice in physical therapy education. *J Phys Ther Educ.* 2002;16:38–53.
16. Karlowicz KA. Development and Testing of a Portfolio Evaluation Scoring Tool. *J Nurs Educ.* 2010;49:78–86.

17. McColgan K, Blackwood B. A systematic review protocol on the use of teaching portfolios for educators in further and higher education. *J Adv Nurs.* 2009;65:2500–2507.

18. Elstein A, Shulman L, Sprafka S. Medical problem solving: a ten-year retrospective study. *Eval Health Prof.* 1990;13:5.

19. May BJ, Dennis JK. Teaching clinical decision-making. In: Higgs J, Jones M, eds. *Clinical Reasoning in the Health Professions.* Boston: Butterworth-Heinemann; 1995:301.

20. Trede F, Higgs J. Collaborative decision making. In: Higgs J, Jones MA, Loftus S, Christiensen N, eds. *Clinical Reasoning in the Health Professions.* 3 rd ed. Philadelphia: Elsevier; 2008:43–54.

21. Grant R, Jones M, Maitland GD. Clinical decision making in upper quarter dysfunction. In: Grant R, ed. *Physical Therapy of the Cervical and Thoracic Spine.* New York: Churchill Livingstone; 1988:51.

22. Grant J, Marsden P. The structure of memorized knowledge in students and clinicians: an explanation for diagnostic expertise. *Med Educ.* 1987;21:92.

23. Higgs J, Jones MA. Clinical decision making and multiple problem spaces. In: Higgs J, Jones MA, Loftus S, eds. *Clinical Reasoning in the Health Professions.* 3rd ed Philadelphia: Elsevier; 2008:3–17.

24. Edwards I, Jones M. Clinical Reasoning and Expert Practice. In: Jensen GM, Gwyer J, Hack LM, Shepard KF, eds. *Expertise in Physical Therapy Practice.* 2nd ed St. Louis: Saunders Elsevier; 2007 [chapter 10].

25. Gale J, Marsden P. Clinical problem solving: the beginning of the process. *Med Educ.* 1982;16:22.

26. Sackett DL, Strauss SE, Richardson WS, et al. *Evidence-Based Medicine.* 2nd ed. New York: Churchill Livingstone; 2000.

27. Schön DA. *The Reflective Practitioner.* New York: Basic Books; 1983.

28. Schon DA. *Educating the Reflective Practitioner.* San Francisco: Jossey-Bass; 1987.

29. Benner P. Uncovering the knowledge embedded in clinical practice. *Image J Nurs Sch.* 1983;15:36.

30. Benner P. *From Novice to Expert: Excellence and Power in Clinical Nursing.* Menlo Park, CA: Addison Wesley; 1984.

31. Benner P, Hooper-Kyriakidis P, Stannard D. *Clinical Wisdom and Interventions in Critical-Care.* Philadelphia: WB Saunders; 1999.

32. Benner PE, Tanner CA, Chesla CA. *Expertise in Nursing Practice: Caring, Clinical Judgment and Ethics.* 2nd ed. New York: Springer; 2009.

33. Dreyfus HI, Dreyfus SE, Athanasiou T. *Mind Over Machine: The Power of Human Intuition and Expertise in the Era of the Computer.* New York: Free Press; 1986.

34. Obura T, Brant WE, Miller F, et al. Participation in community of learners enhances resident perceptions of learning in an e-mentoring program: proof of concept. *BMC Med Educ.* 2011;11:1–6.

35. Carraccio CL, Bradley JB, Nixon J, et al. From the educational bench to the clinical bedside: translating the Dreyfus Developmental Model to the Learning of Clinical Skills. *Acad Med.* 2008;83:761–767.

36. Schmidt HG, Norman GR, Boshuizen HP. A cognitive perspective on medical expertise: theory and implications. *Acad Med.* 1990; 65:611–621.

37. Jensen GM, Gwyer J, Hack LM, et al. *Expertise in Physical Therapy Practice.* 2nd ed. St. Louis: Saunders Elsevier; 2007 [chapters 2 and 12].

38. Bowen JL. Educational strategies to promote clinical diagnostic reasoning. *N Engl J Med.* 2006;355:2217–2235.

39. McKenna AM, Straus SE. Charting a professional course: a review of mentorship in medicine. *J Am Coll Radiol.* 2011;8:109–112.

40. Jensen GM. Expert Practice in Orthopedics: Competence, Collaboration, and Compassion. In: Jensen GM, Gwyer J, Hack LM, eds. *Expertise in Physical Therapy Practice.* Boston: Butterworth-Heinemann; 1999 [chapter 8].

41. Hengeveld E, Banks K, eds. *Maitland's Peripheral Manipulation.* 4th ed London: Elsevier; 2005:3.

42. Graffam B, Bowers L, Keen KN. Using observations of clinician's teaching practices to build a model of clinical instruction. *Acad Med.* 2008;83:768–774.

43. Higgs J, McAllister L. Educating clinical educators: using a model of the experience of being a clinical educator. *Med Teach.* 2007; 29:51–57.

44. Kilminster S, Cottrell D, Grant J, et al. Effective educational and clinical supervision. *Med Teach.* 2007;29:2–19.

45. Black LL, Jensen GM, Mostrom E, et al. The first year of practice: an investigation of the professional learning and development of promising novice physical therapists. *Phys Ther.* 2010;90:1758–1773.

46. Jones M. Clinical reasoning in physical therapy. *Phys Ther.* 1992;72:875.

47. Eva K. What every teacher needs to know about clinical reasoning. *Med Educ.* 2004;39:98–106.

48. Cross V. Introducing physiotherapy students to the idea of "reflective practice. *Med Teach.* 1993;15:293.

49. Ajjawi R, Higgs J. Learning to reason: a journey of professional socialisation. *Adv Health Sci Educ Theory Pract.* 2008;13:133–150.

50. Mezirow J. Learning to think like an adult: core concepts of transformation theory. In: Mezirow J, ed. *Learning as transformation: critical perspectives on a theory in progress.* San Francisco: Jossey-Bass; 2000:6–7.

51. Ness V, Duffy K, McCallum J, Price L. Supporting and mentoring nursing students in practice. *Nurs Stand.* 2010;25:41–46.

52. Benner P, Wrubel J. Skilled clinical knowledge: the value of perceptual awareness. *Nurse Educ.* 1982;7:11.

53. Clouder L. Becoming professional. Exploring the complexities of professional socialization in health and social care. *Learn Health Social Care.* 2003;2:213–222.

54. Edwards H, Franke M, McGuiness B. Using simulated patients to teach clinical reasoning. In: Higgs J, Jones M, eds. *Clinical Reasoning in the Health Professions.* Boston: Butterworth-Heinemann; 1995:269.

55. Rivett D, Higgs J. Experience and expertise in clinical reasoning. *N Z J Physiother.* 1995;23:16.

56. Henry BW, Malu KF. Coaching, mentoring and supervision for workplace learning. In: Hafler JP, ed. *Extraordinary Learning in the Workplace.* New York: Springer Science; 2011:78.

APPENDIX 16-A SUPPLEMENTARY RESOURCES TO AID IN DEVELOPING RESIDENCY CURRICULA

The website of the American Physical Therapy Association (http://www.apta.org) contains extensive resources for developing and existing programs. These resources include a directory and map of residency and fellowship programs across the country, a broad range of resources for starting a program and steps for a program to become credentialed, program models, curriculum development recommendations, courses and other events to aid developing programs, and faculty members.

The following documents can be obtained from the American Physical Therapy Association (APTA), 1111 North Fairfax Street, Alexandria, VA 22314-1488. Phone: 703-684-2782, 1-800-999-2782; Fax: 703-684-7343; website: http://www.apta.org/Educators/ResidencyFellowship/.

- American Board of Physical Therapy Residency and Fellowship Education: Application for Credentialing of Residency and Fellowship Programs. Alexandria, VA: American Physical Therapy Association Residency & Fellowship Credentialing, 2010.
- American Board of Physical Therapy Residency and Fellowship Education: Application Resource Manual. Alexandria, VA: American Physical Therapy Association Clinical Residency and Fellowship Program Credentialing, 2011. Document includes examples for developing program mission, goals, objectives, performance outcomes, and rationale for organization and sequencing of curriculum components. Document also includes examples of procedures and assessment instruments for evaluating performance of the resident and graduate.
- A Normative Model for Physical Therapist Professional Education: Version 2004. Available through APTA Online Store: http://iweb.apta.org/Purchase/SearchCatalog.aspx. Various matrices presented in this document include primary content area, examples of terminal behavioral objectives, and examples of instructional objectives. These materials can be used to develop residency program objectives and performance outcomes.
- Descriptions of Specialty Practice (DSPs) or Descriptions of Advanced Clinical Practice (DACPs) are available for American Board of Physical Therapy Specialty areas and are available at http://www.abpts.org/Resources/SpecialtyPracticeDescriptions/. The DSP or DACP defines the practice dimensions and competencies governing advanced clinical practice within a specialty area. The competencies defined in each document should be used to help develop program objectives and performance outcomes and to design residency curricula.

APPENDIX 16-B WEEKLY MENTORING PROGRESS SUMMARY

Resident's name:

_____

Week _____ beginning:

_____

Date(s) of mentoring:

_____

Total number of hours spent mentoring with this resident during this week:

_____

Mentor's name:

_____

Mentoring occurred in the following setting(s) (circle):
Rehab Hospital SNF/ECF Outpatient LTC Other (list):

_____

Type(s) of patient(s) seen (diagnostically):

_____

_____

_____

Specific areas in which the resident performs well:

_____

_____

_____

Specific areas in which the resident needs to improve:

_____

_____

_____

TO BE COMPLETED BY RESIDENT:
Resident's comments/action plan (use other side if needed):

_____

_____

_____

APPENDIX 16-C PEDIATRIC PHYSICAL THERAPY RESIDENCY MENTORING GUIDE

1. Following the chart review, history, and child/family interview, address the following. *If this is an intervention session, list changes that have occurred below*:
   - Health condition:
   - Body structure/function:
   - Activity limitations:
   - Participation restrictions:
   - Personal factors:
   - Environmental factors:

2. Discuss plans for the Physical Examination or POC Update/reassessment—prioritize plans for the PT exam and prioritize areas of the exam that will be most important and why you feel these are important.

3. Following the Session:
   - What are the LTG/functional activities to focus on? Have they changed?
   - Has the POC changed (if an update/reassessment)? If so, how?
   - Is there a change in the PT prognosis for this child and why?

   - Based on the above and today's performance, what is your specific plan for next week?
     - Specific intervention:
     - Decrease difficulty:
     - Increase difficulty:
     - Activity limitation addressed:
     - Participation restriction addressed:
   - Other ideas: Plans for family/caregiver/child education (including a home program or home activity ideas).

4. Reflection
   - Would you do anything differently with a similar child in the future? Why or why not?
   - Following this child encounter/intervention, what techniques were successful? Why? What techniques were unsuccessful? Why?
   - Key question about the major take-home point: Did you meet the needs of your patient and his/her family today? If yes, how? If no, then what was missing?

APPENDIX 16-D RETROSPECTIVE CASE ANALYSIS

Date:_____
Patient initials: _____
Referring Dx:_____

1. What did I do well during today's sessions with the patient?
2. What do I need to improve on from today's session with this patient?
3. Are there gaps or inconsistent information from the day 1 interview that I need to clarify on day 2?
4. What are the patient's key impairments and how do they relate to the patient's functional limitations?

5. What additional testing do I need to do during the next session?
6. What will I plan to do if the patient comes back better, worse, or the same?
7. What is the patient's prognosis, including the expected level of recovery and associated favorable or unfavorable factors that may affect progress?
8. What additional referrals need to be made to other practitioners?

INDEX

Note: Page numbers followed by *b* indicate boxes, *f* indicate figures, and *t* indicate tables.